Tumors
of the
Upper Aerodigestive Tract
and Ear

Atlas
of
Tumor Pathology

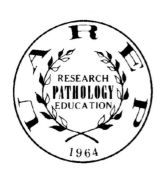

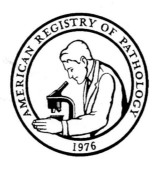

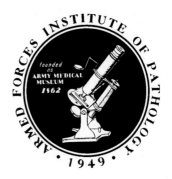

ATLAS OF TUMOR PATHOLOGY

Third Series
Fascicle 26

TUMORS OF THE UPPER AERODIGESTIVE TRACT AND EAR

by

Stacey E. Mills, M.D.
Professor of Pathology
Associate Chair, Surgical Pathology and Cytology
University of Virginia Medical Center
Charlottesville, Virginia

Michael J. Gaffey, M.D. (deceased)
Associate Professor of Pathology
University of Virginia Medical Center
Charlottesville, Virginia

Henry F. Frierson, Jr., M.D.
Professor of Pathology
University of Virginia Medical Center
Charlottesville, Virginia

Published by the
ARMED FORCES INSTITUTE OF PATHOLOGY
Washington, D.C.

Under the Auspices of
UNIVERSITIES ASSOCIATED FOR RESEARCH AND EDUCATION IN PATHOLOGY, INC.
Bethesda, Maryland
2000

Accepted for Publication
1997

_____

Available from the American Registry of Pathology
Armed Forces Institute of Pathology
Washington, D.C. 20306-6000
ISSN 0160-6344
ISBN 1-881041-57-3

ATLAS OF TUMOR PATHOLOGY

EDITOR
JUAN ROSAI, M.D.
Department of Pathology
Memorial Sloan-Kettering Cancer Center
New York, New York 10021-6007

ASSOCIATE EDITOR
LESLIE H. SOBIN, M.D.
Armed Forces Institute of Pathology
Washington, D.C. 20306-6000

EDITORS' NOTE

The Atlas of Tumor Pathology has a long and distinguished history. It was first conceived at a Cancer Research Meeting held in St. Louis in September 1947 as an attempt to standardize the nomenclature of neoplastic diseases. The first series was sponsored by the National Academy of Sciences-National Research Council. The organization of this Sisyphean effort was entrusted to the Subcommittee on Oncology of the Committee on Pathology, and Dr. Arthur Purdy Stout was the first editor-in-chief. Many of the illustrations were provided by the Medical Illustration Service of the Armed Forces Institute of Pathology, the type was set by the Government Printing Office, and the final printing was done at the Armed Forces Institute of Pathology (hence the colloquial appellation "AFIP Fascicles"). The American Registry of Pathology purchased the Fascicles from the Government Printing Office and sold them virtually at cost. Over a period of 20 years, approximately 15,000 copies each of nearly 40 Fascicles were produced. The worldwide impact that these publications have had over the years has largely surpassed the original goal. They quickly became among the most influential publications on tumor pathology ever written, primarily because of their overall high quality but also because their low cost made them easily accessible to pathologists and other students of oncology the world over.

Upon completion of the first series, the National Academy of Sciences-National Research Council handed further pursuit of the project over to the newly created Universities Associated for Research and Education in Pathology (UAREP). A second series was started, generously supported by grants from the AFIP, the National Cancer Institute, and the American Cancer Society. Dr. Harlan I. Firminger became the editor-in-chief and was succeeded by Dr. William H. Hartmann. The second series Fascicles were produced as bound volumes instead of loose leaflets. They featured a more comprehensive coverage of the subjects, to the extent that the Fascicles could no longer be regarded as "atlases" but rather as monographs describing and illustrating in detail the tumors and tumor-like conditions of the various organs and systems.

Once the second series was completed, with a success that matched that of the first, UAREP and AFIP decided to embark on a third series. A new editor-in-chief and an associate editor were selected, and a distinguished editorial board was appointed. The mandate for the third series remains the same as for the previous ones, i.e., to oversee the production of an eminently practical publication with surgical pathologists as its primary audience, but also aimed at other workers in oncology. The main purposes of this series are to promote a consistent, unified, and biologically sound nomenclature; to guide the surgical pathologist in the diagnosis of the various tumors and tumor-like lesions; and to provide relevant histogenetic, pathogenetic, and clinicopathologic information on these entities. Just as the second series included data obtained from ultrastructural (and, in the more recent Fascicles, immunohistochemical) examination, the third series will, in addition, incorporate pertinent information obtained with the newer molecular biology techniques. As in the past, a continuous attempt will be made to correlate, whenever possible, the nomenclature used in the Fascicles with that proposed by the World Health Organization's International Histological Classification of Tumors. The format of the third series has been changed in order to incorporate additional items and to ensure a consistency of style throughout. Close cooperation between the various authors and their respective liaisons from the editorial board will be emphasized to minimize unnecessary repetition and discrepancies in the text and illustrations.

To its everlasting credit, the participation and commitment of the AFIP to this venture is even more substantial and encompassing than in previous series. It now extends to virtually all scientific, technical, and financial aspects of the production.

The task confronting the organizations and individuals involved in the third series is even more daunting than in the preceding efforts because of the ever-increasing complexity of the matter at hand. It is hoped that this combined effort—of which, needless to say, that represented by the authors is first and foremost—will result in a series worthy of its two illustrious predecessors and will be a suitable introduction to the tumor pathology of the twenty-first century.

Juan Rosai, M.D.
Leslie H. Sobin, M.D.

PREFACE AND ACKNOWLEDGMENTS

We have tried to create a worthy successor to the second series Fascicle, *Tumors of the Upper Respiratory Tract and Ear,* by Drs. Vincent J. Hyams, John G. Batsakis, and Leslie Michaels. It is an honor to have been chosen to follow in their footsteps. That we have borrowed multiple illustrations from their earlier work, published over a decade ago, is a testament to the high quality of their publication.

Most of the pathologic material in this Fascicle is derived from the files of our own institution. Needless to say, we would not have many such specimens without the longstanding presence of an outstanding department of Otolaryngology - Head and Neck Surgery at the University of Virginia. Drs. G. Slaughter Fitz-Hugh, Robert W. Cantrell, Michael E. Johns, Paul A. Levine, W. Copley McClean, and James F. Reibel, among others, have been instrumental in developing and maintaining this prestige over the last three decades, which has, in turn, attracted a high volume of clinically and pathologically interesting cases to our files. Indeed, without their efforts, it is doubtful that any of us would have developed and maintained interest or expertise in this area.

We are likewise greatly indebted to our colleagues, here and elsewhere, Drs. E. Leon Barnes, Mark Bernstein, John K.C. Chan, Robert D. Collins, Robert E. Fechner, Douglas R. Gnepp, Allen M. Gown, Kenneth E. Greer, Donald J. Innes, Jr., Silloo B. Kapadia, Ernest E. Lack, Carlos Manivel, Mark H. Stoler, Jerome B. Taxy, John L. Ward, and Lawrence M. Weiss who graciously supplied additional illustrative material for this work. It is impossible to track the origins of every illustration in our collections. If we have inadvertently failed to acknowledge a resident or colleague whose material appears in this work, we apologize for the oversight. In particular, we thank the many colleagues who have sent us material in consultation, as these often challenging cases have provided insight into morphologic variations and diagnostic dilemmas that we have tried to emphasize in this text.

To our co-workers, residents, fellows, and family members who endured often protracted periods of mental distraction or physical absence during the lengthy production and editing of this work, we thank you for your patience with us.

Tragically, our co-author, colleague, and friend, Dr. Michael J. Gaffey, died the day after the first draft of this Fascicle was submitted for publication. This profound loss to his family, friends, colleagues, and the pathology community in general remains strongly with us almost two years later. Mike was a unique individual and his terrific sense of humor, high energy, great academic productivity, and often "larger than life" persona are greatly missed. We take some comfort in the knowledge that he died indulging his great passion for motorcycling and did not suffer in his death. It is with a deep sense of loss that we dedicate this work to him. May it serve as a small memorial to an outstanding pathologist lost in the prime of his career.

Stacey E. Mills, M.D.
Henry F. Frierson, Jr., M.D.

Permission to use copyrighted illustrations has been granted by:

American Academy of Otolaryngology:
  Embryology of the Head and Neck in Relation to the Practice of Otolaryngology, 1957. For figure 16-2.

American Medical Association:
  Arch Otolaryngol 1971;94:351–5. For figures 7-1 and 7-2.

American Society of Clinical Pathologists:
  Pathology of the Larynx, 1985. For figures 1-9, 1-10, 1-11, 1-13, 1-15, 1-16, 5-2, 7-92, and 9-35.

Charles C. Thomas:
  Meningiomas Involving the Temporal Bone, 1964. For figure 16-91.

Lippincott-Raven:
  Diagnostic Surgical Pathology. For figures 1-5 and 5-23.
  Histology for Pathologists, 2nd ed., 1997. For figures 1-8, 1-9, and 1-12.
  Laryngoscope 1981;91:2071–94. For figure 3-2.

Scandanavian University Press:
  Acta Otolaryngol 1968;66:181–98, 515–32. For figure 16-7.

W.B. Saunders:
  Atlas of Otorhinolaryngology and Broncho-esophagology, 1969. For figure 16-31.

Contents

TUMORS OF THE UPPER AERODIGESTIVE TRACT AND EAR

1
ANATOMY, HISTOLOGY, AND EMBRYOLOGY

An understanding of the anatomic divisions of the head and neck, as well as their associated normal histologic features, is of considerable importance when dealing with head and neck pathology. The large number of disease processes that can involve this area is a reflection of the many specialized tissues present and at risk for specific diseases. Many neoplasms show a sharp predilection for specific anatomic locations, and virtually never occur outside these regions. For instance, knowing the location of normal olfactory mucosa allows visualization of the sites of origin of olfactory neuroblastoma. An understanding of the boundaries of the nasopharynx and its distinction from the nasal cavity is particularly important. This junction, perhaps because it marks the interface of endodermally and ectodermally derived tissues, is a critical watershed in neoplasm distribution. Angiofibromas and lymphoepitheliomas almost exclusively arise on the nasopharyngeal side of the interface, whereas schneiderian papillomas, lobular capillary hemangiomas, and sinonasal intestinal-type adenocarcinomas almost entirely arise anteriorly, in the nasal cavity.

NASAL CAVITY

Anatomy

Although usually referred to as a single structure, the nasal cavity actually consists of paired midfacial nares divided into two more or less mirror images by the nasal septum and at its extreme anterior, the columella (figs. 1-1, 1-2). Midline asymmetry of the nasal septum is common and results in considerable variation in the contour and volume of the left and right chambers. Each cavity is bounded anteriorly by the external naris, marking the junction of the nasal cavity with the external world. It is bounded posteriorly by the nasal choana, which forms the

junction with the nasopharynx. The medial border is the smooth-surfaced nasal septum. Beneath the mucosa, the septum is formed by one cartilaginous and two osseous supporting structures. Posteriorly and inferiorly, it is composed of the vomer. This bone extends from the region of the sphenoid sinus posteriorly and superiorly, to the anterior edge of the hard palate. Superior to the vomer, the septum is formed by the perpendicular plate of the ethmoid bone. The most anterior portion of the septum is septal cartilage, which articulates with both the vomer and the ethmoidal plate. The supporting structure of the lateral border of the nasal cavity is complex. Portions of the nasal, ethmoid, and sphenoid bones all contribute to its formation. The lateral nasal wall is distinguished from the smooth septal surface by its "scroll-shaped" superior, middle, and inferior turbinates. The small superior turbinate and larger middle turbinate are formed from the ethmoid bone (19). The lower turbinate is a distinct, separate bone (19).

There are multiple openings along the lateral wall of the nasal cavity, primarily to the adjacent paranasal sinuses. The frontal sinus ostium is located in the frontal recess at the anterior region of the middle turbinate. The sphenoid sinus opening is in the sphenoethmoid recess located behind the superior turbinate. The opening to the posterior ethmoid air cells is located under the superior turbinate, with openings for the middle and anterior cells located in the ethmoid bulla and hiatus semilunaris of the middle turbinate (19). The primary maxillary antrum ostium is also located in the hiatus semilunaris, and there may be an accessory ostium located posterior to the primary maxillary ostium.

The most superior portion of the nasal cavity consists of the cribriform plate with its specialized olfactory mucosa (fig. 1-3). This merges with the remainder of the cavity roof which slopes downward posteriorly to form the superior portion of the

1

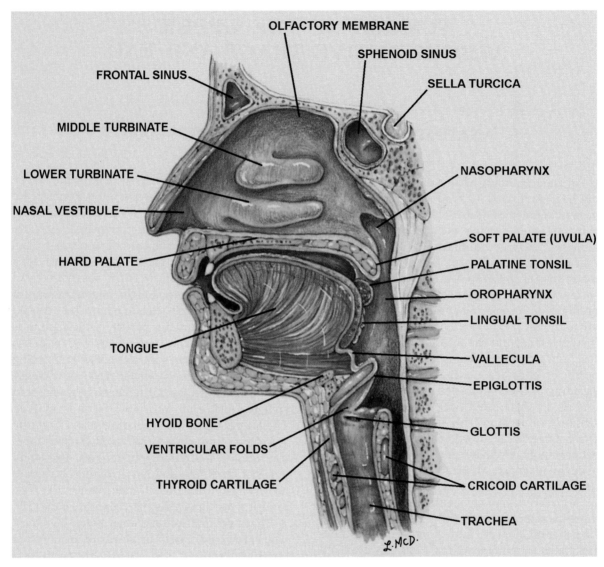

Figure 1-1
A SAGITTAL VIEW OF THE ANATOMY OF THE UPPER RESPIRATORY AND ORAL TRACT
A midline, sagittal section showing the major structures of the nasal cavity, pharynx, and larynx. (Plate I from Fascicle 25, 2nd Series.)

choana. The floor of the nasal cavity is formed by a combination of the hard and soft palates.

Histology

The most anterior portion of the nasal cavity or nasal vestibule is an inward extension of the skin of the external nose. It is lined by keratinized squamous epithelium with associated dermal adnexae, including hair follicles, sebaceous glands, and sweat glands. This inward cutaneous extension averages 1 to 2 cm in depth, after

which there is a gradual loss of adnexal structures and replacement of the keratinized squamous epithelium by so-called schneiderian epithelium (19). The schneiderian epithelium, which lines the nasal cavity and paranasal sinuses, is denoted with this eponym primarily to emphasize its ectodermal origin, as distinct from the endodermal origin of the mucosa lining the pharynx and larynx. With the exception of olfactory mucosa, schneiderian epithelium lacks any histologic distinction from the linings of

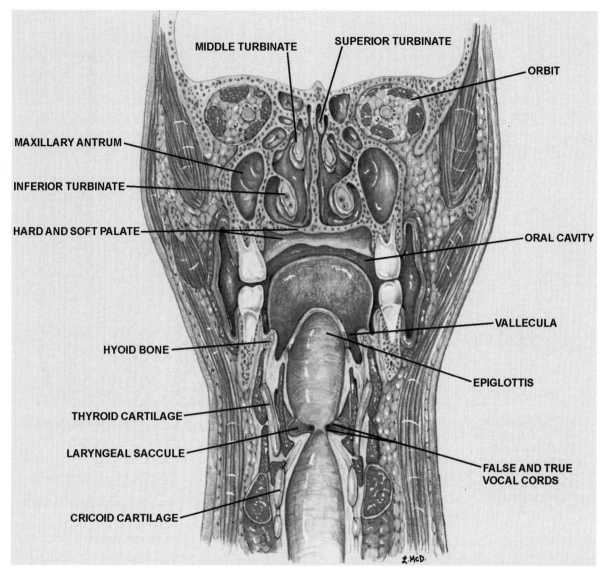

Figure 1-2
A CORONAL VIEW OF THE SINONASAL TRACT, ORAL CAVITY, AND LARYNX
A coronal section through the head at the level of the molar teeth displays the anatomy of the nasal cavity, as well as the pharynx, larynx, and some of the paranasal sinuses. (Plate II from Fascicle 25, 2nd Series.)

these latter structures. It is primarily composed of a mixture of nonkeratinizing squamous cells, ciliated respiratory cells, scattered mucus-containing goblet cells, and intermediate cells. The mucosa varies in thickness from more prominent pseudostratified columnar cells overlying the portions of the middle and inferior turbinates in direct contact with airflow, to thinner layers of cuboidal cells lining recesses of the nasal cavity and the paranasal sinuses (19). Areas of squamous metaplasia may occasionally be found, primarily on the anterior surfaces of the middle and lower turbinates and the anterior portion of the nasal septum (35). Beneath the mucosal surface is a normally thin basal lamina with underling loose stroma containing variably prominent seromucinous glands. Deep to the glands is a prominent erectile-type vascular tissue which should not be confused with a vascular neoplasm.

The olfactory mucosa is normally confined to the cribriform plate, the medial surface of the superior turbinate, and the superior one third of

3

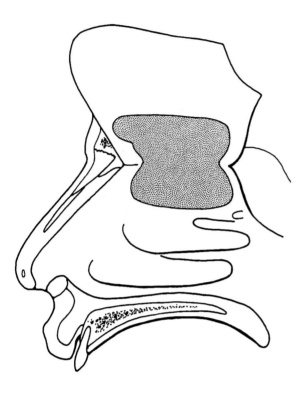

Figure 1-3
NASAL CAVITY

The olfactory mucosa is confined to the superior most portion of the nasal cavity. It involves the superior portion of the superior turbinate, the cribriform plate, and the superior approximately one third of the nasal septum. In adults the distribution becomes somewhat patchy, due to multifocal replacement by nonolfactory mucosa. (Fig. 4 from Fascicle 25, 2nd Series.)

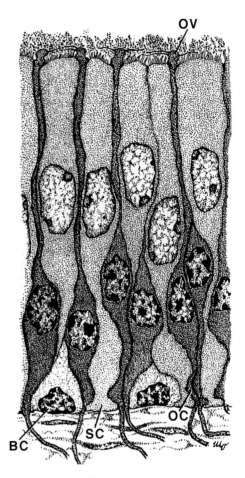

Figure 1-4
NASAL CAVITY

Specialized olfactory mucosa is composed of a mixture of olfactory cells (OC) with neuronal processes penetrating the cribriform plate, sustentacular epithelial cells (SC), and regenerative basal cells (BC). (Fig. 6 from Fascicle 25, 2nd Series.)

the nasal septum. The total surface area in adults is approximately 1.5 cm^2. Over time, areas of olfactory mucosa may be partially replaced by schneiderian epithelium, resulting in a patchy distribution that presumably accounts for the generally diminishing sense of smell with advancing age. Whether olfactory neurons can regenerate in humans is unclear, but this has been demonstrated in other mammals (21). Rarely, ectopic foci of olfactory mucosa lower in the nasal cavity have been described. Several studies using an olfactory marker protein have allowed for relatively easy mapping of the mucosal distribution (16,22,23).

The specialized olfactory mucosa is composed of three cell types (fig. 1-4). Most common are epithelial sustentacular cells, tall columnar eosinophilic cells anchored to the basement mem-

brane but extending upward to the surface where they form microvilli. Interdigitated between the sustentacular cells are the elongated neuronal olfactory cells. At the surface, these cells form widened peripheral processes containing olfactory vesicles. These are embedded in a protective mucus blanket. Proximally, the neuronal cells form thin cytoplasmic processes containing unmyelinated nerve fibers which penetrate the cribriform plate to synapse in the olfactory bulb. Small basal cells just above the basement membrane differentiate to form replacement sustentacular cells and may also form replacement neuronal cells. Just beneath the olfactory mucosa is a distinctive group of simple

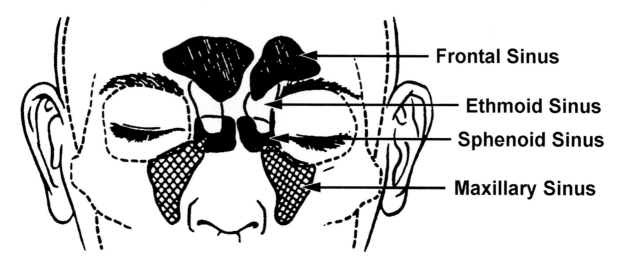

Figure 1-5
PARANASAL SINUSES
The paranasal sinuses as seen projected onto the face. The frontal sinuses are most anterior, the maxillary sinuses are beneath the cheek, the ethmoids occupy the interorbital region, and the sphenoid sinuses are most posterior, just beneath the base of the brain. (Fig. 2 from Mills SE, Fechner RE. The nose, paranasal sinuses, and nasopharynx. In: Sternberg SS, ed. Diagnostic surgical pathology, 2nd ed., New York: Raven Press, 1994:851–91.)

serous glands referred to as the glands of Bowman. The distinctive appearance of these glands and, particularly, their lack of mucin can be an aid in distinguishing olfactory mucosa from normal schneiderian epithelium.

Embryology

The nasal cavity is of ectodermal origin. During the fourth week of embryologic development, a proliferation of ectoderm forms beneath the forebrain and develops a hollow invagination known as the olfactory pit. Cells within this pit acquire neural features and send dendritic processes through the region of the subsequent cribriform plate to synapse with the developing forebrain. While this neuronal differentiation is proceeding, adjacent mesodermal tissues form the structure of the nasal cavity and paranasal sinuses. During the sixth week, the nasal pit deepens considerably, and is initially separated from the primitive oral cavity by the oronasal membrane (15). This ruptures, placing the primitive nasal cavity in continuity with the developing oral cavity. With the fusion of the primitive palate and the lateral palatine shelves of the secondary palate, the nasal and oral cavities become sepa-

rated in the eighth week of development (14). During this process, the definitive nasal choanae form, separating the nasal cavity from the nasopharynx, and the nasal septum grows downward to join the newly fused palate (14).

PARANASAL SINUSES

Anatomy

The paranasal sinuses are diverticula of the nasal cavity (10). The maxillary, frontal, and sphenoid sinuses are relatively large, paired structures (fig. 1-5). The ethmoid sinuses consist of varying numbers of closely apposed air-filled spaces known as the ethmoid air cells. All of the sinuses are small or vestigial structures at birth that progressively enlarge during childhood and adolescence. The frontal sinuses reach full size after puberty. They may vary considerably in size and the larger may cross the midline to impinge on its smaller contralateral twin. The ostium of the frontal sinus is located beneath the anterior end of the middle turbinate. The maxillary sinuses do not reach full development until late adolescence with the acquisition of full permanent dentition. Much of the change in facial contour associated with adolescent growth is due to enlargement of the maxillary sinuses.

The ethmoid air cells vary in number from approximately 3 to 18 cells. The anterior ethmoid air cells are more numerous and are closely related to the frontal sinus. Occasionally, they bulge into the frontal sinus (11). These air cells open beneath the middle turbinate near the opening of the frontal sinus. The middle ethmoid air cells form the ethmoidal bulla and open at varying spots along the middle turbinate. The posterior ethmoid air cells may be absent, but if present they open around the superior turbinate. The posterior ethmoid air cells are closely associated with the sphenoid sinus and may bulge into it; they also are closely associated with the optic nerve and separated from it by only a thin lamina of bone.

The maxillary sinus or antrum lies behind the prominence of the cheek. Its lateral wall, roof, and floor are formed primarily from the maxillary bone, and its medial wall is the lateral wall of the nasal cavity. It opens high on the medial wall of the sinus into the so-called infundibulum. An accessory maxillary ostium, more posterior beneath the middle turbinate, also is common.

The paired sphenoid sinuses lie close together within the body of the sphenoid bone, just below the pituitary gland. On either side of the sinuses are a considerable number of vital structures including the carotid arteries, cavernous sinus, and the ophthalmic and maxillary branches of the trigeminal nerve (11). There may also be a close association with the optic canal if the sinuses extend forward and upward into this region.

It should be noted that of the large paranasal sinuses, only the frontal have gravity drainage in an erect posture (11). Thus, under normal conditions most drainage from these sinuses is by ciliary action. Gravity drainage of the maxillary sinus is best achieved by lying on the side opposite the affected sinus. The sphenoid sinuses are best drained by lying face down. The openings of the ethmoid sinuses are so variable that no position allows complete drainage.

Histology

The lining epithelium of the paranasal sinuses is similar to that of the nasal cavity and consists predominantly of ciliated respiratory cells and scattered mucinous cells. The mucosa is typically only about half as thick as that lining the nasal cavity, and many of the lining cells may be cuboidal or even flattened, rather than columnar. The loose, richly vascular submucosal tissue seen in the nasal cavity is absent. Only a thin layer of fibrous tissue separates the epithelial lining from the underlying periosteum. Seromucinous glands are rare in the lamina propria of the sinuses, and, when present, are primarily located close to the sinus ostia (32).

ORAL CAVITY

Anatomy

The oral cavity or mouth is bounded externally by the internal mucosa of the cheeks and the vermillion border of the lips. It is formed superiorly by the hard and soft palate, and inferiorly by the anterior two thirds of the tongue with the attached mucous membranes of the floor of the mouth (fig. 1-1). The posterior boundary of the oral cavity, at its junction with the oropharynx, is called the fauces. This is defined superiorly by the posterior edge of the soft palate and uvula and laterally by the tonsillar pillars. The inferior margin corresponds to a line across the circumvallate papillae of the tongue.

Histology

At the vermillion border of the lips, the skin of the outer lip junctions with the squamous mucosa of the oral cavity. Most of the oral cavity is lined by nonkeratinizing squamous epithelium. Portions directly involved in chewing, including the hard palate and parts of the gingiva, are lined by squamous mucosa with varying degrees of orthokeratotic and parakeratotic surface epithelium. This is associated with considerable thickening of the underlying rete ridges. Identical histologic changes develop in areas of chronic irritation, most often associated with poorly fitting dentures. The tongue is covered by specialized filiform, fungiform, and circumvallate papillae involved in chewing and taste. Scattered melanocytes are normally present in the squamous mucosa of the oral cavity. On hematoxylin and eosin (H&E)-stained sections they are difficult to spot and appear as clear cells in the basal epithelial layer. Their elongated cell processes interdigitating between mucosal epithelial cells are much better appreciated with immunohisto-chemistry for S-100 protein. The lamina propria of the oral cavity is filled with seromucinous glands. These are especially prominent in the lamina propria of the hard palate. The stroma around teeth often contains epithelial rests of apparent odontogenic origin and the large epithelial nests of the "organ of Chievitz" are present in lamina propria from the region of the retromolar trigone. These rests are discussed in chapter 15.

PHARYNX

Anatomy

The pharynx has three functionally and structurally diverse components: the nasopharynx, oropharynx, and hypopharynx (12). The nasopharynx is that portion of the pharynx located above the soft palate (fig. 1-1) (20). The anterior edge of the nasopharynx is demarcated, and perforated, by the nasal choana. The roof and posterior wall form an arch lying just below the base of the skull. The posterior wall extends downward to the point where it is intersected by a horizontal line from the soft palate, demarcating the superior border of the oropharynx. The anterior border of the oropharynx is partially defined by the fauces at the posterior extreme of the oral cavity, and below this by the dorsum of the tongue. The inferior margin is marked by the tip of the epiglottis. Below this lies the hypopharynx which spreads out laterally around the body of the larynx as the pyriform sinuses. The aryepiglottic folds mark the junction of the larynx and hypopharynx. Moving inferiorly, the hypopharynx rapidly narrows and ends at its junction with the esophagus.

Because of their location and intrinsically difficult surgical access, resection specimens from the nasopharynx and oropharynx are virtually never encountered. The pharynx has a complex musculature and innervation, which is reviewed elsewhere (12,20). It is important for pathologists to be aware of the normal distribution of lymphoid tissue in this region, as well as the location and histologic features of several "landmarks." The pharyngeal tonsil or adenoid is a convoluted mass of lymphoid tissue located in the roof of the nasopharynx in children; it typically atrophies in adults (20). The palatine tonsils lie along the anterolateral border of the oropharynx; they vary markedly in size depending upon the state of reactivity. The tonsillar surface is covered with a large number of epithelial-lined pits which penetrate the tonsillar lymphoid tissue to form the tonsillar crypts. The immobile base of the tongue in the anterior oropharynx contains abundant lymphoid tissue, constituting the so-called lingual tonsil. Along with the pharyngeal and palatine tonsils, this oblique wreath of normal pharyngeal lymphoid tissue constitutes Waldeyer's ring.

The pharyngeal recess or fossa of Rosenmüller is a mucosal-lined depression in the posterior, lateral wall of the nasopharynx. Just anterior to this recess is the eustachian tube opening which is partially surrounded by mucosal-covered cartilage from the wall of the eustachian tube (20).

Histology

A slight majority of the nasopharynx is lined by squamous epithelium, with about 40 percent covered by ciliated respiratory mucosa (1). The respiratory component preferentially lines the region of the choanae and the roof of the nasopharynx. Squamous epithelium predominantly covers the lower portions of the nasopharynx. Alternating islands of squamous and respiratory epithelium are present, particularly in the midregions of the nasopharynx. As in the larynx, the junction between these zones may be sharp or there may be an area of intermediate epithelium representing progressive maturation of immature to mature squamous metaplasia. As in the larynx, the disorganization and basaloid appearance of these regions may lead to confusion with dysplasia or carcinoma in situ.

The epithelium covering the adenoid and palatine tonsils extends downward into the tonsillar crypts were it blurs into the underlying lymphoid tissue (fig. 1-6). At this interface, the epithelial cells typically assume a more basaloid appearance with uniform, vesicular nuclei (fig. 1-7). There also may be areas of abrupt keratinization with keratin "pearl" formation. Invariably, microscopic sections through these regions show disorganized, apparently isolated nests of basaloid squamous cells with abrupt keratinization. These features should not be confused with carcinoma (20).

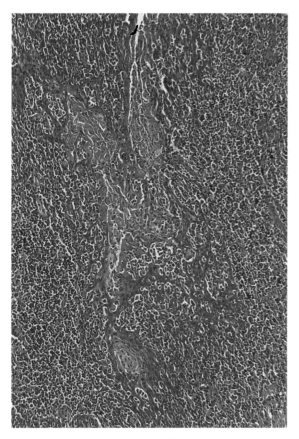

Figure 1-6
NORMAL TONSIL
The squamous mucosa overlying the lymphoid tissue of Waldeyer's ring forms crypt-like invaginations into the lymphoid stroma, with considerable disruption of the epithelium by the lymphoid cells.

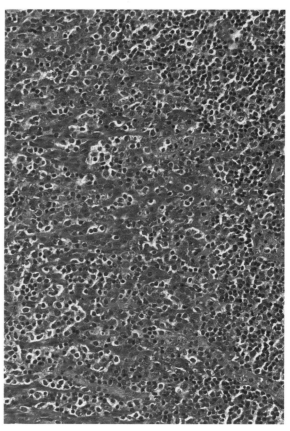

Figure 1-7
NORMAL TONSIL
Basal epithelial cells from a tonsillar crypt are intermingled with the associated lymphoid component. The resultant image, at high magnification, can be confused with carcinoma.

In addition to the larger pharyngeal, palatine, and lingual tonsils, less prominent aggregates of lymphoid tissue may be present in the lamina propria throughout the nasopharynx. These should not be overinterpreted as chronic inflammation. Aggregates of lymphoid follicles are particularly prominent in the rim of the eustachian tube opening (Gerlach's tonsil) (20).

Seromucinous glands and their associated ducts are located throughout the lamina propria of the nasopharynx. Mucin production is prominent in these glands, and they may undergo oncocytic metaplasia with increasing age (20). Microscopic remnants of Rathke's pouch epithelium are present in the roof of the nasopharynx in virtually all individuals (4,17,18). These nests of epithelial cells, referred to as the pharyngeal pituitary, measure 0.2 to 6.0 mm in size and are located in the deep mucosa or underlying periosteum (18,20). Usually, these cell nests appear undifferentiated, but occasionally they have distinctly basophilic or eosinophilic cytoplasm.

The pharyngeal bursa normally forms posterior to Rathke's pouch and remnants of this bursa may be found in the roof of the nasopharynx in about 3 percent of individuals (10,31). Cysts of this bursa occasionally develop and are located adjacent to but distinct from the adenoid (25). Cysts may also develop from the median pharyngeal recess, a nasopharyngeal indentation closely associated with the adenoid. These cysts are located within the adenoid and are removed with it.

The oropharynx and hypopharynx are lined by squamous epithelium. The mucosa is nonkeratinizing, except in areas of chronic irritation, where it may be covered with a layer of

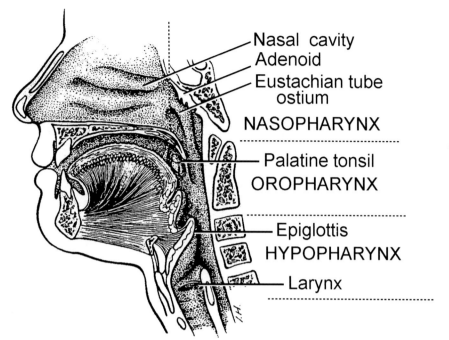

Figure 1-8
SAGITTAL SECTION
OF PHARYNX

The boundaries of the nasal cavity, nasopharynx, oropharynx, and hypopharynx are delineated in this sagittal view. (Fig. 21 from Mills SE, Fechner RE. Larynx and pharynx. In: Sternberg SS, ed. Histology for pathologists, 2nd. ed. New York: Raven Press, 1997:398.)

orthokeratin or parakeratinized cells. The lamina propria of the oropharynx and hypopharynx normally contains scattered lymphoid aggregates and follicles, as well as large numbers of seromucinous glands.

LARYNX

Anatomy

The larynx is bordered superiorly by the tip of the epiglottis and the aryepiglottic folds (figs. 1-8, 1-9). The inferior border and junction with the trachea is formed by the inferior margin of the cricoid cartilage. The anterior border consists of the lingual edge of the epiglottis, the thyroid cartilage, the anterior arch of the cricoid cartilage, the thyrohyoid membrane, and the cricothyroid membrane (20). Posteriorly, the larynx is bounded by the posterior portion of the cricoid cartilage and the arytenoid region. The pyriform fossa is not part of the larynx but represents an outpouching of the hypopharynx located on each lateral border of the larynx (fig. 1-9). It serves as a conduit for food and water rather than air (20).

The structural integrity of the larynx is derived from its major cartilages (figs. 1-10, 1-11). These include the cricoid, thyroid, and paired arytenoid cartilages, all of which are of hyaline cartilage type. Ossification of the thyroid and cricoid cartilages, complete with the formation of bone marrow elements, begins in adulthood. Importantly, ossified cartilage lacks the resistance to the spread of cancer manifest by unaltered hyaline cartilage. The remaining major laryngeal cartilage, the epiglottic cartilage, is of elastic type and never undergoes ossification. However, it contains numerous fenestrations which allow for easy invasion and penetration by carcinoma.

Primarily from a surgical point of view, and partially related to embryology (see below), the larynx is typically divided into three major compartments: supraglottic, glottic, and subglottic. The supraglottic larynx begins superiorly at the tip of the epiglottis and extends downward to the superior edge of the true vocal cord (30). Included in the supraglottic larynx are the epiglottis, aryepiglottic folds, the false vocal cords, and the laryngeal ventricles. The glottic larynx includes the vocal cords and the anterior commissure which bridges them at their anterior point of attachment (fig. 1-12) (2,28). It also includes the small portion of the posterior mucosal wall at the level of the vocal cords located between the arytenoid cartilages. This area is sometimes referred to as the "posterior commissure," but a

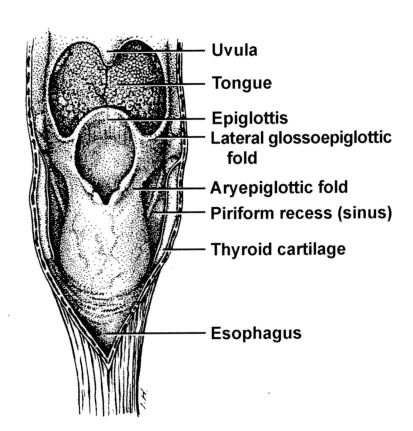

Uvula

Tongue

Epiglottis
Lateral glossoepiglottic fold

Aryepiglottic fold
Piriform recess (sinus)

Thyroid cartilage

Esophagus

Figure 1-9
PIRIFORM SINUSES
The piriform recesses or sinuses are lateral to the larynx and part of the hypopharynx, forming a conduit from the oropharynx to the esophagus. (Fig. 22 from Mills SE, Fechner RE. Larynx and pharynx. In: Sternberg SS, ed. Histology for pathologists, 2nd ed. New York: Raven Press, 1997:399.)

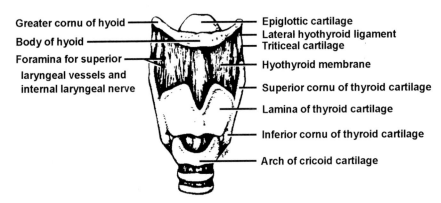

Greater cornu of hyoid
Body of hyoid
Foramina for superior laryngeal vessels and internal laryngeal nerve

Epiglottic cartilage
Lateral hyothyroid ligament
Triticeal cartilage
Hyothyroid membrane
Superior cornu of thyroid cartilage
Lamina of thyroid cartilage
Inferior cornu of thyroid cartilage
Arch of cricoid cartilage

Figure 1-10
THE LARYNGEAL CARTILAGES, VIEWED ANTERIORLY
The lamina of the thyroid cartilage, cricoid arch, and hyothyroid membrane are the major anterior supporting structures. (Fig. 1 from Mills SE, Fechner RE. Pathology of the larynx. Chicago: ASCP 1985:1.)

Figure 1-11
UNOPENED LARYNX, POSTERIOR VIEW
Posteriorly, the major structural support for the larynx is derived from the lamina of the cricoid cartilage. The location of the speech-critical arytenoid cartilages can be clearly visualized. (Fig. 2 from Mills SE, Fechner RE. Pathology of the larynx. Chicago: ASCP 1985:1.)

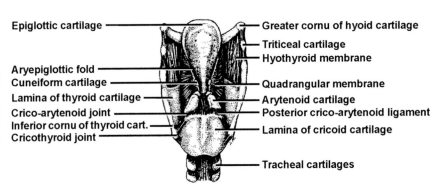

Epiglottic cartilage
Aryepiglottic fold
Cuneiform cartilage
Lamina of thyroid cartilage
Crico-arytenoid joint
Inferior cornu of thyroid cart.
Cricothyroid joint

Greater cornu of hyoid cartilage
Triticeal cartilage
Hyothyroid membrane
Quadrangular membrane
Arytenoid cartilage
Posterior crico-arytenoid ligament
Lamina of cricoid cartilage
Tracheal cartilages

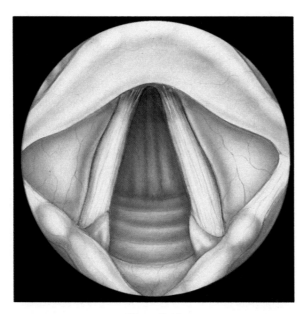

Figure 1-12
VOCAL CORDS

This endoscopic view of the larynx shows the epiglottis anteriorly, and the vocal cords with their posterior attachments to the arytenoids. The false cords are just above and lateral to the true cords. (Fig. 3 from Mills SE, Fechner RE. Larynx and pharynx. In: Sternberg SS, ed. Histology for pathologists, 2nd ed. New York: Raven Press, 1997:393.)

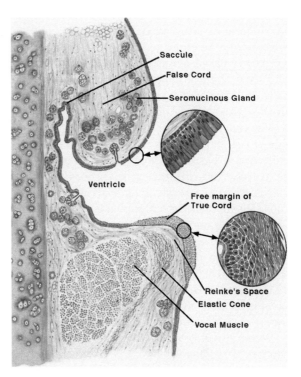

Figure 1-13
TRUE AND FALSE VOCAL CORDS

A coronal section through one side of the larynx shows false vocal cord with abundant seromucinous glands, the laryngeal ventricle and saccule, and the true vocal cord with underlying vocalis muscle. (Slide 2 from Mills SE, Fechner RE. Pathology of the larynx. Chicago: ASCP 1985:3.)

true posterior commissure does not exist (9). The subglottic larynx extends inferiorly from the lower border of the true vocal cords to the region of the inferior border of the cricoid cartilage and the first tracheal cartilage (29).

Histology

In newborns, the larynx is entirely lined by ciliated, respiratory epithelium, with the exception of the true vocal cords which are covered by stratified squamous epithelium (fig. 1-13) (13). Patches of squamous epithelium begin to appear on the false vocal cords at about 6 months of age, but large areas of ciliated epithelium may remain (27,34). The anterior or lingual surface of the epiglottis is not functionally part of the larynx and is invariably covered with squamous epithelium. In adults, the posterior surface is covered by stratified squamous mucosa at its upper end, but this merges with ciliated respiratory epithelium inferiorly. In nonsmoking adults, the supraglottic and infraglottic portions of the larynx are typically lined by irregular patches of squamous epithelium, alternating

with ciliated respiratory epithelium. In smokers, the entire larynx, along with large portions of the remainder of the tracheobronchial tree, may be lined by squamous epithelium.

The ciliated respiratory epithelium of the larynx varies markedly in thickness (20). It may consist of a flattened basal cell layer overlain by a second, modest layer of ciliated respiratory cells with minor variation in nuclear positioning. Alternately, the ciliated layer may be thickened and exhibit prominent pseudostratification of nuclei. Mucous cells vary from rare to numerous. The junction between areas of respiratory and squamous epithelium may be abrupt, but often there is a 1- to 2-mm transitional zone in which columnar cells are gradually replaced by somewhat disorganized immature squamous or basaloid cells. This zone of immature squamous metaplasia is analogous to the junctional changes frequently encountered in the uterine cervix. This pattern can be confused with dysplasia or carcinoma in situ, particularly when dealing with frozen sections or otherwise suboptimal preparations. Closer attention to cytologic detail will show that, although disorganized, the cells have uniform nuclei, with mitotic figures confined to the basal cell layer.

The mature squamous epithelium of the larynx varies in thickness and consists of a mitotically active basal cell layer which may contain scattered, interdigitating melanocytes (5,7), overlain by progressively maturing squamous cells. The most superficial component consists of 2 to 3 small, flattened squamous cells with smaller nuclei. The overall thickness of the squamous epithelium is highly variable and may range from 5 to 25 cells in thickness (20). Normally, a well-formed parakeratotic or orthokeratotic cell layer is lacking, although these changes are commonly present in biopsies from chronic smokers.

Seromucinous glands are present, with one exception, throughout the larynx. They connect to the overlying surface epithelium via ducts lined by mixtures of squamous and columnar epithelia (24). The glands are particularly numerous beneath the false vocal cords. They also are numerous in the epiglottis and often fill the fenestrations in the epiglottic cartilage. In tangential sections, squamous-lined ducts from these glands may appear as apparently isolated squamous nests. Distinction from invasive carcinoma is usually straightforward given sections of adequate quality, but the situation becomes more difficult when dysplastic changes from overlying surface mucosa extend into these ducts.

Seromucinous glands are absent or very sparse beneath the mobile portions of the true vocal cords (figs. 1-13, 1-14). In this region, the lamina propria is composed of loose to dense connective tissue filling the space between the surface epithelium and the underlying vocal ligament (Reinke's space) (20). This area has limited vascular and lymphatic access. The poor lymphatic drainage probably contributes to the development of vocal cord nodules and polyps when edema fluid is trapped in this space. The poor vascular access of the vocal cords may also account for the excellent prognosis associated with carcinomas confined to the true cords, since the chance of spread to regional or distant sites is minimal.

The vocal process of the arytenoid cartilage deserves special mention because this structure

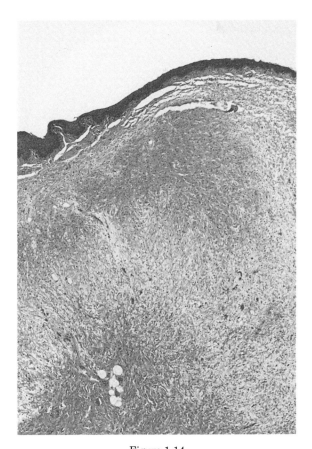

Figure 1-14
TRUE VOCAL CORD
The loose fibromyxoid tissue beneath the vocal cord epithelium is devoid of seromucinous glands.

may cause considerable consternation in biopsies from the posterior portion of the vocal cord (fig. 1-15). The vocal process is a sharply demarcated nodule of elastic cartilage, often surrounded by a narrow, condensed, concentric layer of fibrous tissue. It's elastic nature distinguishes it from chondroid neoplasms, which are composed of hyaline cartilage. Chondroid metaplasia of the vocal cords is present in 1 to 2 percent of autopsies (7, 13). It has been said to preferentially affect the middle and posterior portions of the vocal cords, placing it near the vocal process. Microscopically, it consists of small, somewhat ill-defined nodules of chondrocytes associated with aggregates of elastic fibers (fig. 1-16). The surrounding stroma is often rich in acid mucopolysaccharides (14). Chondroid metaplasia can occur elsewhere in the larynx, particularly in the false vocal cords.

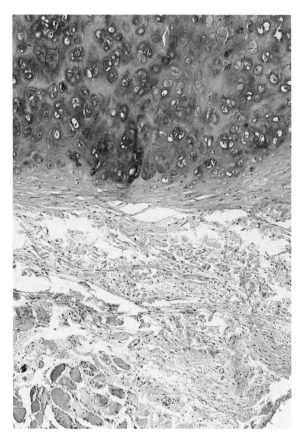

Figure 1-15
ARYTENOID CARTILAGE

Sections from the posterior portion of the vocal cords may include the vocal process of the arytenoid cartilage. This should not be confused with chondroid metaplasia or neoplasia. A portion of vocalis muscle is present at the lower left. (Slide 7 from Mills SE, Fechner RE. Pathology of the larynx. Chicago: ASCP 1985:4.)

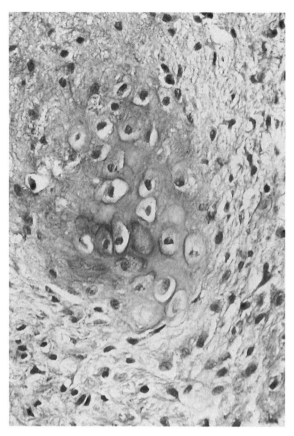

Figure 1-16
CHONDROID METAPLASIA

Chondroid metaplasia forms small, somewhat ill-defined cartilaginous nodules. (Slide 81 from Mills SE, Fechner RE. Cartilagenous tumors. Pathology of the larynx. Chicago: ASCP, 1985:60.)

Embryology

The supraglottic portion of the larynx, along with the oral cavity and oropharynx, is derived from the third and fourth branchial arches (3,20). In contrast, the glottis and subglottic larynx are derived from the sixth branchial arch which also gives rise to the trachea and lungs. Thus, as Bocca et al. (3) demonstrated, the larynx has two embryologically distinct components that form superior and inferior "hemilarynges" with distinct and largely independent lymphatic drainage.

Modes of local and regional spread are, accordingly, quite different for supraglottic as compared to glottic and subglottic neoplasms.

The first portion of the larynx to form during embryogenesis is the epiglottis, and this structure is well formed by the fifth week of embryologic development (26,33). The beginning form of a larynx is recognizable in a 6-mm embryo and by 60 to 70 days, at the 30-mm embryo stage, the vocal cords begin to differentiate. The larynx is a complex structure and subject to varied embryologic anomalies. Over 30 different malformations of the larynx have been described (6).

REFERENCES

1. Ali MY. Histology of the human nasopharyngeal mucosa. J Anat 1965;99:657–72.

2. Andrea M, Guerrier Y. The anterior commissure of the larynx. Clin Otolaryngol 1981;6:259–64.

3. Bocca E, Pignataro O, Mosciaro O. Supraglottic surgery of the larynx. Ann Otol Rhinol Laryngol 1968;77:1005–26.

4. Boyd JD. Observations on the human pharyngeal hypophysis. J Endocrinol 1956;14:66–77.

5. Busuttil A. Dendritic pigmented cells within human laryngeal mucosa. Arch Otolaryngol 1976;102:43–4.

6. Cotton A, Reilly JS. Congenital malformations of the larynx. In: Bluestone CD, Stool SE, eds. Pediatric otolaryngology. Philadelphia: WB Saunders, 1983:1215–24.

7. Goldman JL, Lawson W, Zak FG, Roffman JD. The presence of melanocytes in the human larynx. Laryngoscope 1972;82:824–35.

8. Hill MJ, Taylor CL, Scott GB. Chondromatous metaplasia in the human larynx. Histopathology 1980;4:205–14.

9. Hirano M, Kurita S. Histological structure of the vocal fold and its normal and pathological variations. In: Kirchner JA, ed. Vocal fold histopathology. A symposium. San Diego: College-Hill Press, 1986:17–24.

10. Hollender AR. The nasopharynx. A study of 140 autopsy specimens. Laryngoscope 1946;56:282–304.

11. Hollinshead WH. The ear, orbit, and nose. In: Anonymous, ed. Textbook of anatomy. Hagerstown: Harper & Row, 1967:886–932.

12. Hollinshead WH. Pharynx and larynx. In: Anonymous, ed. Textbook of anatomy. Hagerstown: Harper and Row, 1967:933–54.

13. Hopp ES. The development of the epithelium of the larynx. Laryngoscope 1955;65:475–99.

14. Iyer PV, Rajagopalan PV. Cartilaginous metaplasia of the soft tissues of the larynx. Case report and literature review. Arch Otolaryngol 1981;107:573–5.

15. Langman J. Face, nose and palate. In: Anonymous, ed. Medical embryology. Baltimore: Williams & Wilkins, 1969:354–63.

16. Margolis FL. Olfactory marker protein (OMP). Scand J Immunol 1982;15 (Suppl 9):181–99.

17. McGrath P. Extrasellar adenohypophyseal tissue in the female. Australas Radiol 1970;14:241–7.

18. Melchionna RH, Moore RA. The pharyngeal pituitary gland. Am J Pathol 1938;14:763–72.

19. Michaels L. The normal nose and paranasal sinuses. In: Anonymous, ed. Ear, nose, and throat histolopathology. New York: Springer-Verlag, 1987:131–6.

20. Mills SE, Fechner RE. Larynx and pharynx. In: Sternberg SS, ed. Histology for pathologists, 2nd ed. Philadelphia: Lippincott-Raven, 1997:391–403.

21. Monti-Graziadei GA, Graziadei PP. Neurogenesis and neuron regeneration in the olfactory system of mammals: II. Degeneration and reconstitution of the olfactory sensory neurons after axotomy. J Neurocytol 1979;8:197–213.

22. Nakashima T, Kimmelman CP, Snow JB Jr. Structure of human fetal and adult olfactory neuroepithelium. Arch Otolaryngol 1984;110:641–6.

23. Nakashima T, Kimmelman CP, Snow JB Jr. Olfactory marker protein in the human olfactory pathway. Arch Otolaryngol 1985;111:294–7.

24. Nassar VH, Bridger GP. Topography of the laryngeal mucous glands. Arch Otolaryngol 1971;94:490–8.

25. Nicolai P, Luzzago F, Maroldi R, Falchetti M, Antonelli AR. Nasopharyngeal cysts. Report of seven cases with review of the literature. Arch Otolaryngol Head Neck Surg 1989;115:860–4.

26. O'Rahilly R, Tucker JA. The early development of the larynx in staged human embryos. I. Embryos of the first five weeks (to stage 15). Ann Otol Rhinol Laryngol 1973;82(Suppl 7):1–27.

27. Scott GB. A quantitative study of microscopical changes in the epithelium and subepithelial tissue of the laryngeal folds, sinus and saccule. Clin Otolaryngol 1976;1:257–64.

28. Stell PM, Gregory I, Watt J. Morphometry of the epithelial lining of the human larynx. I. The glottis. Clin Otolaryngol 1978;3:13–20.

29. Stell PM, Gregory I, Watt J. Morphology of the human larynx. II. The subglottis. Clin Otolaryngol 1980;5:389–95.

30. Stell PM, Gudrun R, Watt J. Morphology of the human larynx. III. The supraglottis. Clin Otolaryngol 1981;6:389–93.

31. Toomey JM. Cysts and tumors of the pharynx. In: Paparella MM, Shumrick DA, eds. Otolaryngology. Philadelphia: WB Saunders, 1980.

32. Toppozada HH, Talaat MA. The normal human maxillary sinus mucosa. Arch Otolaryngol 1980;89:204–13.

33. Tucker JA, O'Rahilly R. Observations on the embryology of the human larynx. Ann Otol Rhinol Laryngol 1972;81:520–3.

34. Tucker JA, Vidic B, Tucker GF Jr, Stead J. Survey of the development of the laryngeal epithelium. Ann Otol Rhinol Laryngol 1976;85(Suppl 30):3–16.

35. Walike JW. Anatomy of the nasal cavities. Otolaryngol Clin North Am 1973;6:609–21.

2
STAGING FOR SQUAMOUS CELL CARCINOMA

INTRODUCTION AND BACKGROUND: THE TNM SYSTEM

Clinical staging for squamous cell carcinoma of the head and neck is performed in accordance with the TNM classification proposed by the American Joint Committee on Cancer (AJCC) (1) and the International Union Against Cancer (UICC) (2). The TNM system stages squamous cell carcinoma and other malignant tumors based on the size of the untreated tumor (T), spread to regional lymph nodes (N), and distant metastases (M). The resultant TNM assessment provides a shorthand method for indicating the extent of disease at a particular point in time during tumoral progression. The TNM system is concerned with the anatomic extent of disease only; other factors, such as tumor grade, patient age, and biologic marker expression are usually not considered.

The three components (namely, T, N, and M) are, by definition, assessed on clinical examination prior to therapy. Occasionally, regional lymph node spread and distant metastases may be present but are not yet detectable by clinical examination. Accordingly, the clinical stage (cTNM) established at the time of surgery may differ from the pathologic stage (pTNM) determined following the pathologic examination of the resected tissues. The pathologic results may be utilized for staging purposes, but the pathologic stage should be identified separately from the clinical classification.

Therapeutic procedures, such as chemotherapy, may alter the biologic properties or behavior of any given tumor. Tumors that recur after therapy are staged with the same markers as those used in pretreatment staging. The recurrent or retreatment stage (rTNM) may not be the same as the original assessment, however, and should be distinguished from the original cTNM. Similarly, staging performed after the death of the patient and the postmortem examination should be designated as the autopsy stage (aTNM).

In summary, TNM tumor staging provides an indication of the extent of the tumor and indirectly reflects the natural history and prognosis of the disease. The cTNM is considered essential for treatment selection, whereas the pTNM is regarded as the best indicator of prognosis. The TNM system also facilitates the transfer of information between clinicians or treatment centers, and assists in therapeutic decisions. It is important to remember, however, in addition to the anatomic extent of disease, histologic grade and other pathologic variables, such as assessment of surgical margin and vascular invasion, are also important factors in tumor evaluation. Thus, clinical staging does not preclude careful and complete microscopic examination and reporting.

The current system allows for four levels of T, three levels of N, and two levels of M, for a total of 24 different TNM categories. For computational purposes, it is often necessary to condense these 24 potential categories into a smaller number of TNM stage groupings. By definition, carcinoma in situ is regarded as stage 0, whereas cases with distant metastases are categorized as stage IV. Groupings into stages I, II, and III differ somewhat by tumor type and anatomic site.

GENERAL RULES OF REPORTING

As stated above, the TNM system is based on the assessment of the following variables: T, the extent of the primary (untreated) tumor; N, the presence or absence of regional lymph node metastases; and M, the presence or absence of distant metastases.

The addition of numbers to these three variables provides an indication of the extent of the variable, generally with increasing numbers indicating progressively increasing tumor size or extent of metastases:

TX	primary tumor cannot be assessed
Tis	carcinoma in situ
T0	no evidence of primary tumor
T1, T2, T3, T4	increasing size of primary tumor
NX	regional lymph nodes cannot be assessed
N0	no regional lymph node metastases

N1, N2, N3 increasing involvement of
regional lymph nodes

MX Presence of distant metastases
cannot be assessed

M0 No distant metastases identified

M1 Distant metastases identified

It is recognized that multiple, simultaneous primary tumors may occur in a single organ. In such a circumstance, the largest tumor should be identified, with either "m" (for multiplicity) or the number of tumors present indicated in parentheses (i.e., T2 [m] or T2 [4]). In certain classifications, subgroups (a, b, c) may be used to precisely categorize tumor extent; the use of these subgroups is encouraged but not required.

Direct extension of tumor into a lymph node is classified as a metastasis. Metastases in any lymph node other than regional nodes are classified as distant metastases. Nodal metastases should also be measured. It is recognized that most nodal metastases 3 cm in dimension or larger are not single nodes but rather confluent nodes or soft tissue metastases. Many classifications contain subgroups of regional lymph node metastases, designated a, b, and c; the use of the latter subgroups is recommended but not required.

HISTOPATHOLOGIC GRADE

The predominant cancer of the upper aerodigestive tract is squamous cell carcinoma. The following classification largely assumes that the carcinoma is an epithelial lesion, most likely squamous in type. Nonepithelial tumors, such as sarcomas, melanomas, and lymphomas, are not included. Histologic confirmation of the tumor is required, and grading is recommended. The histopathologic grade is admittedly subjective and does not enter into the staging of the tumor; nonetheless, it should be recorded. In all sites, the histopathologic grade of the tumor is as follows: GX, grade cannot be assessed; G1, well differentiated; G2, moderately differentiated; and G3, poorly differentiated.

SPECIFIC ANATOMIC SITES

The TNM categories for the oral cavity, the pharynx (including the base of tongue, soft palate, and uvula), the larynx, and the paranasal sinuses (maxillary and ethmoid sinuses) are listed below. The nasal cavity has yet to be defined, and tu-

mors of the sphenoid and frontal sinuses are sufficiently rare that a formal staging classification is not warranted. For the specific definitions of the anatomic sites listed, please consult the AJCC Cancer Staging Manual (1).

Oral Cavity

The oral cavity includes the mucosal lip, buccal mucosa, lower alveolar ridge, upper alveolar ridge, retromolar trigone, floor of mouth, hard palate, and the anterior two thirds of the tongue. All the latter structures receive the same T, N, and M assessments as follows:

Primary Tumor (T): Oral Cavity

TX Primary tumor cannot be assessed

T0 No evidence of primary tumor

Tis Carcinoma in situ

T1 Tumor 2 cm or less in dimension

T2 Tumor more than 2 cm but not more than 4 cm in dimension

T3 Tumor greater than 4 cm in dimension

T4 Tumor invades adjacent structures (bone, skin, etc.)

Regional Lymph Nodes (N): Oral Cavity

NX Regional lymph nodes cannot be assessed

N0 No regional lymph node metastasis

N1 Metastasis in a single ipsilateral lymph node, 3 cm or less in greatest dimension

N2 Metastasis in a single ipsilateral lymph node more than 3 cm but less than 6 cm in greatest dimension; or multiple ipsilateral lymph nodes, none more than 6 cm in greatest dimension; or in bilateral or contralateral lymph nodes, none more than 6 cm in greatest dimension.

N2a Metastasis in single ipsilateral lymph node more than 3 cm but not more than 6 cm in greatest dimension

N2b Metastasis in multiple ipsilateral lymph nodes, none more than 6 cm in greatest dimension

N2c Metastasis in bilateral or contralateral lymph nodes, none more than 6 cm in greatest dimension

N3 Metastasis in a lymph node more than 6 cm in greatest dimension

Distant Metastases (M): Oral Cavity

MX Presence of distant metastases cannot be assessed

M0   No distant metastases
M1   Distant metastases present

Pharynx

The pharynx is composed of the base of tongue, soft palate, and uvula and may be divided into three regions: the oropharynx, nasopharynx, and hypopharnx. Tumor size (T) assessment is different for each region. Regional lymph node (N) classification for the nasopharynx is different from that of the oropharynx and hypopharynx, the latter two of which are identical. Distant metastasis (M) assessment is identical for all three pharyngeal regions.

Tumor Size (T): Nasopharynx, Oropharynx, Hypopharynx
TX   Primary tumor cannot be assessed
T0   No evidence of primary tumor
Tis Carcinoma in situ

T - Nasopharynx
T1   Tumor confined to the nasopharynx
T2   Tumor extends to soft tissues of oropharynx and/or nasal fossa
  T2a without parapharyngeal extension
  T2b with parapharyngeal extension
T3   Tumor invades nasal cavity and/or oropharynx
T4   Tumor with intracranial extension and/or involvement of cranial nerves

T - Oropharynx
T1   Tumor 2 cm or less in dimension
T2   Tumor more than 2 cm but not more than 4 cm in dimension
T3   Tumor greater than 4 cm in dimension
T4   Tumor invades adjacent structures

T - Hypopharynx
T1   Tumor limited to one subsite of the hypopharynx and 2 cm or less in dimension
T2   Tumor invades more than one subsite of hypopharynx or an adjacent site, measures more than 2 cm but less than 4 cm in dimension without fixation of hemilarynx
T3   Tumor measures more than 4 cm in dimension or with fixation of hemilarynx
T4   Tumor invades adjacent structures

Regional Lymph Nodes (N)
N - Nasopharynx
NX   Regional lymph nodes cannot be assessed

N0   No regional lymph node metastasis
N1   Unilateral metastasis in lymph node(s), 6 cm or less in dimension, above the supraclavicular fossa.
N2   Bilateral metastasis in lymph node(s), 6 cm or less in dimension, above the supraclavicular fossa
N3   Metastasis in a lymph node(s)
  N3a greater than 6 cm in dimension
  N3b extension to the supraclavicular fossa

N - Oropharynx and Hypopharynx
NX   Regional lymph nodes cannot be assessed
N0   No regional lymph node metastasis
N1   Metastasis in a single ipsilateral lymph node, 3 cm or less in greatest dimension
N2   Metastasis in a single ipsilateral lymph node more than 3 cm but less than 6 cm in greatest dimension; or multiple ipsilateral lymph nodes, none more than 6 cm in greatest dimension; or in bilateral or contralateral lymph nodes, none more than 6 cm in greatest dimension.
  N2a Metastasis in single ipsilateral lymph node more than 3 cm but not more than 6 cm in greatest dimension
  N2b Metastasis in multiple ipsilateral lymph nodes, none more than 6 cm in greatest dimension
  N2c Metastasis in bilateral or contralateral lymph nodes, none more than 6 cm in greatest dimension
N3   Metastasis in a lymph node more than 6 cm in greatest dimension

Distant Metastases (M): Nasopharynx, Oropharynx, Hypopharynx
MX   Presence of distant metastases cannot be assessed
M0   No distant metastases
M1   Distant metastases present

Larynx

Similar to the pharynx, the larynx is divided into several regions, including the supraglottis, glottis, and subglottis. The tumor size (T) designation differs for the latter three regions, whereas the regional lymph node (N) and distant metastasis (M) assessments remain the same.

Tumor Size (T): Supraglottis, Glottis, Subglottis
TX   Primary tumor cannot be assessed

T0   No evidence of primary tumor
Tis   Carcinoma in situ

T - Supraglottis

T1   Tumor confined to one subsite of the supraglottis with normal vocal cord mobility
T2   Tumor invades mucosa of more than one adjacent subsite of supraglottis or region outside the supraglottis (i.e. base of tongue, vallecula) without fixation of the larynx
T3   Tumor limited to larynx with vocal cord fixation and/or invades the postcricoid area or pre-epiglottic soft tissues
T4   Tumor invades through the thyroid cartilage and/or extends beyond the larynx

T - Glottis

T1   Tumor limited to the vocal cords (may involve the commissures) with normal mobility.
    T1a   Tumor may be limited to one vocal cord
    T1b   Tumor involves both vocal cords
T2   Tumor extends to the supraglottis and /or subglottis, and/or with impaired cord mobility
T3   Tumor limited to larynx with vocal cord fixation
T4   Tumor invades through the thyroid carti lage and/or extends beyond the larynx

T - Subglottis

T1   Tumor limited to subglottis
T2   Tumor extends to the vocal cord(s) with normal or impaired cord mobility
T3   Tumor limited to larynx with vocal cord fixation
T4   Tumor invades through the cricoid or thyroid cartilage and/or extends beyond the larynx

Regional Lymph Nodes (N): Supraglottis, Glottis, Subglottis

NX   Regional lymph nodes cannot be assessed
N0   No regional lymph node metastasis
N1   Metastasis in a single ipsilateral lymph node, 3 cm or less in greatest dimension
N2   Metastasis in a single ipsilateral lymph node more than 3 cm but less than 6 cm in greatest dimension; or multiple ipsilateral lymph nodes, none more than 6 cm in greatest dimension; or in bilateral or contralateral lymph nodes, none more than 6 cm in greatest dimension

N2a   Metastasis in single ipsilateral lymph node more than 3 cm but not more than 6 cm in greatest dimension
N2b   Metastasis in multiple ipsilateral lymph nodes, none more than 6 cm in greatest dimension
N2c   Metastasis in bilateral or contralateral lymph nodes, none more than 6 cm in greatest dimension
N3   Metastasis in a lymph node more than 6 cm in greatest dimension

Distant Metastases (M): Supraglottis, Glottis, Subglottis

MX   Presence of distant metastases cannot be assessed
M0   No distant metastases
M1   Distant metastases present

Paranasal Sinuses

This includes the maxillary sinuses and the ethmoid sinuses. Tumors of the sphenoid and frontal sinuses are sufficiently rare that staging is considered unnecessary. The primary tumor (T) assessment is different for the maxillary and ethmoid sinuses, whereas the regional lymph node (N) and distant metastasis (M) assessments are the same.

Tumor Size (T): Maxillary and Ethmoid Sinuses

TX   Primary tumor cannot be assessed
T0   No evidence of primary tumor
Tis   Carcinoma in situ

T - Maxillary Sinus

T1   Tumor limited to antral mucosa with no erosion or destruction of bone
T2   Tumor causing erosion or destruction, except for the posterior antral wall, including extension into the hard palate and/or middle nasal meatus
T3   Tumor invades any of the following structures: bone of posterior wall of maxillary sinus, skin of cheek, floor or medial wall of orbit, infratemporal fossa, pterygoid plates, ethmoid sinuses
T4   Tumor invades orbital contents beyond the medial wall including any of the following structures: orbital apex, cribiform plate, base of skull, nasopharynx, sphenoid, frontal sinuses

T - Ethmoid Sinus

T1   Tumor confined to the ethmoid with or without bone erosion

T2   Tumor extends into the nasal cavity

T3   Tumor extends to the anterior orbit and/ or maxillary sinus

T4   Tumor with intracranial extension, orbital extension, or involving the sphenoid, frontal sinus, and/or skin of external nose

Regional Lymph Nodes (N): Maxillary and Ethmoid Sinus

NX   Regional lymph nodes cannot be assessed

N0   No regional lymph node metastasis

N1   Metastasis in a single ipsilateral lymph node, 3 cm or less in greatest dimension

N2   Metastasis in a single ipsilateral lymph node more than 3 cm but less than 6 cm in greatest dimension; or multiple ipsilateral lymph nodes, none more than 6 cm in greatest dimension; or in bilateral or contralateral lymph nodes, none more than 6 cm in greatest dimension

N2a Metastasis in single ipsilateral lymph node more than 3 cm but not more than 6 cm in greatest dimension

N2b Metastasis in multiple ipsilateral lymph nodes, none more than 6 cm in greatest dimension

N2c Metastasis in bilateral or contralateral lymph nodes, none more than 6 cm in greatest dimension

N3   Metastasis in a lymph node more than 6 cm in greatest dimension

Distant Metastases (M): Maxillary and Ethmoid Sinus

MX   Presence of distant metastases cannot be assessed

M0   No distant metastases

M1   Distant metastases present

Stage Grouping

Following TNM classification, tumors are usually placed into one of four clinical stages. The stage grouping for the oral cavity, pharynx, larynx, and maxillary sinus is identical and is summarized below:

Stage 0:	Tis	N0	M0
Stage I:	T1	N0	M0
Stage II:	T2	N0	M0
Stage III:	T3	N0	M0
	T1	N1	M0
	T2	N1	M0
	T3	N1	M0
Stage IV:	T4	N0	M0
	T4	N1	M0
	Any T	N2	M0
	Any T	N3	M0
	Any T	Any N	M1

REFERENCE

1. American Joint Committee on Cancer. Staging of cancer at specific anatomic sites: head and neck sites. In: Fleming ID, Cooper JS, Henson DE, et al., eds. Manual for staging of cancer, 5th ed. Philadelphia: JB Lippincott Co., 1997:21–3.

2. International Union Against Cancer. TNM classification of malignant tumors. Sobin LH, Wittekind C, eds. 5th ed. New York: Weiley-Liss, 1997:17–43.

3
BENIGN SQUAMOUS PROLIFERATIONS

The upper respiratory tract may give rise to a wide variety of papillomas and other benign squamous epithelial proliferations which should be distinguished from more aggressive lesions (Table 3-1). Papillomas are, by definition, benign neoplasms and may occur anywhere along the length of the upper respiratory tract. Papillomas of the nasal vestibule, schneiderian membrane, oropharynx, larynx, and trachea are often encountered in clinical practice. The upper respiratory tract also contains several non-neoplastic squamous proliferations that may clinically or histologically be confused with neoplasia; these include ordinary keratosis, verrucous hyperplasia, pseudoepitheliomatous hyperplasia, and leukoplakia. Finally, verruca vulgaris, a viral-driven papillary squamous proliferation identical to those that occur on cutaneous surfaces may arise in the larynx and should be distinguished from the above entities.

SQUAMOUS PAPILLOMAS OF THE NASAL VESTIBULE

Definition. Squamous papillomas of the nasal vestibule are benign, exophytic lesions arising from the keratinizing squamous epithelium lining the nasal vestibule.

Clinical Features. These are benign, exophytic lesions which, in contrast to squamous papillomas of the lower respiratory tract, are unassociated with human papillomavirus (HPV). Whether these lesions represent hyperplastic or neoplastic proliferations is unclear.

Pathologic Findings. Typical lesions are composed of variably sized fibrovascular cores covered by mature, stratified, keratinizing squamous epithelium (fig. 3-1). The epithelial cells are bland, without evidence of pronounced nuclear atypia or mitotic activity. Hyperkeratosis and parakeratosis of the lining epithelium may be seen.

Differential Diagnosis. Squamous papillomas of the nasal vestibule should be distinguished from those arising from the schneiderian membrane within the nasal cavity and paranasal sinuses. In addition to the difference in anatomic location, schneiderian papillomas

are not solely composed of mature squamous cells but contain transitional cells and interspersed mucinous cells (mucocytes) as well.

Treatment and Prognosis. Squamous papillomas of the nasal vestibule are benign lesions cured by simple excision.

SCHNEIDERIAN PAPILLOMAS

Most of the nasal cavity and paranasal sinuses are lined by ciliated columnar epithelium referred to as the schneiderian membrane; the exceptions are the nasal vestibule, which is lined by stratified squamous epithelium, and the uppermost portion of the nasal cavity (superior one third of the nasal septum, the superior turbinate, and the cribriform plate) which is covered by olfactory mucosa.

Three benign, neoplastic papillomatous lesions arise from the schneiderian membrane, namely the inverted papilloma, fungiform papilloma, and oncocytic (cylindrical cell) papilloma.

Table 3-1

BENIGN SQUAMOUS PROLIFERATIONS OF THE UPPER RESPIRATORY TRACT

Papillomas

    Squamous papilloma of the nasal vestibule

    Schneiderian papillomas of the nose and paranasal sinuses

        Inverted

        Fungiform

        Oncocytic

Inverted ductal papilloma of minor salivary glands

Squamous papillomas of the oropharynx, larynx, and trachea

Epithelial tumor-like lesions

    Keratosis

    Verrucous hyperplasia

    Pseudoepitheliomatous hyperplasia

    Leukoplakia

Verruca vulgaris

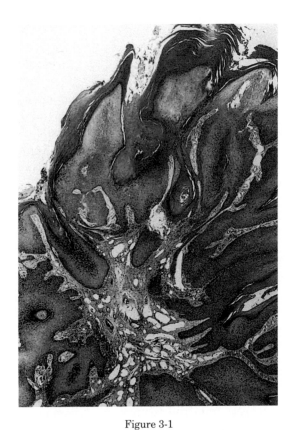

Figure 3-1
PAPILLOMA OF NASAL VESTIBULE
An exophytic, keratinizing, squamous cell papilloma of the anterior vestibule of the nose. (Fig. 41, Fascicle 25, 2nd Series.)

It is important to understand that inverted papillomas may have a minor, exophytic component; similarly, fungiform papillomas may have rare inverted areas. Therefore, categorization is according to the predominant pattern. Most schneiderian papillomas are readily classified as one of the latter types, but mixed forms also occur.

Occasional publications refer to all three schneiderian lesions as "papillomatosis" or lump all three types under the collective heading of "inverted papilloma" (18,21). Recent evidence indicates, however, that these lesions are clinically and pathologically distinct (11). Using in situ hybridization and the polymerase chain reaction, several studies have reported the presence of HPV types 6, 11, 16, or 18 in 69 to 100 percent of fungiform papillomas and up to 50 percent of inverted lesions; all oncocytic papillomas examined to date have been HPV negative

(2,8,16). Several authors have suggested that HPV may be involved in the pathogenesis of fungiform schneiderian papillomas but not the other variants (2,8). The precise histogenesis of these lesions, however, remains unknown.

In general, schneiderian papillomas occur in patients between 30 and 50 years of age, with a male to female ratio of approximately 2 to 1 (6). In the study of Hyams (6), which included all three papilloma types, 20 percent involved the nasal cavity, 40 percent arose in the paranasal sinuses, and 40 percent involved both the nasal cavity and sinuses. Of those lesions involving the paranasal sinuses, the maxillary antrum is involved in most cases; papillomas present in the ethmoid sinuses in a much smaller proportion, whereas the frontal and sphenoid sinuses are rarely, if ever, involved. Schneiderian-type papillomas have also been described in the nasopharynx, oropharynx, nasolacrimal duct, lacrimal duct, middle ear, and mastoid. The pertinent features of each schneiderian papilloma variant are presented below.

Inverted Schneiderian Papilloma

Definition. This is a benign, predominantly inverted neoplastic proliferation arising from the sinonasal tract (schneiderian) mucosa and composed of dilated duct-like structures lined by multiple layers of squamous, ciliated columnar, or transitional epithelium.

General Features. Inverted schneiderian papillomas (ISP) comprised 47 percent of the 315 schneiderian papillomas studied by Hyams (6). They almost exclusively occur on the lateral nasal wall and in the paranasal sinuses, although cases arising on the nasal septum and in the oropharynx, nasopharynx, and middle ear have been reported (7,12,13,15,19,22). ISPs are further distinguished by their strong association with carcinoma; approximately 5 percent occur in association with an invasive carcinoma, which may be seen within or adjacent to the papilloma or may develop later in the same area (4,14,17,18, 21). Associated carcinomas are predominantly squamous, although spindle cell, transitional cell, clear cell, and high-grade mucoepidermoid carcinomas have also been described (1,4,6,14, 18,21). There are no histologic criteria to predict which papillomas will recur or be followed by

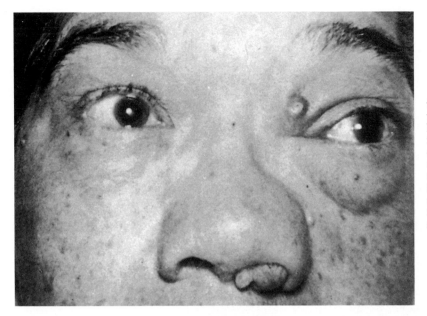

Figure 3-2
SCHNEIDERIAN PAPILLOMA
A clinical picture of an inverted type papilloma associated with proptosis, protruding from the nose. The histologically benign papillomatosis involving the left sinonasal area caused pressure erosion of the frontal sinus bony wall and invaded the cranial cavity. (Fig. 1a from Myers EN, Schramm VL Jr, Barnes EL Jr. Management of inverted papilloma of the nose and paranasal sinuses. Laryngoscope 1981;91:2071–94.)

Figure 3-3
SCHNEIDERIAN PAPILLOMA
A gross specimen of a papillomatous mass arising from the lateral nasal wall in a 45-year-old man. (Fig. 44, Fascicle 25, 2nd Series.)

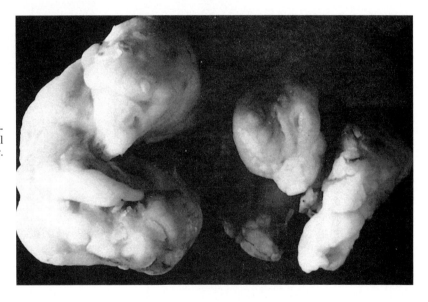

carcinoma; thus all tissue removed from patients with inverted or oncocytic variants should be thoroughly and completely examined to exclude the possibility of a coexistent carcinoma.

Clinical Features. ISPs commonly present as polypoid protuberances on the lateral nasal wall or within the maxillary or ethmoid sinuses. They may be multifocal but bilaterality is extremely uncommon. Patients commonly complain of nasal obstruction, or, less frequently, of epistaxis, facial pain, or a nasal mass (fig. 3-2). Bony erosion may occur.

Gross Findings. Inverted papillomas are usually firm, occasionally bulky, polypoid lesions covered by intact nasal mucosa (fig. 3-3). Lesions may be attached to the underlying nasal/paranasal wall by a broad base.

Microscopic Findings. There is predominantly (but not exclusively) an inverted pattern of growth in which cords and nests of epithelium endophytically project into the underlying stroma. Dilated ductal-like structures, lined by multiple layers of epithelium and terminating in smaller cellular nests, are often present (figs.

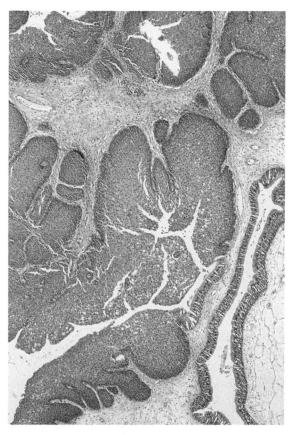

Figure 3-4
INVERTED SCHNEIDERIAN PAPILLOMA
Most inverted papillomas arise from the lateral nasal wall and are composed of epithelial-lined, duct-like structures that endophytically project into the underlying stroma.

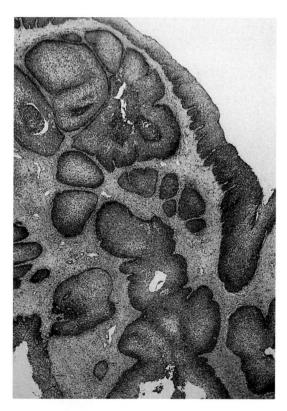

Figure 3-5
INVERTED SCHNEIDERIAN PAPILLOMA
Another inverted papilloma with inverting cords, nests, and duct-like structures of neoplastic epithelium. The overlying respiratory epithelium of the nasal wall has been replaced by metaplastic squamous epithelium. (Fig. 45, Fascicle 25, 2nd Series.)

3-4, 3-5) (11). Inverted papillomas are lined by 5 to 30 layers of squamous, ciliated columnar, or intermediate (transitional) epithelium with interspersed mucus-secreting cells (6,9). The surface is often lined by a single layer of ciliated cells, irrespective of the epithelial type underneath (fig. 3-6). In all epithelial types, nuclei are generally small and uniform, with darkly staining chromatin and rare nucleoli. Mitoses are few and confined to the lower epithelial levels; atypical forms are not seen. Nuclear pleomorphism is present in about 10 percent of cases. Small microcysts distended with either mucin or neutrophils and scattered throughout the neoplastic epithelium are characteristic. The fibrous stroma often contains scattered chronic inflammatory cells and occasional lymphoid follicles (11). A proportion of ISPs may show a coexisting

or underlying carcinoma, which is usually squamous in type (figs. 3-7, 3-8).

Differential Diagnosis. The primary differential diagnostic consideration is squamous cell carcinoma. ISPs are readily distinguished from the latter by a lack of atypical mitoses, significant nuclear pleomorphism, and foci of aberrant keratinization deep within the epithelial layer; also, they do not exhibit single cell stromal invasion or a desmoplastic response.

Treatment and Prognosis. ISPs have a recurrence rate of up to 75 percent if treated by local excision alone. Lateral rhinotomy and medial maxillectomy are recommended for optimal management of lateral nasal wall lesions (3,6,17). ISPs with associated carcinomas are biologically aggressive lesions. In the study of Hyams (6), of 12 patients with ISP and associated carcinoma on

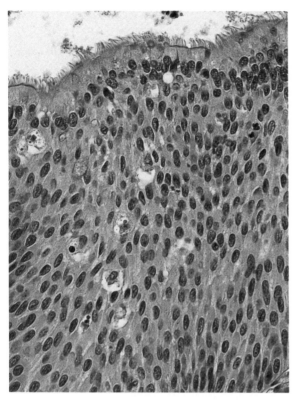

Figure 3-6
INVERTED SCHNEIDERIAN PAPILLOMA

Most inverted papillomas are predominantly composed of small, intermediate "transitional" cells with monotonous, bland nuclei and scant eosinophilic cytoplasm. Small microcystic structures containing basophilic mucin or polymorphonuclear leukocytes are often present and characteristic of this lesion. The surface is typically covered by a single layer of ciliated, respiratory-type columnar cells.

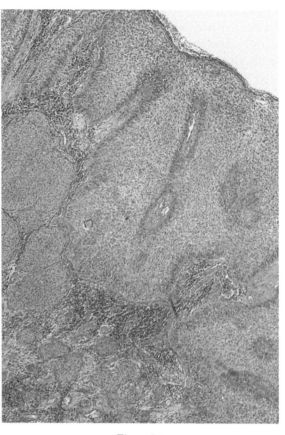

Figure 3-7
INVERTED SCHNEIDERIAN PAPILLOMA WITH AN ASSOCIATED SQUAMOUS CELL CARCINOMA

Some of the carcinoma may be seen in the lower left portion of the lesion. (Figures 3-7 and 3-8 are from the same patient.)

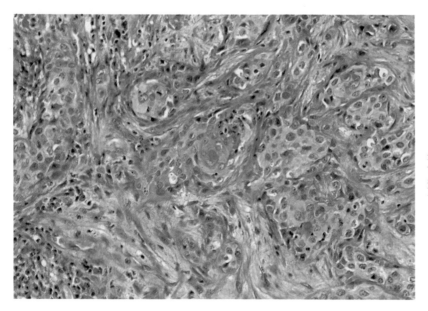

Figure 3-8
INVERTED SCHNEIDERIAN PAPILLOMA WITH AN ASSOCIATED CARCINOMA

Most carcinomas associated with inverted papillomas are invasive, well to moderately differentiated squamous cell carcinomas with foci of keratinization.

whom follow-up was available, 3 died of tumor, 1 was alive with systemic metastases, and 2 died of unknown causes; only the remaining 2 patients were alive without known disease 5 years after surgery.

Fungiform Schneiderian Papillomas

Definition. This benign exophytic neoplastic proliferation arises from the schneiderian mucosa and is composed of arborizing fibrovascular fronds covered by multiple layers of squamous, ciliated columnar, or transitional epithelium.

General Features. In some series, fungiform schneiderian papillomas (FSP) comprise up to 50 percent of all schneiderian papillomas (6, 11). Of the three schneiderian lesions, FSP best fulfills the concept of papilloma. In contrast to inverted variants, FSPs are not associated with malignancy and arise almost exclusively on the nasal septum; the lateral nasal walls and paranasal sinuses are rarely involved (6).

Clinical Features. Most FSPs appear as tan-gray polypoid growths on the nasal septum. Neither side is predilected and bilaterality is rare. They appear to involve younger patients more often than the other two variants, and most patients are between the ages of 20 and 40 years (6).

Gross Findings. FSPs have been described as gray-pink, raised, cauliflower-like, verrucous, or mulberry-appearing exophytic lesions with a firm consistency (6). Lesions are often attached to the underlying mucosa by a narrowed stalk.

Microscopic Findings. These are predominantly exophytic lesions with branching, fibrovascular fronds covered by 5 to over 30 layers of epithelium (fig. 3-9). In a minority of cases occasional invaginations may be seen. Cytologically, the epithelium is identical to that of the inverted variant, and includes squamous, ciliated columnar, and intermediate epithelial types (fig. 3-10). Admixed mucous cells with peripherally displaced nuclei are also present, either individually or in small groups. Occasional microcysts filled with mucin may be seen. FSPs may be composed of one, two, or all three epithelial types. Nuclear pleomorphism is typically absent and mitotic figures, when present, are restricted to the basal or parabasal layers. The underlying stroma is composed of vascular fibrous tissue with rare chronic inflammatory cells. Seromucinous glands may

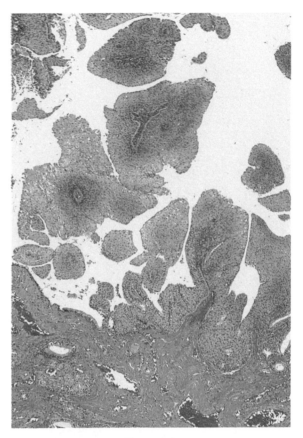

Figure 3-9
FUNGIFORM SCHNEIDERIAN PAPILLOMA

A representative fungiform papilloma arising from the nasal septum. The lesion is composed of thin, branching, fibrovascular papillations covered by up to 30 layers of epithelial cells. (Figures 3-9 and 3-10 are from the same patient.)

be seen in cases in which the underlying lamina propria has been sampled (11).

Differential Diagnosis. The differential diagnosis of FSP, particularly those with invaginations and mitotic activity, includes papillary squamous carcinoma. In contrast to FSP, however, papillary carcinomas usually show nuclear pleomorphism, mitotic activity in the middle or upper epithelial layers, foci of dyskeratosis, and stromal invasion.

Treatment and Prognosis. FSPs have the lowest recurrence rate of the three schneiderian lesions. One study of 156 FSPs reported a recurrence rate of 22 percent, compared to recurrence rates of 46 and 40 percent for inverted (146 cases) and oncocytic (10 cases) schneiderian papillomas, respectively (6). Of those patients with recurrence, approximately half have multiple

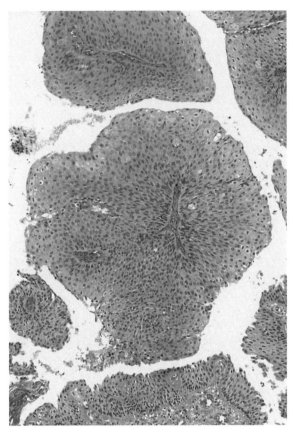

Figure 3-10
FUNGIFORM SCHNEIDERIAN PAPILLOMA
Similar to inverted papillomas, fungiform papillomas may be composed of squamous cells, or intermediate or ciliated columnar cells. The papilloma depicted is covered by cytologically bland intermediate cells with superficial maturation. Microcysts containing inflammatory cells are also present.

episodes. Lesions confined to the septum are best managed by wide local excision (17).

Oncocytic Schneiderian Papillomas

Definition. This is a benign, mixed exophytic-endophytic neoplastic proliferation arising from the schneiderian mucosa and characterized by short fibrovascular papillae and inverting epithelial cords covered by several layers of tall columnar, oncocytic epithelial cells.

General Features. Oncocytic schneiderian papillomas (OSPs), also referred to as *cylindrical cell papillomas,* are rare lesions and comprise 3 to 8 percent of all schneiderian papillomas (1,6, 11). Approximately 53 cases of OSP have been

reported to date (1,5,6,9,11,20,23). Similar to ISPs, OSPs typically involve the lateral nasal wall, and maxillary and ethmoid paranasal sinuses (6). Dissimilar to the fungiform and inverted variants, however, the epithelial lining cells of OSP have the features of oncocytes; thus the term oncocytic, as opposed to cylindrical cell, schneiderian papilloma is preferred (1).

Clinical Features. Lesions typically appear as single or multifocal polypoid areas involving the lateral nasal wall or paranasal sinuses (6, 11). Bilaterality or involvement of the sphenoid and frontal sinuses has not been described. To the best of our knowledge, 12 of the 53 reported OSPs (23 percent) were associated with an invasive carcinoma of the squamous cell, high-grade mucoepidermoid, or undifferentiated type (1,6,9,20,23).

Gross Findings. Specimens usually consist of curetted material with soft, pink-tan tissue fragments admixed with blood and, on occasion, spicules of bone (1). Specimens are usually small although lesions up to 10 x 6 x 2 cm in aggregate dimension have been described (1).

Microscopic Findings. Most OSPs exhibit both inverted and exophytic patterns of growth (1,6,11,20). Exophytic areas are characterized by thin, fibrovascular tissue cores covered by 3 to 8 layers of epithelial cells, whereas inverted areas are typified by cords and islands of epithelium which grow into the underlying stroma (fig. 3-11). The lesional cells are tall columnar and resemble oncocytes, with abundant, granular, eosinophilic cytoplasm and distinct cell borders (fig. 3-12) (1,6). The nuclei are round to oval and uniform, with dark chromatin and rare inconspicuous nucleoli. Nuclear pleomorphism is minimal and mitoses are infrequent. Cilia may occasionally be seen on the surface epithelial layer (6). The underlying stroma is composed of loose fibrous tissue with scattered chronic inflammatory cells.

Immunohistochemical Findings. Only eight OSPs have been studied immunohistochemically (5,23). Yang and Abraham (23) reported that the neoplastic cells in a single OSP as well as an associated squamous cell carcinoma were positive for both cytokeratin and carcinoembryonic antigen. Cunningham et al. (5) reported that the epithelial cells in all of seven OSPs stained for mitochondrial enzyme cytochrome C oxidase.

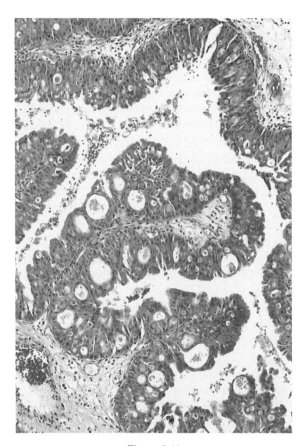

Figure 3-11
ONCOCYTIC SCHNEIDERIAN PAPILLOMA
Oncocytic papillomas are exophytic/endophytic lesions often with a thin, fibrovascular tissue core covered by several layers of oncocytic epithelial cells. Numerous microcysts containing mucoid material or inflammatory cells are evident, even at scanning magnification.

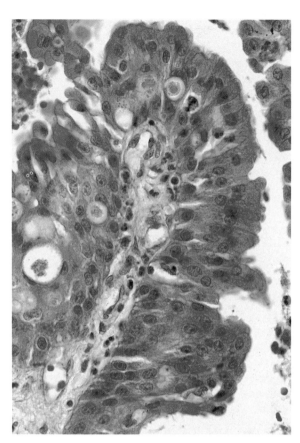

Figure 3-12
ONCOCYTIC SCHNEIDERIAN PAPILLOMA
Oncocytic papillomas are invariably composed of large, polygonal to columnar cells with copious amounts of granular, eosinophilic cytoplasm. The nuclei are round, dark, and uniform, with little to no evidence of pleomorphism. The tall columnar appearance of the cells is responsible for the older term of cylindrical cell papilloma that was once applied to these lesions.

Electron Microscopic Findings. The few OSPs studied ultrastructurally were predominantly composed of polyhedral cells with numerous intracytoplasmic mitochondria (1). These oncocytic cells also contained sparse numbers of other organelles and oval nuclei with finely dispersed chromatin. The plasma membranes showed short microvilli and well-formed desmosomes. Typical ciliated respiratory cells were present. Cells with features intermediate between the oncocytes and respiratory cells were also seen.

Differential Diagnosis. Due to the numerous microcystic structures found within the epithelial layer, OSPs may be mistaken for sporangia of the fungus *Rhinosporidium seeberi,* the etiologic agent of rhinosporidiosis. Rhinosporidiosis is endemic in Central and South America, Sri Lanka,

and India but rare in the United States. As indicated by Barnes et al. (10), at least one reported case of rhinosporidiosis in fact represents an OSP. The infection is easily distinguished from OSP by the absence of oncocytic change in the adjacent epithelium, the presence of true intraepithelial endospores, and the presence of organisms in the underlying stroma.

OSP may also be misdiagnosed as adenocarcinoma, particularly in necrotic and/or maloriented specimens (18). The low-grade and intestinal-type adenocarcinomas typical of the nasal and paranasal regions, however, show variable degrees of nuclear atypia, mitotic activity, and true lumen formation with cribriforming, back-to-back glands, and stromal invasion, features absent in OSP (20).

Treatment and Prognosis. In the series of Hyams et al. (6), 4 of 10 OSPs recurred locally within an average of 1 year. One patient each had two and three recurrences, whereas two patients experienced four recurrences, all at the site of previous tumor removal. Details regarding surgical treatment in the latter cases were not supplied, but in general, surgical excision with wide margins is recommended over simple curettage to minimize recurrence. Of nine OSPs with associated carcinoma, extended follow-up showed that six patients died of uncontrolled local disease from 3 months to 4 years after excision; two patients were alive without disease at 18 months and 7 years; and the final patient died after 8 years of an unrelated cause (1,9,20).

INVERTED DUCTAL PAPILLOMA OF MINOR SALIVARY GLANDS

Definition. This benign, endophytic, minor salivary gland lesion is composed of duct-like structures lined by basaloid epithelial cells which appear to converge upon, and open into, a central cystic cavity.

General Features. Inverted ductal papillomas (IDP) are rare lesions that, with the sole exception of a single case reported in the parotid gland, exclusively arise in the minor salivary glands (24–32). These lesions were first recognized by Batsakis et al. in 1981 (31), who designated them as "epidermoid papillary adenomas." One year later White et al. (31) reported four additional cases and proposed the more descriptive term "inverted ductal papilloma," due to the resemblance of these lesions to inverted papillomas of the nose, paranasal sinuses, and urinary bladder. Assuming that the three cases originally reported by Batsakis et al. at the Armed Forces Institute of Pathology (AFIP) were included in the six cases subsequently reported by Ellis et al. (26) (while at the AFIP), 18 cases of IDP have been reported in the English literature (24–32). The lesions arise in the excretory duct of the minor salivary glands but the pathogenesis is unclear.

Clinical Features. Clinically, IDPs appear as firm, asymptomatic nodules ranging in size from 1.0 to 1.5 cm in diameter. Those lesions reported have all occurred in adults, with an age range of 32 to 66 years. There is no apparent sexual predilection. Virtually all lesions have arisen within the oral cavity, with the lip and buccal mucosa as the most common sites (24–32). Most tumors are interpreted clinically as mucoceles, lipomas, or fibromas (25,31).

Pathologic Findings. On gross examination IDPs appear as firm, white-tan mucosal nodules measuring up to 1.5 cm in greatest diameter. On cut section most lesions are homogeneous and show a small but grossly visible central cystic cavity.

Histologically, IDPs are strikingly similar to ISPs of the nose and paranasal sinuses. On scanning magnification IDPs appear as well-circumscribed, cup-shaped lesions composed of radially oriented, broad epithelial projections that endophytically extend into the underlying stroma (fig. 3-13) (28–32). In most lesions the epithelial projections contain narrow, duct-like structures which, on serial sectioning, appear to open into a centrally located crater or cystic cavity (fig. 3-14) (32). The central cavity is thought to represent the terminus of the minor salivary gland excretory duct from which these lesions arise. Occasional IDPs appear entirely solid (31). The epithelial projections are predominantly composed of small basaloid cells with dark nuclei and scant basophilic cytoplasm (fig. 3-15). In contrast, the luminal surface is often lined by cuboidal to columnar, duct-type cells with basally located nuclei and moderate amounts of eosinophilic cytoplasm. Interspersed ciliated or mucous cells containing a periodic acid–Schiff (PAS)- and mucicarmine-positive substance are usually present. Small microcysts containing either mucous material or polymorphonuclear leukocytes are commonly seen throughout the epithelial layer. Nuclear pleomorphism and mitotic figures are rare or absent.

The lesion arises in excretory ducts and is typically based in the lamina propria. In most lesions the endophytic epithelial component is contiguous with the stratified squamous epithelium of the overlying oral mucosa. The tumor appears to grow by centripetal expansion rather than stromal invasion; hence, IDPs show well-circumscribed, broad, "pushing" margins. Peripherally, IDPs are often surrounded by minor salivary glands separated from the tumoral mass by thin strands of connective tissue (25).

Immunohistochemical Findings. Only one IDP has been studied immunohistochemically (29). The neoplastic cells were strongly

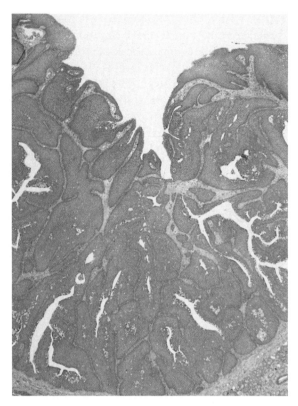

Figure 3-13
INVERTED DUCTAL PAPILLOMA
OF MINOR SALIVARY GLAND

Inverted ductal papillomas of minor salivary gland origin are circumscribed, cup-shaped, endophytic epithelial proliferations radially arranged around a centrally placed crater or cystic cavity. The central defect is thought to represent the excretory duct of an underlying minor salivary gland from which these lesions arise. (Courtesy of Dr. D.R. Gnepp, Providence, RI.)

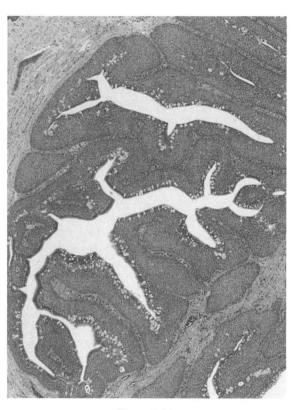

Figure 3-14
INVERTED DUCTAL PAPILLOMA
OF MINOR SALIVARY GLAND

Peripherally the lesion contains lobulations of neoplastic cells surrounding a duct-like structure. On serial sections the ductal structures often open into the overlying central defect. (Courtesy of Dr. D.R. Gnepp, Providence, RI.)

Figure 3-15
INVERTED DUCTAL
PAPILLOMA OF MINOR
SALIVARY GLAND

Similar to inverted papillomas of the nasal cavity and paranasal sinuses, inverted ductal papillomas of minor salivary gland origin are composed of small basaloid ("intermediate") epidermoid cells with bland nuclei and scant amounts of eosinophilic cytoplasm. (Courtesy of Dr. D.R. Gnepp, Providence, RI.) (Figures 3-13–3-15 are from the same patient.)

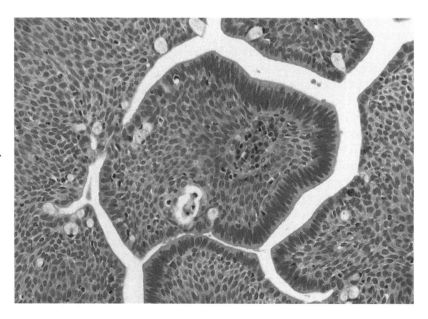

immunoreactive for cytokeratin, moderately positive for epithelial membrane antigen, and weakly reactive for carcinoembryonic antigen (29). Staining for vimentin, S-100 protein, desmin, and muscle-specific actin was negative.

Differential Diagnosis. Due to their histologic similarities but differing biologic potential, IDP should be distinguished from ISP of the nose and paranasal sinuses. Both lesions are endophytic epithelial proliferations composed of basaloid, squamous, and columnar cells with interspersed mucous and inflammatory cells. ISPs of the nose and paranasal sinuses, however, are haphazard, noncircumscribed lesions that may assume a large size and lack an association with a central duct-like structure or crater. In contrast, IDPs are small, circumscribed lesions with a centripetal growth pattern oriented about a central defect. Unlike ISPs of the nose, 5 to 20 percent of which have an associated malignancy, all IDPs described to date have been uniformly benign (24–32).

IDPs are distinguished from sialadenoma papilliferum by the absence of a double cell layer and a plasma cell–predominant inflammatory infiltrate. The absence of cellular pleomorphism and stromal invasion distinguish IDP from potentially similar-appearing malignant epithelial lesions such as mucoepidermoid carcinoma or basaloid squamous cell carcinoma.

Treatment and Prognosis. The treatment of choice is surgical excision. None of the lesions reported to date have recurred or metastasized.

PAPILLOMAS OF THE LARYNX AND TRACHEA

Definition. Benign, exophytic squamous epithelial papillomas may arise from the true vocal cords and other sites within the larynx, as well as the oropharynx and trachea.

General Features. Squamous papillomas of the oropharynx, larynx, and trachea, often referred to in aggregate as *laryngeal papillomatosis*, are histologically benign but clinically troublesome lesions characterized by frequent recurrences, occasional airway obstruction, and a tendency to spread throughout the respiratory tract (33–49). In 1986 Lindeberg et al. (44) classified laryngeal papillomas into four groups: I, multiple juvenile papillomas; II, solitary juvenile papillomas; III, multiple adult papillomas; and IV, solitary adult papillomas.

Juvenile papillomas were defined as those that presented before the age of 20 years, whereas adult cases were those that presented after that age. Cases were also grouped as either solitary if no more than two papillomas were present, or multiple if three or more lesions were identified. The authors admitted that the 20-year cut-off was arbitrary and could cause problems in classifying patients who developed papillomas between the ages of 16 and 20 years. Notably, at least one author defined adult papillomata as those that first occurred in patients over 16 years of age (49). Yet another author classified these lesions according to the number of papillomas present without regard to age (45). Thus, to date, there is not complete concordance on the classification of these lesions.

Many studies have reported an association of laryngeal papillomas with the human papilloma virus (HPV). As in other sites, the frequency of HPV detection in laryngeal papillomas depends on the sensitivity of the methodology used. It is currently clear, however, that most, if not all, laryngeal papillomas are associated with, and probably caused by, HPV types 6 and 11 (33,35, 36,38,41,47,49). Using immunohistochemical techniques, Costa et al. (35) found HPV antigens in 11 of 19 multiple juvenile variants but in none of 5 adult multiple papillomas. Using in situ hybridization, Terry et al. (49) detected HPV 6 and 11 in 13 of 13 juvenile multiple papillomas and 3 of 3 juvenile solitary lesions, compared to 2 of 11 adult solitary papillomas and 5 of 14 adult multiple papillomas. Using a combination of in situ hybridization and the polymerase chain reaction, Gale et al. (38) found HPV in 28 of 29 multiple juvenile papillomas, 26 of 30 multiple adult papillomas, and 17 of 20 solitary adult lesions. Levi et al. (41) found HPV in 10 of 13 juvenile multiple lesions and 2 of 6 adult solitary lesions using in situ hybridization, however, examination of the same lesions by the polymerase chain reaction increased the positivity to 100 percent. These results suggest that adult papillomas contain lower copy numbers of the virus compared to juvenile lesions and therefore exhibit a lower detection rate with conventional hybridization methods.

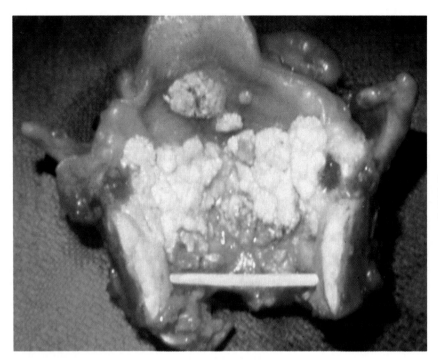

Figure 3-16
LARYNGEAL
PAPILLOMATOSIS
Gross laryngectomy specimen from a patient with multiple juvenile papillomas showing diffuse involvement of the true vocal cords, and supraglottic and subglottic larynx.

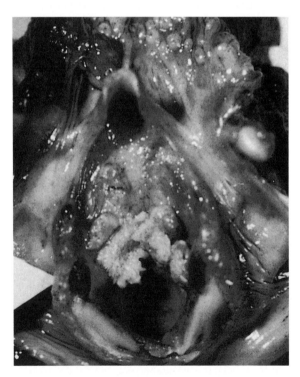

Figure 3-17
LARYNGEAL PAPILLOMATOSIS

An autopsy specimen from a 2-year-old boy with a history of recurrent vocal cord papillomas since the 6th month of life. Regrowth and neglect caused airway obstruction and death. (Fig. 60, Fascicle 25, 2nd Series.)

Clinical Features. The clinical behavior of upper aerorespiratory tract papillomas, both juvenile and adult, is that of multiple, unpredictable recurrences and a small but definite association with squamous cell carcinoma. Clinically and grossly, papillomas appear as glistening, nodular to pedunculated, white to pink exophytic masses (figs. 3-16, 3-17). They may develop at any age, from several months to over 80 years, and most patients present with hoarseness, stridor, or respiratory distress (34). Juvenile papillomas have a nearly equal distribution between males and females whereas adult variants are much more common in men (ratio of 5 to 2) (43). In one study of 231 cases, 111 (48 percent) were classified as solitary adult, 67 (29 percent) were multiple juvenile variants, 46 (20 percent) were multiple adult, and 7 (3 percent) were solitary juvenile papillomas (43). Primary lesions invariably involve the true vocal cords or ventricular bands (44). Multiple papillomas may also involve the epiglottis, subglottic area, uvula, or palate. Recurrences often develop near the original excisional site and may extend distally to involve the trachea or major bronchi.

The development of squamous cell carcinoma in nonirradiated, nonsmoking patients with laryngeal papillomas is rare but well documented

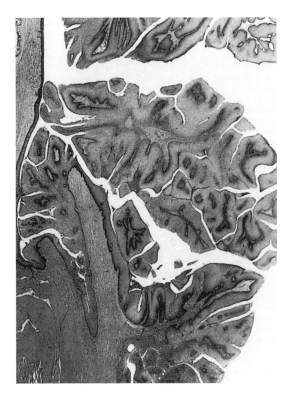

Figure 3-18
LARYNGEAL PAPILLOMATOSIS
A scanning microscopic view of a juvenile squamous cell papilloma in a 12-year-old girl. This represents a recurrence that required laryngectomy because of diffuse involvement. (Fig. 61, Fascicle 25, 2nd Series.)

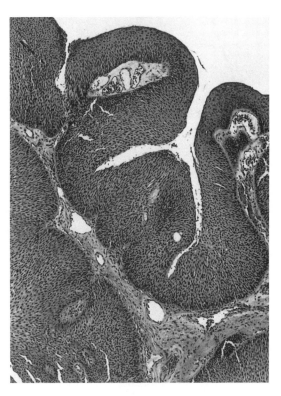

Figure 3-19
LARYNGEAL
PAPILLOMATOSIS
A high-power magnification of figure 3-18 supports a benign, nonkeratinizing, epidermoid neoplastic element. (Fig. 62, Fascicle 25, 2nd Series.)

(37,39,40). Guillou et al. (39) located 18 pathologically documented cases of squamous cell carcinoma arising in patients with such a history and multiple laryngeal papillomatosis, and added an additional case of their own. The carcinomas originated in the upper respiratory tract in only 4 patients, whereas the remaining 14 carcinomas arose in the lung. In the latter review, all patients had multiple papillomas with pulmonary extension and developed a squamous cell carcinoma an average of 15 years after presentation (range, 4 to 26 years).

Pathologic Findings. Pathologically, laryngeal papillomas consist of a variably sized, but usually thin, fibrovascular core covered by multiple layers of squamous epithelium (fig. 3-18). Additional secondary or tertiary branching may be seen. Most papillomas show an orderly epithelial arrangement with proper maturation and little to no atypia (fig. 3-19). Several studies

have shown that juvenile multiple, adult multiple, and adult solitary papillomas are histologically indistinguishable (fig. 3-20) (33,38,42). Mild, moderate, or severe intraepithelial dysplasia, similar in appearance to that seen in the uterine cervix, may be present in a minority of cases (figs. 3-21, 3-22). Prominent keratin production, manifest either as surface or intraepithelial dyskeratosis, is rarely seen, and if present, suggests the possibility of a verrucae vulgaris or verrucous carcinoma.

There is relatively little information on the frequency and extent of intraepithelial dysplasia in laryngeal papillomas. Lindeberg et al. (44) reported the presence of mild or moderate dysplasia in 9 of 21 (43 percent) juvenile multiple papillomas, 12 of 20 (60 percent) adult multiple papillomas, and 6 of 30 (20 percent) adult solitary lesions. Severe dysplasia was noted in 4 additional patients, including 1 juvenile and 3

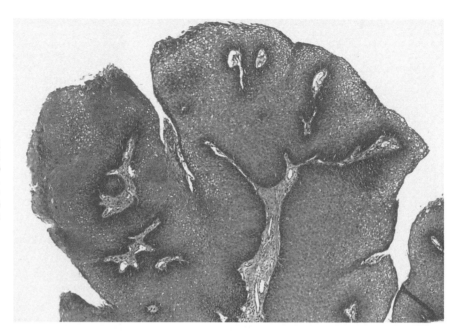

Figure 3-20
LARYNGEAL
PAPILLOMATOSIS

Solitary papilloma excised from the right true vocal cord of a 71-year-old male with no previous laryngeal disease. The specimen is morphologically identical to the multiple juvenile papillomata shown in figure 3-19.

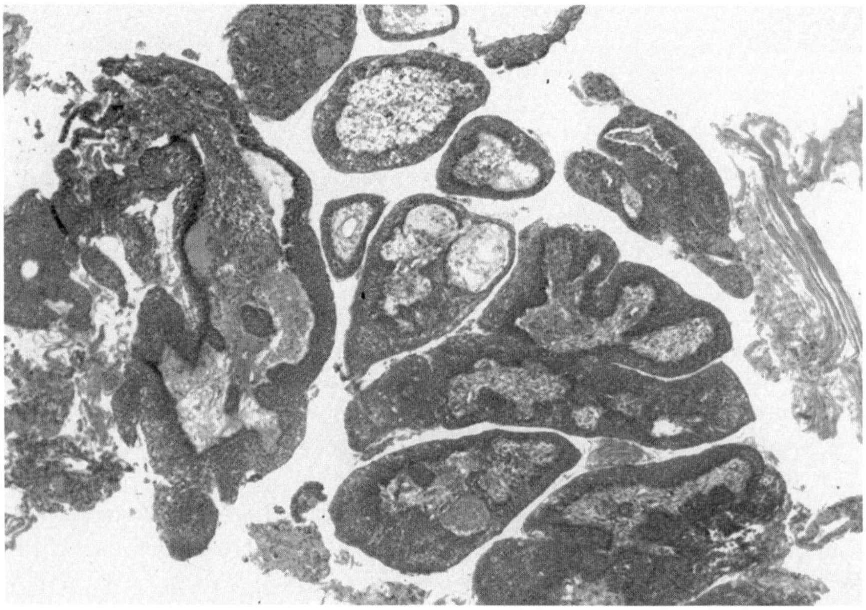

Figure 3-21
LARYNGEAL
PAPILLOMATOSIS

Biopsy specimen of a solitary adult papilloma excised from the anterior commissure of a 76-year-old male. The lesion consists of multiple fibrovascular cores covered by multiple layers of squamous epithelium, the nuclei of which appear hyperchromatic even at low magnification. (Figures 3-21 and 3-22 are from the same patient.)

adults with multiple papillomas, all of whom went on to develop laryngeal carcinoma. Quick et al. (46) reported that of 16 patients with either multiple juvenile or adult solitary papillomas and limited recurrence rates, none showed evidence of dysplasia; in contrast, 16 patients with multiple papillomas and frequent recurrences all had histologically typical papillomas at disease onset but developed evidence of moderate to severe dysplasia on subsequent excisions. Unfortunately, pathologic and photographic documentation in these two series was either sparse (46) or nonexistent (44), thus the true incidence and significance of dysplasia in these lesions is unresolved.

Squamous cell carcinomas arising in association with laryngeal papillomatosis are usually associated with juvenile lesions and are often

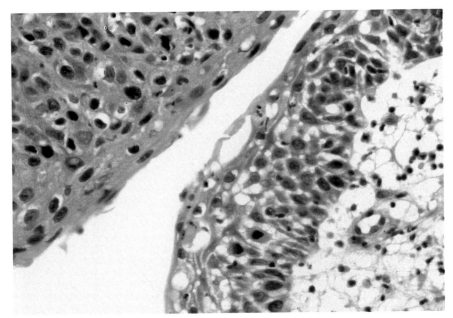

Figure 3-22
LARYNGEAL
PAPILLOMATOSIS
Several foci of moderate to severe dysplasia were identified on higher magnification. Dysplastic papillomata, particularly in adults, should be completely excised to exclude the possibility of an underlying carcinoma.

extraordinarily well-differentiated papillary tumors. Fechner et al. (37) described a case in which benign-appearing squamous papillations histologically identical to the patient's laryngeal papillomas extensively invaded the larynx. To our knowledge, histologic features predictive of the development of squamous cell carcinoma have not been documented, in part due to the rarity of these lesions, the scarcity of pathologic documentation, and the fact that many have occurred in patients with other risk factors, including a history of radiation, tobacco use, or ethanol abuse.

Differential Diagnosis. The problem of distinguishing laryngeal papillomas from verrucous or exophytic squamous cell carcinoma is extremely difficult and may be impossible from superficial biopsy specimens alone. All papillomas with any degree of dysplasia, particularly those arising as solitary variants in adults, should be distinguished from papillary squamous carcinoma by either prolonged clinical follow-up or, preferably, complete surgical excision to exclude the possibility of an underlying invasive lesion.

Treatment and Prognosis. Patients with multiple papillomas have a guarded prognosis, as the clinical behavior (in both juvenile and adult patients) is that of multiple, unpredictable recurrences. Insufficiently or untreated patients may develop partial or complete upper airway obstruc-

tion, and an association with squamous cell carcinoma has been documented. In one series of 113 patients with multiple papillomas, including 67 juvenile and 46 adult variants, only 5 remained free of disease after a single operation (43). The remaining 108 patients underwent a median of seven additional procedures over a period of about 5 years, with intervals between operations of up to 42 years. The possibility of late recurrence has lead at least one author to propose that patients with multiple papillomas should never be considered to be cured of their disease (43). A minority of patients experience at least one episode of acute respiratory distress during the course of their disease, often necessitating a tracheostomy to insure an adequate airway.

In contrast, solitary adult and juvenile papillomas are less aggressive and usually cured after a single excision. Of 111 patients with solitary papillomas in Lindeberg's study (43), 93 (84 percent) were considered cured following a single surgical procedure and a median follow-up of 7.2 years.

Treatment is currently directed towards ablation of all visible papillomas consistent with preservation of the airway (48). Simple surgical (forceps) excision, cryotherapy, or laser-assisted ablation via direct laryngoscopy have all been utilized, with apparently similar degrees of success (33,34,44,48).

TUMOR-LIKE LESIONS

Ordinary Keratosis, Verrucous Hyperplasia, Pseudoepitheliomatous Hyperplasia, and Leukoplakia

Definition, General and Clinical Features.
The upper respiratory tract in general, and the oral cavity and larynx in particular, may give rise to a variety of non-neoplastic, hyperkeratotic epithelial proliferations that may be confused with carcinoma. These include ordinary keratosis, verrucous hyperplasia, pseudoepitheliomatous hyperplasia, and leukoplakia (50-60).

Ordinary keratosis refers to an epithelial area with an abnormally marked degree of orthokeratosis or parakeratosis unassociated with an underlying epithelial proliferation.

Verrucous hyperplasia is a markedly keratotic, papillomatous, noninvasive squamous epithelial proliferation that clinically appears as an elevated, sessile, whitish plaque indistinguishable from verrucous carcinoma. Virtually all patients are 50 years of age or older, with an approximately equal sex distribution (56). Verrucous hyperplasia most commonly occurs in the oral cavity, particularly the gingiva, cheek, and tongue. In one study of 68 cases, 20 (29 percent) had an associated verrucous carcinoma and 7 (10 percent) had an associated squamous cell carcinoma (56).

Pseudoepitheliomatous hyperplasia (PEH) indicates a reactive, downward proliferation of the squamous epithelium into the underlying stroma. It may occur in association with several chronic inflammatory conditions of the upper respiratory tract including tuberculosis, fungal infections, and chronic ulceration (53). Granular cell tumors, which often occur in the tongue, lip, oral cavity, and larynx, are notorious for stimulating PEH in the overlying epithelium (50,52,55,58).

The term leukoplakia was originally used to denote the presence of a white, patch-like lesion on the oral mucosa with histologic evidence of dysplasia. Currently, leukoplakia is considered a clinically descriptive term with no histologic correlate (51,54,57). Lesions diagnosed as leukoplakia typically appear as a white patch or plaque in the oral cavity that cannot be further characterized as any specific disease (59). Most cases involve the mandibular or buccal mucosa of older adults and have been attributed to

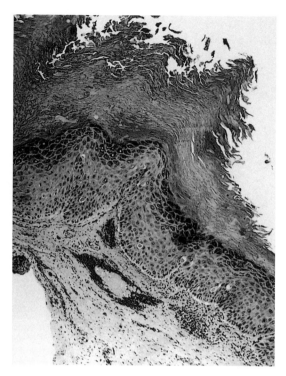

Figure 3-23
KERATOSIS
A 68-year-old man with chronic hoarseness over many years had several biopsies of suspicious clinical areas of the larynx. All had a histology similar to this of a minimal benign squamous hyperplasia of the mucosa, but with marked hyperkeratosis and a prominent stratum granulosum cell layer. (Fig. 67, Fascicle 25, 2nd Series.)

chronic mechanical (such as poorly fitting dentures) or chemical (tobacco abuse) irritation (59).

Pathologic Findings. Histologically, ordinary keratosis appears as an area of marked, often uneven hyperkeratosis with a variably hyperplastic underlying squamous epithelium (fig. 3-23). The underlying epithelium should appear normal without papillations, upward projections, or extension into the underlying mucosa.

Areas of verrucous hyperplasia may be grossly evident as mucosal-based, white-colored plaques, nodules, or papillations (fig. 3-24). Microscopically, verrucous hyperplasia is composed of hyperplastic squamous epithelium with regularly spaced, verrucous epithelial projections alternating with thick columns of orthokeratin. Shear and Pindborg (56) described both sharp and blunt varieties, based on whether the verrucous processes were narrow or blunt, respectively (figs. 3-25, 3-26). The sharp variety is typically

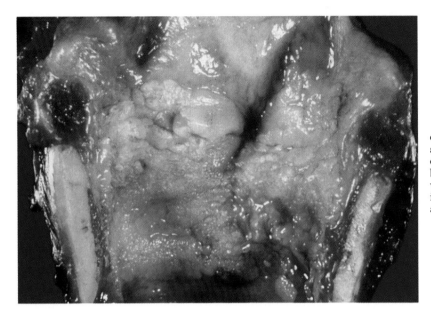

Figure 3-24
VERRUCOUS HYPERPLASIA
Gross photograph of an unusually extensive case of verrucous hyperplasia involving the larynx. Multiple biopsies were correctly interpreted as benign hyperplasia but laryngectomy was performed to exclude the possibility of carcinoma. (Figures 3-24–3-27 are from the same patient.)

Figure 3-25
VERRUCOUS HYPERPLASIA
OF THE ORAL CAVITY
An example of the sharp variety, in which the verrucous processes are elongated, narrow, and heavily keratinized.

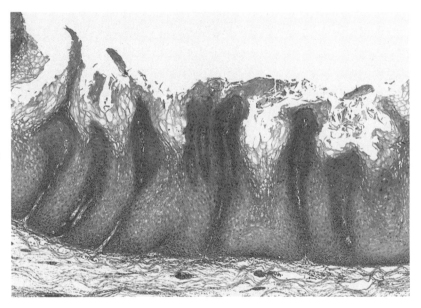

heavily keratinized, whereas blunt types usually show only a thin keratotic layer. Intraepithelial dysplasia may be present. By definition the process is sharply defined and superficial, such that the entire lesion remains on a plane above the surrounding normal epithelium (fig. 3-27).

PEH is a squamous epithelial proliferation that sends irregular tongues and rete pegs of epithelium deep into the underlying stroma. The overall appearance is not dissimilar from a well-differentiated squamous cell carcinoma (fig. 3-28).

PEH associated with a granular cell tumor may be sufficiently extensive to obscure the underlying tumor (figs. 3-29, 3-30). Mild nuclear pleomorphism, abrupt keratinization (horn-pearl formation), and numerous mitotic figures may be seen (50,52,60). Marked nuclear pleomorphism, hyperchromasia, and abnormal mitotic figures are absent.

Leukoplakia is a clinical term with no histologic correlate, thus biopsied lesions may show ordinary or verrucous keratosis, epithelial dysplasia, or

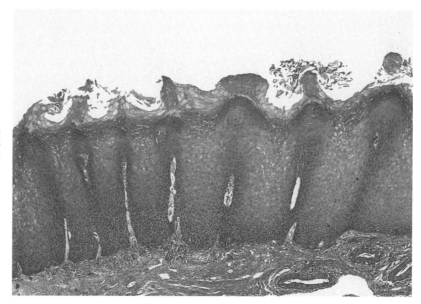

Figure 3-26
VERRUCOUS HYPERPLASIA
OF THE ORAL CAVITY
Verrucous hyperplasia of the blunt
variety, with verrucous processes that
are broader, shorter, and more rounded
than those seen in the sharp variety.

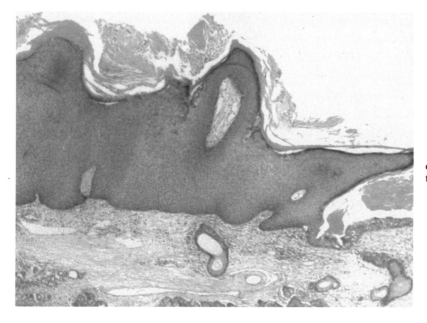

Figure 3-27
VERRUCOUS HYPERPLASIA
OF THE ORAL CAVITY
The lesion is superficial and lo-
cated above the adjacent normal epi-
thelium, which is seen on the right.

invasive squamous cell carcinoma (51,54,59). Histologically, most lesions submitted as "leukoplakia" (i.e., cannot clinically be attributed to another, more specific entity) show hyperkeratosis without dysplasia (54).

Differential Diagnosis. Ordinary keratotic lesions should not cause diagnostic difficulty on adequate biopsy specimens. Superficial biopsies showing a hyperkeratotic lesion, however, should be interpreted with caution if the base of the proliferation cannot be assessed.

Verrucous hyperplasia is distinguished from verrucous carcinoma solely on the depth of invasion. As suggested by Shear and Pindborg (56), verrucous proliferations that remain on a plane above the surrounding normal epithelium constitute verrucous hyperplasia, whereas those that extend below the plane represent verrucous carcinoma. A proportion of lesions, however, contain a coexisting verrucous or frankly invasive squamous cell carcinoma, thus verrucous hyperplasia and the latter diagnoses are not mutually exclusive (56).

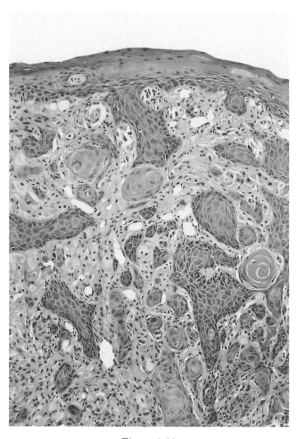

Figure 3-28
PSEUDOEPITHELIOMATOUS HYPERPLASIA
Prominent pseudoepitheliomatous hyperplasia associated with an underlying granular cell tumor of the tongue.

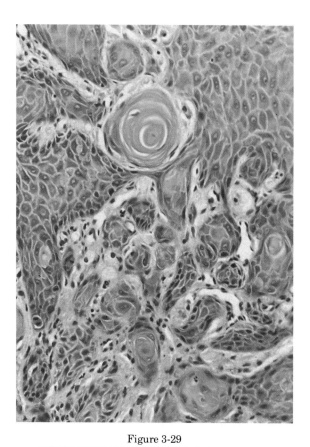

Figure 3-29
PSEUDOEPITHELIOMATOUS HYPERPLASIA
Situated between the granular cells are irregular, infiltrative nests of squamous cells mimicking squamous cell carcinoma. The underlying granular cell tumor is almost totally obscured in the field shown. (Figures 3-29 and 3-30 are from the same patient.)

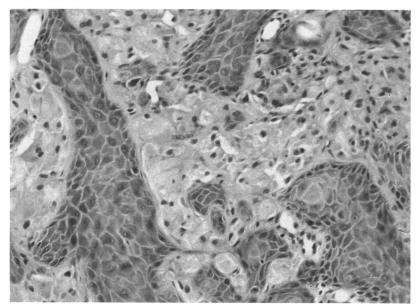

Figure 3-30
PSEUDOEPITHELIOMATOUS
HYPERPLASIA
Typical granular cell tumor is associated with the epithelial proliferation in the deeper portion of the lesion.

PEH is distinguished from verrucous carcinoma in that it lacks the superficial, verrucous hyperkeratotic component typical of the latter lesion. The deep epithelial border of verrucous carcinoma is rounded and bulbous, whereas the deep projections of PEH are often irregular and sharp. Distinction from squamous cell carcinoma may be difficult (60). PEH lacks marked nuclear pleomorphism, individual cell keratinization, and abnormal mitotic figures, but these features may be absent in squamous cancers as well. In certain cases PEH may be indistinguishable from a well-differentiated squamous cell carcinoma on superficial biopsy specimens. Identification of the associated condition, such as an underlying granular cell tumor, and repeat biopsy showing the base of the lesion may be necessary to make the distinction (60).

Treatment and Prognosis. Treatment for these lesions is either surgical excision or, particularly in cases of PEH, resolution or excision of the associated process.

Verruca Vulgaris of the Larynx and Oral Cavity

Definition. This is a benign, circumscribed, squamous epithelial proliferation arising from the oral cavity or laryngeal mucosa and characterized by hyperkeratosis, acanthosis, papillomatosis, koilocytic epithelial cells, and prominent keratohyaline granules (61–71).

General and Clinical Features. Verruca vulgaris is a common cutaneous epithelial lesion strongly associated with the human papillomavirus (HPV). Verrucae are most commonly found on the dorsal aspect of the fingers and hands, but may occur anywhere on the skin surface. Rarely, verruca vulgaris may develop in the oral mucosa and larynx as well. Oral cavity verrucae are uncommon but not rare; one study found 96 cases in the files of two oral pathology laboratories (67). In contrast, laryngeal verrucae are vanishingly rare; only eight cases have been reported in the literature to date (63,66).

On cutaneous or mucosal surfaces, verruca vulgaris clinically appears as circumscribed, firm, exophytic nodules with a papillomatous, hyperkeratotic surface. Almost all lesions are single, although rare patients with multiple oral verrucae have been described (67). Patients with oral cavity or laryngeal lesions commonly present with

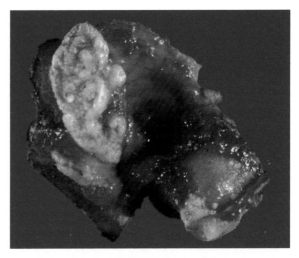

Figure 3-31
VERRUCA VULGARIS OF LARYNX
A hemilaryngectomy specimen of a verruca vulgaris of the larynx misinterpreted as a verrucous carcinoma on biopsy. The lesion is circumscribed, exophytic, and keratotic. (Courtesy of Dr. R.E. Fechner, Charlottesville, VA; figures 3-31–3-35 are from the same patient.)

hoarseness of variable duration. Patients with verrucae in the oral cavity range in age from 7 to 72 years, with an average of 35 years; the male to female ratio is 1.5 to 1 (67). The eight reported patients with laryngeal verrucae include seven males and one female ranging in age from 37 to 70 years, with an average of 56 years. About half of oral verrucae involve the lips; the next most common location is the palate, which accounts for about one fifth of lesions, followed by the alveolus, gingiva, tongue, and buccal mucosa. All laryngeal lesions reported to date have been localized to the true vocal cords.

The precise etiology of cutaneous verrucae is unknown but most, if not all lesions are presumed to be of viral etiology. Similar to their cutaneous counterparts, oral and laryngeal verrucae are associated with HPV. Studies using electron microscopy, immunohistochemistry, or in situ hybridization have detected HPV types 2, 6, or 11 in 55 to 100 percent of examined lesions (62,63,65–68,70,71).

Pathologic Findings. Pathologically, verrucae vulgaris from the oral cavity and larynx are virtually identical to their cutaneous counterparts. Those few lesions in which a gross description is available are multiple, soft, white tissue fragments, some of which have a papillary, hyperkeratotic appearance (fig. 3-31). Specimens commonly

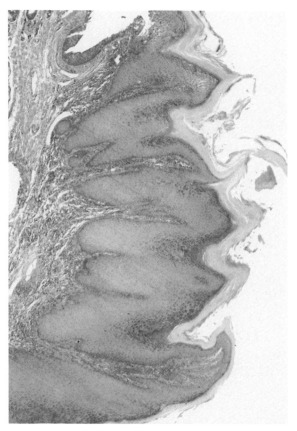

Figure 3-32
VERRUCA VULGARIS OF LARYNX
On low power, verruca vulgaris is characterized by hyperkeratosis, acanthosis, and papillomatosis. Lesions are typically superficial and situated predominantly or entirely above the level of the surrounding epithelium.

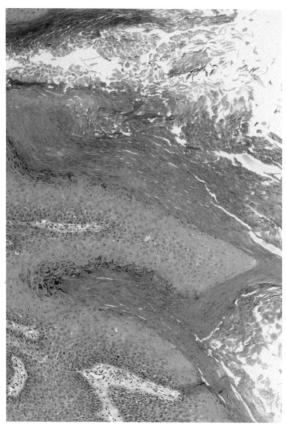

Figure 3-33
VERRUCA VULGARIS OF LARYNX
Verruca consist of thin fibrovascular cores covered by multiple layers of squamous epithelium with a dense layer of orthokeratosis.

measure less than 0.5 cm in largest dimension (63). On scanning magnification, the lesions are superficial epithelial proliferations often located above the level of the surrounding epithelium. They are characterized by hyperkeratosis, acanthosis, and papillomatosis (fig. 3-32). The acanthotic rete pegs are elongated, thin, and often sharp. The rete pegs at the periphery of the lesion are unusually elongated and typically bend inwards, pointing towards the center of the lesion. The surface is covered by a thick layer of orthokeratin with occasional vertical columns of parakeratotic cells (figs. 3-33, 3-34). Just beneath the keratin is a prominent granular cell layer, predominantly composed of flattened squamous cells with large vesicular nuclei, eosinophilic nucleoli, and numerous intracytoplas-

mic keratohyaline granules. The granular cell layer also contains vertical tiers and nests of koilocytic squamous cells with hyperchromatic nuclei and cleared (vacuolated) cytoplasm (fig. 3-35). The keratohyaline granular cells are usually concentrated in the lesional troughs (or "valleys"), whereas the koilocytic cells are mostly located on the papillary peaks, underneath vertical columns of parakeratotic cells. There is typically no evidence of epithelial dysplasia. Mitoses are infrequent and confined to the basal layer of the epithelium.

Differential Diagnosis. Laryngeal and oral cavity verrucae should be distinguished from squamous papillomas, verrucous hyperplasia, and verrucous carcinoma. Laryngeal squamous papillomas of both the juvenile and adult type lack the

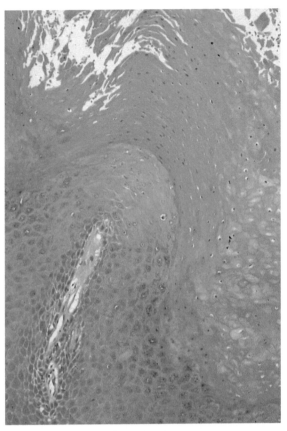

Figure 3-34
VERRUCA VULGARIS OF LARYNX
Vertical tiers of parakeratotic cells are usually found originating from the papillary peaks. The granular cell layer is focally present on either side.

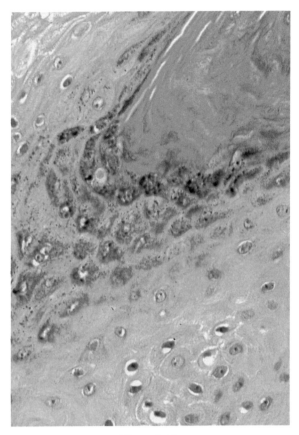

Figure 3-35
VERRUCA VULGARIS OF LARYNX
The sine qua non of verruca vulgaris is the presence of a prominent granular layer, the cells of which contain numerous, irregularly sized, basophilic keratohyaline granules. These areas are typically located in the lesional "valleys" between the papillary peaks. Koilocytic change is focally present as well.

dense, keratohyaline cell layer, irregular acanthosis, and periodicity typical of verrucae. Verrucous hyperplasia and carcinoma are also characterized by large, uniform squamous cells and bulbous, blunt-ending acanthotic rete pegs but lack the prominent keratohyaline granular layer, parakeratosis, and sharp acanthotic pegs of verrucous vulgaris (61,64,69).

Treatment and Prognosis. The treatment of choice is local excision which is curative in almost all cases. We are not aware of local recurrence being documented in oral verrucae following excision. Of the eight patients with laryngeal verrucae, follow-up was available on six, one of whom developed two local recurrences at 5 and 7 years after surgery (66).

REFERENCES

Schneiderian Papillomas

1. Barnes L, Bedetti C. Oncocytic schneiderian papilloma: a reappraisal of cylindrical cell papilloma of the sinonasal tract. Hum Pathol 1984;15:344–51.
2. Buchwald C, Franzmann MB, Jacobsen GK, Lindeberg H. Human papillomavirus (HPV) in sinonasal papillomas: a study of 78 cases using in situ hybridization and the polymerase chain reaction. Laryngoscope 1995;105:66–71.
3. Calceterra TC, Thompson JW, Paglia DE. Inverting papillomas of the nose and paranasal sinuses. Laryngoscope 1980;90:53–8.
4. Christensen WN, Smith RL. Schneiderian papillomas: a clinicopathologic study of 67 cases. Hum Pathol 1986;17:393–400.
5. Cunningham MJ, Brantley S, Barnes L, Schramm VL. Oncocytic Schneiderian papilloma in a young adult: a rare diagnosis. Otolaryngol Head Neck Surg 1987;97:47–51.
6. Hyams VJ. Papillomas of the nasal cavity and paranasal sinuses. A clinicopathologic study of 315 cases. Ann Otol Rhinol Laryngol 1971;80:192–206.
7. Hyams VJ, Batsakis JG, Michaels L. Tumors of the upper respiratory tract and ear. Atlas of Tumor Pathology, 2nd Series, Fascicle 25. Washington D.C.: Armed Forces Institute of Pathology, 1986:320.
8. Judd R, Zaki SR, Coffield LM, Evatt BL. Sinonasal papillomas and human papillomavirus: human papillomavirus 11 detected in fungiform schneiderian papillomas by in situ hybridization and the polymerase chain reaction. Hum Pathol 1991;22:550–6.
9. Kapadia SB, Barnes L, Pelzman K, Mirani N, Heffner DK, Bedetti C. Carcinoma ex oncocytic Schneiderian (cylindrical cell) papilloma. Am J Otolaryngol 1993;14:332–8.
10. Lasser A, Smith HW. Rhinosporidiosis. Arch Otolaryngol 1976;102:308–10.
11. Michaels L, Young M. Histogenesis of papillomas of the nose and paranasal sinuses. Arch Pathol Lab Med 1995;119:821–6.
12. Nosanchuk JS. Oropharyngeal inverted papilloma. Arch Otolaryngol 1974;100:71–2.
13. O'Reilly BJ, Zuk R. Transitional type papilloma of the nasopharynx. J Laryngol Otol 1989;103:528–30.
14. Ridolfi RL, Liberman PH, Erlandson RA, Moore OS. Schneiderian papillomas: a clinicopathologic study of 30 cases. Am J Surg Pathol 1977;1:43–53.
15. Roberts WH, Dinges DL, Hanly MG. Inverted papilloma of the middle ear. Ann Otol Rhinol Laryngol 1993;102:890–2.
16. Sarkar FH, Visscher DW, Kintanar EB, Zarbo RJ, Crissman JD. Sinonasal schneiderian papillomas: human papillomavirus typing by polymerase chain reaction. Mod Pathol 1992;5:329–32.
17. Smith O, Gullane PJ. Inverting papilloma of the nose: analysis of 48 patients. J Otolaryngol 1987;16:154–6.
18. Snyder RN, Perzin KH. Papillomatosis of nasal cavity and paranasal sinuses (inverted papilloma; squamous papilloma). A clinicopathologic study. Cancer 1972;30:668–90.
19. Stone DM, Berktold RE, Ranganathan C, Wiet RJ. Inverted papilloma of the middle ear and mastoid. Otolaryngol Head Neck Surg 1987;97:416–8.
20. Weissler MC, Montgomery WW, Montgomery SK, Turner PA, Joseph MP. Inverted papilloma. Ann Otol Rhinol Laryngol 1986;95:215–21.
21. Wenig BM. Schneiderian-type mucosal papillomas of the middle ear and mastoid. Ann Otol Rhinol Laryngol 1996;105:226–33.
22. Ward BE, Fechner RE, Mills SE. Carcinoma arising in oncocytic Schneiderian papilloma. Am J Surg Pathol 1990;14:364–9.
23. Yang YJ, Abraham JL. Undifferentiated carcinoma arising in oncocytic Schneiderian (cylindrical cell) papilloma. J Oral Maxillofac Surg 1997;55:289–94.

Inverted Ductal Papilloma of Minor Salivary Glands

24. Batsakis JG, Brannon RB, Sciubba JJ. Monomorphic adenomas of major salivary glands: a histologic study of 96 tumors. Clin Otolaryngol 1981;6:129–43.
25. Clark DB, Priddy RW, Swanson AE. Oral inverted ductal papilloma. Oral Surg Oral Med Oral Pathol 1990;69:487–90.
26. Ellis GL, Auclair PL, Gnepp DR. Ductal papillomas. In: Surgical pathology of the salivary glands. Philadelphia: WB Saunders, 1991:238–51.
27. Gardiner GW, Briant TD, Sheman L. Inverted ductal papilloma of the parotid gland. J Otolaryngol 1984;13:23–6.
28. Hegarty DJ, Hopper C, Speight PM. Inverted ductal papilloma of minor salivary glands. J Oral Pathol Med 1994;23:334–6.
29. Koutlas IG, Jessrun J, Iamaroon A. Immunohistochemical evaluation and in situ hybridization in a case of oral inverted papilloma. J Oral Maxillofac Surg 1994;52:503–6.
30. Regezi JA, Lloyd RV, Zarbo RJ, McClatchey KD. Minor salivary gland tumors. A histologic and immunohistochemical study. Cancer 1985;55:108–15.
31. White DK, Miller AS, McDaniel RK, Rothman BN. Inverted ductal papilloma: a distinctive lesion of minor salivary gland. Cancer 1982;49:519–24.
32. Wilson DF, Robinson BW. Oral inverted ductal papilloma. Oral Surg 1984;57:520–3.

Papillomas of the Larynx and Trachea

33. Abramson AL, Steinberg BM, Winkler B. Laryngeal papillomatosis: clinical, histopathologic, and molecular studies. Laryngoscope 1987;97:678–85.
34. Cohen SR, Seltzer S, Geller KA, Thompson JW. Papilloma of the larynx and tracheo-bronchial tree in children. A retrospective study. Ann Otol 1980;89:497–503.
35. Costa J, Howley PM, Bowling MC, Howard R, Bauer WC. Presence of human papilloma viral antigens in juvenile multiple laryngeal papilloma. Am J Clin Pathol 1981;75:194–7.
36. Crissman JD, Kessis T, Shah KV, et al. Squamous papillary neoplasia of the adult upper aerodigestive tract. Hum Pathol 1988;19:1387–96.

37. Fechner RE, Goepfert H, Alford BR. Invasive laryngeal papillomatosis. Arch Otolaryngol 1974;99:147–51.
38. Gale N, Poljak M, Kambic V, Ferluga D, Fischinger J. Laryngeal papillomatosis: molecular, histopathological, and clinical evaluation. Virchows Arch 1994;425:291–5.
39. Guillou L, Sahli R, Chaubert P, Monnier P, Cuttat JF, Costa J. Squamous cell carcinoma of the lung in a nonsmoking, nonirradiated patient with juvenile laryngotracheal papillomatosis. Am J Surg Pathol 1991;15:891–8.
40. Helmuth RA, Strate RW. Squamous carcinoma of the lung in a nonirradiated, nonsmoking patient with juvenile laryngotracheal papillomatosis. Am J Surg Pathol 1987;11:643–50.
41. Levi J, Delcelo R, Alberti VN, Torloni H, Villa LL. Human papillomavirus DNA in respiratory papillomatosis detected by in situ hybridization and the polymerase chain reaction. Am J Pathol 1989;135:1179–84.
42. Lindeberg H, Laryngeal papillomas: histomorphometric evaluation of multiple and solitary lesions. Clin Otolaryngol 1991;16:257–60.
43. Lindeberg H, Elbrond O. Laryngeal papillomas: clinical aspects in a series of 231 patients. Clin Otolaryngol 1989;14:333–42.
44. Lindeberg H. Oster S, Oxlund I, Elbrond O. Laryngeal papillomas: classification and course. Clin Otolaryngol 1986;11:423–9.
45. Nikolaidis ET, Trost D, Buchholz C, Wilkinson E. The relationship of histologic and clinical factors in laryngeal papillomatosis. Arch Pathol Lab Med 1985;109:24–9.
46. Quick CA, Foucar E, Dehner LP. Frequency and significance of epithelial atypia in laryngeal papillomatosis. Laryngoscope 1979;89:550–60.
47. Steinberg BM, Topp WC, Schneider PS, Abramson AL. Laryngeal papillomavirus infection during clinical remission. N Engl J Med 1983;308:1261–4.
48. Strong MS, Vaughan CW, Cooperbrand SR, Healy GB, Clemente MA. Recurrent respiratory papillomatosis. Management with the CO2 laser. Ann Otol 1976;85:508–16.
49. Terry RM, Lewis FA, Robertson S, Blythe D, Wells M. Juvenile and adult laryngeal papillomata: classification by in-situ hybridization for human papillomavirus. Clin Otolaryngol 1989;14:135–9.

Keratosis, Verrucous Hyperplasia, Pseudoepitheliomatous Hyperplasia, and Leukoplakia

50. Compagno J, Hyams VJ, Ste-Marie P. Benign granular cell tumors of the larynx: a review of 36 cases with clinicopathologic data. Ann Otol 1975;84:308–14.
51. Gassenmaier A, Hornstein OP. Presence of papillomavirus DNA in benign and precancerous oral leukoplakias and squamous cell carcinomas. Dermatologica 1988;176:224–33.
52. Lack EE, Worsham F, Callihan MD, et al. Granular cell tumor: a clinicopathologic study of 110 patients. J Surg Oncol 1980;13:301–16.
53. Michaels L. Infections. In: Ear, nose, and throat histopathology. London: Springer-Verlag, 1987:315–33.
54. Pindborg JJ. Pathology of oral leukoplakia. Am J Dermatopathol 1980;2:277–8.
55. Regezi JA, Batsakis JG, Courtney RM. Granular cell tumors of the head and neck. J Oral Surg 1979;37:402–6.
56. Shear M, Pindborg JJ. Verrucous hyperplasia of the oral mucosa. Cancer 1980;46:1855–62.
57. Shklar G. Modern studies and concepts of leukoplakia in the mouth. J Dermatol Surg Oncol 1981;7:996–1003.
58. Strong EW, McDivitt RW, Brasfield RD. Granular cell myoblastoma. Cancer 1970;25:415–22.
59. Waldron CA, Shafer WG. Leukoplakia revisited. A clinicopathologic study of 3256 leukoplakias. Cancer 1975;36:1386–92.
60. Wolber RA, Talerman A, Wilkinson EJ, Clement PB. Vulvar granular cell tumors with pseudocarcinomatous hyperplasia: a comparative analysis with well-differentiated squamous cell carcinoma. Int J Gynecol Pathol 1991;10:59–66.

Verruca Vulgaris of the Larynx and Oral Cavity

61. Ackerman LV. Verrucous carcinoma of the oral cavity. Surgery 1948;23:670–8.
62. Adler-Storthz K, Newland JR, Tessin BA, Yeudall WA, Sillitoe EJ. Identification of human papillomavirus in oral verruca vulgaris. J Oral Pathol 1986;15:230–3.
63. Barnes L, Yunis EJ, Krebs FJ, Sonmez-Alpan E. Verruca vulgaris of the larynx. Demonstration of human papillomavirus types 6/11 by in situ hybridization. Arch Pathol Lab Med 1991;115:895–9.
64. Biller HF, Ogura JH, Bauer WC. Verrucous cancer of the larynx. Laryngoscope 1971;81:1323–9.
65. Eversole LR, Laipis PJ, Green TL. Human papillomavirus type 2 DNA in oral and labial verruca vulgaris. J Cutan Pathol 1987;14:319–25.
66. Fechner RE, Mills SE. Verruca vulgaris of the larynx: a distinctive lesion of probable viral origin confused with verrucous carcinoma. Am J Surg Pathol 1982;6:357–62.
67. Green TL, Eversole LR, Leider AS. Oral and labial verruca vulgaris: clinical, histologic and immunohistochemical evaluation. Oral Surg Oral Med Oral Pathol 1986;62:410–6.
68. Miller CS, Zeuss MS, White DK. In situ detection of HPV DNA in oral mucosal lesions: a comparison of two hybridization kits. J Oral Pathol Med 1991;20:403–8.
69. Shear M, Pindborg JJ. Verrucous hyperplasia of the oral mucosa. Cancer 1980;46:1855–62.
70. Wysocki GP, Hardie J. Ultrastructural studies of intraoral verruca vulgaris. Oral Surg Oral Med Oral Pathol 1979;47:58–62.
71. Zeuss MS, Miller CS, White DK. In situ hybridization analysis of human papillomavirus DNA in oral mucosal lesions. Oral Surg Oral Med Oral Pathol 1991;71:714–20.

4
CONVENTIONAL SQUAMOUS CELL CARCINOMA

KERATOSIS / DYSPLASIA / SQUAMOUS CELL CARCINOMA IN SITU

The progression from increasing dysplasia of the surface epithelium to the development of invasive squamous cell carcinoma is well documented in a variety of anatomic sites, most notably the uterine cervix. There are, however, some significant differences between the cervical model and the squamous mucosa of the head and neck, particularly in regard to the microscopic appearance of the dysplasia and the grading criteria applied to these changes.

Keratosis

Keratosis without associated dysplastic change may be seen throughout the head and neck mucosa, most often in areas of preexistent squamous epithelium, but occasionally superimposed on metaplastic squamous mucosa. Typically, there is an identifiable, long-term irritant such as ill-fitting dentures or chronic use of tobacco products. In the larynx, hyperkeratosis is strongly associated with smoking and predilects the vocal cords. Clinically, the mucosa has a white, thickened appearance (fig. 4-1), perhaps with visible increased vascularity in the underlying stroma. The clinical terms, leukoplakia and erythroplakia, have been applied to patches of white and more vascularized, keratotic mucosa. These terms do not have distinct microscopic counterparts as both nondysplastic and dysplastic lesions may have this appearance. It has been suggested that in the oral cavity, the clinical presence of erythroplakia is more likely to be associated with significant dysplasia (24,32). In the larynx there appears to be no difference in the frequency of dysplasia with clinical leukoplakia or erythroplakia (32,62).

Grasping thickened, keratotic mucosa with forceps and gently pulling typically leads to its easy removal, particularly from the vocal cords. The junction of the basal cells and underlying stroma is usually the fracture line for this separation. The presence of an intact layer of basal cells is a useful feature for excluding invasive carcinoma when dealing with dysplastic strips of keratotic mucosa.

Microscopically, nondysplastic keratosis is characterized by a squamous mucosa of normal or increased thickness, often with a prominent granular cell layer, and overlying layers of ortho-keratin, often admixed with parakeratotic cells (fig. 4-2). Distinction between anuclear keratotic cells (orthokeratin) and flattened keratotic cells with pyknotic nuclei (parakeratin) is of no significance. The cell layers may be thickened, but maturation is orderly, with mitotic figures confined to the basal cell layer. Aberrant keratinization of individual cells (dyskeratosis) is not present.

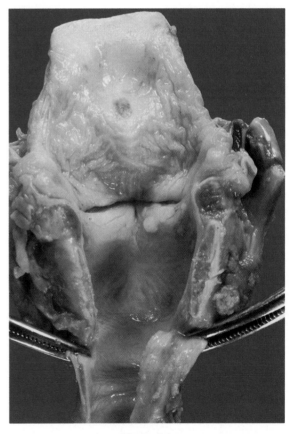

Figure 4-1
HYPERKERATOSIS
The right vocal cord is involved by a zone of hyperkeratosis. This was an incidental finding at autopsy.

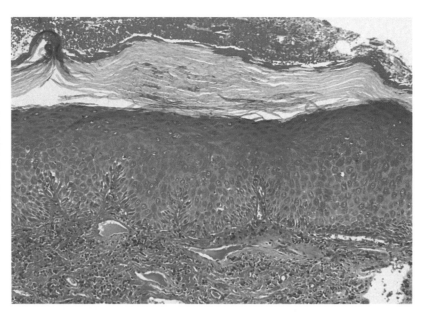

Figure 4-2
HYPERKERATOSIS
This area of hyperkeratosis consists of a thick band of orthokeratin overlying a thickened layer of squamous mucosa with some stromal chronic inflammation. Although the nuclei in the basal cell layer are enlarged and "active" appearing, there is normal maturation with no evidence of dysplasia.

It has been documented that keratosis without dysplasia carries a minimal risk for subsequent carcinoma. Norris and Peale (106) studied 30 patients with laryngeal keratosis devoid of dysplasia and noted that only 1 developed subsequent invasive carcinoma; in contrast, 11 of 86 patients with dysplastic lesions developed subsequent carcinomas, although in some instances invasive versus in situ lesions were not clearly distinguished. Gabriel and Jones (49) studied 13 patients with nondysplastic laryngeal keratoses, none of whom developed subsequent carcinoma. In a larger series of 225 patients having laryngeal keratoses without atypia (8), 2.7 percent were subsequently diagnosed as having carcinoma from 9 to 32 months after initial diagnosis. Approximately 6 to 10 percent of patients with nondysplastic keratoses later develop a dysplastic component, with the associated increased risk for invasive carcinoma (63,106).

Dysplasia

The association of keratosis containing varying degrees of dysplasia with the subsequent development of invasive squamous cell carcinoma was first recognized in the 1930s and has been the subject of numerous subsequent publications. McGavran (103), in a study of 87 patients with keratotic laryngeal lesions followed for 5 to 15 years, noted that the presence of dysplasia not only correlated with an increased

risk for subsequent carcinoma, but also correlated with more frequent recurrences of the keratosis. In a more recent study of 92 patients with laryngeal keratoses followed for a minimum of 5 years, Crissman (30) noted that 3 patients developed subsequent carcinoma, all of whom had severe dysplasia in their initial specimens. Others have noted a general correlation between the degree of dysplastic change and the frequency of subsequent carcinoma: in a symposium on this topic, rates of 7 to 36 percent were noted for oral cavity lesions, and 8 to 29 percent for laryngeal involvement (32).

It is important to note, however, that the presence of severely dysplastic mucosa, particularly in the larynx, should lead to the careful search for a synchronous invasive tumor. Invasive carcinomas discovered within 6 months of the initial dysplastic lesion almost certainly were present and undiagnosed at the time of initial presentation. Such cases should not be considered to represent "rapidly progressing" dysplasias. Inclusion of such cases may result in artifactual inflation of risk of subsequent invasive carcinoma.

Whether preinvasive dysplasias are "reversible" lesions, following removal of instigating factors (i.e., cessation of smoking) was the subject of a large autopsy study by Auerbach and colleagues (3). They noted that almost 16 percent of 644 cigarette smoking patients had severe dysplasia or carcinoma in situ of the larynx,

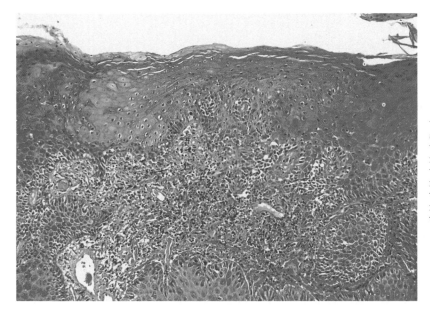

Figure 4-3
HYPERKERATOSIS
In this example of hyperkeratosis, the biopsy specimen is folded such that surface epithelium is present both at the top and bottom of the field. There is a layer of surface parakeratin with the underlying epithelium showing rare hyperchromatic and dyskeratotic cells. There is considerable stromal inflammation and we consider the changes to be reactive.

whereas no ex-smokers had carcinoma in situ and only 25 percent had mild atypia. The findings in the ex-smokers were similar to those in never-smokers, supporting the circumstantial conclusion that similar lesions in the former smokers had regressed, at least at the light microscopic level, following smoking cessation.

Various grading systems have been applied to squamous dysplasias of the head and neck. Although these are somewhat similar to systems applied to the uterine cervix, dominance of the dysplastic process by a basaloid cell component associated with loss of cytoplasmic differentiation, as is typical in the cervix, is not frequently encountered in the head and neck. Dysplastic lesions arising in the latter locations often retain a major component of keratinized cells, even in high-grade lesions (16). These keratinizing dysplasias are much less common in the gynecologic tract. The potential value of grading dysplasias was noted in a study by Hellquist et al. (62). In a large series of mild, moderate, and severe laryngeal dysplasias, subsequent invasive carcinoma was documented in 2 percent, 13 percent, and 23 percent of patients, respectively.

We prefer a three-part grading system for head and neck squamous dysplasia which recognizes mild, moderate, and severe dysplasia. We avoid the term, carcinoma in-situ, and include these lesions under the rubric of severe dysplasia. Mild dysplasia is characterized, microscopically, by nuclear irregularity with nuclear crowding, primarily in the basal cell layer. Nuclear chromatin is essentially normal (figs. 4-3, 4-4) (32). Moderate dysplasia is characterized by the presence of larger, irregular nuclei, often with peripherally condensed chromatin, resulting in central clearing. Nucleoli are focally prominent. Mitotic figures are increased in the basal cell layer, but do not extend into the more superficial epithelial layers (figs. 4-5, 4-6). Severe dysplasia is characterized by the presence of aberrant cell maturation with dyskeratotic cells, mitotic figures focally present above the basal cell layer, and the presence of atypical mitotic figures (figs. 4-7, 4-8) (32). These anomalies often occur in a setting of partial or complete maturation, with keratinization of the overlying surface mucosa (fig. 4-9). In our experience, the presence of individually keratinized (dyskeratotic) cells is an important low-power microscopic clue to the presence of significant dysplasia. The lack of importance of surface keratinization in assessing laryngeal dysplasia was emphasized by Blackwell et al. (16). In an evaluation of 125 laryngeal biopsies from 62 patients with laryngeal squamous dysplasia and long-term follow-up, factors associated with a progression to invasive carcinoma included: mitotic activity, abnormal mitotic figures, maturation level, and nuclear pleomorphism. Notably, the presence of surface keratinization did not suggest an improved prognosis or lessened risk for subsequent invasive carcinoma.

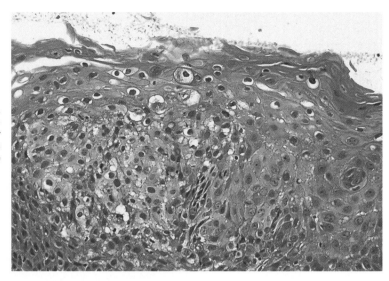

Figure 4-4
MILD DYSPLASIA
In this biopsy the surface layer of keratin is relatively thin and the underlying squamous cells show disorganization in the lower layers, with some "koilocyte-like" cleared cells located superficially. Areas of this type may be considered to represent mild dysplasia.

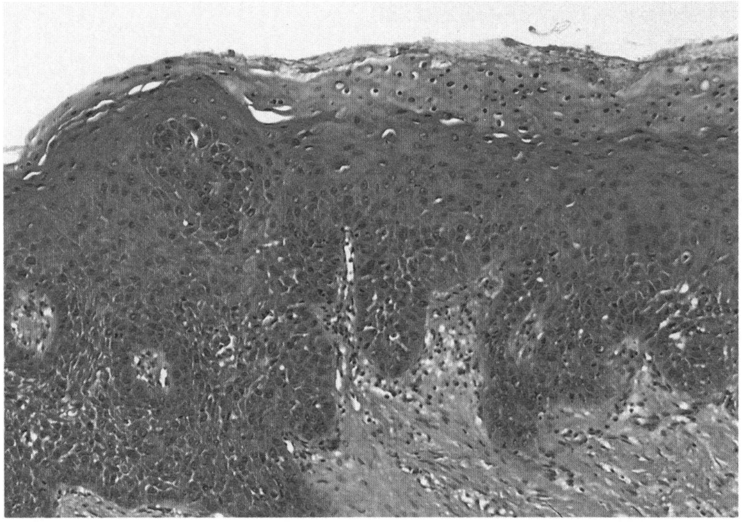

Figure 4-5
MODERATE DYSPLASIA
This example of hyperkeratosis with underlying moderate dysplasia shows considerable irregular thickening of the squamous epithelium.

Figure 4-6
MODERATE DYSPLASIA
A higher power magnification of the moderate dysplasia seen in figure 4-5 shows considerable nuclear enlargement with scattered dyskeratotic cells.

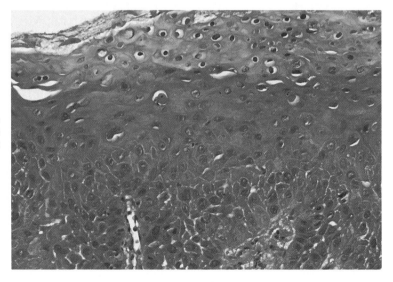

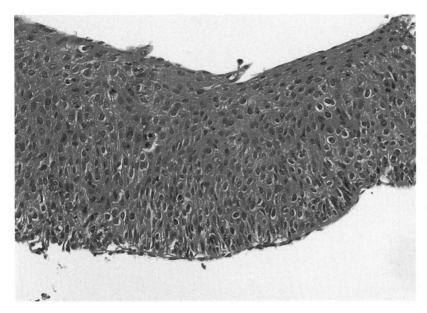

Figure 4-7
SEVERE DYSPLASIA
In this example of severe dysplasia there is some flattening of the surface epithelium, but the remainder shows disorganization, marked nuclear pleomorphism, and nuclear hyperchromasia. The presence of a sharp "fracture line" at the basal cell-stromal interface suggests that there is no underlying invasion.

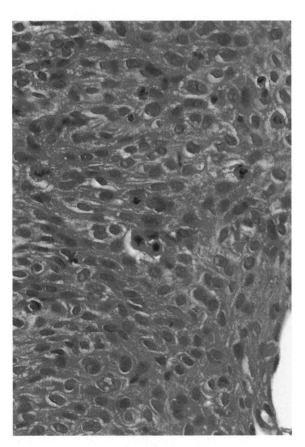

Figure 4-8
SEVERE DYSPLASIA
A higher magnification of figure 4-7 shows nearly full thickness cellular disorganization, scattered dyskeratotic or apoptotic cells, and multiple mitotic figures located well above the basal cell layer.

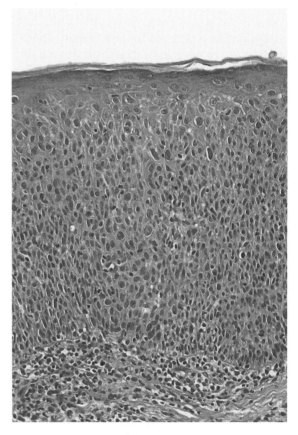

Figure 4-9
SEVERE DYSPLASIA
In this example of severe dysplasia, the epithelium shows a thin layer of surface maturation and keratosis. However, below this is a markedly thickened zone of disorganized and highly dysplastic squamous cells. The surface maturation should not prevent an interpretation of severe dysplasia for such cases.

Squamous dysplasia in many locations in the head and neck may extend for considerable distances into underlying seromucinous ducts. This is analogous to glandular involvement in dysplasia of the uterine cervix. Involvement of seromucinous ducts by dysplasia must be distinguished from invasive carcinoma, as this process does not represent true invasion. The distinction may be difficult, particularly in frozen sections where the ducts are incompletely sectioned and appear as isolated nests of dysplastic cells in the underlying stroma. As in the uterine cervix, keys to the recognition of dysplasia include the sharp circumscription of the nests, the lack of surrounding stromal response, and the nearby presence of more easily recognized seromucinous ducts.

The evaluation of keratotic lesions using immunohistochemical markers for differentiation and proliferation has been the subject of several studies. The goal of these efforts, like their light microscopic, hematoxylin and eosin (H&E) stain-based counterparts, has been the reliable recognition of dysplastic changes. Studies using squamous differentiation markers, most notably cytokeratins and involucrin, have documented variably aberrant expression in dysplastic, as compared to nondysplastic, keratotic lesions (16,27,81,124,147). Proliferation markers such as proliferating cell nuclear antigen (PCNA) have also shown promise in this regard (27). PCNA is confined to the basal cell layer in normal and keratotic mucosa. In one study, suprabasal reactivity for PCNA was invariably present in dysplasia and carcinoma in situ (27). It has been suggested that expression of p53, assessed immunohistochemically, also correlates with dysplasia (27). Although these studies may occasionally be of value when dealing with small, distorted biopsies, it remains to be shown that they provide information beyond that obtainable by careful examination of an adequate H&E-stained slide.

INVASIVE SQUAMOUS
CELL CARCINOMA

The diagnosis of typical squamous cell carcinoma is seldom problematic. Non-neoplastic diagnostic pitfalls such as necrotizing sialometaplasia, median rhomboid glossitis, pseudoepitheliomatous hyperplasia, and the juxtaoral organ of Chievitz are discussed in the chapter dealing

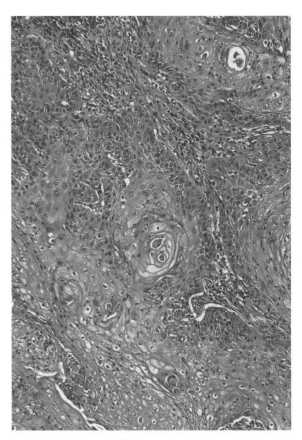

Figure 4-10
SQUAMOUS CELL CARCINOMA
Invasive, well-differentiated squamous cell carcinoma consists of large, interconnecting nests of overtly squamous cells. A keratin "pearl" is present in the center of the field.

with tumor-like lesions. Distinct, often diagnostically problematic variants of squamous cell carcinoma are discussed in the next chapter.

Most squamous cell carcinomas of the head and neck region are obviously malignant and show obvious squamous differentiation. Well-differentiated forms are typically composed of large, closely apposed cell nests. Keratinization is prominent, often with keratin "pearl" formation (fig. 4-10). When encountering tumors of this type, the differential diagnosis includes verrucous carcinomas and non-neoplastic hyperplasias due to a variety of causes. Moderately differentiated squamous cell carcinomas consist of smaller nests of more pleomorphic cells with increased mitotic activity and clear-cut but often less prominent squamous differentiation (figs. 4-11, 4-12). Poorly differentiated squamous cell carcinomas consist of highly mitotically active

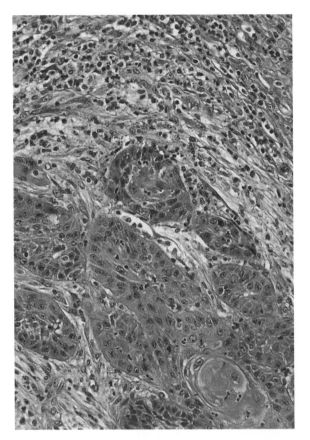

Figure 4-11
SQUAMOUS CELL CARCINOMA
This moderately differentiated squamous cell carcinoma consists of small nests of squamous cells with some central keratinization. As is the case in many carcinomas of the head and neck, there is an associated prominent component of inflammation.

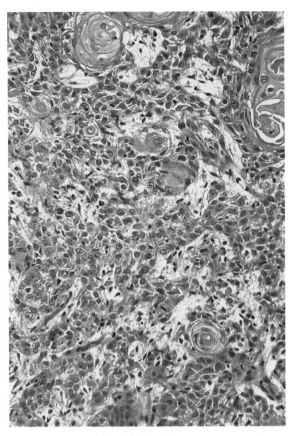

Figure 4-12
SQUAMOUS CELL CARCINOMA
Moderately differentiated squamous cell carcinoma consists of anastomosing cords of neoplastic cells with areas of abrupt keratinization.

cells growing singly and in small nests, and showing ragged or diffuse rather than "pushing" infiltration. Squamous differentiation is focal and often poorly developed (fig. 4-13). The differential diagnostic considerations include poorly differentiated carcinoma variants such as undifferentiated carcinoma (lymphoepithelioma) and basaloid squamous cell carcinoma, as well as nonsquamous malignancies. Moderately and poorly differentiated squamous cell carcinomas may demonstrate prominent intralymphatic invasion (fig. 4-14), and in our experience, this finding is associated with an increased incidence of both local and regional recurrences. We do not routinely employ immunohistochemical markers for endothelial cells to aid in the assessment of vascular involvement, but we do believe that

clear-cut examples of vascular invasion in H&E-stained sections should be reported.

The association between dysplasia and the subsequent development of an invasive squamous cell carcinoma is well established in the head and neck region. Nonetheless, it should be recognized that occasional carcinomas will appear to "drop off" the basal cell layer, with the overlying mucosa showing no evidence of dysplasia (figs. 4-15, 4-16). For ease of communication in our own practices, we have applied the term "drop down carcinoma" to such tumors, although this should not be viewed as a specific entity. These squamous cell carcinomas may cause considerable diagnostic difficulty, clinically, because they are overlain by essentially normal mucosa. This makes them difficult to localize grossly or endoscopically, and biopsy specimens must be deep enough to extend

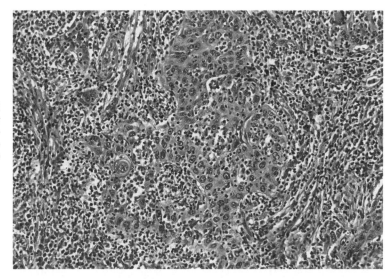

Figure 4-13
SQUAMOUS CELL CARCINOMA
This poorly differentiated squamous cell carcinoma has a prominent inflammatory stroma. Rare cells show squamous-like features. The appearance of the tumor approaches that of a lymphoepithelioma-like carcinoma.

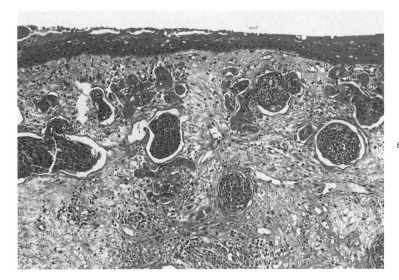

Figure 4-14
SQUAMOUS CELL CARCINOMA
OF THE LARYNX
There is extensive involvement of the subepithelial lymphatics.

Figure 4-15
SQUAMOUS CELL CARCINOMA
This small focus of well-differentiated squamous cell carcinoma appears to "drop down" from the basal cell layer of the otherwise normal-appearing surface mucosa.

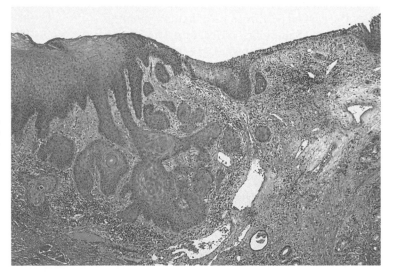

through the surface layer of normal mucosa. Once deep biopsies are obtained, the diagnosis is usually straightforward. "Drop down carcinomas" are often well differentiated, but they have cytologic features of malignancy and, hence, are not variants of verrucous carcinoma.

SITE-SPECIFIC INVASIVE SQUAMOUS CELL CARCINOMA

Lip

General Features. The lip is the single most common site for oral cavity squamous cell carcinoma, accounting for up to 40 percent of tumors (89). Both tobacco use, particularly pipe smoking, and solar damage have been associated with the development of these neoplasms.

Clinical Features. Over 90 percent of labial carcinomas arise from the lower lip (45,89), usually near the vermillion border and lateral to the midline (fig. 4-17) (157). Historically, male patients have predominated. Patients are middle-aged or elderly. Grossly, these are typically ulcerated, indurated, crusted, or even fungating masses.

Microscopic Findings. Although most of the variants of squamous cell carcinoma can occur in the lip, the vast majority are conventional, moderately differentiated neoplasms. Occasionally, verrucous carcinomas arise from the lip, and rarely there may be spindle cell, adenoid squamous cell, or other poorly differentiated variants.

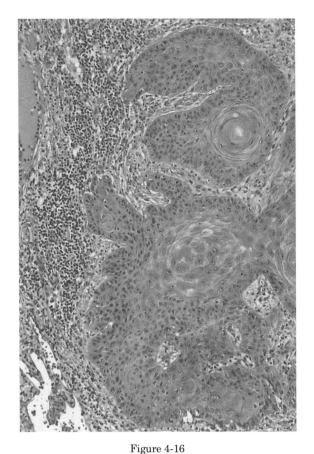

Figure 4-16
SQUAMOUS CELL CARCINOMA
A higher magnification of the lesion seen in figure 4-15 shows nests of well-differentiated squamous cell carcinoma infiltrating an inflamed stroma.

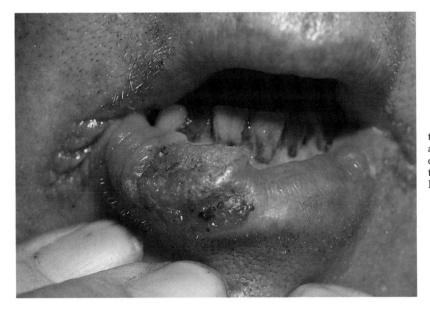

Figure 4-17
SQUAMOUS CELL CARCINOMA
This squamous cell carcinoma of the right portion of the lower lip forms an obvious, partially exophytic, crusted mass. The tumor does not extend to the midline. (Courtesy of Dr. K.E. Greer, Charlottesville, VA.)

Spread and Metastasis. Squamous cell carcinomas of the lower lip are typically slow-growing, indolent neoplasms. Metastases usually occur late in the clinical course and involve ipsilateral submandibular lymph nodes, submental lymph nodes, or more rarely spread to remote sites. The overall rate of metastasis has been approximately 16 percent (45,107,122,157,160). The rare squamous cell carcinomas that arise from the upper lip have been said to be more aggressive lesions with "early" metastasis to periparotid lymph nodes (157).

Treatment and Prognosis. Most squamous cell carcinomas of the lip are treated by complete surgical excision, usually in the form of a wedge resection. Larger lesions may be treated by radiation therapy. The 5-year survival rate is approximately 75 percent (45,157). In a study of 188 squamous cell carcinomas of the lower lip, Frierson and Cooper (45) found that a tumor thickness of 6 mm was a valuable prognostic cutoff point. Of patients with tumors 6 mm or more in thickness, 75 percent developed metastases; in contrast, less than 4 percent of patients with thinner tumors developed metastatic disease, as did only 1 of 121 patients with tumors less than 3 mm in thickness. Other factors associated with an increased risk of metastasis include perineural invasion and a dispersed cell growth pattern at the infiltrating margin. Once metastases to cervical lymph nodes develop the overall survival drops to approximately 50 percent.

Oral Cavity (General)

General Features. Oral cavity squamous cell carcinoma has historically been a male affliction, related to the association of these tumors with prolonged tobacco and alcohol use. However, behavioral changes have resulted in an increased incidence of these tumors in women in the last few decades (135). All forms of tobacco use, including snuff and "smokeless tobacco" have been strongly associated with oral cavity squamous cell carcinoma. Alcohol intake is also associated with the development of these tumors and probably plays a synergistic role in combination with tobacco (117,118). It has been suggested that tobacco and alcohol have slight differing predilections for tumor development. One study of 690 patients noted that the risk associated with smoking, adjusted for alcohol use, was highest in the region of the retromolar trigone, followed by the floor of the mouth, and was lowest for the mucosa of the cheek (79). For alcohol drinking, adjusted for smoking, the risk was highest for involvement of the floor of the mouth, followed by the tongue. This study also noted that the relative risks associated with smoking were greater than for those associated with alcohol consumption. Another study noted that the strongest association with cigarette smoking and oral cavity squamous cell carcinoma was seen with lesions involving the floor of the mouth, in which 97 percent of the patients were smokers (7). This study, however, did not control for the effects of alcohol consumption. The peculiar South American, Caribbean, and Indian practice of putting the lighted end of a "chutta" cigarette in the mouth ("reverse smoking"), is associated with a high incidence of carcinomas involving the palate (113,114,146).

More recently, studies have examined the potential role of human papillomavirus (HPV) and Epstein-Barr (EBV) virus in the development of oral cavity squamous cell neoplasms and their precursor lesions. In one study of 84 squamous proliferations of the oral cavity, HPV type 16 was found by polymerase chain reaction (PCR) in 2 of 4 hyperplasias, 2 of 5 inflammatory lesions, 9 of 36 dysplasias, and 7 of 39 carcinomas (67). However, virus was also detected in 1 of 6 normal mucosal biopsies. Another study examined 79 oral squamous proliferations for EBV using PCR, in situ hybridization, and immunohistochemistry (68). By PCR, 19 of 36 squamous cell carcinomas contained EBV DNA. Using in situ hybridization for both EBV DNA and EBV messenger RNA, 10 of these cases showed positivity in the epithelial cells and in 3 additional cases positivity was noted in associated lymphocytes. Although initial studies of this type may suggest a possible role for these known carcinogenic viruses, multiple additional studies will be necessary before any causative association with oral cavity squamous cell carcinoma can be accepted.

Clinical Features. Excluding the lip and tongue, the most common site for squamous cell carcinoma is the floor of the mouth (88,135). Crissman et al. (31) suggested that the predilection for this region might be due to pooling of carcinogens in saliva, acting on a thin, susceptible squamous mucosa. Patients often present with advanced disease at the time of initial diagnosis, and over half have involvement of regional lymph nodes (37,144). Delays in diagnosis may be related to misconceptions by the patient, and occasionally by the clinician, that the lesion is an inflammatory process. Enlargement of regional lymph nodes is a common finding at the time of presentation, but this may be due to inflammatory hyperplasia. Conversely, metastases to these nodes may not be clinically apparent (6,31, 86). Submandibular gland enlargement secondary to associated inflammation or duct obstruction may also lead to confusion with metastases.

The incidence of squamous cell carcinoma of the buccal mucosa varies regionally in the United States, in part related to geographic variation in the use of smokeless (chewing) tobacco and snuff. Squamous cell carcinomas typically arise at or below the line of dental occlusion, in the middle or posterior segments of the mucosa (28,148). Over half extend beyond the buccal mucosa into surrounding structures such as the mucosa overlying the mandible or maxilla, retromolar trigone, tonsil, palate, or lips. Extension into the maxilla or mandible may also occur (109).

Squamous cell carcinoma arising from the palate is relatively uncommon, accounting for about 2 to 5 percent of all oral carcinomas (74,88,128). Most of these tumors arise from the soft palate or the uvula. As noted above, palatal carcinomas are much more common in cultures practicing "reverse smoking."

Microscopic Findings. With rare exception, these tumors are moderately differentiated or well-differentiated squamous cell carcinomas that, as discussed above, often arise in a setting of preexistent keratosis with associated dysplasia.

Spread and Metastasis. Lymphatics in the floor of the mouth have numerous anastomoses that cross the midline. Accordingly, tumors in this portion of the oral cavity metastasize to bilateral or contralateral, as well as ipsilateral, lymph nodes. Histologic grading may be of some value in predicting the presence and extent of nodal metastases from oral cavity tumors. One study noted that the prevalence of metastases to regional lymph nodes did not significantly correlate with primary tumor site or size, but did correlate with histologic grade (145). In a series of 60 patients, those with grade I to II tumors had limited metastases to level I to II lymph nodes, whereas those with grade III to IV malignancy often had metastases that extended beyond level III nodes, regardless of the size and extent of the primary tumor. Others have also noted a correlation between high-grade malignancy, aneuploidy, and tumor size, and the development of regional lymph node metastases (144). In a review of 31 patients with oral cavity squamous cell carcinoma, Horiuchi et al. (69) noted that tumors expressing human leukocyte antigen (HLA)-DR and showing prominent tumor associated eosinophilia had an unfavorable prognosis. In a separate review of 126 patients with oral cavity squamous cell carcinoma undergoing neck dissections, Martinez-Gimeno et al. (102) noted that the following factors correlated with the presence of lymph node metastases: microvascular invasion, tumor grade, tumor size as manifest by "T" category, tumor thickness, inflammatory infiltration, and perineural spread.

Treatment and Prognosis. Surgical resection, radiation therapy, or a combination has been the therapeutic mainstay for oral cavity squamous cell carcinomas (28,148). Chemotherapy may aid in initial remissions, but may not influence long-term survival (64). The overall prognosis is dependent on the location of the lesion, its local extent, and the presence or absence of lymph node metastases. Not surprisingly, tumors of the palate are often low stage at the time of presentation; about three fourths are stage I or II (38). At other anatomic sites in the oral cavity there is a much greater dispersal of disease stage at the time of presentation, with many patients having locally advanced disease.

Patients with oral cavity squamous cell carcinomas are at significant risk for the development of additional carcinomas of the upper aerodigestive tract. This relative risk has been stated to be as high as 74.7-fold in males and 190.4-fold in females (80). These patients also have significantly increased risks for carcinoma of the esophagus (25-fold in males; 45-fold in females), as well as tumors of the lungs (80).

Tongue

General Features. The anterior two thirds or the mobile portion of the tongue is of a different embryologic origin than the posterior, immobile one third. The line of the circumvallate papillae forms a row just anterior to this junction. Squamous cell carcinomas of the tongue proportionately involve these two general regions, such that two thirds arise from the anterior, mobile component. Depending on the study, this is either the most common site or the second most common site (following lip) for oral cavity neoplasia. As with other sites in the oral cavity, smoking and alcohol consumption are causally associated with these tumors. The possible association with HPV also has been initially examined with regard to tongue lesions (132). One study of 24 cases found HPV DNA in 8 tumors, using the PCR methodology. Given the high sensitivity of the PCR reaction with the associated concerns regarding contamination, and the noted presence in other reports of HPV DNA in normal mucosa, the significance of this finding requires additional study.

Clinical Features. The middle third of the tongue is the single most common site; origin from the dorsal surface of the tongue is very uncommon (fig. 4-18). As with other ear, nose, and throat (ENT) squamous cell carcinomas, historically there has been a strong male predilection (44). The typical presentation is of a painless, infiltrative and indurated, or exophytic mass. Surface ulceration is common. With extension into the tongue musculature, tongue mobility may be compromised. There is wide variation in the extent of disease at the time presentation. Nyman et al. (108) noted that the frequency of tumor size at presentation in 289 cases, as measured by "T" category was: T1, 26 percent; T2, 32 percent; T3, 30 percent; and T4, 13 percent. In a separate study of 75 carcinomas of the tongue, Levy et al. (94) noted that 29 percent were stage I, 36 percent were stage II, 27 percent were stage III, and 8 percent were stage IV.

Lesions involving the base of the tongue less often produce a symptomatic mass and may present with complaints of a protracted "sore throat."

Microscopic Findings. Tumors involving the anterior, mobile portion of the tongue are typically well-differentiated or moderately differentiated squamous cell carcinomas, although higher grade variants including adenoid and spindle cell subtypes have been identified (50,51,137). There is a tendency for higher grade carcinomas to involve the base of the tongue, and included in this category are the basaloid squamous cell carcino-

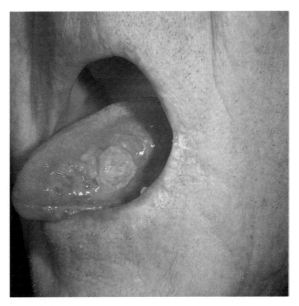

Figure 4-18
SQUAMOUS CELL CARCINOMA OF TONGUE
A large squamous cell carcinoma involves the left lateral aspect of the mobile portion of the tongue. The more anterior portion of the tumor is ulcerated, and the posterior portion is exophytic, without ulceration. (Courtesy of Dr. K.E. Greer, Charlottesville, VA.)

mas that frequently involve this area. Associated areas of adjacent dysplasia or "carcinoma in situ" are less frequent than with tumors at other ENT locations, such as the larynx (44).

Spread and Metastasis. Tumors of the mobile portion of the tongue usually metastasize first to the subdigastric lymph nodes on the side of the tumor, followed by involvement of submaxillary triangle region nodes and midjugular lymph nodes. Extension to lower and more posterior node groups is rare (96). Base of tongue tumors have a similar pattern of nodal spread (96). Centrally located tumors are frequently associated with bilateral lymph node involvement. Distant metastases are relatively uncommon and occur late in the clinical course. In about 80 percent of patients dying of disease, death is due to locoregional disease (133).

Treatment and Prognosis. Treatment is typically based on surgical resection, radiation therapy, or a combination of the two. Some authors have advocated surgical resection for T1 and T2 disease, followed by postoperative radiation therapy, with primary radiation therapy and possible postradiation resection for patients with larger lesions (39). In a series of 289 patients with carcinoma of the "oral" portion of the tongue, Nyman et al. (108) noted that 5-year survival was 61 percent for patients with T1 tumors, 51 percent for those with T2, 19 percent for T3, and 0 percent for T4. In a separate study of oral tongue lesions, Levy et al. (94) documented 5-year survivals for patients with stages I, II, III, and IV of 90 percent, 84 percent, 43 percent, and 0 percent. Although multiple studies have suggested a worse prognosis for base of tongue carcinomas, perhaps because of their tendencies to be more poorly differentiated and to present at a higher clinical stage, this has not invariably been the case, at least when controlling for tumor stage at presentation. In a series of 100 patients with base of tongue carcinomas treated primarily by surgical resection, Kraus et al. (87) noted 5-year disease-specific survival rates for patients with stages I/II, III, and IV tumors of 77 percent, 64 percent, and 59 percent, respectively. In a separate study of 134 patients with base of tongue tumors treated primarily by external beam radiation therapy, with or without neck dissection, relapse-free 5-year survival rates were 100 percent for stages I and II, 68 percent for stage III, 81 percent for stage IVA, and 37 percent for stage IVB (65). These survival rates are comparable to those of stage-matched carcinomas from the mobile portion of the tongue.

Whether regional lymph node dissections should be performed on clinically low-stage lesions is controversial. Lydiatt et al. (101) studied 156 patients with T1 and T2 lesions. Intraoral resection alone was performed on 102 patients and 16.5 percent of these subsequently developed clinically apparent cervical lymph node metastases. The remaining 54 patients received elective radical neck dissections at the time of tumor resection and 20.4 percent had clinically occult nodal metastases.

Factors reported to influence prognosis have included location on the tongue, tumor size, histologic grade, depth of invasion, perineural invasion, and status of regional lymph nodes. Gomez et al. (52) studied 38 squamous cell carcinomas from the mobile portion of the tongue and examined a series of factors including tumor size, depth of invasion, histologic differentiation, ploidy pattern, and S-phase fraction, all of which were shown to correlate with prognosis in univariate analysis. A multifactorial regression analysis identified S-phase fraction and depth of tumor invasion as independent prognostic factors. Assays for tumor angiogenesis and p53 antigen are not useful for predicting T1 and T2 tumors more likely to spread nodally (92).

Nasal Cavity / Paranasal Sinuses

General Features. About 3 percent of head and neck carcinomas arise in the sinonasal region. The approximate distribution of these tumors is: maxillary antrum, 58 percent; nasal cavity, 30 percent; ethmoid sinuses, 10 percent; and frontal and sphenoid sinuses, 1 percent each (95). Sinonasal squamous cell carcinoma has been strongly associated with cigarette smoking (14,20), as well as the mining and refining of nickel ore (84,150). Occupational contact with chromium, isopropyl alcohol, and radium has also been implicated (119). Formaldehyde has been suggested as a sinonasal carcinogen, although a recent case control study noted no increased risk of sinonasal squamous cell carcinoma due to occupational contact with this substance (99). A possible association with sinonasal adenocarcinoma and a synergistic effect with exposure to wood dust could not be excluded, however (99). Though not in use for decades, cases of Thorotrast-related carcinoma continue to arise and have been described in the maxillary antrum (53).

As in other anatomic sites in the head and neck region, the possible role of HPV in the development of sinonasal squamous cell carcinoma remains to be clarified. By PCR, 14 percent of sinonasal squamous cell carcinomas were said to contain HPV types 16 and 18 DNA (47). However, the high sensitivity of this technique raises concerns regarding contamination and the presence of the viral DNA cannot, of course, be equated with causation.

Squamous cell carcinomas of the nasal cavity have been noted to be associated with second primary tumors in up to one fourth of cases (9,20). About 40 percent of the associated carcinomas involve other sites in the head and neck. The remainder occur in anatomically dispersed locations including lung, breast, and gastrointestinal tract (9). This tendency for multiplicity is not seen with squamous cell carcinoma of the maxillary antrum (131). These tumors show only a 5 percent incidence of bilateral involvement and no associated increase in neoplasia at other anatomic sites (131).

Clinical Features. Sinonasal squamous cell carcinomas have historically shown a male predominance of approximately 2 to 1 (9). At the time of presentation, most patients are in their sixth decade of life or older; occurrence in patients under 40 years of age is rare. Nasal lesions typically present with more obvious localizing symptoms including obstruction, rhinorrhea, epistaxis, and pain. As noted by Barnes (9), there is some controversy regarding the most common site for nasal cavity tumors. Batsakis and colleagues (10) consider the lateral nasal wall to be the most common location; other authors consider the nasal septum, particularly its anterior portion near the mucocutaneous junction of the vestibule, to be the most common site (4,111).

Carcinomas arising in the paranasal sinuses are rare, accounting for only about 0.2 percent of all human malignancies (9). Over three fourths arise in the maxillary antrum. If one excludes the intestinal-type adenocarcinomas occurring in the ethmoid sinuses, the predilection of squamous cell carcinoma for the maxillary antrum is even more striking. Tumors arising in this region typically produce signs and symptoms of chronic sinusitis (95). Because of this, they often go undiagnosed for a protracted period of time (95, 123). Other signs and symptoms suspicious for malignancy include radiographic displacement of the lateral nasal wall, continuous bloody or blood-tinged nasal secretions, exophthalmos, or a mass involving the zygomatic bone, maxillary tuberosity, or canine fossa (9,123). Larger tumors erode bony boundaries and extend into adjacent structures, producing obvious facial disfigurement and a mass typically visible within the nasal cavity.

Gross Findings. The tumors typically appear as friable, papillary, polypoid, or sessile thickenings of the mucosa. There may be areas of associated surface ulceration. Larger tumors may completely fill the involved sinus or nasal cavity with a yellow-gray, often partially necrotic mass.

Microscopic Findings. The majority of sinonasal squamous cell carcinomas are well or moderately differentiated, focally keratinizing neoplasms that are easily diagnosed. Rarely, un-

differentiated carcinomas (lymphoepitheliomas), spindle cell carcinomas (112), verrucous carcinomas (55), and basaloid squamous cell carcinomas (152) may occur in this region. In addition, there may be undifferentiated neoplasms distinct from undifferentiated carcinoma of lymphoepithelioma type (sinonasal undifferentiated carcinoma) that arise in this region (2,46,54,61). The microscopic features of all these distinctive variants are discussed with each tumor type.

Nonkeratinizing carcinomas lacking the microscopic features of undifferentiated carcinoma of lymphoepithelioma type also occur in this region and have been referred to by a variety of terms including transitional cell carcinoma, intermediate cell carcinoma, and schneiderian carcinoma. We consider these tumors to be variants of squamous cell carcinoma rather than a distinct pathologic entity. The nonkeratinizing tumors tend to grow in nests and broad cellular cords that may superficially resemble a schneiderian papilloma, particularly if the cellular pleomorphism is minimal, as is often the case. At higher magnification, however, these tumors have a higher mitotic rate, more nuclear pleomorphism, and often a higher nuclear to cytoplasmic ratio than is typical of schneiderian papillomas. In addition, the central portions of larger nests may show comedo-like necrosis.

Spread and Metastasis. Only about 15 percent of patients with nasal lesions develop lymph nodal metastases (9). Because of their central location, nasal cavity lesions may involve ipsilateral or contralateral lymph nodes. Lymphatic drainage is primarily to the submental and submandibular nodes, followed by the facial, superficial parotid, and deep cervical lymph node groups (9).

Spread of paranasal sinus carcinoma to regional lymph nodes has been generally considered uncommon when the tumor is confined to the sinus cavity. Once there is extension outside the confines of the cavity, access to lymphatics is more readily available, and both regional and distant metastases may occur (1). It has been argued that metastases from carcinomas of the maxillary antrum and other sinuses are more common than generally recognized because of the tendency to involve difficult to palpate retropharyngeal nodes and the clinical dominance of local disease (26,142).

Treatment and Prognosis. Treatment is typically by a combination of surgical resection and radiation therapy, with or without the addition of chemotherapy. There is controversy regarding the relative efficacy of preoperative versus postoperative radiation therapy. Because few nasal cavity carcinomas metastasize to regional lymph nodes, elective resection or radiation of regional lymph nodes is not typically employed. Many tumors within the paranasal sinuses are not resectable at the time of presentation, although intranasal lesions can more often be surgically removed (42). The orbital contents are generally preserved at the time of surgery, unless there is extension into the orbital periosteum. Regardless of the treatment modalities employed, local recurrences are common and death is usually due to local extension into vital structures.

Prognosis varies with location and clinical stage at the time of diagnosis (9). Nasal cavity carcinomas have a better prognosis than tumors involving the sinuses. Five-year survival for patients with tumors confined to the nasal cavity is over 50 percent (20); in contrast, 5-year survival for those with maxillary antrum carcinoma is approximately 25 percent (90).

Nasopharynx

General Features. In western civilizations, about 85 percent of nasopharyngeal carcinomas are nonglandular neoplasms (129), classified as keratinizing squamous cell carcinoma, nonkeratinizing carcinoma, and undifferentiated carcinoma (lymphoepithelioma) (129,164). Undifferentiated carcinomas have distinct clinical, epidemiologic, and pathologic features and are discussed in the next chapter dealing with variants of squamous cell neoplasia. This section considers squamous cell carcinoma of the nasopharynx in general with emphasis on the keratinizing and nonkeratinizing subtypes.

EBV, as well as genetic factors, has been associated with the development of nonkeratinizing and especially undifferentiated nasopharyngeal carcinoma. These factors also are discussed in the section in the next chapter dealing with lymphoepithelioma.

Clinical Features. Unlike undifferentiated carcinoma of the nasopharynx, keratinizing and nonkeratinizing carcinomas are rare in childhood, and typically occur after 40 years of age (35,129). All forms show a male predominance of approximately 2.53 to 1 (29,35,129). Many nasopharyngeal carcinomas arise near the fossa of Rosenmüller and present with complaints referable to middle ear congestion due to obstruction of the eustachian tube opening. The most common complaint is unilateral hearing loss. Epistaxis, headaches, and deficits of the fifth cranial nerve are also frequent findings. Involvement of cervical lymph nodes suggests an undifferentiated or high-grade nonkeratinizing neoplasm.

Gross Findings. Gross descriptions of resection specimens are almost nonexistent given the reliance on radiation therapy. One classic autopsy study of 31 Chinese patients noted that only 4 tumors filled the nasopharynx (143). Most were of moderate size with superficial ulceration, and some were quite small, appearing as only a small granular patch of nasopharyngeal mucosa.

Microscopic Findings. By definition, keratinizing squamous cell carcinoma of the nasopharynx exhibits overt squamous differentiation in the form of cytoplasmic or extracellular keratinization and intercellular bridge formation (129). With the exception of rare "adenoid" variants (166), these tumors rarely cause diagnostic difficulty. Nonkeratinizing carcinomas exhibit varying degrees of cellular maturation, but lack light microscopically discernable keratin formation. The cells vary considerably in nuclear size, shape, and chromatin distribution. Both hyperchromatic and vesicular nuclei are typically present. Cell borders are easily discernible and the cells "mesh" or interdigitate in a pattern superficially resembling pavement stones. The growth pattern and microscopic appearance resembles a transitional cell carcinoma of the urinary tract. Mucin production or glandular differentiation is absent by definition (129). The stroma surrounding keratinizing and nonkeratinizing carcinomas of the nasopharynx may contain variable numbers of inflammatory cells including lymphocytes, plasma cells, and eosinophils (97,129). The presence of these elements cannot be used to distinguish these tumors from undifferentiated carcinomas.

Spread and Metastasis. Keratinizing carcinomas tend to remain localized within the nasopharynx. Nonkeratinizing carcinomas, like undifferentiated carcinomas, tend to disseminate to regional lymph nodes as well as distant sites.

Lymph nodes most often involved are in the upper cervical region, and are clinically located near the angle of the jaw and posterior to the sternocleidomastoid muscle.

Treatment and Prognosis. Nasopharyngeal carcinomas of all types are virtually never amenable to surgical resection and require treatment primarily by radiation therapy. Adjuvant chemotherapy protocols for advanced disease are under continued investigation. Traditionally, keratinizing carcinomas have the poorest response to radiation therapy and, correspondingly, the poorest prognosis. In some studies, there have been no 5-year survivors (17). Overall, however, 5-year survival for patients with keratinizing nasopharyngeal carcinoma is approximately 20 percent (9). Depending on the study, non-keratinizing carcinoma has a prognosis intermediate between keratinizing and undifferentiated carcinomas (17), or behaves like the latter carcinoma (129). In our experience, as well as that of Barnes et al. (9), those with nonkeratinizing carcinomas have an intermediate prognosis, with a 5-year survival of approximately 35 percent as compared to the above and a 60 percent 5-year survival for undifferentiated carcinoma.

Oropharynx

General Features. The oropharynx is typically divided, clinically, into the palatine arch and the oropharynx proper. The latter includes the base of the tongue, a relatively common site of disease, as well as the remaining oropharyngeal boundaries. There is confusion regarding where the palatine tonsils fit in this system (125, 149). If one includes carcinoma of the tonsil in the group of oropharyngeal malignancies, then this site accounts for up to 75 percent of all such tumors (149,165). Some authors even include tumors of the retromolar trigone, a portion of the posterior oral cavity, as lesions of the palatine arch and hence within the oropharynx. As with carcinomas from many other head and neck sites, oropharyngeal squamous cell carcinomas are causally associated with smoking and alcohol abuse (149).

Clinical Features. Oropharyngeal carcinomas are historically more common in males by a factor of approximately 3 to 1. Patients are typically in their sixth decade of life or older at the time of presentation. Complaints include difficulty swallowing, sore throat, a neck mass, and weight loss (121,149). Bleeding is uncommon. Pain in the ear may indicate involvement of the glossopharyngeal nerve, a sign of advanced disease (149).

Microscopic Findings. In general, squamous cell carcinoma of the oropharynx tends to be more poorly differentiated than oral cavity tumors (121). In our experience, this is largely due to the predilection of basaloid squamous cell carcinoma, a poorly differentiated microscopic subtype of squamous cell carcinoma, for the base of tongue portion of the oropharynx. In addition, the palatine tonsils are a relatively common site for lymphoepithelioma-like undifferentiated carcinomas arising outside the nasopharynx (85). These distinctive variants are discussed in the next chapter.

Spread and Metastasis. Tumors of the oropharynx proper are twice as likely to produce regional metastases as carcinomas of the palatine arch (149). The lymphatic drainage from the oropharynx is primarily towards the jugulodigastric lymph nodes, followed by the parapharyngeal and retropharyngeal lymph nodes (126). Tumors arising from the palatine arches, primarily from the tonsils, typically extend inferiorly, and often involve the base of the tongue. They may also extend laterally into the retromolar trigone region, posteriorly into the wall of the lateral oropharynx, or grow deeply to invade the underlying angle of the mandible (149).

Treatment and Prognosis. Surgical resection and radiation therapy, separately or in combination, are the mainstays of treatment (40,60, 75). The overall 5-year survival for all oropharyngeal sites is 35 to 40 percent (76,149,154). Death is usually at least partially due to persistent local disease, often in association with significant other medical problems such as malnutrition. Approximately 25 percent of patients with oropharyngeal squamous cell carcinoma develop second primary malignancies elsewhere in the head and neck region, the lung, or the esophagus (60,76,125,141,149,154).

Hypopharynx

General Features. Squamous cell carcinoma of the hypopharynx is strongly associated with smoking and alcohol abuse (8,82). Partially as a corollary to the latter, it is also associated with cirrhosis of the liver (82). Carcinomas developing in a setting of long-term hypochromic, iron deficiency anemia (Plummer-Vinson syndrome, sideropenic dysphagia) also predilect this region (163). Tumors in this location are about one third as common as those arising in the larynx (8,23,33,71,78,115).

Clinical Features. As with other squamous cell carcinomas, these tumors have historically occurred in men in their sixth decade of life and older. Because of their location, tumors involving the hypopharynx may reach considerable size before becoming symptomatic. Many patients have locally advanced lesions extending into adjacent structures at the time of diagnosis. Up to three fourths have involvement of regional lymph nodes at the time of presentation (34,56,70,83, 138). Newer radiographic techniques such as magnetic resonance imaging (MRI) hold promise for more completely delineating the extent of hypopharyngeal neoplasia. Wenig et al. (156) noted that this technique improved the staging in 40 percent of 25 patients, and correctly predicted cartilage invasion in 6 of 6 patients, with a single false positive (156). Patients with hypopharyngeal carcinoma typically complain of difficulty swallowing, the sensation of a mass in the throat, sore throat, pain referred to the ear, and hemoptysis (8). In one study, 17 percent of patients surviving 2 or more years developed additional primary carcinomas (66).

Microscopic Findings. Excluding basaloid squamous cell carcinomas which predilect the hypopharynx and are discussed in the next chapter, most squamous cell carcinomas of the hypopharynx are moderately differentiated neoplasms causing no diagnostic difficulty.

Spread and Metastasis. Tumors involving the pyriform sinus portion of the hypopharynx often grow medially to invade the lateral portion of the supraglottic larynx. From that point they often extend downward to cross the glottis, unlike primary supraglottic carcinomas (83). Lateral growth of a pyriform sinus carcinoma may result in permeation of the (ossified) thyroid cartilage and extension into the thyroid gland (8,83). Extension into the base of the tongue is indicative of advanced disease. Involvement of the esophagus is rare (8,83). Lymphatic drainage is primarily to the upper jugular lymph nodes (127).

Tumors arising from the posterior wall of the hypopharynx often cross the midline and are therefore associated with a high frequency of bilateral regional lymph node metastases (71, 153). Lymphatic drainage is to the upper and middle jugular lymph nodes and also to the retropharyngeal nodes (8). In one study, 42 percent of lesions involved the retropharyngeal lymph nodes (5).

In a series of 239 patients with laryngeal and hypopharyngeal carcinomas, Wenig and Applebaum (155) noted that involvement of the submandibular triangle lymph nodes was uncommon (2 of 95 patients with nodal disease), suggesting that this region could be spared during neck dissections.

Treatment and Prognosis. When possible, the primary treatment modality for hypopharyngeal carcinoma is surgical resection. In a study of 109 patients with hypopharyngeal carcinoma treated surgically, stage of disease and lymph node status strongly predicted 5-year survival (66). Survival rates at 5 years according to stage were: stage I, 74 percent; stage II, 63 percent; stage III, 32 percent; and stage IV, 14 percent. Five-year survival rates according to preoperative lymph node assessment were: N0, 57 percent; N1, 28 percent; N2, 6 percent; and N3, 0 percent.

Postoperative radiation therapy appears to considerably improve prognosis. In one series of 110 patients treated with resection, with and without postoperative radiation therapy, the stage-adjusted 5-year survival rates were 48 percent and 18 percent, respectively (43). The role of retropharyngeal lymph node dissection for hypopharyngeal carcinoma has been controversial. Hasegawa and Matsuura (58) noted that 8 of 13 patients with stage III/IV squamous cell carcinoma of the hypopharynx had involvement of retropharyngeal lymph nodes in resection specimens. Based on this finding, they recommended elective resections in patients with stage III/IV disease. The site of origin in the hypopharynx may also influence the necessity and extent of nodal dissection. In particular, approximately 14 percent of patients with medial wall pyriform sinus involvement develop metastases to contralateral lymph nodes; only about 5 percent of patients with involvement of the lateral pyriform sinus develop contralateral metastases (77).

The role of histologic grading in predicting tumor prognosis has been the subject of multiple studies. Elaborate grading systems for squamous cell carcinoma have been developed and applied to varying degrees. These are discussed in more detail in the section below on carcinoma of the larynx. Although clinical stage remains the most significant predictor of survival, degree of differentiation continues to provide independent prognostic information for hypopharyngeal tumors (158). In one large review of over 1,300 patients with tumors of larynx or hypopharynx, tumor grading made a significant contribution to prediction of prognosis, even when clinical stage was taken into account in a multivariant analysis (158). In particular, patients with well-differentiated tumors had significantly better survival and tumor-free rates than did those with anaplastic tumors.

Larynx

General Features. In the United States in 1995, carcinoma of the larynx accounted for 1.3 percent of carcinomas in men and 0.4 percent in women (159). During that year, there were 11,600 newly diagnosed laryngeal malignancies and over 4,000 individuals died from this disease (159). The development of laryngeal carcinoma is strongly associated with smoking and heavy alcohol ingestion. It has been suggested that smoking nonfiltered cigarettes, a form of smoking found predominantly in males, leads to an even greater risk (162). This, perhaps, accounts for the continued high incidence of this tumor in men while lung cancer frequencies in women have continuously increased. Lowry (98) suggested that the heavy use of alcohol was strongly associated with supraglottic carcinomas, but not with glottic tumors. Heavy alcohol intake appears to be required for substantially increased risk, as Lowry noted that many of his patients drank more than a fifth of distilled liquor per day for over a decade. Occasional, "social" intake does not appear to significantly increase risk (161). Although some authors have suggested a causal association between occupational contact with asbestos and carcinoma of the larynx (130,134,139), others have indicated no statistically significant association (25,167). Many of the case control studies purporting to show an association with asbestos

exposure fail to control for the important confounding variables of smoking and alcohol consumption. In our opinion, a causal association with asbestos has not been convincingly demonstrated. A variety of other substances including nickel and wood dusts have been suggested as possible laryngeal carcinogens, but likewise have not been clearly shown to be causative (22,162,167).

Carcinomas of the larynx are traditionally divided into supraglottic, glottic, and subglottic tumors. There are important clinical and therapeutic reasons for this subdivision, primarily related to the relative abundance and direction of drainage of lymphatics, as well as options for surgical resection. The term transglottic carcinoma is sometimes applied to carcinomas which bridge the laryngeal ventricle and involve both vocal cord and supraglottic structures. The vast majority of such cases appear to represent glottic carcinomas with supraglottic extension. In fact, up to one fourth of glottic carcinomas exhibit such supraglottic involvement (8,105). Thus, transglottic tumors are best viewed as T2 or greater glottic carcinomas.

Clinical Features. Glottic carcinomas account for almost two thirds of laryngeal neoplasms. Most arise somewhat anteriorly on the mobile portion of the vocal cord. Hoarseness or obvious alteration in voice is the most common presenting complaint.

Most of the remaining laryngeal carcinomas (30 to 35 percent) arise from the supraglottic larynx (8,120). Included in this category are tumors arising from the epiglottis, aryepiglottic folds, false cords, and ventricles. Presenting complaints are often related to a change in the quality of the voice, but may include difficulty swallowing or the sensation of a mass. As they enlarge, supraglottic cancers tend to grow upward to involve adjacent structures such as the pyriform sinus and the base of the tongue. Downward growth to involve the glottis is uncommon (18).

Subglottic carcinomas of the larynx are the least common, accounting for 5 percent or less of all laryngeal cancers (8). Because they do not involve the vocal cords, alterations in voice are not common presenting complaints. Instead, the tumors enlarge until they produce symptomatic airway compromise that manifests as stridor or dyspnea. This may be of acute onset, requiring emergency tracheostomy (140).

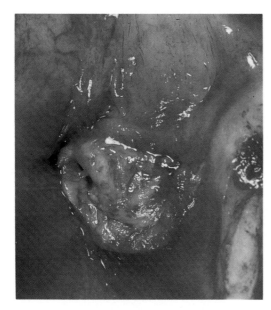

Figure 4-19
SQUAMOUS CELL CARCINOMA
This large squamous cell carcinoma of the right true
vocal cord forms a predominantly intraluminal mass. In
spite of the size of the lesion, there is no invasion of the
ventricle or false cord.

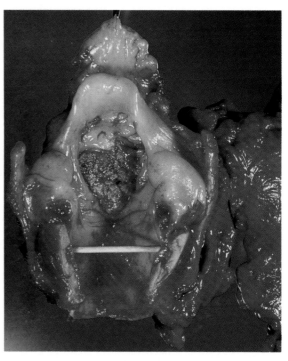

Figure 4-20
SQUAMOUS CELL CARCINOMA
This squamous cell carcinoma of the anterior portion of the
supraglottic larynx extends upward to involve the epiglottis.

The mainstay of diagnosis is laryngoscopy by
direct or indirect (endoscopic) techniques. This
methodology allows assessment of the lateral
extent of disease based on appearance and verified by multiple biopsies. The well-known problem with this technique is the difficulty in assessing depth of invasion or involvement of
difficult to visualize spaces such as the ventricles. As discussed briefly below, MRI and computed tomography (CT) techniques are achieving increasingly better levels of resolution, and
these techniques are finding increasing use in
the evaluation of tumor depth.

Gross Findings. In laryngectomy specimens, squamous cell carcinomas typically appear as partially exophytic or fungating, pink or
tan, focally ulcerated tumors (figs. 4-19–4-22).
They vary tremendously in size from small lesions partially involving the vocal cord, to large
masses substantially compromising the laryngeal lumen. Lesions at the small extreme of size
are not treated with laryngectomy; most laryngectomy specimens are from 1 to 4 cm in size
(104). Often, the edges of the lesion are elevated
or indurated due to submucosal extension. As-

sessment of depth of invasion requires multiple
sections through the neoplasm. Lesions involving the ventricle may not be visible within the
laryngeal lumen as mucosal lesions, and produce
only bulging of the overlying mucosa (fig. 4-23).

Microscopic Findings. Clinically or pathologically distinctive variants of squamous cell
carcinoma are discussed in the next chapter.
Among the subtypes discussed, verrucous,
basaloid squamous cell, and spindle cell carcinomas are relatively common as laryngeal variants. Most laryngeal squamous cell carcinomas
are moderately differentiated tumors with foci of
obvious keratinization. Tumor grading and its
potential clinical value is discussed below in the
section on treatment and prognosis.

Spread and Metastasis. Because of the limited lymphatic supply to the true vocal cords, tumors confined to the cord have an excellent prognosis and are amenable to cure by either radiation
therapy or limited surgical resection. Fortunately,
about half of vocal cord carcinomas are limited to
the cords (T1) at the time of presentation (59). Of

63

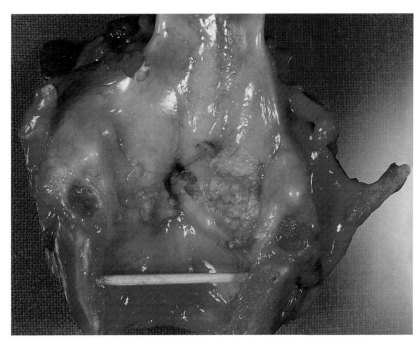

Figure 4-21
BILATERAL SQUAMOUS
CELL CARCINOMA
This laryngectomy specimen contains multifocal, bilateral, squamous cell carcinomas. The lesion on the right involves the true vocal cord with upward extension into the supraglottic larynx.

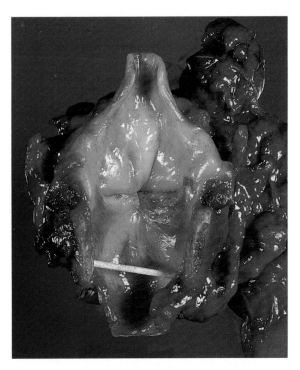

Figure 4-22
SQUAMOUS CELL CARCINOMA OF VOCAL CORD
A hemorrhagic appearing squamous cell carcinoma of the right vocal cord extends downward to involve the subglottic portion of the larynx.

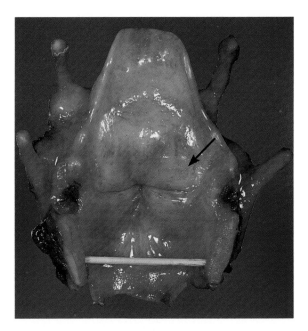

Figure 4-23
LARYNGEAL CARCINOMA
Laryngeal carcinomas involving the ventricle may produce only a slight mass (arrow), as seen on the right side in this laryngectomy specimen, with normal-appearing overlying mucosa.

the remainder, approximately 20 percent exhibit extracord extension or cord fixation (T2), an equal number are of stage T3, and about 5 percent exhibit extralaryngeal extension (T4) at the time of presentation (8,59). The frequency of regional lymph node metastases for glottic carcinoma according to tumor stage is approximately as follows: T1, 2 percent; T2, 17 percent; T3, 25 percent; and T4, 65 percent (93).

Between one quarter and half of patients with supraglottic carcinomas have lymph node metastases at the time of diagnosis (18,19,21,104). About 60 percent of pathologically positive lymph nodes are clinically enlarged; the remainder are clinically occult metastases detected microscopically in neck dissection specimens (21).

Subglottic carcinomas often involve the entire circumference of the subglottic larynx and commonly extend beyond the larynx, usually by penetrating the cricothyroid membrane (8). About 10 percent extend directly into the thyroid gland or its isthmus (8,110). Approximately 20 percent of patients with subglottic carcinomas have cervical lymph node metastases at the time of diagnosis (8,57,104). Involvement of pretracheal (Delphian) lymph node may be clinically apparent. Although only about one fifth of patients have positive cervical lymph nodes, Harrison (57) noted that the paratracheal nodes are involved in half, and are not clinically apparent.

Treatment and Prognosis. Many early stage carcinomas of the glottic larynx are initially treated by radiation therapy. In a review of 39 patients from the Mayo Clinic, 32 had local tumor control following radiation (41). Of the other 7, 3 underwent successful larynx-sparing resections. New radiation sensitizing drugs such as Taxol have shown some experimental promise with regard to squamous cell carcinoma (36). The high resolution of laryngeal structures possible with CT has led to studies evaluating extent of disease prior to radiation therapy. Factors associated with decreased local control following radiation therapy for a series of T3 tumors included involvement of the face of the arytenoid, involvement of the paraglottic space at the level of the false cord, and tumor volume greater than 3.5 cm^3 (91). It has also been suggested that radiation therapy given over a long period of time is associated with a higher recurrence rate (116).

Five-year survival rates for patients with glottic carcinoma according to tumor stage is approximately as follows: T1, 93 percent; T2, 85 percent; T3, 56 percent; and T4, 26 percent (93). In a series of supraglottic carcinomas treated by surgical resection and regional lymph node dissection, Ogura (110) noted 3-year survival rates according to stage: T1, 83 percent; T2, 79 percent; T3, 70 percent; and T4, 67 percent. Using the same surgical approach, Bocca (18) reported an overall (all stages) 5-year survival rate of 79 percent.

Approximately 50 percent of patients with subglottic carcinomas die of local or stomal recurrences (8,57); one third develop distant metastases, usually to lungs or bones (140). Regardless of therapy, the 5-year survival for those with subglottic tumors appears to be no greater than 40 percent (8,57,100).

Excluding the importance of tumor site (discussed above), there are a number of prognostic factors for laryngeal squamous cell carcinoma in general. Not surprisingly, size is an important feature. McGavran and colleagues (8,104) noted that tumors under 2 cm in size had a 14 percent rate of metastasis, compared to 40 percent for larger tumors. A large number of grading systems have been applied to squamous cell carcinomas from differing sites, and some of these have shown prognostic significance when applied to laryngeal lesions (11,12,48). Bennett and colleagues (8,15) compared tumor grade and lymph node metastases and noted that for grades I, II, III, and IV associated rates of metastases were, respectively, 25 percent, 54 percent, 67 percent, and 72 percent.

Jakobsson (72,73) developed an elaborate grading system for squamous cell carcinoma, which was later modified by Crissman (31). This system applies a numerical value of 1 to 4 for each of seven parameters and derives an overall score of 7 to 28 by summation of these values. Because of its somewhat complex approach, the system has not gained widespread use. Nonetheless, it clearly identifies important histologic parameters that may be assessed in a qualitative if not quantitative fashion. Factors evaluated based on the tumor itself include: degree of differentiation, based on the amount of keratin formation (50 percent, 20 to 50 percent, 5 to 20 percent, 0 to 5 percent); nuclear pleomorphism (75 percent mature, 50 to 75 percent mature, 25 to 50 percent mature, and 0 to 25 percent mature); and mitotic rate (0 to 1 per high-power field [HPF], 2 to 3/HPF, 4 to 5/HPF, ≥6/HPF). Factors related to the tumor-host interaction include: pattern of invasion (exophytic pushing border, exophytic infiltrating border, sessile infiltrating border, dissociated cells), vascular invasion (present or absent), lymphoid response (marked, moderate, patchy, none), and stage of invasion (carcinoma in situ, microinvasive, superficial, deep). In Jakobsson's original studies (using eight rather than seven parameters), patients with laryngeal tumors who scored less than 15 had significantly fewer treatment failures than those with higher scores.

The status of the tumor margin remains an important factor for evaluating laryngeal, as well as other carcinomas of the head and neck. Futrell and colleagues (48) noted that patients with tumor more than 5 mm from the resection margin had a 52 percent 5-year survival rate, patients with tumor within 2 mm of a clear resection margin had a 30 percent 5-year survival, and patients with involved surgical margins had a 28 percent 5-year survival rate. Bauer et al. (13) studied partial laryngectomy specimens and noted that when surgical margins were positive, the local recurrence rate was 18 percent, as opposed to 6 percent when surgical margins were negative.

The status of regional lymph nodes is the single most important histologic factor in assessing prognosis. Approximately one in five clinically negative cervical lymph node resections in patients with head and neck squamous cell carcinomas contain metastases (8). Even a single positive lymph node decreases 5-year survival by over 50 percent (48). Whether multiple positive lymph nodes are an additional adverse factor has been controversial, but some authors have noted additional decline in prognosis with multiple metastases (48). Spread beyond the confines of the lymph node capsule also has been suggested to be a strong predictor of recurrent disease in the neck (136,168).

Patients with laryngeal carcinomas, as with tumors at other sites in the head and neck, have an increased risk for secondary malignancies and the latter may be the prognosis-determining factor. Approximately 11 percent of patients develop secondary tumors, and when the primary tumor is in the larynx the secondary malignancy is usually in the lung or elsewhere in the head and neck (151).

REFERENCES

1. Ahmad K, Cordoba RB, Fayos JV. Squamous cell carcinoma of the maxillary sinus. Arch Otolaryngol 1981;107:48–51.
2. Ascaso FJ, Adiego MI, Garcia J, et al. Sinonasal undifferentiated carcinoma invading the orbit. Eur J Ophthalmol 1994;4:234–6.
3. Auerbach O, Hammond EC, Garfinkel L. Histologic changes in the larynx in relation to smoking habits. Cancer 1970;25:92–104.
4. Badib AO, Kurohara SS, Webster JH, Shedd DP. Treatment of cancer of the nasal cavity. Am J Roentgen Rad Ther Nuclear Med 1969;106:824–30.
5. Ballantyne AJ. Principles of surgical management of cancer of the pharyngeal walls. Cancer 1967;20:663–7.
6. Ballard BR, Suess GR, Pickren JW, Green GW Jr, Shedd DP. Squamous cell carcinoma of the floor of the mouth. Oral Surg 1978;45:568–79.
7. Barasch A, Morse DE, Krutchkoff DJ, Eisenberg E. Smoking, gender, and age as risk factors for site-specific intraoral squamous cell carcinoma. A case-series analysis. Cancer 1994;73:509–13.
8. Barnes L, Gnepp DR. Diseases of the larynx, hypopharynx, and esophagus. In: Barnes L, ed. Surgical pathology of the head and neck. New York: Marcel Dekker, 1985:141–226.
9. Barnes L, Verbin RS, Gnepp DR. Diseases of the nose, paranasal sinuses, and nasopharynx. In: Barnes L, ed. Surgical pathology of the head and neck. New York: Marcel Dekker, 1985:403–51.
10. Batsakis JG, Rice DH, Solomon AR. The pathology of head and neck tumors: squamous and mucous-gland carcinomas of the nasal cavity, paranasal sinuses and larynx, part 6. Head Neck Surg 1980;2:497–508.
11. Bauer WC. Varieties of squamous cell carcinoma–biologic behavior. Front Radiation Ther Oncol 1974;9:164–86.
12. Bauer WC, Edwards DL, McGavran MH. Critical analysis of laryngectomy in the treatment of epidermoid carcinoma of the larynx. Cancer 1962;15:263–70.
13. Bauer WC, Lesinski SG, Ogura JH. The significance of positive margins in hemilaryngectomy specimens. Laryngoscope 1975;85:1–13.
14. Beatty CW, Pearson BW, Kern EB. Carcinoma of the nasal septum: experience with 85 cases. Otolaryngol Head Neck Surg 1982;90:90–4.
15. Bennett SH, Futrell JW, Roth JA, Hoye RC, Ketcham AS. Prognostic significance of histologic host response in cancer of the larynx and hypopharynx. Cancer 1971;28:1255–65.

16. Blackwell KE, Fu YS, Calcaterra TC. Laryngeal dysplasia. A clinicopathologic study. Cancer 1995;75:457–63.

17. Bloom SM. Cancer of the nasopharynx: a study of 90 cases. J Mt Sinai Hosp 1969;36:277–98.

18. Bocca E. Supraglottic cancer. Laryngoscope 1975; 85:1318–26.

19. Bocca E, Pignataro O, Mosciaro O. Supraglottic surgery of the larynx. Ann Otol Rhinol Laryngol 1968; 77:1005–26.

20. Bosch A, Vallecillo L, Frias Z. Cancer of the nasal cavity. Cancer 1976;37:1458–63.

21. Bryce DP. The management of laryngeal cancer. J Otolaryngol 1979;8:105–26.

22. Burch JD, Howe GR, Miller AB, Semenciw R. Tobacco, alcohol, asbestos, and nickel in the etiology of cancer of the larynx: a case-control study. JNCI 1981;67:1219–24.

23. Carpenter RJ III, DeSanto LW, Devine KD, Taylor WF. Cancer of the hypopharynx: analysis of treatment and results in 162 patients. Arch Otolaryngol 1976;102:716–21.

24. Cawson RA. Premalignant lesions in the mouth. Br Med Bull 1975;31:164–8

25. Chan CK, Gee JB. Asbestos exposure and laryngeal cancer: an analysis of epidemiologic evidence. J Occup Med 1997;30:23–7.

26. Chaudhry AP, Gorlin RJ, Mosser DG. Carcinoma of the antrum. A clinical and histopathologic study. Oral Surg 1960;13:269–81.

27. Coltrera MD, Zarbo RJ, Sakr WA, Gown AM. Markers for dysplasia of the upper aerodigestive tract. Suprabasal expression of PCNA, p53, and CK19 in alcohol-fixed, embedded tissue. Am J Pathol 1992;141:817–25.

28. Conley J, Sadoyama JA. Squamous cell carcinoma of the buccal mucosa. A review of 90 cases. Arch Otolaryngol 1973;97:330–3.

29. Creely JJ Jr, Lyons GD Jr, Trail ML. Cancer of the nasopharynx: a review of 114 cases. South Med J 1973;66:405–9.

30. Crissman JD. Laryngeal keratosis and subsequent carcinoma. Head Neck Surg 1979;1:386–91.

31. Crissman JD, Gluckman J, Whiteley J, Quenelle D. Squamous-cell carcinoma of the floor of the mouth. Head Neck Surg 1980;3:2–7.

32. Crissman JD, Gnepp DR, Goodman ML, Hellquist H, Johns ME. Preinvasive lesions of the upper aerodigestive tract: histologic definitions and clinical implications (a symposium). Pathol Annu 1987;22(1):311–52.

33. Cunningham MP, Catlin D. Cancer of the pharyngeal wall. Cancer 1967;20:1859–66.

34. DeSanto LW, Carpenter RJ. Reconstruction of the pharynx and upper esophagus after resection for cancer. Head Neck Surg 1980;2:369–79.

35. Easton JM, Levine PH, Hyams VJ. Nasopharyngeal carcinoma in the United States. A pathologic study of 177 US and 30 foreign cases. Arch Otolaryngol 1980;106:88–91.

36. Elomaa L, Joensuu H, Kulmala J, Klemi P, Grenman R. Squamous cell carcinoma is highly sensitive to taxol, a possible new radiation sensitizer. Acta Otolaryngol (Stockh) 1995;115:340–4.

37. Farr HW, Arthur K. Epidermoid carcinoma of the mouth and pharynx 1960–1964. J Laryngol Otol 1972;86:243–53.

38. Fee WE Jr, Schoeppel SL, Rubenstein R, et al. Squamous cell carcinoma of the soft palate. Arch Otolaryngol 1979;105:710–2.

39. Fein DA, Mendenhall WM, Parsons JT, et al. Carcinoma of the oral tongue: a comparison of results and complications of treatment with radiotherapy and/or surgery. Head Neck 1994;16:358–65.

40. Fletcher GH, MacComb WS, Lindberg RD. Cancer of the oropharynx. In: Conley J, ed. Cancer of the head and neck. Washington, D.C.: Butterworths, 1967:317–23.

41. Foote RL, Olsen KD, Kunselman SJ, et al. Early-stage squamous cell carcinoma of the glottic larynx managed with radiation therapy. Mayo Clin Proc 1992;67:629–36.

42. Fradis M, Podoshin L, Gertner R, Sabo E. Squamous cell carcinoma of the nasal septum mucosa. Ear Nose Throat J 1993;72:217–21.

43. Frank JL, Garb JL, Kay S, et al. Postoperative radiotherapy improves survival in squamous cell carcinoma of the hypopharynx. Am J Surg 1994;168:476–80.

44. Frazell EL, Lucas JC. Cancer of the tongue: report of the management of 1,554 patients. Cancer 1962;15:1085–99.

45. Frierson HF Jr, Cooper PH. Prognostic factors in squamous cell carcinoma of the lower lip. Hum Pathol 1986;17:346–54.

46. Frierson HF Jr, Mills SE, Fechner RE, Taxy JB, Levine PA. Sinonasal undifferentiated carcinoma. An aggressive neoplasm derived from schneiderian epithelium and distinct from olfactory neuroblastoma. Am J Surg Pathol 1986;10:771–9.

47. Furuta Y, Takasu T, Asai T, et al. Detection of human papillomavirus DNA in carcinomas of the nasal cavities and paranasal sinuses by polymerase chain reaction. Cancer 1992;69:353–7.

48. Futrell JW, Bennett SH, Hoye RC, Roth JA, Ketcham AS. Predicting survival in cancer of the larynx or hypopharynx. Am J Surg 1971;122:451–7.

49. Gabriel CD, Jones DG. Hyperkeratosis of the larynx. J Laryngol 1962;76:947–57.

50. Gelfman WE, Williams A. Spindle-cell carcinoma of the tongue. Oral Surg 1969;27:659–63.

51. Goldman RL, Klein HZ, Sung M. Adenoid squamous cell carcinoma of the oral cavity. Arch Otolaryngol 1977;103:496–8.

52. Gomez R, El-Naggar AK, Byers RM, Garnsey L, Luna MA, Batsakis JG. Squamous carcinoma of oral tongue: prognostic significance of flow-cytometric DNA content. Mod Pathol 1992;5:141–5.

53. Goren AD, Harley N, Eisenbud L, Levin S, Cohen N. Clinical and radiobiologic features of Thorotrast-induced carcinoma of the maxillary sinus. A case report. Oral Surg Oral Med Oral Pathol 1980;49:237–42.

54. Greger V, Schirmacher P, Bohl J, et al. Possible involvement of the retinoblastoma gene in undifferentiated sinonasal carcinoma. Cancer 1990;66:1954–9.

55. Hanna GS, Ali MH. Verrucous carcinoma of the nasal septum. J Laryngol Otol 1987;101:184–7.

56. Harrison DF. Surgical pathology of hypopharyngeal neoplasms. J Laryngol Otol 1971;85:1215–8.

57. Harrison DF. The pathology and management of subglottic cancer. Ann Otol Rhinol Laryngol 1971;80:6–12.

58. Hasegawa Y, Matsuura H. Retropharyngeal node dissection in cancer of the oropharynx and hypopharynx. Head Neck 1994;16:173–80.

59. Hawkins NV. The treatment of glottic carcinoma: an analysis of 800 cases. Laryngoscope 1975;85:1485–93.

60. Healy GB, Strong MS, Uchmakli A, Vaughan CW, DiTroia JF. Carcinoma of the palatine arch. Am J Surg 1976;132:498–503.

61. Helliwell TR, Yeoh LH, Stell PM. Anaplastic carcinoma of the nose and paranasal sinuses. Light microscopy, immunohistochemistry, and clinical correlation. Cancer 1986;58:2038–45.

62. Hellquist H, Lundgren J, Olofsson J. Hyperplasia, keratosis, dysplasia and carcinoma in situ of the vocal cords—follow-up study. Clin Otolaryngol 1982;7:11–27.

63. Henry RC. The transformation of laryngeal leukoplakia to cancer. J Laryngol Otol 1979;93:447–59.

64. Hill BT, Price LA. Lack of survival advantage in patients with advanced squamous cell carcinomas of the oral cavity receiving neoadjuvant chemotherapy prior to local therapy, despite achieving an initial high clinical complete remission rate. Am J Clin Oncol 1994;17:1–5.

65. Hinerman RW, Parsons JT, Mendenhall WM, Stringer SP, Cassisi NJ, Million RR. External beam irradiation alone or combined with neck dissection for base of tongue carcinoma: an alternative to primary surgery. Laryngoscope 1994;104:1466–70.

66. Ho CM, Lam KH, Wei WI, Yuen PW, Lam LK. Squamous cell carcinoma of the hypopharynx—analysis of treatment results. Head Neck 1993;15:405–12.

67. Holladay EB, Gerald WL. Viral gene detection in oral neoplasms using the polymerase chain reaction. Am J Clin Pathol 1993;100:36–40.

68. Horiuchi K, Mishima K, Ichijima K, Sugimura M, Ishida T, Kirita T. Epstein-Barr virus in the proliferative diseases of squamous epithelium in the oral cavity. Oral Surg Oral Med Oral Pathol Oral Radiol Endod 1995;79:57–63.

69. Horiuchi K, Mishima K, Ohsawa M, Sugimura M, Aozasa K. Prognostic factors for well-differentiated squamous cell carcinoma in the oral cavity with emphasis on immunohistochemical evaluation. J Surg Oncol 1993;53:92–6.

70. Horwitz SD, Caldarelli DD, Hendrickson FR. Treatment of carcinoma of the hypopharynx. Head Neck Surg 1979;2:101–11.

71. Inoue T, Shigematsu Y, Sato T. Treatment of carcinoma of the hypopharynx. Cancer 1973;31:649–55.

72. Jakobsson PA. Histologic grading of malignancy and prognosis in glottic carcinoma of the larynx. In: Alberti PW, Bryce DP, eds. Centennial Conference on Laryngeal Cancer. New York: Appleton-Century-Crofts, 1976:847–54.

73. Jakobsson PA, Eneroth CM, Killander D, Moberger G, Martensen B. Histologic classification and grading of malignancy in carcinoma of the larynx. Acta Radiol Ther Phys Biol 1973;12:1–8.

74. Jaques DA. Epidermoid carcinoma of the palate. Otolaryngol Clinics North Am 1979;12:125–8.

75. Jesse RH, Lindberg RD. The efficacy of combining radiation therapy with a surgical procedure in patients with cervical metastasis from squamous cell cancer of the oropharynx and hypopharynx. Cancer 1975;35:1163–6.

76. Jesse RH, Sugarbaker EV. Squamous cell carcinoma of the oropharynx: why we fail. Am J Surg 1976;132:435–8.

77. Johnson JT, Bacon GW, Myers EN, Wagner RL. Medial vs lateral wall pyriform sinus carcinoma: implications for management of regional lymphatics. Head Neck 1994;16:401–5.

78. Jorgensen K. Carcinoma of the hypopharynx. Therapeutic results in a series of 103 patients. Acta Radiol 1971;10:465–73.

79. Jovanovic A, Schulten EA, Kostense PJ, Snow GB, van der Waal I. Tobacco and alcohol related to the anatomical site of oral squamous cell carcinoma. J Oral Pathol Med 1993;22:459–62.

80. Jovanovic A, van der Tol IG, Schulten EA, et al. Risk of multiple primary tumors following oral squamous-cell carcinoma. Int J Cancer 1994;56:320–3.

81. Kaplan MJ, Mills SE, Rice RH, Johns ME. Involucrin in laryngeal dysplasia. A marker of differentiation. Arch Otolaryngol 1984;110:713–6.

82. Keller AZ. Cirrhosis of the liver, alcoholism, and heavy smoking associated with cancer of the mouth and pharynx. Cancer 1967;20:1015–22.

83. Kirchner JA. Pyriform sinus cancer: a clinical and laboratory study. Ann Otol Rhinol Laryngol 1975;84:793–803.

84. Klein-Szanto AJ, Boysen M, Reith A. Keratin and involucrin in preneoplastic and neoplastic lesions. Distribution in the nasal mucosa of nickel workers. Arch Pathol Lab Med 1987;111:1057–61.

85. Klijanienko J, Micheau C, Azli N, et al. Undifferentiated carcinoma of nasopharyngeal type of tonsil. Arch Otolaryngol Head Neck Surg 1989;115:731–4.

86. Kolson H, Spiro RH, Rosevit B, Lawson W. Epidermoid carcinoma of the floor of the mouth. Analysis of 108 cases. Arch Otolaryngol 1971;93:280–3.

87. Kraus DH, Vastola AP, Huvos AG, Spiro RH. Surgical management of squamous cell carcinoma of the base of the tongue. Am J Surg 1993;166:384–8.

88. Krolls SO, Hoffman S. Squamous cell carcinoma of the oral soft tissues: a statistical analysis of 14,253 cases by age, sex and race of patients. J Am Dent Assoc 1976;92:571–4.

89. Krutchkoff DJ, Chen J, Eisenberg E, Katz RV. Oral cancer: a survey of 566 cases from the University of Connecticut oral pathology biopsy service, 1975-1986. Oral Surg Oral Med Oral Pathol 1990;70:192–8.

90. Larsson LG, Mårtensson G. Maxillary antral cancers. JAMA 1972;219:342–5.

91. Lee WR, Mancuso AA, Saleh EM, Mendenhall WM, Parsons JT, Million RR. Can pretreatment computed tomography findings predict local control in T3 squamous cell carcinoma of the glottic larynx treated with radiotherapy alone? Int J Radiat Oncol Biol Phys 1993;25:683–7.

92. Leedy DA, Trune DR, Kronz JD, Weidner N, Cohen JI. Tumor angiogenesis, the p53 antigen, and cervical metastasis in squamous carcinoma of the tongue. Otolaryngol Head Neck Surg 1994;111:417–22.

93. Leroux-Robert J. A statistical study of 620 laryngeal carcinomas of the glottic region personally operated upon more than five years ago. Laryngoscope 1975;85:1440–52.

94. Levy R, Segal K, Hadar T, Shvero J, Abraham A. Squamous cell carcinoma of the oral tongue. Eur J Surg Oncol 1991;17:330–4.

95. Lewis JS, Castro EB. Cancer of the nasal cavity and paranasal sinuses. J Laryngol Otol 1972;86:255–62.

96. Lindberg R. Distribution of cervical lymph node metastases from squamous cell carcinoma of the upper respiratory and digestive tracts. Cancer 1972;29:1446–9.

97. Looi LM. Tumor-associated tissue eosinophilia in naso-pharyngeal carcinoma. A pathologic study of 422 primary and 138 metastatic tumors. Cancer 1987;59:466–70.

98. Lowry WS. Alcoholism in cancer of the head and neck. Laryngoscope 1975;85:1275–80.

99. Luce D, Gerin M, Leclerc A, Morcet JF, Brugere J, Goldberg M. Sinonasal cancer and occupational exposure to formaldehyde and other substances. Int J Cancer 1993;53:224–31.

100. Lund WS. Classification of subglottic tumors and discussion of their growth and spread. In: Alberti PW, Bryce DP, eds. Centennial conference on laryngeal carcinoma. New York: Appleton-Century-Crofts, 1976:63–5.

101. Lydiatt DD, Robbins KT, Byers RM, Wolf PF. Treatment of stage I and II oral tongue cancer. Head Neck 1993;15:308–12.

102. Martinez-Gimeno C, Rodriguez EM, Vila CN, Varela CL. Squamous cell carcinoma of the oral cavity: a clinicopathologic scoring system for evaluating risk of cervical lymph node metastasis. Laryngoscope 1995;105:728–33.

103. McGavran MH, Bauer WC, Ogura JH. Isolated laryngeal keratosis. Its relation to carcinoma of the larynx based on a clinico-pathologic study of 87 consecutive cases with long-term follow-up. Laryngoscope 1960;70:932–51.

104. McGavran MH, Bauer WC, Ogura JH. The incidence of cervical lymph node metastases from epidermoid carcinoma of the larynx and their relationship to certain characteristics of the primary tumor: A study based on the clinical and pathologic findings for 96 patients treated by primary en bloc laryngectomy and radical neck dissection. Cancer 1961;14:55–66.

105. Medonca DR, Bryce DP. Transglottic cancer of the larynx–a case presentation. Can J Otolaryngol 1973;2:271–6.

106. Norris CM, Peale AR. Keratosis of the larynx. J Laryngol 1963;77:635–47.

107. Nuutinen J, Kärjä J. Local and distant metastases in patients with surgically treated squamous cell carcinoma of the lip. Clin Otolaryngol 1981;6:415–9.

108. Nyman J, Mercke C, Lindstrom J. Prognostic factors for local control and survival of cancer of the oral tongue. A retrospective analysis of 230 cases in western Sweden. Acta Oncol 1993;32:667–73.

109. O'Brien PH. Cancer of the cheek (mucosa). Cancer 1965;18:1392–8.

110. Ogura JH. Surgical pathology of cancer of the larynx. Laryngoscope 1955;65:867–926.

111. Parker RG. Carcinoma of the nasal fossa. Am J Roentgen Rad Ther Nuclear Med 1958;80:766–74.

112. Piscioli F, Aldovini D, Bondi A, Eusebi V. Squamous cell carcinoma with sarcoma-like stroma of the nose and paranasal sinuses: report of two cases. Histopathology 1984;8:633–9.

113. Quigley LF, Cobb CM, Schoenfeld S, Hunt EE, Williams P. Reverse smoking and its oral consequences in Caribbean and South American peoples. J Am Dent Assoc 1964;69:427–42.

114. Ramulu C, Ramju MV, Venkatarathnam G, Reddy CR. Nicotine stomatitis and its relation to carcinoma of the hard palate in reverse smokers of chuttas. J Dent Res 1973;52:711–8.

115. Razack MS, Sako K, Marchetta FC, Calamel P, Bakamjian V, Shedd DP. Carcinoma of the hypopharynx: success and failure. Am J Surg 1977;134:489–91.

116. Rezvani M, Fowler JF, Hopewell JW, Alcock CJ. Sensitivity of human squamous cell carcinoma of the larynx to fractionated radiotherapy. Br J Radiol 1993;66:245–55.

117. Rothman K. The effect of alcohol consumption on risk of cancer of the head and neck. Laryngoscope 1978;88:51–5.

118. Rothman KJ, Keller A. The effect of joint exposure to alcohol and tobacco on risk of cancer of the mouth and pharynx. J Chron Dis 1972;25:711–6.

119. Rousch GC. Epidemiology of cancer of the nose and paranasal sinuses: current concepts. Head Neck Surg 1979;2:3–11.

120. Rowley NJ, Boles R. Supraglottic carcinoma: a ten year review at the University Hospital. Laryngoscope 1972;82:1264–72.

121. Rubin P. Cancer of the head and neck. Oropharynx. JAMA 1971;217:940–2.

122. Sack JG, Ford CN. Metastatic squamous cell carcinoma of the lip. Arch Otolaryngol 1978;104:282–5.

123. Sakai S, Shigematzu Y, Fuchihata H. Diagnosis and TNM classification of maxillary sinus carcinoma. Acta Otolaryngol (Stockh) 1972;74:123–9.

124. Schulz J, Ermich T, Kasper M, Raabe G, Schumann D. Cytokeratin pattern of clinically intact and pathologically changed oral mucosa. Int J Oral Maxillofac Surg 1992;21:35–9.

125. Schulz MD. Tonsil and palatine arch cancer–treatment by radiotherapy. Laryngoscope 1965;75:958–67.

126. Schumrick DA, Gluckman JL. Suen JY, Myers EN, eds. Cancer of the head and neck. New York: Churchill Livingstone, 1981:342–71.

127. Sessions DG. Surgical pathology of the larynx and hypopharynx. Laryngoscope 1976;86:814–39.

128. Seydel HG, Scholl H. Cancer of the soft palate and uvula. Am J Roentgen Rad Ther Nuclear Med 1974;120:603–7.

129. Shanmugaratnam K, Chan SH, de-The G, et al. Histopathology of nasopharyngeal carcinoma: correlations with epidemiology, survival rates and other biological characteristics. Cancer 1979;44:1029–44.

130. Shettigara PT, Morgan RW. Asbestos, smoking, and laryngeal carcinoma. Arch Environ Health 1975;30:517–9.

131. Shibuya H, Amagasa T, Hanai A, Horiuchi JC, Suzuki S. Second primary carcinomas in patients with squamous cell carcinoma of the maxillary sinus. Cancer 1986;58:1122–5.

132. Shindoh M, Sawada Y, Kohgo T, Amemiya A, Fujinaga K. Detection of human papillomavirus DNA sequences in tongue squamous-cell carcinoma utilizing the polymerase chain reaction method. Int J Cancer 1992;50:167–71.

133. Skolnik EM, Saberman MN. Cancer of the tongue. In: Ogura JH, ed. Otolaryngologic Clinics of North America, Symposium on cancer of the head and neck. Philadelphia: WB Saunders, 1969:603–15.

134. Smith AH, Handley MA, Wood R. Epidemiologic evidence indicates asbestos causes laryngeal cancer. J Occup Med 1990;32:499–507.

135. Smith EM. Epidemiology of oral and pharyngeal cancers in the United States: review of recent literature. JNCI 1979;63:1189–98.

136. Smith RR, Caulk RM, Russell WO, Jackson CL. End results of 600 laryngeal cancers using the American Joint Committee's proposed method of stage classification and end result reporting. Surg Gynecol Obstet 1961;113:435–44.

137. Someren A, Karcioglu Z, Clairmont AA. Polypoid spindle-cell carcinoma (pleomorphic carcinoma): report of a case occurring on the tongue and review of the literature. Oral Surg 1976;72:474–89.

138. Stefani S, Eells RW. Carcinoma of the hypopharynx–a study of distant metastases, treatment failures, and multiple primary cancers in 215 male patients. Laryngoscope 1971;81:1491–8.

139. Stell PM, McGill T. Asbestos and laryngeal carcinoma. Lancet 1973;2:416–7.

140. Stell PM, Tobin KE. The behavior of cancer affecting the subglottic space. Can J Otolaryngol 1975;4:612–7.

141. Strong MS, DiTroia JF, Vaughan CW. Carcinoma of the palatine arch. A review of 73 patients. Trans Am Acad Ophthalmol Otolaryngol 1971;75:957–67.

142. Tabb HG, Barranco SJ. Cancer of the maxillary sinus: an analysis of 108 cases. Laryngoscope 1971;81:818–27.

143. Teoh TB. Epidermoid carcinoma of the nasopharynx among Chinese: a study of 31 necropsies. J Pathol Bact 1957;73:451–65.

144. Tytor M, Olofsson J. Prognostic factors in oral cavity carcinomas. Acta Otolaryngol (Stockh) 1992;492:75–8.

145. Umeda M, Yokoo S, Take Y, Omori A, Nakanishi K, Shimada K. Lymph node metastasis in squamous cell carcinoma of the oral cavity: correlation between histologic features and the prevalence of metastasis. Head Neck 1992;14:263–72.

146. van der Eb MM, Leyten EM, Gavarasana S, Vandenbroucke JP, Kahn PM, Cleton FJ. Reverse smoking as a risk factor for palatal cancer: a cross-sectional study in rural Andhra Pradesh, India. Int J Cancer 1993;54:754–8.

147. van der Velden LA, Schaafsma HE, Manni JJ, Ramaekers FC, Kuijpers W. Cytokeratin expression in normal and (pre)malignant head and neck epithelia: an overview. Head Neck 1993;15:133–46.

148. Vegers JW, Snow GB, van der Waal I. Squamous cell carcinoma of the buccal mucosa. A review of 85 cases. Arch Otolaryngol 1979;105:192–5.

149. Verbin RS, Bouquot JE, Guggenheimer J, Barnes L, Peel RL. Cancer of the oral cavity and oropharynx. In: Barnes L, ed. Surgical pathology of the head and neck. New York: Marcel Dekker, 1985:333–401.

150. Virtue JA. The relationship between the refining of nickel and cancer of the nasal cavity. Can J Otolaryngol 1972;1:37–42.

151. Vrabec DP. Multiple primary malignancies associated with index cancers of the oral, pharyngeal, and laryngeal areas. Trans Pa Acad Ophthalmol Otolaryngol 1979;32:177–81.

152. Wan SK, Chan JK, Tse KC. Basaloid-squamous carcinoma of the nasal cavity. J Laryngol Otol 1992;106:370–1.

153. Wang CC. Radiotherapeutic management of carcinoma of the posterior pharyngeal wall. Cancer 1971;27:894–6.

154. Weller SA, Goffinet DR, Goode RL, Bagshaw MA. Carcinoma of the oropharynx. Results of megavoltage radiation therapy in 305 patients. Am J Roentgen Rad Ther Nuclear Med 1976;126:236–47.

155. Wenig BL, Applebaum EL. The submandibular triangle in squamous cell carcinoma of the larynx and hypopharynx. Laryngoscope 1991;101:516–8.

156. Wenig BL, Ziffra KL, Mafee MF, Schild JA. MR imaging of squamous cell carcinoma of the larynx and hypopharynx. Otolaryngol Clinics North Am 1995;28:609–19.

157. Wenig BM. Neoplasms of the oral cavity, nasopharynx, tonsils, and neck. In: Anonymous, ed. Atlas of head and neck pathology. Philadelphia: WB Saunders, 1993:143–99.

158. Wiernik G, Millard PR, Haybittle JL. The predictive value of histological classification into degrees of differentiation of squamous cell carcinoma of the larynx and hypopharynx compared with the survival of patients. Histopathology 1991;19:411–7.

159. Wingo PA, Tong T, Bolden S. Cancer statistics, 1995. CA Cancer J Clin 1995;45:8–30.

160. Wurman LH, Adams GL, Meyerhoff WL. Carcinoma of the lip. Am J Surg 1975;130:470–4.

161. Wynder E. Toward the prevention of laryngeal cancer. Laryngoscope 1975;85:1190–6.

162. Wynder EL, Covey LS, Mabuchi K, Mushinski M. Environmental factors in cancer of the larynx. A second look. Cancer 1976;38:1591–601.

163. Wynder EL, Hultberg S, Jacobson F, Bross IJ. Environmental factors in cancer of the upper alimentary tract: a Swedish study with special reference to Plummer-Vinson (Paterson-Kelly) syndrome. Cancer 1957;10:470–87.

164. Yeh S. A histological classification of carcinomas of the nasopharynx with critical review as to the existence of lymphoepitheliomas. Cancer 1962;15:895–920.

165. Young JL, Percy CL, Asire AJ, et al. Cancer incidence and mortality in the United States, 1973-77. National Cancer Institute Monograph 57. NCI, 1979.

166. Zaatari GS, Santoianni RA. Adenoid squamous cell carcinoma of the nasopharynx and neck region. Arch Pathol Lab Med 1986;110:542–6.

167. Zagraniski RT, Kelsey JL, Walter SD. Occupational risk factors for laryngeal carcinoma: Connecticut, 1975–1980. Am J Epidemiol 1986;124:67–76.

168. Zoller M, Goodman ML, Cummings CW. Guidelines for prognosis in head and neck cancer with nodal metastasis. Laryngoscope 1978;88:135–40.

◇◇◇

5

SQUAMOUS CELL CARCINOMA:
DIAGNOSTICALLY PROBLEMATIC VARIANTS

VERRUCOUS CARCINOMA

Definition. This wart-like, heavily keratinized, exquisitely well-differentiated squamous cell neoplasm lacks conventional cytologic features of malignancy, but exhibits a locally destructive growth pattern. Provided there is no associated conventional squamous cell carcinoma, the tumor has no metastatic potential. Nonetheless, local control may be difficult, and there may be considerable destruction of invaded tissues.

General Features. Although examples were included in earlier studies of oral tobacco-related squamous carcinomas (13), verrucous carcinoma was first recognized by Ackerman in 1948 (2) as a distinct, diagnostically problematic squamous cell neoplasm involving the oral cavity. Because of this, some authors have referred to this lesion as "Ackerman's tumor" (12,20). There is considerable variation in the frequency with which verrucous carcinoma is diagnosed, but in our opinion a narrow definition is correct, and these tumors account for about 1 percent of squamous neoplasms involving the head and neck region. One of the earliest recorded and more famous examples of verrucous carcinoma appears to have been an oral tumor excised from United States President Grover Cleveland in 1893 (5).

Verrucous carcinoma of the oral cavity and larynx shows a strong association with tobacco product usage. The oral cavity lesions, in particular, are strongly associated with the chronic use of smokeless tobacco (13,19). In their review of 104 patients with verrucous carcinoma of the oral cavity, Luna and Tortoledo (19) noted that 84 percent used tobacco products, including 32 percent who dipped snuff and 26 percent who chewed tobacco (19). Oral cavity verrucous carcinoma may also be associated with the practice of chewing betel nuts (6). Several studies have suggested a potential role for human papillomavirus (HPV) as a cofactor in tumor development based on its detection in tissue specimens (1,4,14,29). However, HPV also has been detected by polymerase chain reaction (PCR) in 25 percent of normal larynges (24), and a causal role has not yet been clearly demonstrated.

The diagnosis of verrucous carcinoma is exclusionary and often extremely difficult. The associated difficulties fall into two major categories. First, superficial biopsies contain only keratotic debris and benign-appearing squamous cells. Without tissue showing the margin of the lesion and evidence of invasive growth, distinction from benign squamous proliferations (see differential diagnosis) cannot be made. Conversely, without adequate biopsy specimens or, optimally, a complete resection, it is not possible to completely exclude an underlying conventional squamous cell carcinoma. In our experience, the presence of any areas of cytologically typical squamous cell carcinoma should place the lesion outside the diagnostic category of verrucous carcinoma because of the associated potential for metastatic disease not seen with pure verrucous lesions.

A second major area of controversy regarding verrucous carcinoma relates to the role and effect of radiation therapy on these neoplasms, with specific regard to the frequency of postradiation anaplastic transformation (25). The literature is confusing in this regard because some studies lump patients receiving primary radiation therapy along with those treated for salvage following failure of initial surgical resection. In a review of the literature Hagen et al. (14) noted that of 37 patients with verrucous carcinoma of the larynx treated initially with radiation therapy, 18 (49 percent) were cured of disease, and 19 (51 percent) were treatment failures either due to lack of initial response or recurrence. Of the later group, 4 patients (11 percent overall, 21 percent of failures) developed anaplastic transformation of their tumors and ultimately died of disease. In a separate study of verrucous carcinoma from all head and neck sites, anaplastic transformation was documented in 7 percent of irradiated tumors (31). Anaplastic transformation has been said to often

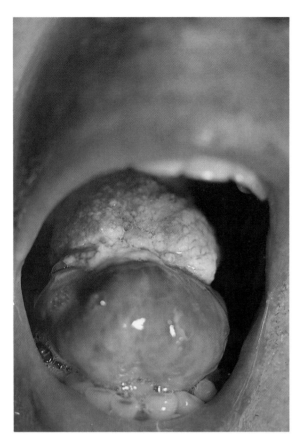

Figure 5-1
VERRUCOUS CARCINOMA
The "cauliflower-like" surface of a large verrucous carcinoma involving the posterior portion of the oral cavity is easily visualized behind the tongue. (Courtesy of Dr. K. E. Greer, Charlottesville, VA.)

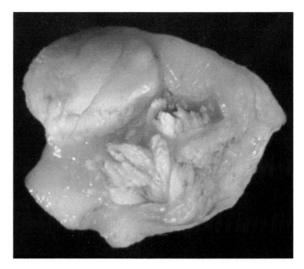

Figure 5-2
VERRUCOUS CARCINOMA
This hemilaryngectomy specimen shows the wart-like surface features of a verrucous carcinoma. (Slide 57 from Mills SE, Fechner RE. Anatomy of the larynx. Chicago: ASCP 1985:40.)

occur with "explosive swiftness," manifesting 2 to 8 months following radiation therapy (14). This is far more rapid than radiation-related secondary neoplasia, which typically takes 7 or more years to develop. It has been postulated that radiation-induced DNA breaks may facilitate integration of HPA DNA into host nuclear DNA, leading to malignant (anaplastic) transformation (1,30). Currently, however, this is only an interesting hypothesis. It has been noted that dedifferentiation rarely may occur following surgery alone (31).

Clinical Features. Verrucous carcinoma is a disease of later life, typically occurring in the seventh and eighth decades. It is rare in patients under 40 years of age (19). Almost all studies of oral verrucous carcinoma have shown a strong male predominance, in keeping with the generally much greater use of oral "smokeless" tobacco

products by males (2,12,18). As an exception, older studies from the southeastern United States include larger numbers of women because of the historically common practice of snuff dipping by women in this geographic area (19,21).

In the head and neck region, verrucous carcinomas most commonly involve the oral cavity (2,3,6, 13,17,18,21,29) and larynx (1,3,4,7,11,12,14,20, 27). In a review of 105 verrucous carcinomas from all anatomic sites, Kraus and Perez-Mesa (18) noted that 73 percent arose in the oral cavity, 11 percent involved the larynx, 4 percent involved the sinonasal region, and the remainder occurred outside of the head and neck, primarily involving the genitalia. Within the oral cavity, the buccal mucosa is by far the most common site, followed by the mandibular alveolar ridge, hard and soft palate, tongue, and lip (fig. 5-1) (19). Within the larynx, most verrucous carcinomas arise from the vocal cords (12). These tumors also involve the nasopharynx, oropharynx, sinonasal region, and esophagus (3,8,16).

As a pure lesion, verrucous carcinoma is uncommon. Even in the oral cavity, its most common site, it has been estimated to account for only 2 to 4.5 percent of squamous neoplasms (3, 15); in the larynx, it comprises 1 to 4 percent of squamous carcinomas (12). It has been suggested that approximately 20 percent of oral cavity neoplasms with an appearance of verrucous carcinoma in superficial biopsy specimens have an underlying component of more conventional squamous cell carcinoma (19), removing them from this pure diagnostic category. This phenomenon also occurs with laryngeal lesions.

Verrucous carcinomas are typically slowly growing neoplasms, and they may reach considerable size before being brought to medical attention. They appear as a papillary or "cobblestone" surfaced, usually nonulcerated mass with a broad base of attachment to the underlying mucosa. The surface ranges in color from graywhite to red depending on the thickness of the surface keratin layer. Invasion of underlying tissues is required by definition, but is often less than the extensive lateral growth of the lesion would suggest (19). Regional lymph nodes are often slightly enlarged, but provided the tumor is a pure verrucous carcinoma, this is due to infection-associated lymphoid hyperplasia rather than metastases.

Gross Findings. Resected specimens typically show a tan to gray, rough, bulky exophytic mass with a shaggy or overtly papillary wart-like surface (fig. 5-2). On sectioning through the tumor, the margin of invasion is sharp and pushing. The tan-white edge of the invasive carcinoma is usually easy to distinguish from the adjacent tissue (fig. 5-3).

Microscopic Findings. Verrucous carcinoma is characterized by dense superficial keratinization, often forming "church spires" of orthokeratotic and parakeratotic squamous cells extending upward from the surface. The result is a distinctly wart-like or verrucoid appearance (figs. 5-4, 5-5). The neoplastic cells typically have vesicular nuclei with small nucleoli. Nuclear pleomorphism is absent or minimal and mitotic activity is confined to the basal cell layer. Cells have abundant eosinophilic cytoplasm, which generally undergoes uniform keratinization as the cells migrate toward the surface. Individual cell keratinization (dyskeratosis) and keratin "pearl" formation may be focally present. At the base of the lesion, downgrowth is in the form of broad, bulbous, sharply demarcated ridges of well-differentiated, benign-appearing squamous cells (fig. 5-6). This is usually associated with a prominent lymphoplasmacytic infiltrate at the

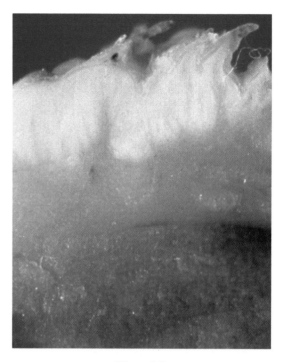

Figure 5-3
VERRUCOUS CARCINOMA
A cut section through the specimen seen in figure 5-2 shows verrucous carcinoma invading below adjacent normal mucosa (right) as a sharply demarcated, pushing border.

base of the lesion (fig. 5-7), occasionally with granulomatous inflammation in response to "escaped" keratin debris (19). Ragged infiltration by small, irregular nests of cells, vascular invasion, or perineural invasion are not seen.

Ultrastructural Findings. Not surprisingly, the ultrastructural features of verrucous carcinoma are strikingly similar to those of normal squamous mucosa (26). There is a basal layer of less differentiated cells, with progressive maturation to larger cells with abundant intracytoplasmic tonofilament bundles and well-formed desmosomal attachments (26). At the stromal interface, there is often fragmentation and reduplication of the basal lamina (28).

Other Special Techniques. Verrucous carcinoma exhibits characteristic cell kinetics that are more akin to those of normal mucosa than conventional squamous cell carcinoma (9,11,19,26,33). In particular, DNA synthesis (S-phase) is confined to the basal cell layer, along with the more conventionally detected mitotic activity. The lack of S-phase cells above the basal cell layer is quite

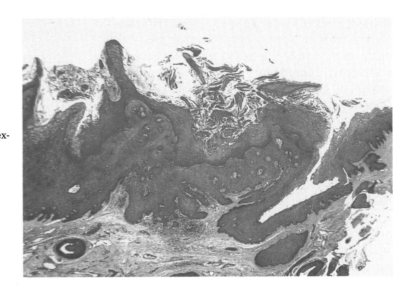

Figure 5-4
VERRUCOUS CARCINOMA
Microscopically, verrucous carcinoma exhibits abundant surface keratinization.

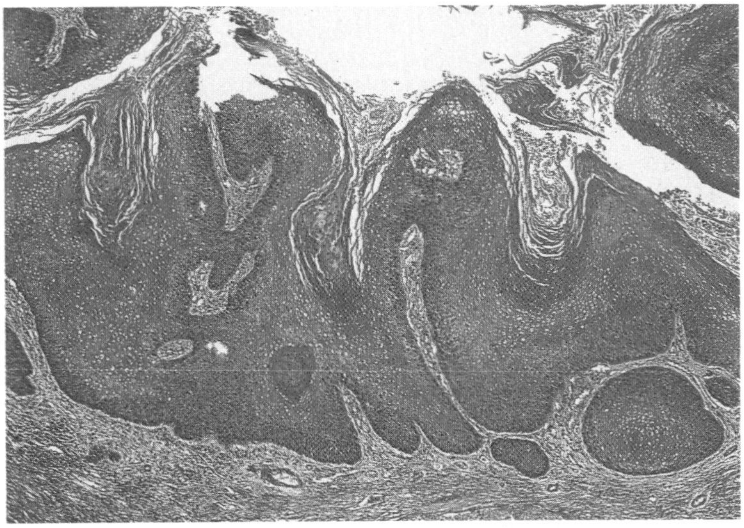

Figure 5-5
VERRUCOUS CARCINOMA
This example of laryngeal verrucous carcinoma has characteristic "spires" of surface keratinization and underlying well-differentiated squamous epithelium which invades the stroma in a broad, pushing border.

Figure 5-6
VERRUCOUS CARCINOMA
This deeply invasive verrucous carcinoma consists of sharply demarcated nests of well-differentiated squamous cells lacking conventional features of malignancy.

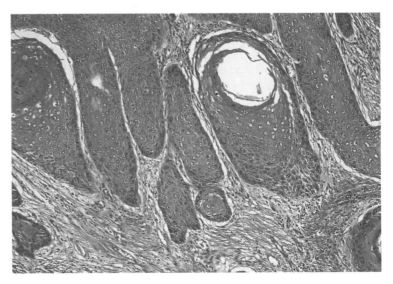

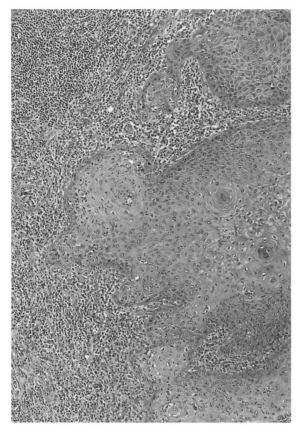

Figure 5-7
VERRUCOUS CARCINOMA
Frequently, the deeper portions of verrucous carcinoma are associated with considerable inflammation. The squamous nests remain sharply demarcated and lack conventional features of malignancy.

unlike the findings in conventional squamous cell carcinomas (11,26,33). By flow cytometry, verrucous carcinomas are diploid lesions (33).

Differential Diagnosis. There are three broad categories of diagnostic difficulty associated with verrucous carcinoma. The lesion must be distinguished from conventional squamous cell carcinoma and from benign keratotic proliferations, and it must be verified to be a pure lesion without an associated high-grade component. Distinction from conventional squamous cell carcinoma is a more common problem for clinicians confronted by the often extensive nature of the lesion. Pathologists, examining microscopic sections of an exquisitely bland, benign-appearing squamous proliferation are more likely to confuse the lesion with a benign process. Indeed, this

problem was the root of Dr. Ackerman's interest in this lesion. An anecdote that he related to the authors and many others during his extensive travels dealt with his early experience at the Ellis Fischel Cancer Center and a patient who had multiple biopsies of an oral cavity lesion which Dr. Ackerman had repeatedly labeled as "keratosis." Finally, in desperation the surgeon demanded that Dr. Ackerman personally examine the patient and confronted him with an obviously invasive lesion extending through the oral cavity and involving the skin of the cheek. "What kind of keratosis is that?" asked the surgeon. "The bad kind!" replied Dr. Ackerman, and not long thereafter his seminal article on verrucous carcinoma was published (2).

Because verrucous carcinomas are, by definition, cytologically benign, their distinction from so-called verrucous hyperplasia cannot be based on cytologic features. This often makes the diagnosis of verrucous carcinoma difficult or impossible on limited biopsies. Without knowledge at the microscopic level of the tumor interface in relation to the surrounding normal tissues, the invasive nature of the lesion cannot be ascertained. Histologically identical lesions lacking invasion are considered to represent verrucous hyperplasia (23,28). It should be noted that some authors consider verrucous hyperplasia to be irreversible, with a strong tendency to progress to verrucous carcinoma (23). In the original description by Shear and Pindborg (28), 20 of 68 patients with verrucous hyperplasia had synchronous verrucous carcinoma and 7 had coexistent typical squamous cell carcinoma.

We have described keratotic laryngeal lesions which differed somewhat in their microscopic appearance from verrucous hyperplasia or carcinoma and, instead, had features of verruca vulgaris (10). Like verrucous hyperplasia, verruca vulgaris is an exophytic, noninvasive lesion. It differs from verrucous hyperplasia in that the troughs of the papillae contain cells with large, dense keratohyaline granules identical to those seen in common cutaneous warts. The basal portion of the lesion is composed of more variable rete ridges, ranging from narrow to broad downgrowths. As with verrucous hyperplasia and carcinoma, the underlying stroma may show prominent chronic inflammation. HPV has been associated with verruca vulgaris (10), but has also been described in verrucous hyperplasia and carcinoma (32). Distinction of verruca vulgaris from verrucous hyperplasia may be difficult or impossible in small biopsy specimens and is of less clinical importance than the distinction from an invasive verrucous carcinoma.

The deep component of all apparent verrucous carcinomas should be carefully examined microscopically to exclude a hybrid neoplasm containing a more conventional-appearing squamous cell carcinoma component (19,22). Such foci may be present in up to 20 percent of cases (22), and their presence excludes a diagnosis of verrucous carcinoma. Any lymph nodes included with a resection specimen should be carefully examined microscopically to exclude such a possibility.

Spread and Metastasis. We agree with others that pure verrucous carcinomas do not metastasize (3,19), although they may, rarely, involve regional lymph nodes by direct extension (2). Regional lymph nodes may be enlarged due to follicular hyperplasia. Accordingly, radical neck dissections are not performed for pure verrucous carcinomas.

Treatment and Prognosis. Surgical resection is the treatment of choice for verrucous carcinoma anywhere in the head and neck region. This is not primarily related to concerns about radiation-induced anaplastic transformation, but because of the widely acknowledged greater local control associated with surgical treatment (14,31). Hagen et al. (14) recommended the following approach for laryngeal tumors: stage T1, carbon dioxide laser excision; stage T2, hemilaryngectomy or laryngofissure with cordectomy; stages T3 and T4, total laryngectomy. As noted above, neck dissection is not indicated for any pure verrucous carcinoma of the head and neck region, given the absence of nodal metastases. Radiotherapy can be utilized in selected clinical settings in which surgical resection is not possible (31).

SPINDLE CELL CARCINOMA

Definition. This variant of squamous cell carcinoma often has a grossly fungating or polypoid growth pattern. It is characterized, microscopically, by a usually prominent spindle cell, sarcoma-like stroma and a minor component of conventional squamous cell carcinoma or in situ carcinoma. Mucosal-based, purely spindle cell neoplasms demonstrating immunohistochemical reactivity for cytokeratin or ultrastructural features of epithelial differentiation and lacking evidence of other differentiation are also included in this group. Mucosal-associated spindle cell neoplasms without demonstrable epithelial differentiation and lacking features of specific sarcomatous differentiation (muscle markers, melanocytic markers, etc) are more problematic, but probably belong in this group as well, based in part on their clinical features and biologic behavior. Other terms applied to these tumors have included: *spindle cell squamous carcinoma, sarcomatoid carcinoma, pseudosarcoma, carcinosarcoma,* and *collision tumor.*

General Features. The nature of these neoplasms has been controversial, at least in the past, and this is reflected in the varying terminology. Some authors have considered them to represent carcinomas with a benign, reactive spindle cell stroma (pseudosarcoma) (45). Others have viewed them as collisions between carcinomas and distinct sarcomas (carcinosarcomas). More recently, however, the use of electron microscopy and immunohistochemistry has strongly supported the concept that these are fundamentally carcinomatous neoplasms that have acquired divergent, mesenchymal differentiation (spindle cell carcinoma). This conclusion was originally based on ultrastructural studies showing residual epithelial features in the spindled cells (36, 48). Subsequently, immunohistochemical studies demonstrated focal reactivity for epithelial markers, primarily cytokeratin, in a high percentage of the spindle cell components (41,56).

Because of the above and their biologic behavior, we believe these tumors should be labeled as spindle cell carcinomas. The term, pseudosarcoma, should particularly be avoided because of possible confusion with benign sarcoma-like processes. Spindle cell carcinomas of the head and are clearly associated with cigarette smoking or use of other tobacco products (47,55). In some series, over 90 percent of patients used tobacco products (47), although it has been suggested by others that this association may not be as strong as for typical squamous carcinomas (37). Some patients with spindle cell carcinomas, particularly those with tumors outside the larynx, have a history of radiation therapy, raising the possibility of radiation-induced neoplasia (46,47).

Clinical Features. The clinical features of spindle cell carcinomas of the head and neck are similar to those of their conventional squamous counterparts (34,36–38,41–44,46–48,52,55,56). Common sites of involvement, from most to least frequent, include the larynx, oral cavity, hypopharynx, and nasal cavity (38). In the Armed Forces Institute of Pathology–Otolaryngic Tumor Registry (AFIP-OTR) encompassing the years 1939 to 1976, there are 81 spindle cell carcinomas of the larynx, accounting for 1.3 percent of tumors in that location (42). The same registry includes 18 spindle cell carcinomas of the sinonasal region (0.6 percent of tumors in this region), and 3 spindle cell carcinomas of the pharynx (0.006 percent) (42). Other series have suggested a somewhat higher frequency of pharyngeal involvement (41,56). Within the larynx, up to 72 percent of cases have involved the vocal cords with almost all of the remainder equally distributed between the hypopharynx and supraglottic larynx (43,44). Subglottic lesions are uncommon (44). Complaints are nonspecific and related to tumor location. Common symptoms include dyspnea, dysphagia, hoarseness, bleeding, otalgia, swelling, loosening of teeth, and a persistent ulceration (55).

At all locations in the head and neck, spindle cell carcinomas show a male predominance (42, 44,47). Lambert et al. (44) reviewed 111 cases of laryngeal spindle cell carcinoma and found a male to female ratio of 10 to 1. Weidner (55) noted that most studies have reported a 4:1 to 2:1 male predominance. Some studies have shown a tendency for spindle cell carcinoma to primarily affect older individuals (mean age, 70 years) (38), whereas other reviews have noted a broader age distribution, from 14 to 94 years with a median of approximately 60 years (55).

Gross Findings. At least two thirds of spindle cell carcinomas have a distinctly polypoid appearance (38,43,44,55). Lesions may range from 1 to 6 cm in size, with polypoid lesions tending to be larger (fig. 5-8) (47). The surface may be intact or ulcerated and covered with a fibrinopurulent exudate. Polypoid lesions have an obvious attenuated stalk. Infiltrating, nonpolypoid variants are grossly indistinguishable from conventional squamous cell carcinomas. On sectioning of the polypoid variant, the mass is typically firm and tan or white. Central necrosis is not a common feature (55).

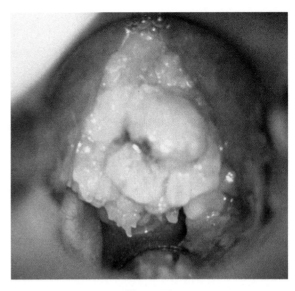

Figure 5-8
SPINDLE CELL CARCINOMA
Spindle cell carcinomas of the larynx are often exophytic, distinctly polypoid masses.

Microscopic Findings. The spindle cell element is virtually always predominant and varies considerably in its microscopic appearance (43). It may exhibit obvious differentiation in the form of collagen production or, occasionally, an osteoid or cartilaginous matrix (44,46). Most lesions labeled as osteosarcoma of the larynx are probably spindle cell carcinomas with osteoid production by the metaplastic tumor cells. The cellularity and pleomorphism of the spindle component may be quite variable. In some instances the spindled cells are thin and dispersed in a myxoid matrix, a pattern resembling so-called myxoid malignant fibrous histiocytoma. There may be microcyst formation within the stroma (47). The myxoid areas contain variable numbers of inflammatory cells, mainly of acute type. There may be prominent xanthoma cells containing abundant lipidized cytoplasm or hyaline-like globules (47). In these cases, the major diagnostic question relates to whether the stromal cells are reactive or a portion of the neoplasm. Even in these relatively hypocellular areas, mitotic activity is easily demonstrated, and atypical forms are common (47). In other instances, the spindle cell component is obviously malignant and composed of densely cellular, enlarged pleomorphic cells with little intervening stroma (figs. 5-9, 5-10). Widely dilated, branching blood vessels may

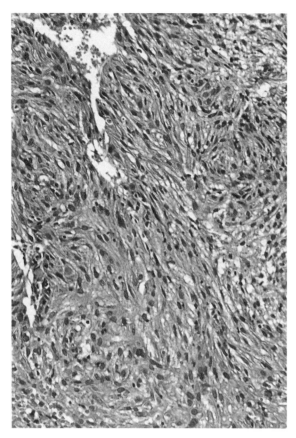

Figure 5-9
SPINDLE CELL CARCINOMA
This spindle cell carcinoma of the larynx could easily be mistaken for a sarcoma. Clear-cut epithelial differentiation is not present.

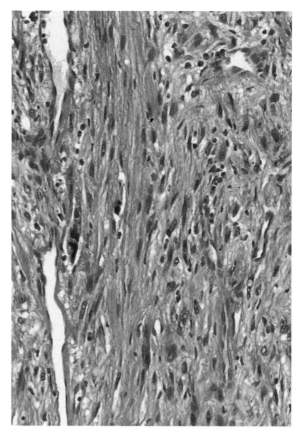

Figure 5-10
SPINDLE CELL CARCINOMA
The neoplastic cells of this laryngeal spindle cell carcinoma grow in "sarcoma-like" fascicles. Epithelial features are not present in this microscopic field.

create the appearance of an hemangiopericytoma. Highly pleomorphic stromal cells may intersect in a storiform pattern suggestive of a malignant fibrous histiocytoma. Areas of overt osteoid or cartilage formation by neoplastic cells are common (46). The osteoid may be well-formed and benign or reactive appearing, or it may have the "lace-like" appearance of osteoid seen in osteosarcomas. These areas of osteoid or chondroid have been said to be more common in patients with prior radiation therapy (55).

The overtly squamous elements may be abundant and evenly distributed throughout the tumor (fig. 5-11). More often, however, they are a minor component in an overwhelmingly sarcoma-like neoplasm. The squamous elements may be located superficially, in association with high-grade surface dysplastic changes (47), or

they may be present deep within the lesion at the base or stalk, making them difficult or impossible to obtain in superficial biopsy specimens (43). The junction between the overtly squamous and spindle cell components is sometimes abrupt, but more often the interface is blurred.

Immunohistochemical Findings. Zarbo et al. (56) noted that 8 of 13 patients with biphasic spindle cell carcinomas had spindle cell components that were immunoreactive for cytokeratin. In 3 of the cases the reactivity was focal, and in the remaining 5 it was diffuse (fig. 5-12). Four of 7 pure spindle cell tumors with surface ulceration were also reactive for cytokeratin. Spindle cells expressing both cytokeratin and vimentin have been occasionally identified. In a separate study of 21 cases, Ellis et al. (41) documented reactivity for cytokeratin in the spindle cell component of

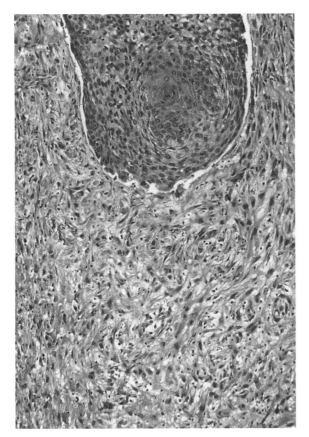

Figure 5-11
SQUAMOUS CELL CARCINOMA
WITH SPINDLE CELL COMPONENT
A nest of conventional squamous cell carcinoma is sharply demarcated from the adjacent neoplastic spindle cell carcinomatous component. When present these nests allow ready diagnosis of spindle cell carcinoma. In their absence, additional studies may be required to confirm the diagnosis.

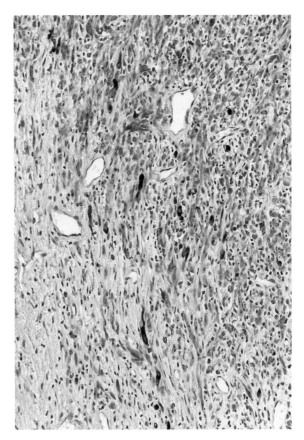

Figure 5-12
SPINDLE CELL CARCINOMA
The spindled cells in this spindle cell carcinoma show focal strong positivity for cytokeratin (anticytokeratin, hematoxylin).

13. The spindle cells lacked reactivity for S-100 protein, but were reactive for alpha-1-antitrypsin and alpha-1-antichymotrypsin. A potentially confusing factor with regard to the immunohistochemical findings in spindle cell carcinoma is the occasional presence of myogenous markers (50,51). One study documented pan-muscle actin in 42 percent of spindle cell neoplasms with an associated conventional squamous cell carcinoma component (50). In 25 percent of these cases, both cytokeratin and actin were expressed. Only one of the tumors expressed desmin and none expressed sarcomeric actin. Other studies have documented desmin in a minority of these tumors (40,51).

Ultrastructural Findings. Electron microscopic studies have confirmed at least focal epithelial features in the spindle cell component of these neoplasms. Zarbo et al. (56) performed ultrastructural studies on the spindle cell elements in 13 tumors. Of 5 biphasic tumors that were nonreactive for cytokeratin, 3 showed ultrastructural evidence of epithelial differentiation. Of 4 monophasic spindle cell tumors that were reactive for cytokeratin, 1 showed epithelial features ultrastructurally. Thus, in comparison to immunohistochemistry, electron microscopy is a somewhat less sensitive, but complementary technique for identifying epithelial features. The early ultrastructural study by Battifora (36) demonstrated apparent modulation of the neoplastic cells from epithelioid to mesenchymal features, supporting their fundamentally epithelioid lineage.

Differential Diagnosis. The diagnostic approach to pure spindle cell neoplasms of the head and neck has been problematic. In the past, as noted above, when such lesions showed focal osteoid or chondroid production, they were invariably labeled as osteosarcoma or chondrosarcoma. Pure spindle cell lesions without an obvious osteoid or chondroid matrix were interpreted as fibrosarcoma or malignant fibrous histiocytoma. It is generally (but not universally) accepted that when these neoplasms exhibit at least focal cytokeratin production or ultrastructural evidence of epithelioid differentiation, they should be considered as spindle cell carcinomas (56). Even in the absence of demonstrable epithelioid differentiation, we believe most, if not all such neoplasms behave as spindle cell carcinomas.

It is important to consider a mucosal malignant melanoma in the differential diagnosis of any spindle cell neoplasm involving the mucosal membranes of the head and neck. Immunohistochemical studies for S-100 protein and with HMB-45, coupled with epithelial markers, greatly aid in this distinction. Rhabdomyosarcoma may also be a consideration and, if necessary, immunohistochemical studies for myogenous markers may be added to the diagnostic panel. As discussed above, however, pan-actin markers are often focally positive in spindle cell carcinomas and desmin may be focally positive as well. Strong positivity for desmin or, more importantly, for sarcomeric actin would support a diagnosis of rhabdomyosarcoma.

Spread and Metastases. The metastatic rate to regional (cervical) lymph nodes is 15 percent for tumors arising from the vocal cords, 30 percent for supraglottic lesions, and 66 percent for hypopharyngeal tumors (44). Initial studies suggested that only the carcinomatous component was capable of metastasis, but metastasis of the sarcoma-like, spindle cell elements has been well documented (39,43,49,53,54). The tendency to involve regional lymph nodes with later systemic dissemination is further evidence of the carcinomatous nature of these neoplasms.

Treatment and Prognosis. Radiation therapy as a primary treatment modality has been of questionable value (38). Lambert et al. (44) noted that four patients with glottic tumors (3 of T1N0, 1 of T2N0) all had persistent or recurrent disease 1 year after radiation therapy, necessitating total laryngectomy. Of 10 additional patients of unknown clinical stage who received radiation therapy, 8 had recurrent or persistent disease. The role of radiation as adjuvant therapy is even less understood (38).

In a review of 23 patients treated by local resection, with or without adjuvant radiation therapy, 13 demonstrated no evidence of recurrence with a minimum follow-up of 3 years; 10 patients developed recurrences requiring additional surgery (44). The overall 3-year survival rate for glottic polypoid tumors was 90 percent, but was only 44 percent for the less frequent sessile glottic lesions. Patients with supraglottic and hypopharyngeal spindle cell tumors did poorly, regardless of gross features. Only one of the 3-year survivors had cervical lymph node metastases at the time of diagnosis. Berthelet et al. (38) noted 2-year and 5-year disease-free survival rates of 52 percent and 45 percent, respectively, for a series of 17 patients with tumors from all head and neck sites, treated primarily by surgical resection, with or without radiation therapy. Batsakis et al. (35), in a review of 154 cases, noted a 34 percent overall mortality for patients with laryngeal tumors, a 60 percent mortality for those with oral cavity tumors, and a 77 percent mortality for those with sinonasal tract tumors. Other studies have not shown an improved survival for patients with laryngeal tumors (38). Leventon and Evans (47) noted that the overall size of the lesions did not correlate with survival, and they suggested that local invasion was the key to prognostication: of 10 patients with polypoid, superficial tumors, none died of disease, whereas 9 of 10 patients with invasive tumors died as a result of their tumors. This is a potentially important point because many large tumors of the larynx are exophytic with no invasion at the point of stalk attachment. These should not be labeled as T2 tumors, but should be staged based on the degree of invasion at their attachment site.

BASALOID SQUAMOUS CELL CARCINOMA

Definition. This variant of squamous cell carcinoma is characterized by nests of small basaloid cells with a high nuclear to cytoplasmic ratio and little visible cytoplasm. Central necrosis within the cell nests is often prominent. Areas of more conventional squamous cell carcinoma are present but are usually a minor component. Stage for stage, biologic behavior appears to be analogous to that of poorly differentiated, conventional squamous cell carcinoma. However, the basaloid variant often presents as an advanced stage lesion, with an associated poor prognosis. This variant should also be recognized because of its associated distinct diagnostic problems.

General Features. This form of squamous cell carcinoma was first described as a distinct entity in the head and neck region by Wain et al. in 1986 (83). Histologically identical tumors had been recognized at other anatomic sites, such as the anus (64), thymus (84), and esophagus (81), and had been referred to by a variety of terms including cloacogenic carcinoma or basaloid carcinoma. As discussed under Differential Diagnosis, these tumors in the head and neck region had been previously placed in a variety of diagnostic categories including small cell undifferentiated carcinoma, adenoid cystic carcinoma, and adenosquamous carcinoma (83). The clinical features and biologic behavior of such tumors are distinct from those of basaloid squamous cell carcinoma, or stage-matched conventional squamous cell carcinoma, and this distinction is thus important.

Basaloid squamous cell carcinomas show the same strong association with tobacco and alcohol usage seen with conventional squamous cell carcinomas (59). In one review, 24 of 26 patients with known smoking status were smokers; similarly, 22 of 25 were known to drink ethanol (59). Initial studies of this tumor noted its strong predilection for the hypopharynx and supraglottic laryngeal regions (59,72,75,83). More recent studies have continued to document a striking predilection for these areas (65,69,78,80), but have noted smaller numbers of cases from other anatomic sites including the nasopharynx (85), floor of mouth (60,62), oral cavity (63), palate (67,71,82), and nasal cavity (86). Occasional cases have involved the tracheobronchial tree (70,79).

One study of three nasopharyngeal basaloid squamous cell carcinomas noted that all contained Epstein-Barr (EBV) virus RNA by in situ hybridization (85). This is not surprising given the strong association of EBV with several other forms of squamous neoplasia in the nasopharynx (73,77,87). Thus far, Epstein-Barr virus has not been associated with this tumor at other locations in the head and neck (87).

Clinical Features. The clinical features of basaloid squamous cell carcinoma are generally similar to those of conventional squamous cell carcinoma, although there are distinctions. The basaloid tumors show a strong predilection to involve the base of the tongue, pyriform sinus, supraglottic larynx, and palatine tonsil (59,83). They tend to present as advanced lesions. In our series of 40 patients (59), 10 tumors were stage III and 21 were stage IV at the time of presentation; 27 had metastasized to regional lymph nodes at the time of diagnosis.

As with most head and neck carcinomas, at least historically, there is a strong male predominance. In our series of 40 patients, 35 were men and 5 were women. The presenting complaints varied with anatomic site, but typically consisted of sore throat (10 of 40), hoarseness (6 of 40), dysphagia (3 of 40), tinnitus (2 of 40), nasal obstruction (2 of 40), epistaxis (2 of 40), hemoptysis (1 of 40), and night sweats (1 of 40).

Gross Findings. The gross appearance of the tumor is not highly distinctive. However, it has been noted that basaloid squamous cell carcinomas are seldom exophytic, and that they are often centrally ulcerated with considerable induration of the adjacent nonulcerated mucosa (65, 72). The latter feature is due to tumor spread beneath intact surface epithelium. On cross section, the tumors are typically dense, firm, pale, focally ulcerated, infiltrating masses (65,72,78).

Microscopic Findings. These tumors are composed of closely packed, moderately pleomorphic basaloid cells arranged in variably sized nests and cords. Larger nests frequently exhibit central comedonecrosis (fig. 5-13) (59,72,78,83). The smaller nests often feature prominent single-cell necrosis. Cells at the edges of the nests may show nuclear palisading. A cribriform-like pattern within the cell nests, due to the interspersion of mucinous material or hyalinized stroma, is common and mimics the low-power microscopic appearance of adenoid cystic carcinoma (figs. 5-14, 5-15). Smaller gland-like spaces filled with mucin or hyalinized material are sometimes seen in the cell nests. In about two thirds of cases, the stroma between the cell nests has, at least focally, a dense, refractile, hyalinized appearance. In other areas stromal mucin may be prominent, creating a myxoid basophilic background. This material stains for connective tissue mucins,

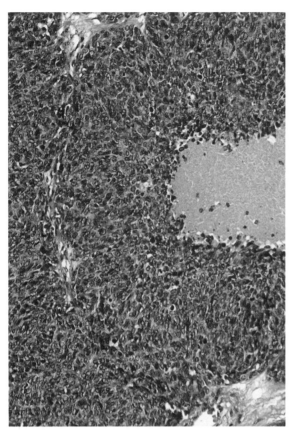

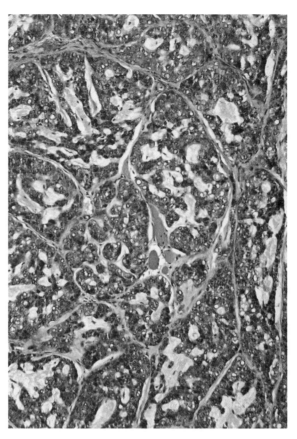

Figure 5-13
BASALOID SQUAMOUS CELL CARCINOMA
This basaloid squamous cell carcinoma contains large nests of basaloid cells, some of which exhibit central comedo-like necrosis.

Figure 5-14
BASALOID SQUAMOUS CELL CARCINOMA
This basaloid squamous cell carcinoma has a cribriform growth pattern with nests of cells surrounding mucoid material. However, the basaloid cells are far more pleomorphic than those of adenoid cystic carcinoma.

but the neoplastic cells are negative for intracytoplasmic epithelial mucins (59).

The basaloid neoplastic cells have a high nuclear to cytoplasmic ratio, often with dense, hyperchromatic nuclei. Occasionally, nuclei may be more vesicular with scattered nucleoli. Mitotic figures are usually numerous, and atypical forms are easily found (59). Foci of overt squamous differentiation consisting of cells with more abundant eosinophilic cytoplasm, intercellular bridges, or keratin pearl formation are invariably present (fig. 5-16). The interface between the nests of squamous cells and the surrounding basaloid cells is abrupt with no transitional cells between the two components. Occasionally, large zones of conventional squamous cell carcinoma may be found outside of but adjacent to the basaloid component (59).

If there is intact surface mucosa overlying a basaloid squamous cell carcinoma, this frequently demonstrates high-grade dysplasia. In one study, 34 of 40 cases showed direct continuity with overlying dysplastic epithelium (59). In many instances, the carcinoma appears to "drop off" from the overlying dysplastic epithelium. Occasionally, the neoplasm appears to "drop off" the basal cell layer with no dysplasia in the overlying surface epithelium (fig. 5-17). Metastases of basaloid squamous cell carcinoma resemble the primary tumors and often have a prominent basaloid component.

Immunohistochemical Findings. Basaloid squamous cell carcinomas show surprisingly weak, focal or absent reactivity for cytokeratin in the basaloid component (59,81). Most examples are reactive, at least focally, for cytokeratin, if one

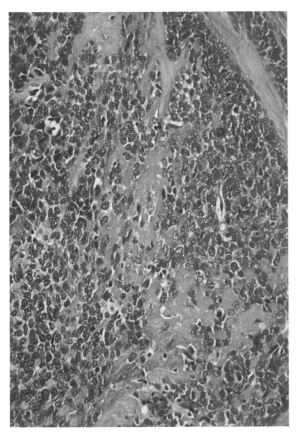

Figure 5-15
BASALOID SQUAMOUS CELL CARCINOMA
This basaloid squamous cell carcinoma has areas of stromal sclerosis surrounded by basaloid cells.

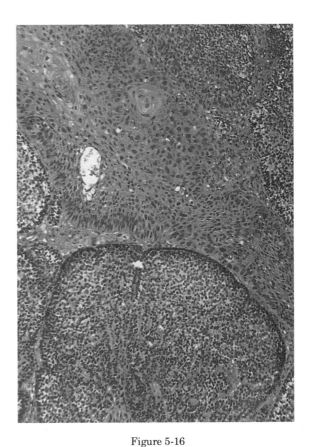

Figure 5-16
BASALOID SQUAMOUS CELL CARCINOMA
A nest of basaloid cells (bottom) is closely apposed to, but distinct from, a nest of conventional squamous cell carcinoma with keratinization (top and center). Foci of conventional squamous cell carcinoma are invariably present in basaloid squamous cell carcinoma.

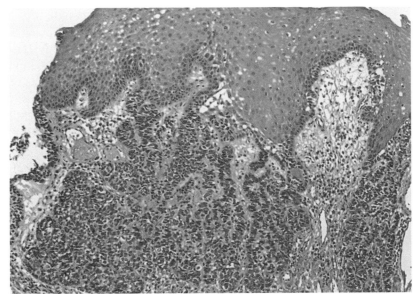

Figure 5-17
NEOPLASTIC BASALOID CELLS
Strands of neoplastic basaloid cells appear to "drop off" from a mucosal basal cell layer. The overlying squamous mucosa appears hyperplastic, but does not show changes of dysplasia.

uses a mixture (cocktail) of antibodies including CAM5.2, AE1/AE3, and 34BE12 (59,81). Our study (59) showed that admixed components of conventional squamous cell carcinoma exhibit much stronger positivity. Punctate cytokeratin positivity of the type encountered in small cell neuroendocrine carcinomas was not seen. In the same study, 83 percent of tumors reacted for epithelial membrane antigen. Although these tumors may display abortive neuroendocrine differentiation, this feature remains to be further studied. In our study, 75 percent of cases showed diffuse, weak reactivity for neuron-specific enolase, but we are uncertain of the significance of this finding. The tumors did not react for synaptophysin or chromogranin. In 16 of 30 cases, the squamous cells in the tumors displayed reactivity for carcinoembryonic antigen, but the basaloid cells did not react for this marker. In 14 of 36 cases, there was focal positivity for S-100 protein in the neoplastic cells, and virtually all tumors contained scattered S-100 protein-positive dendritic cells.

Ultrastructural Findings. Wain et al. (83) studied five basaloid squamous cell carcinomas ultrastructurally. The cytoplasm contained well-formed desmosomes, rare bundles of tonofilaments, and scattered free ribosomes, with few other organelles. The cyst-like spaces seen at the light microscopic level were true extracellular spaces lined by basal lamina. There were no neurosecretory granules, no myofilaments with dense bodies, and no evidence of glandular or secretory differentiation.

Differential Diagnosis. In small biopsy specimens, basaloid squamous cell carcinoma can resemble small cell undifferentiated carcinoma. This distinction is important because the latter tumors are treated with specific radiation therapy and chemotherapy protocols. Small cell undifferentiated carcinomas may contain foci of squamous differentiation, but these are not as extensive as in basaloid squamous cell carcinoma, and they are not associated with dysplasia of the overlying surface mucosa (76). They also lack the stromal mucin and pseudoglandular structures frequently seen in basaloid squamous cell carcinomas (59). Immunohistochemical studies may be of some value in making this distinction. Although both tumors may express neuron-specific enolase, basaloid squamous cell carcinomas lack staining for chromogranin or

synaptophysin. Gnepp and Wick (66) noted that at least one neuroendocrine marker was positive when neuron-specific enolase, chromogranin, synaptophysin, and Leu-7 were applied to a series of small cell undifferentiated carcinomas from the salivary glands of the head and neck. In addition, basaloid squamous cell carcinomas lack the punctate perinuclear cytokeratin positivity that is typical of the other tumor. Ultrastructurally, basaloid squamous cell carcinomas lack evidence of neuroendocrine differentiation (83), whereas dense core granules have been documented in small cell undifferentiated carcinomas from the head and neck region (68,76).

In our experience, basaloid squamous cell carcinomas are also commonly confused with adenoid cystic carcinomas, a mistake of considerable clinical importance. Adenoid cystic carcinomas, although often fatal, are more indolent neoplasms that do not metastasize to regional lymph nodes (57,74). A review of publications dealing with "adenoid cystic carcinomas" from a variety of anatomic sites shows multiple examples better interpreted as basaloid squamous cell carcinoma (81). This distinction is usually straightforward at the light microscopic level if one is familiar with both diagnostic possibilities. Basaloid squamous cell carcinomas often show continuity with overlying surface epithelium, are often associated with dysplasia of the overlying epithelium, and invariably contain foci of squamous differentiation. These features are not found in adenoid cystic carcinomas arising in salivary glands or seromucinous glands of the head and neck region. Cribriform and pseudoglandular structures, as well as connective tissue mucin, may be seen in both tumor types and are of no diagnostic value. Cytologically, the cells of adenoid cystic carcinoma have small uniform nuclei, typically lack nucleoli, and have scant amounts of cytoplasm. The cells of basaloid squamous cell carcinoma are far more pleomorphic and more mitotically active.

Clinical findings are also of value in making this distinction. Basaloid squamous cell carcinoma strongly predilects the hypopharynx, base of tongue, supraglottic larynx, and tonsillar regions (59,65,72,78,83). There are often associated regional lymph node metastases. Embolic lymph node metastases are virtually nonexistent with true adenoid cystic carcinoma, which metastasizes hematogenously and only involves regional lymph nodes by direct extension (57).

Immunohistochemistry is of some qualitative value in distinguishing these two tumor types when confronted with small biopsy specimens. Cytokeratin staining tends to be more prominent in the basaloid cells of adenoid cystic carcinoma. Epithelial membrane antigen is focally present in basaloid squamous cell carcinoma, primarily in the larger squamous cells. In adenoid cystic carcinoma, it is present in the apices of basaloid cells lining duct-like spaces. Likewise, carcinoembryonic antigen (CEA) is present in basaloid squamous cell carcinomas, but is almost exclusively present in the larger squamous cells, rather than the diagnostically problematic basaloid component (59,81). In adenoid cystic carcinoma, CEA reactivity is chiefly present in the cells that line duct-like structures (88). Over 60 percent of adenoid cystic carcinomas with a cribriform growth pattern are immunoreactive for muscle-specific actin (61). In our experience basaloid squamous carcinomas are uniformly negative for this antigen, even in areas with a cribriform growth pattern.

Cytology. In fine needle aspiration specimens, basaloid squamous cell carcinomas have been confused with both small cell undifferentiated carcinomas and adenoid cystic carcinomas (58). The basaloid cells have round or oval, hyperchromatic nuclei with small nucleoli. In one study of nine cases (58), only three tumors had occasional keratinized cells; six contained necrotic debris; pseudoglandular structures with stromal cores, mimicking adenoid cystic carcinoma, were present in four; and nuclear molding was present in seven. Three cases were originally diagnosed as small cell undifferentiated carcinoma. On review, each contained a few fragments of larger, tightly cohesive cells with vesicular nuclei.

Treatment and Prognosis. No approaches to treatment have been systematically studied. Patients usually receive resection, if possible, often followed by adjuvant radiation therapy, chemotherapy, or both. Twenty-six of our 40 patients underwent resection, and 32 received chemotherapy, radiation therapy, or both (59). Local recurrences were documented in 6 patients, and distant metastases developed in 15 patients, most often involving the lung (13 patients). Other sites of distant disease included liver, bone, and central nervous system. Of our 40 patients, 50 percent were alive 1 year postdiagnosis, but 7 of these had persistent disease. Seventeen patients died of disease from 2 months to 4 years (median, 18 months) after diagnosis.

At the time of the initial description of these neoplasms, it was suggested that they had a worse prognosis than conventional squamous cell carcinomas (83). More recent studies have noted that, stage for stage, the prognoses appear to be similar (59,72). However, because of the advanced stage at presentation, the overall prognosis for this group of tumors tends to be poor.

PAPILLARY SQUAMOUS CELL CARCINOMA

Definition. This poorly documented variant of squamous cell carcinoma has a papilloma-like low-power microscopic appearance, but is composed of papillae covered by overtly malignant squamous cells. The latter feature distinguishes these tumors from papillomas, verrucous carcinomas, or mixed verrucous and conventional squamous carcinomas. The neoplasm may be completely exophytic, but often there is an underlying component of nonpapillary, invasive squamous cell carcinoma. Documentation of the underlying invasion can be difficult or impossible with superficial biopsies.

General Features. Papillary squamous cell carcinomas have been described at a variety of anatomic sites, such as the uterine cervix, and are noted for the difficulties associated with assessing invasion (91). In the head and neck region, the relationship of these neoplasms to benign papillary proliferations of the sinonasal region, including schneiderian papillomas, is unclear. Also unclear is any association with HPV. In one in situ hybridization study of a variety of papillary lesions from the head and neck, papillomas routinely expressed HPV types 6 and 11, but six papillary squamous cell carcinomas were uniformly negative for HPV DNA (89). All six of these tumors were also noted to have an aneuploid DNA content. A separate study failed to find HPV DNA by in situ hybridization in three papillary squamous cell carcinomas, but did report HPV type 6 DNA by polymerase chain reaction (PCR) in a single example (90).

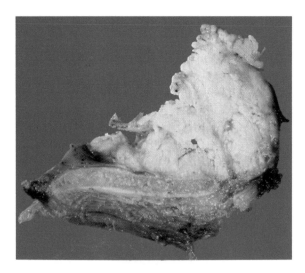

Figure 5-18
PAPILLARY SQUAMOUS CELL CARCINOMA
This papillary squamous cell carcinoma of the larynx produced a large intraluminal "cauliflower-like" mass.

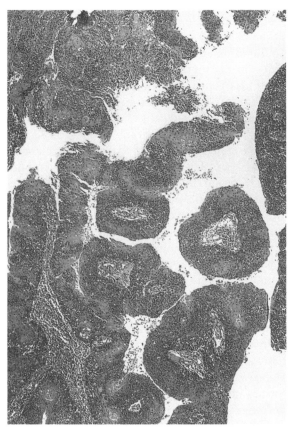

Figure 5-19
PAPILLARY SQUAMOUS CELL CARCINOMA
Microscopically, papillary squamous cell carcinomas are highly complex, with surface papillations often overlying nests of invasive squamous cell carcinoma.

Clinical Features. The small numbers of well-documented cases have shown a strong male predilection (89,90). Sites of involvement have included the larynx, pyriform sinus, oropharynx, nasal cavity, and maxillary antrum.

The natural history of the noninvasive form of papillary squamous cell carcinoma is unclear. Crissman et al. (89) have suggested that the rate of transformation to an invasive lesion is high.

Gross Findings. These tumors often have a grossly papillary appearance similar to that of verrucous carcinoma, but they lack the prominent surface keratinization seen in the latter tumor (fig. 5-18).

Microscopic Findings. Crissman et al. (89) divided papillary squamous carcinomas into two groups: those with underlying invasive carcinoma and those lacking underlying invasion. The noninvasive variant consists entirely of an exophytic proliferation of malignant-appearing squamous cells covering papillae with fibrovascular cores (fig. 5-19). The epithelium varies in thickness and may be of approximately the same thickness as that seen in a papilloma, or thicker or thinner than that. In our experience, the covering epithelium is often paradoxically thinner than in a benign papilloma. The epithelial cells may be immature and basal cell–like, resembling the appearance of "classic" carcinoma in situ as described in the uterine cervix (89). Alternately, there may be marked pleomorphism with prominent nuclear and cytoplasmic variation, individual cell keratinization (dyskeratosis), and surface keratin deposition (fig. 5-20).

The invasive form of the tumor is similar to the above (fig. 5-21), but contains an underlying component of invasive squamous cell carcinoma. In most instances the pattern of the underlying invasive component is that of conventional, nonpapillary squamous cell carcinoma (fig. 5-22). We have encountered examples in which the papillary pattern was at least partially retained in the invasive and metastatic components of the tumor. Reaching or excluding the invasive component can be difficult when endoscopic biopsies

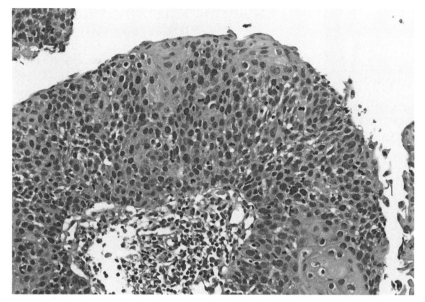

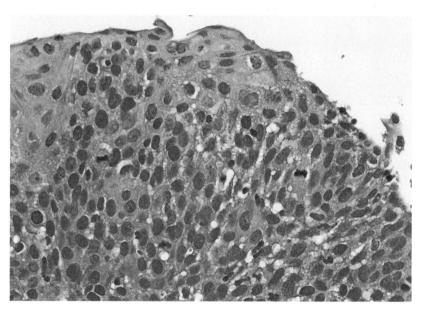

Figure 5-20
PAPILLARY SQUAMOUS
CELL CARCINOMA
Unlike verrucous carcinoma, the papillae of papillary squamous cell carcinoma lack abundant surface keratinization and are composed of variably atypical to overtly malignant cells.

are performed. Typically, the best approach is to obtain multiple biopsies from the same spot, first removing the papillary component and then assessing the underlying stroma.

Differential Diagnosis. As noted above, the major problem associated with these neoplasms is the assessment of underlying invasion. At low-power magnification, papillary squamous cell carcinoma may resemble a schneiderian papilloma. However, at higher magnification, the obvious cellular pleomorphism and mitotic activity allow

ready distinction. Likewise, these lesions should not be confused with verrucous carcinomas because of their cytologic features of malignancy, which are lacking, by definition, in the former tumors.

Treatment and Prognosis. Although the number of well-documented cases is small, the biologic behavior of papillary squamous cell carcinoma with invasion appears to be analogous to that of conventional squamous cell carcinoma of equal stage.

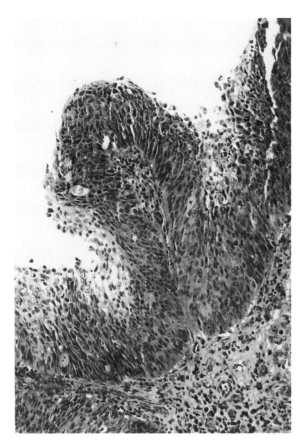

Figure 5-21
PAPILLARY SQUAMOUS CELL CARCINOMA

This papillary squamous cell carcinoma is composed of surface papillae lined by highly dysplastic cells. Edges of cell nests just visible at the lower right suggest underlying invasion.

UNDIFFERENTIATED CARCINOMA (LYMPHOEPITHELIOMA)

Definition. This is a variant of carcinoma most commonly involving the nasopharynx and characterized by a neoplastic proliferation of medium-sized, light microscopically undifferentiated, chromatically uniform cells, usually associated with a prominent reactive lymphoplasmacytic infiltrate. Abortive features of squamous differentiation may be identified at the ultrastructural level. Synonyms for this tumor have included *undifferentiated carcinoma, lymphoepithelioma-like carcinoma, lymphoepithelioma of Regaud or Schmincke, embryonal carcinoma,* and *transitional carcinoma.*

General Features. Understanding of this neoplasm was greatly aided by the adoption of the 1978 World Health Organization (WHO) classification scheme which distinguished three forms of nonglandular nasopharyngeal carcinoma: 1) keratinizing squamous cell carcinoma, 2) non-keratinizing carcinoma, and 3) undifferentiated carcinoma (lymphoepithelioma). The last group of lesions forms the current topic of discussion.

The term lymphoepithelioma is a well-recognized if rather inaccurate designation for this group of neoplasms which is contained, at least parenthetically, in the WHO designation. The word was coined by initial observers who noted the intimate association of the lymphoid and epithelial elements and erroneously concluded

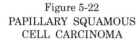

Figure 5-22
PAPILLARY SQUAMOUS
CELL CARCINOMA

Lower magnification of the lesion seen in figure 5-21 shows nests of poorly differentiated, nonpapillary squamous cell carcinoma beneath the surface papillations.

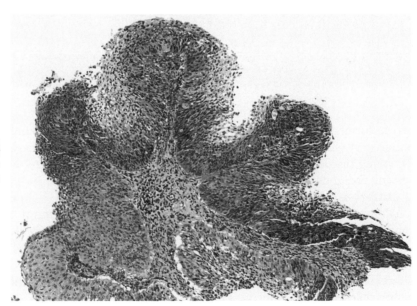

that this was a mixed lymphocytic and epithelial neoplasm. Their misconception was understandable, given the florid lymphoid response associated with these neoplasms, even at sites of distant metastatic disease. We favor the designation of "undifferentiated carcinoma, lymphoepithelioma type," although in practice this is often shortened to simply "lymphoepithelioma." Using the term undifferentiated carcinoma without modifiers leads to confusion with other distinct entities including small cell undifferentiated carcinoma and sinonasal undifferentiated carcinoma.

The epidemiology of these tumors has been intensively examined. Early studies concentrated on environmental and dietary factors, such as the ingestion of dimethylnitrosamine-containing smoked fish by southern Chinese, a group known to have a high incidence of this tumor (140). The role of cigarette smoking remains unclear and does not appear to be as strong as with conventional squamous cell carcinomas at other anatomic sites such as the larynx. Genetic factors have also been examined. In Hong Kong, nasopharyngeal carcinomas account for 18 percent of all malignancies, as compared to 2 percent in the United States (100). It has been noted that racial susceptibility tends to remain constant in those emigrating to other countries. Chinese patients in Singapore with this tumor have a significantly increased frequency of histocompatibility antigens HLA-A2 and HLA-BW46 (133). Other studies have noted that the frequency of nasopharyngeal carcinoma is decreased in patients with blood group A (97).

In the last 10 years, the role of EBV in the pathogenesis of these tumors has undergone considerable research. The association between EBV and nasopharyngeal carcinoma of both undifferentiated and nonkeratinizing types is now well established (95,96,103,105,107,114,116,117,121,125, 131,138,139). Genomic EBV DNA has been repeatedly demonstrated in the proliferating epithelial cells of undifferentiated and some nonkeratinizing carcinomas of the nasopharyngeal region using in situ hybridization (106,131,139). In addition, serum antibodies against viral capsid antigens have been useful in the diagnosis of metastases from occult primaries (121,128,135).

Tumors light microscopically identical to nasopharyngeal lymphoepitheliomas have been described in a variety of anatomic sites, including other areas of the head and neck region. The term *lymphoepithelioma-like carcinoma* has been applied to these neoplasms. In the salivary glands, thymus, larynx, lungs, and stomach an association with EBV has been shown in multiple studies (103,107,138), and one study has suggested the presence of EBV in tumors of this type involving the tonsil (110). Interestingly, in salivary gland and lung, the association with EBV is restricted to Asian patients, whereas in stomach and thymus, the association has been independent of ethnic or geographic factors (107). Microscopically identical tumors occurring in other anatomic sites such as skin, urinary bladder, and uterine cervix, have not been shown to contain EBV DNA, suggesting fundamentally different pathogenetic factors for the evolution of these neoplasms (103,107). Importantly, regardless of anatomic site, the presence or absence of EBV DNA appears to be of no prognostic importance (107).

Clinical Features. Nasopharyngeal undifferentiated carcinomas of lymphoepithelioma type occur in a broad age range and often affect children. There is a distinct, bimodal age distribution with peaks in the second and sixth decades of life (98,101,104,106,130,131). All forms of nasopharyngeal carcinoma (squamous, nonkeratinizing, and lymphoepithelioma) show a male predilection of approximately 2.5 to 1 (98,101,131).

A high percentage of nasopharyngeal carcinomas of lymphoepithelioma type arise near the eustachian tube opening in the fossa of Rosenmüller. Not surprisingly, presenting symptoms are often related to middle ear obstruction, with serous otitis and associated hearing loss. Local invasion may result in headaches, cranial nerve deficits, or epistaxis (93,98,101). Importantly, over half of patients with lymphoepithelioma-type carcinomas of the nasopharynx have clinically apparent cervical lymph node metastases as a presenting sign or symptom, with a much less obvious or clinically occult nasopharyngeal primary; about 25 percent of these individuals have bilateral cervical lymph node metastases (fig. 5-23) (93,98). The involved nodes are typically located posterior to the sternocleidomastoid muscle at the level of the mandibular angle (98). This location is unusual for metastases from more common sites of carcinoma arising in the head and neck, and serves as a clue to strongly consider a primary neoplasm in the nasopharynx.

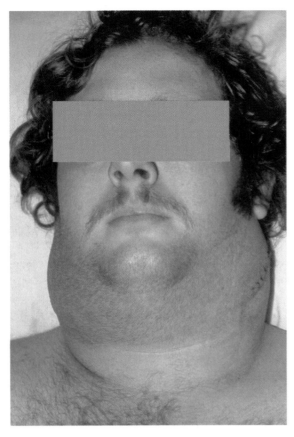

Figure 5-23
NASOPHARYNGEAL
UNDIFFERENTIATED CARCINOMA
Nasopharyngeal undifferentiated carcinoma often has a clinical presentation dominated by metastatic disease from an occult primary. Not infrequently, the metastases are bilateral, mimicking a lymphoma. (Fig. 75 from Collins RD, Casey TT, Glick AD, McCurley TL, Swerdlow SH, Cousar JB. Lymph nodes. In: Sternberg SS. Diagnostic surgical pathology, 2nd ed. New York: Raven Press, 1994:725.)

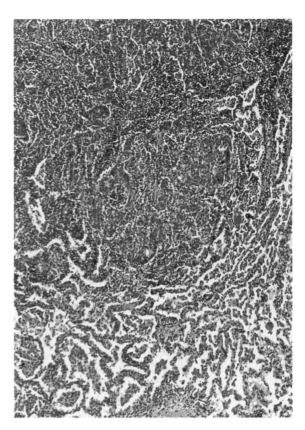

Figure 5-24
METASTASIS FROM A NASOPHARYNGEAL
UNDIFFERENTIATED CARCINOMA
This lung metastasis from a nasopharyngeal undifferentiated carcinoma evokes the same dense reactive lymphoid infiltrate seen at the site of the primary tumor.

On examination, the nasopharynx may appear entirely normal, or there may be fullness or surface granularity; an obvious carcinoma is uncommon. Even when the nasopharynx appears normal, initial biopsies from the region of the fossa of Rosenmüller yield diagnostic tissue in almost three fourths of patients (98). The remaining patients may require rebiopsy.

Gross Findings. Because these tumors are virtually never resected, gross descriptions of primary lesions are rare. Lymph nodes replaced by metastatic lymphoepithelioma-type carcinoma have a uniform, pale tan, lymphoma-like appearance.

Microscopic Findings. Undifferentiated carcinoma of lymphoepithelioma type is charac-

terized, microscopically, by cytologically uniform cells with uniformly vesicular, round to oval nuclei and medium-sized nucleoli. Mitotic figures are typically numerous, usually ranging from 5 to 10 per 10 high-power fields (104). When the neoplastic cells grow in cohesive nests, the cell borders between adjacent cells are indistinct, creating a syncytial cytoplasmic appearance. By definition, keratinization or squamous "pearl" formation, as well as glandular differentiation, are absent. Spindle cells may be present, as well as apoptotic cells with shrunken, hyperchromatic nuclei. An inflammatory infiltrate primarily consisting of lymphocytes and plasma cells, but occasionally with prominent eosinophils (113,115), is a key feature of lymphoepithelioma-type carcinoma. The lymphoid infiltrate is often present in metastases as well as primary tumors (fig. 5-24), although in some cases the metastases

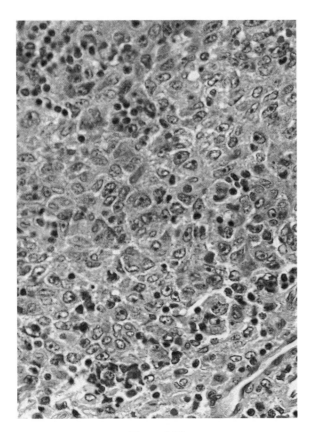

Figure 5-25
NASOPHARYNGEAL
UNDIFFERENTIATED CARCINOMA

Some nasopharyngeal undifferentiated carcinomas have a relatively sparse lymphoid infiltrate. The diagnosis nonetheless remains appropriate provided the neoplastic cells have characteristic, chromatically uniform vesicular nuclei, with no overt evidence of squamous differentiation.

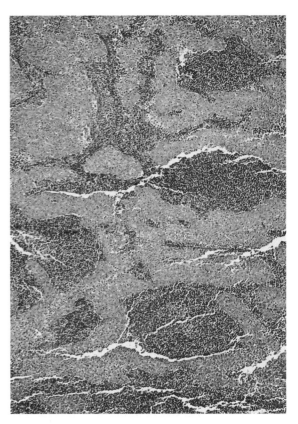

Figure 5-26
NASOPHARYNGEAL
UNDIFFERENTIATED CARCINOMA

The low-power appearance of nasopharyngeal undifferentiated carcinoma metastatic to a regional lymph node may mimic sinus histiocytosis.

may consist only of the neoplastic epithelial component. It should be emphasized that the diagnosis is based on the character of the neoplastic epithelial cells, and may be made even in the absence of a prominent inflammatory component (fig. 5-25).

Two microscopic growth patterns have been identified in these neoplasms and bear eponyms derived from their describers (127,129). The two patterns are often mixed and are of no prognostic importance, but their recognition is vital to an understanding of the differential diagnostic considerations associated with these neoplasms. The patterns may be encountered in the primary site of disease, as well as in metastases. In the *Regaud pattern,* the neoplastic cells form cohesive nests and cords sharply distinct from the

surrounding inflammation (figs. 5-26–5-28). This results in an appearance which is usually readily identified as a carcinoma (104). In the *Schmincke pattern,* the inflammatory infiltrate permeates the cell nests, resulting in more widely separated, smaller nests of epithelial cells, as well as single neoplastic cells in a background of inflammation (figs. 5-29, 5-30). The end result is distinctly noncarcinomatous in appearance and is often confused with lymphoma on initial light microscopic examination (94,104 141). The fact that lymphoepithelioma-type carcinoma may present in children and young adults as cervical lymphadenopathy from an occult primary adds to the potential for confusion with lymphoma. In fact, although there are clues to the correct diagnosis (see Differential Diagnosis, below), a clear distinction from lymphoma

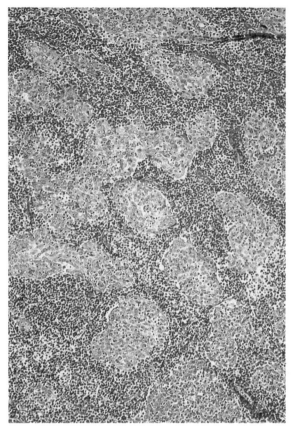

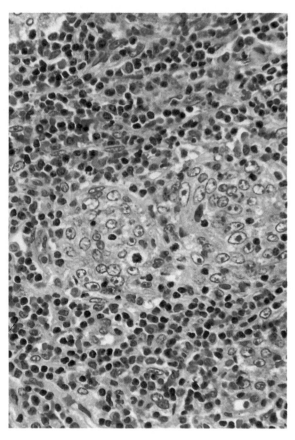

Figure 5-27
NASOPHARYNGEAL UNDIFFERENTIATED
CARCINOMA: REGAUD PATTERN

When the neoplastic cells of undifferentiated carcinoma grow in sharply demarcated nests (Regaud pattern), their epithelial nature is more readily apparent.

Figure 5-28
NASOPHARYNGEAL UNDIFFERENTIATED
CARCINOMA: REGAUD PATTERN

A cell nest of nasopharyngeal undifferentiated carcinoma consists of cells with chromatically uniform, vesicular nuclei, and indistinct cell borders.

Figure 5-29
NASOPHARYNGEAL
UNDIFFERENTIATED
CARCINOMA:
SCHMINCKE PATTERN

When the neoplastic cells of undifferentiated carcinoma are more widely dispersed in the reactive lymphoid infiltrate (Schmincke pattern), their epithelial nature is less apparent.

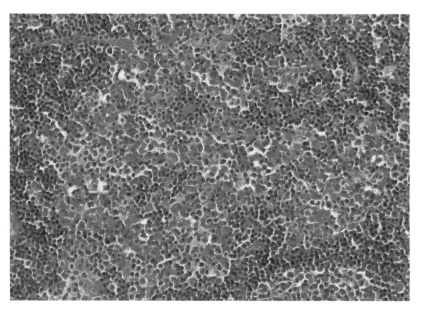

often cannot be made on the basis of light microscopic features alone (94,104,141).

Immunohistochemical and In Situ Hybridization Findings. The advent of sensitive and specific immunohistochemical markers for both epithelial and hematolymphoid differentiation has been the single greatest factor in improving the diagnostic ease and accuracy of these neoplasms (94,108,111,112,118,123,132,134,136,137, 141,142). Lymphoepithelioma-like carcinomas strongly express low molecular weight cytokeratin (118,132,136,142) and epithelial membrane antigen (fig. 5-31) (123,134). The accompanying, reactive lymphoid component strongly expresses leukocyte common antigen (fig. 5-32) (111,112,137). Although not required for diagnostic purposes, in situ hybridization for EBV DNA routinely shows strong labeling of the epithelial cells of nasopharyngeal lymphoepithelioma, without labeling of the lymphoid component (fig. 5-33).

Ultrastructural Findings. Although considerably more time consuming and expensive to perform than immunohistochemistry, and restricted to far smaller sample sizes, electron microscopy is a useful technique for documenting the epithelial nature of the neoplastic cells (104,119,136). The syncytial appearance seen at the light microscopic level is shown ultrastructurally to be due to complex interdigitations of cell membranes, rather than a true membrane-free cytoplasmic syncytium (119). Desmosomal

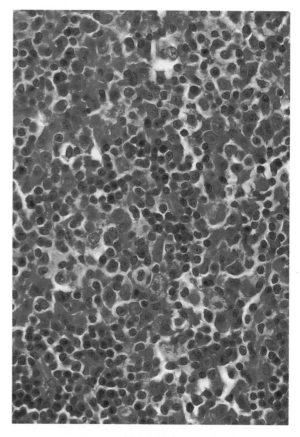

Figure 5-30
NASOPHARYNGEAL UNDIFFERENTIATED
CARCINOMA: SCHMINCKE PATTERN
This Schmincke pattern undifferentiated carcinoma has a distinctly lymphoma-like appearance due to the wide separation of the neoplastic cells in the lymphoid infiltrate.

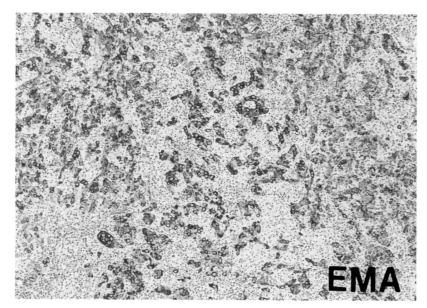

Figure 5-31
NASOPHARYNGEAL
UNDIFFERENTIATED
CARCINOMA:
SCHMINCKE PATTERN
Immunohistochemical reactivity for epithelial membrane antigen (EMA) highlights the widely dispersed neoplastic epithelial cells (anti-EMA, hematoxylin).

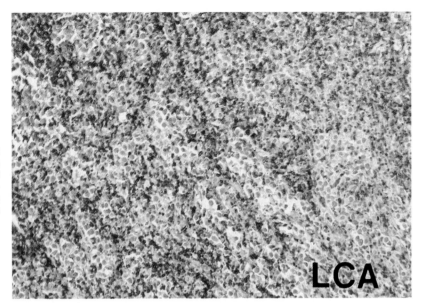

Figure 5-32
NASOPHARYNGEAL
UNDIFFERENTIATED
CARCINOMA:
SCHMINCKE PATTERN
Immunoreactivity for leukocyte
common antigen (LCA) is positive in
the abundant reactive lymphoid cells
but not in the larger neoplastic epithelial cells. The resultant image is
the "reverse" of that seen in figure
5-31 (anti-LCA, hematoxylin).

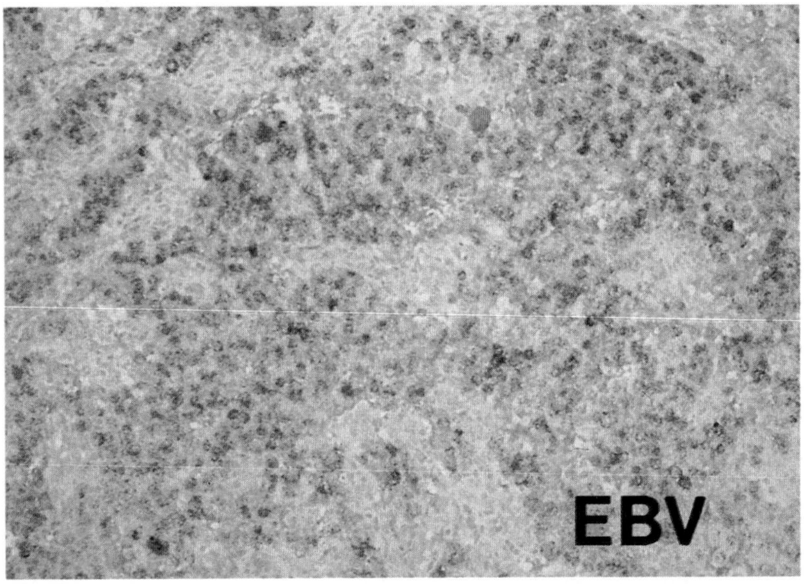

Figure 5-33
NASOPHARYNGEAL
UNDIFFERENTIATED
CARCINOMA
In situ hybridization for Epstein-
Barr virus DNA shows strong labeling
(silver grains) overlying the neoplastic
epithelial cells of nasopharyngeal un-
differentiated carcinoma. (Courtesy of
Dr. L.M. Weiss, Duarte, CA.)

cell junctions are easily discernable between adjacent cells, allowing easy recognition of their
epithelial nature (119,136). Intracytoplasmic
tonofilament bundles may be readily apparent
or absent (136). The absence of demonstrable
tonofilament bundles ultrastructurally does not
correlate with decreased or absent immunohistochemical reactivity for cytokeratin (136).

Differential Diagnosis. The Schmincke pattern of lymphoepithelioma-type carcinoma may
strongly resemble Hodgkin's disease or non-

Hodgkin's lymphoma, particularly when it presents in a cervical lymph node (94,104,141). The
resemblance of the neoplastic cells to the Reed-
Sternberg cells of Hodgkin's disease may be striking (94,106). Fortunately, consideration of carcinoma, and application of epithelial and lymphoid
markers (cytokeratin, epithelial membrane antigen, leukocyte common antigen, etc.) allow ready
distinction. Rare lymphomas have been demonstrated to be focally cytokeratin positive (102),
and some true histiocytic and T-cell lymphomas

may express epithelial membrane antigen (123). However, these lesions lack the diffuse strong reactivity for cytokeratin seen with lymphoepithelioma-type carcinomas. It is instructive to review the standard light microscopic features of these lesions for diagnostic clues. In our experience, diagnosis is usually possible with this technique alone, perhaps adding immunohistochemistry for confirmation. Even in Schmincke pattern metastases, delicate cytoplasmic strands can often be seen connecting widely separated neoplastic cells, and careful searching often reveals more cohesive cell nests (fig. 5-34). The long cytoplasmic strands appear to be due to strong desmosomal junctions connecting epithelial cells which are progressively drawn apart by the intervening inflammation.

Undifferentiated carcinoma of lymphoepithelioma type should be distinguished from nonkeratinizing squamous cell carcinoma because of the clear-cut morphologic distinctions associated with apparent behavioral differences. In some studies these tumors have had a more aggressive behavior than lymphoepithelioma-type carcinomas (93), although others have suggested a similar behavior (131). Unlike lymphoepithelioma-type carcinomas, nonkeratinizing carcinomas are rare in childhood (101,131). Microscopically, they are composed of cells exhibiting, to varying degrees, light microscopic features of squamous carcinoma but lacking evidence of keratinization. Unlike lymphoepithelioma-type carcinoma, nuclei are variable in appearance and are often hyperchromatic. Adjacent cells are typically arranged in a "cobble stone" or "pavement stone" arrangement with distinct cell borders. Rare intercellular bridges may be noted between adjacent cells. Mucin production or glandular differentiation is absent.

Occasionally, lymphoepithelioma-type carcinoma of the Regaud pattern metastatic to a regional lymph node may be mistaken for sinus histiocytosis (fig. 5-26). The chromatic uniformity of the neoplastic cells, with their moderate amounts of eosinophilic cytoplasm and tendency to fill sinusoidal spaces, can create an image which at low magnification clearly resembles sinus histiocytosis. At higher magnification, however, the high nuclear to cytoplasmic ratio, enlarged nuclei, and high mitotic rate of the neoplastic cells allow for easy distinction. If any

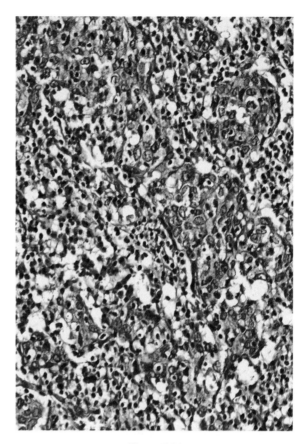

Figure 5-34
NASOPHARYNGEAL UNDIFFERENTIATED
CARCINOMA: SCHMINCKE PATTERN
This predominantly Schmincke pattern undifferentiated carcinoma contains a few cohesive nests of neoplastic cells. In addition, delicate cytoplasmic strands can be seen in the background between dispersed neoplastic cells. These can be better appreciated by focusing up and down through a tissue section.

doubt remains after more careful examination, immunohistochemical reactivity for cytokeratin or epithelial membrane antigen should allow ready recognition.

Spread and Metastasis. As noted above, lymphoepithelioma-type carcinomas show a strong tendency to metastasize to regional lymph nodes, often as the dominant clinical feature. Distant metastases to lung, brain, liver, bone, and other sites are also common (109,122). A striking lymphoplasmacytic reaction may be present at the metastatic site (fig. 5-24). Although bone marrow biopsies have not been routinely performed to evaluate these tumors, one study using iliac crest biopsy in the prechemotherapy work-up of patients with advanced stage locoregional disease noted bone marrow metastases in 21 of 56 patients (120).

Treatment and Prognosis. Nasopharyngeal carcinomas of all types are virtually always treated by radiation therapy, with or without adjuvant chemotherapy. The complex anatomy of the nasopharynx makes complete surgical resection impossible in almost all cases. In an aggregate of several large series published in the 1960s and 1970s using radiation therapy as the primary or sole treatment modality, patients with undifferentiated lymphoepithelioma-type carcinomas of the nasopharynx had the following stage related 5-year survival rates (93,98, 122,131): stage I (confined to nasopharynx), 50 to 60 percent; stage II (cervical lymph node involvement), 20 to 30 percent; and stage III (invasion of surrounding structure), 5 to 20 percent.

More recent studies have suggested an improved prognosis. In a 1988 report based on radiation therapy, Qin et al. (124) noted 5-year survival rates of: stage I, 86 percent; stage II, 59.5 percent; stage III, 45.8 percent; and stage IV, 29.2 percent. Combinations of chemotherapy with a variety of agents may also significantly improve survival (99,126).

In a study of 99 nasopharyngeal carcinomas including 41 "lymphoepitheliomas," Baker and Wolfe (92) noted patients 20 years of age or younger had the best survival. Unfortunately, survival was not specified according to tumor type and the younger patients undoubtedly had a high percentage of radiation-sensitive lymphoepithelioma-type carcinomas. A very large series of 1379 patients from China with nasopharyngeal carcinomas also noted that younger patients had a better prognosis: 67 patients under 19 years of age had a 64 percent 5-year survival (124). Although it could be speculated that this reflects a high percentage of lymphoepithelioma-type tumors in this age group, the authors further noted that the pathologic subtype of nasopharyngeal carcinoma, excluding adenocarcinomas, did not affect prognosis. In addition to age, factors which adversely affected prognosis included high clinical stage, male sex, bony invasion of the skull base, and paralysis of cranial nerves. This study also noted that 5-year survival could not be equated with cure, and that patients continued to die of disease more than 15 years after initial therapy.

"ADENOID" AND "ANGIOSARCOMA-LIKE" SQUAMOUS CELL CARCINOMA

Definition. This microscopic variant of squamous cell carcinoma is characterized by extensive acantholysis resulting in pseudoglandular or pseudovascular spaces. In many instances the low-power microscopic appearance of the tumor may strikingly resemble an angiosarcoma or an adenocarcinoma.

General Features. This variant of squamous cell carcinoma was first recognized in the skin and predilects sun-involved regions including the skin of the head and neck (145,148). Mucosal head and neck lesions have been documented involving the vermillion of the lip (144, 151), oral cavity (150), tongue (143), and nasopharynx (152). This change may be seen focally in otherwise typical squamous cell carcinoma from any anatomic site, but rarely dominates the microscopic appearance. It was suggested in at least one study that the acantholytic change might be the result of radiation therapy (150).

Clinical Features. There have been too few cases of adenoid squamous cell carcinoma arising from mucosal sites in the head and neck to draw firm conclusions regarding any prognostic distinctions. One study of 18 cases from the vermillion of the lip suggested a good prognosis with no metastases or deaths from disease (151). Other studies of oral cavity lesions have noted no apparent behavioral significance to this morphologic subtype (150,152).

Gross Findings. The gross findings are nonspecific in comparison to conventional squamous cell carcinoma. Oral cavity lesions have been described as ulcerated, nodular, indurated, warty, exophytic, keratotic, or crusted (146). Tumors often measure several centimeters in size with a tan or tan-white cut surface (152). Importantly, the purple or violaceous, multinodular pattern of a true angiosarcoma is not present (149).

Microscopic Findings. The microscopic hallmark of these tumors is the presence of alveolar or gland-like spaces lined by a peripheral layer of flattened, cuboidal, or "hobnail" neoplastic cells (fig. 5-35). Exfoliated single cells and cell aggregates are present within the lumen-like spaces (fig. 5-36) (152). Occasionally, the spaces form complex, anastomosing, sinusoidal channels, and this creates a distinctly angiosarcoma-like

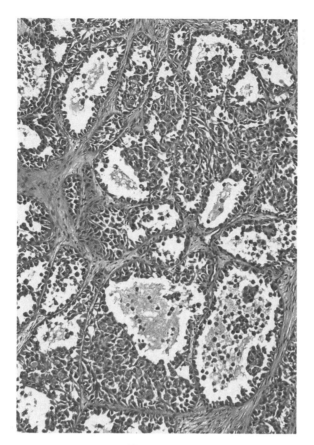

Figure 5-35
SQUAMOUS CELL CARCINOMA
Marked acantholysis in squamous cell carcinoma results in the formation of spaces mimicking glands or vascular lumina.

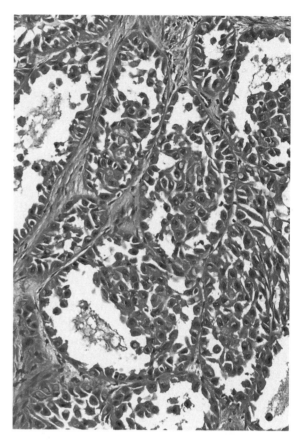

Figure 5-36
ACANTHOLYTIC SQUAMOUS CELL CARCINOMA
Apparently free-floating nests of squamous cells within the lumens of acantholytic squamous cell carcinoma allow distinction from adenocarcinoma or angiosarcoma. Occasionally, immunohistochemical studies may be necessary to make this distinction.

image (147,148). In some instances, papillary structures lined by neoplastic cells protrude into the sinusoidal spaces, which also may contain fresh red blood cells ("blood lakes"), further enhancing the resemblance to angiosarcoma.

The nuclei of the neoplastic cells are pleomorphic and often hyperchromatic, with occasional giant or multinucleated cells. The cytoplasm varies from scant to prominent and when present is typically eosinophilic. Small, pearl-like aggregates of cohesive, overtly squamous cells may be present within the lumen-like spaces and, if seen, greatly aid in diagnosis. Larger areas of overt squamous differentiation also may be seen (148). Mitotic figures are frequent. Staining with periodic acid–Schiff (PAS) shows focal intracytoplasmic glycogen removed with diastase predigestion. Mucin stains (mucarmine, alcian blue) are negative (152). The periphery of the lesion is

usually well demarcated at low-power magnification, but higher magnification shows a clearly invasive growth pattern with lumen-like spaces insinuated for a limited distance between adjacent normal structures.

Immunohistochemical Findings. Immunohistochemical studies of these neoplasms in the oral cavity, as well as analogous tumors involving the skin and lung, have shown strong reactivity for the epithelial markers, cytokeratin and epithelial membrane antigen (146–148). The tumors are uniformly nonreactive for markers of endothelial differentiation including CD34, CD31, and factor VIII-related antigen.

Ultrastructural Findings. The electron microscopic features are typical of squamous cell carcinoma (152). Adjacent cells remain connected by well-formed desmosomes, and intracytoplasmic tonofilament bundles are readily identified. Microvilli are often prominent along the "luminal" cell surface but there is no evidence of true polarization of intracytoplasmic organelles. Free-floating cells exhibit extensive microvillous projections involving all cell surfaces. Features of glandular differentiation are absent (147,148).

Differential Diagnosis. As its names imply, the two lesions that should be distinguished from (pseudovascular) adenoid squamous cell carcinoma are angiosarcoma and adenocarcinoma. In our experience, confusion with adenocarcinoma occurs primarily at low magnification microscopy. At higher power, the lack of cellular polarization or orientation with respect to the luminal spaces and the presence of cells with more prominent eosinophilic cytoplasm or even pearl-like structures usually discourage consideration of an adenocarcinoma. Mucin stains are seldom needed, but if performed, lack of intracytoplasmic positivity supports the correct diagnosis. Distinction from angiosarcoma may be occasionally more problematic, particularly when complex sinusoidal spaces are present. As noted above, the gross appearance lacks the multinodular, violaceous appearance of an angiosarcoma. The surrounding true vascular channels are lined by flattened, normal-appearing endothelial cells with no evidence of the cytologic atypia often seen adjacent to true angiosarcomas. Although seldom required, immunohistochemistry or electron microscopy is confirmatory. Due to the highly aggressive clinical course of angiosarcoma, this is a critically important distinction.

Treatment and Prognosis. As noted above, oral cavity tumors have been associated with a good prognosis (146). In a literature review of 26 adenoid squamous carcinomas from this location, 20 patients were free of disease, 3 died of disseminated disease, and 3 were lost to follow-up (146). It seems likely that the favorable prognosis is primarily due to the relative ease of diagnosis at this location, rather than to any inherent biologic differences in this morphologic subtype . Pattern of disease spread is also analogous to that of conventional squamous cell carcinoma and is dominated early in the clinical course by involvement of regional lymph nodes, with distant dissemination occurring later.

ADENOSQUAMOUS CARCINOMA

Definition. This unusual carcinoma of the head and neck contains components of adenocarcinoma and squamous cell carcinoma in close proximity. Although previously considered by some to be synonymous with salivary-type mucoepidermoid carcinoma, the tumor can and should be distinguished from that neoplasm. Adenosquamous carcinoma is typically high grade and lacks microscopic features of salivary mucoepidermoid carcinoma, more closely resembling a pulmonary adenosquamous carcinoma. In most instances in the head and neck, the tumor appears to arise from salivary or seromucinous glands, but it may also originate from surface mucosa.

General Features. Adenosquamous carcinomas occur at a variety of anatomic sites throughout the body including the gastrointestinal tract, genitourinary tract, female reproductive tract, lung, skin, and upper respiratory tract (161). In the head and neck region, this is a real but poorly defined tumor variant. Perusal of published illustrations suggests that many purported examples of these tumors might be better interpreted as adenoid (acantholytic) squamous cell carcinoma, basaloid squamous cell carcinoma, salivary duct carcinoma, squamous cell carcinoma entrapping non-neoplastic seromucinous glands, or squamous cell carcinoma with necrosis-related pseudoglandular spaces (154,158,159,161). Nonetheless, well-documented examples do exist (153,155,160,162). Perhaps just as common as overdiagnosis is the problem of underdiagnosing these tumors as a mucoepidermoid carcinoma. As discussed below, we agree with Evans that this is an important distinction, given the more aggressive behavior of adenosquamous carcinoma (156,157).

Clinical Features. Within the head and neck region, tumor has been reported in the oral cavity (161,162), and more commonly in the larynx and paranasal sinuses (153,155,159,160). Presenting symptoms and complaints are similar to those associated with squamous cell carcinoma at analogous locations. In one review of patients with involvement of the larynx and hypopharynx, the typical presentation was hoarseness or, less commonly, hemoptysis, dysphagia, or a neck mass (155). Average duration of symptoms was

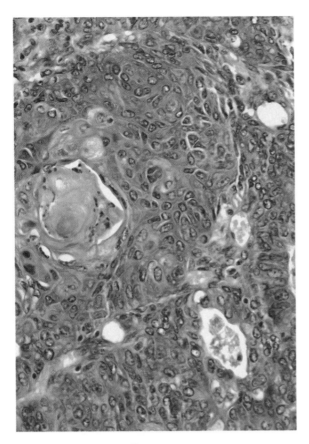

Figure 5-37
ADENOSQUAMOUS CARCINOMA
This adenosquamous carcinoma shows overt keratinization. Small, gland-like spaces are also present. At the extreme right of the field is the edge of a larger gland surrounded by more elongated, radially arranged cells.

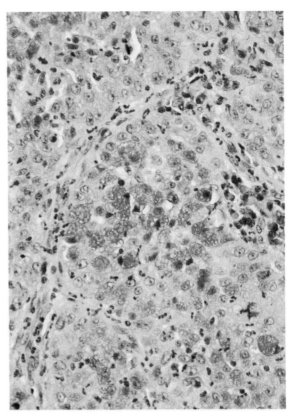

Figure 5-38
ADENOSQUAMOUS CARCINOMA
A mucicarmine stain documents the presence of prominent
epithelial mucin within this adenosquamous carcinoma.

9 months. One third of these patients had palpa-
bly enlarged regional lymph nodes.

Gross Findings. Grossly, these tumors are
indistinguishable from conventional squamous
cell carcinoma.

Microscopic Findings. These are cytologically high-grade neoplasms composed of mixtures
of squamous cell carcinoma and adenocarcinoma
(fig. 5-37). The squamous component usually predominates and often demonstrates overt keratinization. The adenocarcinomatous component is always closely associated with the squamous
elements and lacks the characteristic features of a
distinctive form of salivary-type adenocarcinoma.
Instead, it typically consists of a moderately or
poorly differentiated "generic" adenocarcinoma, as
evidenced by gland formation or the production of
intracellular epithelial-type mucin (fig. 5-38). The
overall appearance of the tumor is indistinguishable from an adenosquamous carcinoma of the
lung, uterine cervix, or elsewhere.

Immunohistochemical Findings. The glandular elements of these tumors express carcinoembryonic antigen and low molecular weight
cytokeratins (160). High molecular weight
cytokeratins are present in both the squamous
and glandular components (160).

Differential Diagnosis. We agree with
Evans that adenosquamous carcinomas should
be distinguished from high-grade mucoepidermoid carcinomas of salivary type because of
the more aggressive biologic behavior of the former tumors (156,157). True mucoepidermoid
carcinomas typically consist of multiple cell
types, including mucous, intermediate, epidermoid, and clear cell (156). Even high-grade
mucoepidermoid carcinomas of salivary type
show only mild nuclear pleomorphism, and have

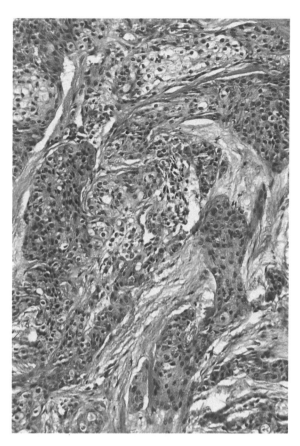

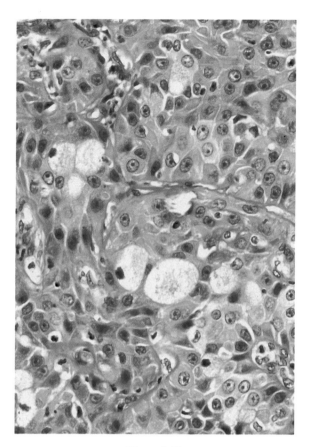

Figure 5-39
SALIVARY-TYPE MUCOEPIDERMOID CARCINOMA
This high-grade salivary-type mucoepidermoid carcinoma consists of cords and strands of squamoid cells, clear cells, and rare mucinous cells exhibiting only mild nuclear pleomorphism. Mitotic figures are not identified. There is no obvious keratinization.

Figure 5-40
SALIVARY-TYPE MUCOEPIDERMOID CARCINOMA
The high-grade salivary-type mucoepidermoid carcinoma of figure 5-39 is seen at higher magnification. It contains scattered mucinous cells with small uniform nuclei. The squamoid cells have atypical but relatively uniform nuclei without keratinization. Mitotic figures are not identified.

low mitotic rates with absent or only focal necrosis (figs. 5-39, 5-40) (156). Cystic areas filled with extracellular mucin are prominent in low-grade mucoepidermoid carcinomas, but are often present in the higher grade tumors as well. In contrast, adenosquamous carcinomas usually exhibit striking nuclear pleomorphism, high mitotic rates, and areas of necrosis. The tumors typically form solid cell nests with scattered, poorly formed glandular structures. A "salivary appearance" is absent and the tumors are indistinguishable from adenosquamous carcinomas arising in the lung or elsewhere. Adenosquamous carcinoma should also be distinguished from basaloid squamous cell carcinoma in which the basaloid cells assume a pattern reminiscent of adenoid cystic carcinoma (fig. 5-41). The latter

tumors lack true glandular structures but consist of pleomorphic basaloid cells haphazardly arranged around extracellular spaces filled with connective tissue mucin or hyaline material.

Spread and Metastasis. Of 21 patients with tumors of the larynx and hypopharynx, 7 developed local recurrences in cervical lymph nodes and 2 developed distant metastases to lung, brain, and elsewhere (155). As with many studies dealing with these tumors, it is impossible to be certain which tumors were salivary-type high-grade mucoepidermoid carcinomas and which were adenosquamous carcinomas. The overall 5-year survival rate of 77 percent suggests that some were more indolent salivary-type mucoepidermoid carcinomas.

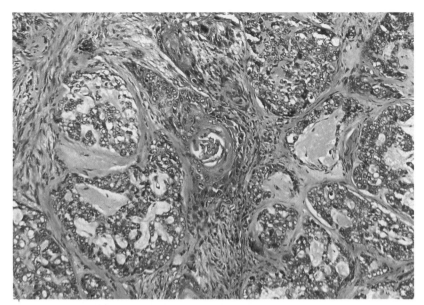

Figure 5-41
BASALOID SQUAMOUS
CELL CARCINOMA
The adenoid cystic-like regions in
this basaloid squamous cell carcinoma,
in combination with the obvious squamous differentiation, may lead to confusion with adenosquamous carcinoma.

Treatment. Therapy for adenosquamous carcinoma should be identical to that for analogous
stage squamous cell carcinomas. Both surgical
resection and high-dose radiation therapy have
been shown to be effective treatment regimens
(155).

REFERENCES

Verrucous Carcinoma

1. Abramson AL, Brandsma JL, Steinberg BM, Winkler B. Verrucous carcinoma of the larynx: possible human papillomavirus etiology. Arch Otolaryngol Head Neck Surg 1985;111:709–15.
2. Ackerman LV. Verrucous carcinoma of the oral cavity. Surgery 1948;23:670–8.
3. Batsakis JG, Hybels R, Crissman JD, Rice DH. The pathology of head and neck tumors: verrucous carcinoma, part 15. Head Neck Surg 1982;5:29–38.
4. Brandsma JL, Steinberg BM, Abramson AL, Winkler B. Presence of HPV-16 related sequences in verrucous carcinoma of the larynx. Cancer Res 1986;46:2185–8.
5. Brooks JJ, Enterline HT, Apontet GE. The final diagnosis of president Cleveland's lesion. Trans Stud Coll Phys Phila 1980;2:1–25.
6. Cooke RA. Verrucous carcinoma of the oral mucosa in Papua - New Guinea. Cancer 1969;24:397.
7. Edstrom S, Johannson S, Lindström J, et al. Verrucous squamous cell carcinoma of the larynx: evidence for increased metastatic potential after irradiation. Otolaryngol Head Neck Surg 1987;97:381–4.
8. Elliott GB, Macdougall JA, Elliott JD. Problems of verrucous squamous carcinoma. Ann Surg 1973;177:21–9.
9. Eversole LR, Papanicolaou SJ. Papillary and verrucous lesions of the oral mucous membranes. J Oral Med 1983;38:3–13
10. Fechner RE, Mills SE. Verruca vulgaris of the larynx. A distinctive lesion of probable viral origin confused with verrucous carcinoma. Am J Surg Pathol 1997;6:357–62.
11. Ferlito A, Antonutto G, Silvestri F. Histological appearances and nuclear DNA content of verrucous squamous cell carcinoma of the larynx. ORL J Otorhinolaryngol Relat Spec 1976;38:65–85.
12. Ferlito A, Recher G. Ackerman's tumor (verrucous carcinoma) of the larynx: a clinicopathologic study of 77 cases. Cancer 1980;46:1617–30.

13. Fridell HL, Rosenthal LN. The etiologic role of chewing tobacco in cancer of the mouth. JAMA 1941;116:2130

14. Hagen P, Lyons GD, Haindel C. Verrucous carcinoma of the larynx: role of human papillomavirus, radiation, and surgery. Laryngoscope 1993;103:253–7.

15. Jacobson S, Shear M. Verrucous carcinoma of the mouth. J Oral Pathol 1972;1:66–75.

16. Jahn AF, Walter JB, Farkashidy J. Verrucous carcinoma of the nasopharynx—a clinicopathologic case report. J Otolaryngol 1980;9:84–9.

17. Kahn JL, Blez P, Gasser B, Weill-Bousson M, Vetter JM, Champy M. [Carcinoma cuniculatum. Apropos of 4 cases with orofacial involvement]. Rev Stomatol Chir Maxillofac 1991;92:27–33.

18. Kraus FT, Perez-Mesa C. Verrucous carcinoma. Clinical and pathologic study of 105 cases involving oral cavity, larynx, and genitalia. Cancer 1966;19:26–38.

19. Luna MA, Tortoledo ME. Verrucous carcinoma. In: Gnepp DR, ed. Pathology of the head and neck. New York: Churchill Livingstone, 1988:497–515.

20. Lundgren JA, Van Norstrand AW, Harwood AR, Cullen RJ, Bryce DP. Verrucous carcinoma (Ackerman's tumor) of the larynx: diagnostic and therapeutic considerations. Head Neck Surg 1986;9:19–26.

21. McCoy JM, Waldron CA. Verrucous carcinoma of the oral cavity. A review of 49 cases. Oral Surg Oral Med Oral Pathol 1981;52:623–9.

22. Medina JE, Dichtel W, Luna MA. Verrucous squamous carcinoma of the oral cavity. A clinicopathologic study of 104 cases. Arch Otolaryngol 1984;110:437–40.

23. Murrah VA, Batsakis JG. Proliferative verrucous leukoplakia and verrucous hyperplasia. Ann Otol Rhinol Laryngol 1994;103:660–3.

24. Nunez DA, Astley SM, Lewis FA, Wells M. Human papilloma viruses: a study of their prevalence in the normal larynx. J Laryngol Otol 1994;108:319–20.

25. Perez CA, Kraus FT, Evans JC, Powers WE. Anaplastic transformation in verrucous carcinoma of the oral cavity after radiation therapy. Radiology 1966;26:108–15.

26. Prioleau PG, Santa Cruz DJ, Meyer JS, Bauer WC. Verrucous carcinoma: a light and electron microscopic, autoradiographic, and immunofluorescence study. Cancer 1980;45:2849–57.

27. Ryan RE Jr, DeSanto LW, Devine KD, Weiland LH. Verrucous carcinoma of the larynx. Laryngoscope 1977;87:1989–95.

28. Shear M, Pindborg JJ. Verrucous hyperplasia of the oral mucosa. Cancer 1980;46:1855–62.

29. Shroyer KR, Greer RO, Fankhouser CA, McGuirt WF, Marshall R. Detection of human papillomavirus DNA in oral verrucous carcinoma by polymerase chain reaction. Mod Pathol 1993;6:669–72.

30. Sllamniku B, Bauer W, Painter C, Sessions D. Clinical and histopathological considerations for the diagnosis and treatment of verrucous carcinoma of the larynx. Arch Otorhinolaryngol 1989;246:126–32.

31. Tharp ME Jr, Shidnia H. Radiotherapy in the treatment of verrucous carcinoma of the head and neck. Laryngoscope 1995;105:391–6.

32. Young SK, Min KW. In-situ DNA hybridization analysis of oral papillomas, leukoplakias and carcinomas for human papillomavirus. Oral Surg Oral Med Oral Pathol 1991;71:276–9.

33. Youngberg GA, Thornthwaite JT, Inoshita T, Franzus D. Cytologically malignant squamous cell carcinoma arising in verrucous carcinoma of the penis. J Dermatol Surg Oncol 1983;9:474–9.

Spindle Cell Carcinoma

34. Alguacil-Garcia A, Alonso A, Pettigrew NM. Sarcomatoid carcinoma (so-called pseudosarcoma) of the larynx simulating malignant giant cell tumor of soft parts. A case report. Am J Clin Pathol 1984;82:340–3.

35. Batsakis JG, Rice DH, Howard DR. The pathology of head and neck tumours: spindle cell lesions (sarcomatoid carcinomas, nodular fasciitis and fibrosarcoma) of the aerodigestive tract, part 14. Head Neck Surg 1982;4:499–513.

36. Battifora HA. Spindle cell carcinoma. Cancer 1976;37:2275–82.

37. Benninger MS, Kraus D, Sebek B, Tucker HM, Lavertu P. Head and neck spindle cell carcinoma: an evaluation of current management. Cleve Clin J Med 1992;59:479–82.

38. Berthelet E, Shenouda G, Black MJ, Picariello M, Rochon L. Sarcomatoid carcinoma of the head and neck. Am J Surg 1994;168:455–8.

39. Cornes JS, Lewis MS. Polypoid carcinomas of the pharynx with sarcomatous or pseudosarcomatous stroma. Br J Surg 1966;53:340–4.

40. Ellis GL, Langloss JM, Enzinger FM. Coexpression of keratin and desmin in a carcinosarcoma involving the alveolar ridge. Oral Surg Oral Med Oral Pathol 1985;60:410–6.

41. Ellis GL, Langloss JM, Heffner DK, Hyams VJ. Spindle-cell carcinoma of the areodigestive tract. An immunohistochemical analysis of 21 cases. Am J Surg Pathol 1987;11:335–42.

42. Howell JH, Hyams VJ, Sprinkle PM. Spindle cell carcinoma of the nose and paranasal sinuses. Surg Forum 1978;29:565–8.

43. Hyams VJ. Spindle cell carcinoma of the larynx. Can J Otolaryngol 1975;4:307–13.

44. Lambert PR, Ward PH, Berci G. Pseudosarcoma of the larynx. Arch Otolaryngol 1980;106:700–8.

45. Lane N. Pseudosarcoma (polypoid sarcoma-like masses) associated with squamous cell carcinoma of the mouth, fauces, and larynx. Cancer 1957;10:19–41.

46. Lasser KH, Naeim F, Higgins J, Cove H, Waisman J. "Pseudosarcoma" of the larynx. Am J Surg Pathol 1979;3:397–404.

47. Leventon GS, Evans HL. Sarcomatoid squamous cell carcinoma of the mucous membranes of the head and neck: a clinicopathologic study of 20 cases. Cancer 1981;48:994–1003.

48. Lichtiger B, Mackay B, Tessmer CF. Spindle-cell variant of squamous carcinoma. A light and electron microscopic study. Cancer 1970;26:1311–20.

49. Minckler DS, Meligro CH, Norris HT. Carcinosarcoma of the larynx. Cancer 1970;26:195–200.

50. Nakhleh RE, Zarbo RJ, Ewing S, Carey JL, Gown AM. Myogenic differentiation in spindle cell (sarcomatoid) carcinomas of the upper aerodigestive tract. Appl Immunohistochem 1993;1:58–68.

51. Ophir D, Marshak G, Czernobilsky B. Distinctive immunohistochemical labeling of epithelial and mesenchymal elements in laryngeal pseudosarcoma. Laryngoscope 1987;97:490–4.

52. Piscioli R, Aldovini D, Bondi A, Eusebi V. Squamous cell carcinoma with sarcoma-like stroma of the nose and paranasal sinuses: report of two cases. Histopathology 1984;8:633–9.

53. Randall G, Alonso WA, Ogura JH. Spindle cell carcinoma (pseudosarcoma) of the larynx. Arch Otolaryngol 1975;101:63–6.

54. Staley CJ, Ujiki GT, Yokoo H. "Pseudosarcoma" of the larynx. Independent metastasis of carcinomatous and sarcomatous elements. Arch Otolaryngol 1971;94:458–65.

55. Weidner N. Sarcomatoid carcinoma of the upper aerodigestive tract. Semin Diagn Pathol 1987;4:157–68.

56. Zarbo RJ, Crissman JD, Venkat H, Weiss MA. Spindle-cell carcinoma of the upper aerodigestive tract mucosa. An immunohistologic and ultrastructural study of 18 biphasic tumors and comparison with seven monophasic spindle-cell tumors. Am J Surg Pathol 1986;10:741–53.

Basaloid Squamous Cell Carcinoma

57. Allen MS Jr, Marsh WL Jr. Lymph node involvement by direct extension in adenoid cystic carcinoma. Absence of classic embolic lymph node metastasis. Cancer 1976;38:2017–21.

58. Banks ER, Frierson HF Jr, Covell JL. Fine needle aspiration cytologic findings in metastatic basaloid squamous cell carcinoma of the head and neck. Acta Cytol 1992;36:126–31.

59. Banks ER, Frierson HF Jr, Mills SE, George E, Zarbo RJ, Swanson PE. Basaloid squamous cell carcinoma of the head and neck. A clinicopathologic and immunohistochemical study of 40 cases. Am J Surg Pathol 1992;16:939–46.

60. Campman SC, Gandour-Edwards RF, Sykes JM. Basaloid squamous carcinoma of the head and neck. Report of a case occurring in the anterior floor of the mouth. Arch Pathol Lab Med 1994;118:1229–32.

61. Chen JC, Gnepp DR, Bedrossian CW. Adenoid cystic carcinoma of the salivary glands: an immunohistochemical analysis. Oral Surg Oral Med Oral Pathol 1988;65:316–26.

62. Coppola D, Catalano E, Tang CK, Elfenbein IB, Harwick R, Mohr R. Basaloid squamous cell carcinoma of floor of mouth. Cancer 1993; 72:2299–305.

63. de Araujo VC, Biazolla ER, Moraes NP, Furuse TA, Melhado RM. Basaloid squamous carcinoma of the oral cavity. Report of a case. Oral Surg Oral Med Oral Pathol 1993;75:622–5.

64. Dougherty BG, Evans HL. Carcinoma of the anal canal: a study of 79 cases. Am J Clin Pathol 1985;83:159–64.

65. Ereno C, Lopez JI, Sanchez JM, Toledo JD. Basaloid-squamous cell carcinoma of the larynx and hypopharynx. A clinicopathologic study of 7 cases. Pathol Res Pract 1994;110:186–93.

66. Gnepp DR, Wick MR. Small cell carcinoma of the major salivary gland. An immunohistochemical study. Cancer 1990;66:185–92.

67. Hellquist HB, Dahl F, Karlsson MG, Nilsson C. Basaloid squamous cell carcinoma of the palate. Histopathology 1994;25:178–80.

68. Johnson GD, Mahataphongse VP, Abt AB, Conner GH. Small cell undifferentiated carcinoma of the larynx. Ann Otol 1979;88:774–8.

69. Larner JM, Malcolm RH, Mills SE, Frierson HF Jr, Banks ER, Levine PA. Radiotherapy for basaloid squamous cell carcinoma of the head and neck. Head Neck 1993;15:249–52.

70. Lin O, Harkin TJ, Jagirdar J. Basaloid-squamous carcinoma of the bronchus. Report of a case with review of the literature. Arch Pathol Lab Med 1995;119:1167–70.

71. Lovejoy HM, Matthews BL. Basaloid-squamous carcinoma of the palate. Otolaryngol Head Neck Surg 1992;106:159–62.

72. Luna MA, El-Naggar A, Parichatikanond P, Weber RS, Batsakis JG. Basaloid squamous carcinoma of the upper aerodigestive tract. Clinicopathologic and DNA flow cytometric analysis. Cancer 1990;66:537–42.

73. Lung ML, Sham JS, Lam WP, Choy DT. Analysis of Epstein-Barr virus in localized nasopharyngeal carcinoma tumors. Cancer 1993;71:1190–2.

74. Marsh WL Jr, Allen MS Jr. Adenoid cystic carcinoma. Biologic behavior in 38 patients. Cancer 1979;43:1463–73.

75. McKay MJ, Bilous AM. Basaloid-squamous carcinoma of the hypopharynx. Cancer 1989;63:2528–31.

76. Mills SE, Cooper PH, Garland TA, Johns ME. Small cell undifferentiated carcinoma of the larynx. Report of two patients and review of 13 additional cases. Cancer 1983;51:116–20.

77. Raab-Traub N. Epstein-Barr virus and nasopharyngeal carcinoma. Semin Cancer Biol 1992;3:297–307.

78. Raslan WF, Barnes L, Krause JR, Contis L, Killeen R, Kapadia SB. Basaloid squamous cell carcinoma of the head and neck: a clinicopathologic and flow cytometric study of 10 new cases with review of the English literature. Am J Otolaryngol 1994;15:204–11.

79. Saltarelli MG, Fleming MV, Wenig BM, Gal AA, Mansour KA, Travis WD. Primary basaloid squamous cell carcinoma of the trachea. Am J Clin Pathol 1995;104:594–8.

80. Seidman JD, Berman JJ, Yost BA, Iseri OA. Basaloid squamous carcinoma of the hypopharynx and larynx associated with second primary tumors. Cancer 1991;68:1545–9.

81. Tsang WY, Chan JK, Lee KC, Leung AK, Fu YT. Basaloid-squamous carcinoma of the upper aerodigestive tract and so-called adenoid cystic carcinoma of the oesophagus: the same tumour type? Histopathology 1991;11:35–46.

82. van der Wal JE, Snow GB, Karim AB, van der Waal I. Adenoid cystic carcinoma of the palate with squamous metaplasia or basaloid-squamous carcinoma? Report of a case. J Oral Pathol Med 1994;23:461–4.

83. Wain SL, Kier R, Vollmer RT, Bossen EH. Basaloid-squamous carcinoma of the tongue, hypopharynx, and larynx: report of 10 cases. Hum Pathol 1986;17:1158–66.

84. Walker AN, Mills SE, Fechner RE. Thymomas and thymic carcinomas. Semin Diagn Pathol 1990;7:250–65.

85. Wan SK, Chan JK, Lau WH, Yip TT. Basaloid-squamous carcinoma of the nasopharynx. An Epstein-Barr virus-associated neoplasm compared with morphologically identical tumors occurring in other sites. Cancer 1995;76:1689–93.

86. Wan SK, Chan JK, Tse KC. Basaloid-squamous carcinoma of the nasal cavity. J Laryngol Otol 1992;106:370–1.

87. Weiss LM, Movahed LA, Butler AE, et al. Analysis of lymphoepithelioma and lymphoepithelioma-like carcinomas for Epstein-Barr viral genomes by in-situ hybridization. Am J Surg Pathol 1989;13:625–31.

88. Wick MR, Abenoza P, Manivel JC. Diagnostic immunohistopathology. In: Gnepp DR, ed. Pathology of the head and neck. New York: Churchill Livingstone, 1988:191–260.

Papillary Squamous Cell Carcinoma

89. Crissman JD, Kessis T, Shah KV, et al. Squamous papillary neoplasia of the adult upper aerodigestive tract. Hum Pathol 1988;19:1387–96.

90. Judd R, Zaki SR, Coffield LM, Evatt BL. Human papillomavirus type 6 detected by the polymerase chain reaction in invasive sinonasal papillary squamous cell carcinoma. Arch Pathol Lab Med 1991;115:1150–3.

91. Randall ME, Andersen WA, Mills SE, Kim JA. Papillary squamous cell carcinoma of the uterine cervix: a clinicopathologic study of nine cases. Int J Gynecol Pathol 1986;5:1–10.

Undifferentiated (Lymphoepithelioma-like) Carcinoma

92. Baker SR, Wolfe RA. Prognostic factors of nasopharyngeal malignancy. Cancer 1982;49:163–9.

93. Bloom SM. Cancer of the nasopharynx: a study of 90 cases. J Mt Sinai Hosp 1969;36:277–98.

94. Carbone A, Micheau C. Pitfalls in microscopic diagnosis of undifferentiated carcinoma of nasopharyngeal type (lymphoepithelioma). Cancer 1982;50:1344–51.

95. Chao TY, Chow KC, Chang JY, et al. Expression of Epstein-Barr virus-encoded RNAs as a marker for metastatic undifferentiated nasopharyngeal carcinoma. Cancer 1996;78:24–9.

96. Choi PH, Suen MW, Huang DP, Lo KW, Lee JC. Nasopharyngeal carcinoma: genetic changes, Epstein-Barr virus infection, or both. A clinical and molecular study of 36 patients. Cancer 1993;72:2873–8.

97. Clifford P. Blood groups and nasopharyngeal carcinoma. Lancet 1970;2:48–9.

98. Creely JJ Jr, Lyons GD Jr, Trail ML. Cancer of the nasopharynx: a review of 114 cases. South Med J 1973;66:405–9.

99. Crissman JD, Pajak TF, Zarbo RJ, Marcial VA, Al-Sarraf M. Improved response and survival to combined cisplatin and radiation in non-keratinizing squamous cell carcinomas of the head and neck. An RTOG study of 114 advanced stage tumors. Cancer 1987;59:1391–7.

100. Digby KH, Fook WL, Che YT. Nasopharyngeal malignancy. Br J Surg 1941;28:517–37.

101. Easton JM, Levine PH, Hyams VJ. Nasopharyngeal carcinoma in the United States. A pathologic study of 177 US and 30 foreign cases. Arch Otolaryngol 1980;106:88–91.

102. Frierson HF Jr, Bellafiore FJ, Gaffey MJ, McCary WS, Innes DJ Jr, Williams ME. Cytokeratin in anaplastic large cell lymphoma. Mod Pathol 1994;7:317–21.

103. Gaffey MJ, Weiss LM. Association of Epstein-Barr virus with human neoplasia. Pathol Annu 1992;27(Pt. 1):55–74.

104. Giffler RF, Gillespie JJ, Ayala AG, Newland JR. Lymphoepithelioma in cervical lymph nodes of children and young adults. Am J Surg Pathol 1977;1:293–302.

105. Hamilton-Dutoit SJ, Therkildsen MH, Neilsen NH, Jensen H, Hansen JP, Pallesen G. Undifferentiated carcinoma of the salivary gland in Greenlandic Eskimos: demonstration of Epstein-Barr virus DNA by in situ nucleic acid hybridization. Hum Pathol 1991;22:811–5.

106. Hawkins EP, Krischer JP, Smith BE, Hawkins HK, Finegold MJ. Nasopharyngeal carcinoma in children—a retrospective review and demonstration of Epstein-Barr viral genomes in tumor cell cytoplasm: a report of the Pediatric Oncology Group. Hum Pathol 1990;21:805–10.

107. Iezzoni JC, Gaffey MJ, Weiss LM. The role of Epstein-Barr virus in lymphoepithelioma-like carcinomas. Am J Clin Pathol 1995;103:308–15.

108. Kamino H, Huang SJ, Fu YS. Keratin and involucrin immunohistochemistry of nasopharyngeal carcinoma. Cancer 1988;61:1142–8.

109. Khor TH, Tan BC, Chua EJ, Chia KB. Distant metastases in nasopharyngeal carcinoma. Clin Radiol 1978;29:27–30.

110. Klijanienko J, Micheau C, Azli N, et al. Undifferentiated carcinoma of nasopharyngeal type of tonsil. Arch Otolaryngol Head Neck Surg 1989;115:731–4.

111. Kurtin PJ, Pinkus GS. Leukocyte common antigen—a diagnostic discriminant between hematopoietic and nonhematopoietic neoplasms in paraffin sections using monoclonal antibodies: correlation with immunologic studies and ultrastructural localization. Hum Pathol 1985;16:353–65.

112. Lauder I, Holland D, Mason DY, Gowland G, Cunliffe WJ. Identification of large cell undifferentiated tumours in lymph nodes using leucocyte common and keratin antibodies. Histopathology 1984;8:259–72.

113. Leighton SE, Teo JG, Leung SF, Cheung AY, Lee JC, van Hasselt CA. Prevalence and prognostic significance of tumor-associated tissue eosinophilia in nasopharyngeal carcinoma. Cancer 1996;77:436–40.

114. Leung SY, Yuen ST, Chung LP, Kwong WK, Wong MP, Chan SY. Epstein-Barr virus is present in a wide histological spectrum of sinonasal carcinomas. Am J Surg Pathol 1995;11:994–1001.

115. Looi LM. Tumor-associated tissue eosinophilia in nasopharyngeal carcinoma. A pathologic study of 422 primary and 138 metastatic tumors. Cancer 1987;59:466–70.

116. Lopategui JR, Gaffey MJ, Frierson HF Jr, et al. Detection of Epstein-Barr viral RNA in sinonasal undifferentiated carcinoma from Western and Asian patients. Am J Surg Pathol 1994;18:391–8.

117. Lung ML, Sham JS, Lam WP, Choy DT. Analysis of Epstein-Barr virus in localized nasopharyngeal carcinoma tumors. Cancer 1993;71:1190–2.

118. Madri JA, Barwick KW. An immunohistochemical study of nasopharyngeal neoplasms using keratin antibodies: epithelial versus nonepithelial neoplasms. Am J Surg Pathol 1982;6:143–9.

119. Michaels L, Hyams VJ. Undifferentiated carcinoma of the nasopharynx: a light and electron microscopical study. Clin Otolaryngol 1977;2:105–14.

210. Micheau C, Boussen H, Klijanienko J, et al. Bone marrow biopsies in patients with undifferentiated carcinoma of nasopharyngeal type. Cancer 1987;60:2459–64.

121. Pearson GR, Weiland LH, Neel HBI, et al. Application of Epstein-Barr virus (EBV) serology to the diagnosis of North American nasopharyngeal carcinoma. Cancer 1983;51:260–8.

122. Perez CA, Ackerman LV, Mill WB, Ogura JH, Powers WE. Cancer of the nasopharynx. Factors influencing prognosis. Cancer 1969;24:1–17.

123. Pinkus GS, Kurtin PJ. Epithelial membrane antigen—a diagnostic discriminant in surgical pathology: immuno-histochemical profile in epithelial, mesenchymal, and hematopoietic neoplasms using paraffin sections and monoclonal antibodies. Hum Pathol 1985;16:929–40.

124. Qin D, Hu Y, Yan J, et al. Analysis of 1379 patients with nasopharyngeal carcinoma treated by radiation. Cancer 1988;61:1117–24.

125. Raab-Traub N. Epstein-Barr virus and nasopharyngeal carcinoma. Semin Cancer Biol 1992;3:297–307.

126. Rahima M, Rakowsky E, Barzilay J, Sidi J. Carcinoma of the nasopharynx. An analysis of 91 cases and a comparison of differing treatment approaches. Cancer 1986;58:843–9.

127. Regaud C, Reverchon L. Sur un cas d'epithelioma epidermoide developpe dans le massif maxillaire superieur. Rev Laryngol Otol Rhinol (Bord) 1921; 42:369-78.

128. Ringborg U, Henle W, Henle G, et al. Epstein-Barr virus-specific serodiagnostic tests in carcinomas of the head and neck. Cancer 1983;52:1237–43.

129. Schmincke A. Uber lympho-epitheliale Geschwulste. Beitr Pathol Anat Allg Pathol 1921;68:161–70.

130. Sham JS, Poon YF, Wei WI, Choy D. Nasopharyngeal carcinoma in young patients. Cancer 1990;65:2606–10.

131. Shanmugaratnam K, Chan SH, de-The G, et al. Histopathology of nasopharyngeal carcinoma: correlations with epidemiology, survival rates and other biological characteristics. Cancer 1979;44:1029–44.

132. Shi SR, Goodman ML, Bhan AK, Pilch BZ, Chen LB, Sun TT. Immunohistochemical study of nasopharyngeal carcinoma using monoclonal keratin antibodies. Am J Pathol 1984;117:53–63.

133. Simons MJ, Wee GB, Goh EH, et al. Immunogenetic aspects of nasopharyngeal carcinoma in young patients. JNCI 1976;57:977–80.

134. Sloane JP, Ormerod MG. Distribution of epithelial membrane antigen in normal and neoplastic tissues and its value in diagnostic tumor pathology. Cancer 1981;47:1786–95.

135 Tamada A, Makimoto K, Yamabe H, et al. Titers of Epstein-Barr virus-related antibodies in nasopharyngeal carcinoma in Japan. Cancer 1984;53:430–40.

136. Taxy JB, Hidvegi DF, Battifora H. Nasopharyngeal carcinoma: antikeratin immunohistochemistry and electron microscopy. Am J Clin Pathol 1985;83:320–5.

137. Warnke RA, Gatter KC, Falini B, et al. Diagnosis of human lymphoma with monoclonal antileukocyte antibodies. N Engl J Med 1983;309:1275–81.

138. Weiss LM, Gaffey MJ, Shibata D. Lymphoepithelioma-like carcinoma and its relationship to Epstein-Barr virus [Editorial]. Am J Clin Pathol 1991;96:156–8.

139. Weiss LM, Movahed LA, Butler AE, et al. Analysis of lymphoepithelioma and lymphoepithelioma-like carcinomas for Epstein-Barr viral genomes by in-situ hybridization. Am J Surg Pathol 1989;13:625–31.

140. Yu MC, Ho JH, Lai SH, Henderson BE. Cantonese-style salted fish as a cause of nasopharyngeal carcinoma: report of a case-control study in Hong Kong. Cancer Res 1986;46:956–61.

141. Zarate-Osorno A, Jaffe ES, Medeiros LJ. Metastatic nasopharyngeal carcinoma initially presenting as cervical lymphadenopathy. A report of two cases that resembled Hodgkin's disease. Arch Pathol Lab Med 1992;116:862–5.

142. Ziegels-Weissman J, Nadji M, Penneys NS, Morales AR. Prekeratin immunohistochemistry in the diagnosis of undifferentiated carcinoma of the nasopharyngeal type. Arch Pathol Lab Med 1984;108:588–9.

Adenoid (Angiosarcoma-like) Squamous Cell Carcinoma

143. Goldman RL, Klein HZ, Sung M. Adenoid squamous cell carcinoma of the oral cavity: report of the first case arising in the tongue. Arch Otolaryngol Head Neck Surg 1977;103:496–8.

144. Jacoway JR, Nelson JF, Boyers RC. Adenoid squamous cell carcinoma of the oral labial mucosa. A clinicopathologic study of 15 cases. Oral Surg 1971;32:444–9.

145. Johnson WC, Helwig EB. Adenoid squamous cell carcinoma (adenoacanthoma). A clinicopathologic study of 155 patients. Cancer 1966;19:1639–50.

146. Jones AC, Freedman PD, Kerpel SM. Oral adenoid squamous cell carcinoma: a report of three cases and review of the literature. J Oral Maxillofac Surg 1993;51:676–81.

147. Nappi O, Swanson PE, Wick MR. Pseudovascular adenoid squamous cell carcinoma of the lung: clinicopathologic study of three cases and comparison with true pleuropulmonary angiosarcoma. Hum Pathol 1994;25:373–8.

148. Nappi O, Wick MR, Pettinato G, Ghiselli RW, Swanson PE. Pseudovascular adenoid squamous cell carcinoma of the skin. A neoplasm that may be mistaken for angiosarcoma. Am J Surg Pathol 1992;16:429–38.

149. Ritter JH, Mills SE, Nappi O, Wick MR. Angiosarcoma-like neoplasms of epithelial organs: true endothelial tumors or variants of carcinoma? Semin Diagn Pathol 1995;12:270–82.

150. Takagi M, Sakota Y, Takayama S, Ishikawa G. Adenoid squamous cell carcinoma of the oral mucosa: report of two autopsy cases. Cancer 1977;40:2250–5.

151. Weitzner S. Adenoid squamous cell carcinoma of the vermillion mucosa of lower lip. Oral Surg Oral Med Oral Pathol 1974; 37:589–93.

152. Zaatari GS, Santoianni RA. Adenoid squamous cell carcinoma of the nasopharynx and neck region. Arch Pathol Lab Med 1986;110:542–6.

Adenosquamous Carcinoma

153. Aden KK, Niehans G, Adams GL, Abdel-Fattah HM. Adenosquamous carcinoma of the larynx and hypopharynx with five new case presentations. Trans Am Laryngol Assoc 1988;109:216–21.

154. Bombi JA, Riverola A, Bordas JM, Cardesa A. Adenosquamous carcinoma of the esophagus. A case report. Pathol Res Pract 1991;187:514–9.

155. Damiani JM, Damiani KK, Hauck K, Hyams VJ. Mucoepidermoid-adenosquamous carcinoma of the larynx and hypopharynx: a report of 21 cases and a review of the literature. Otolaryngol Head Neck Surg 1981;89:235–43.

156. Evans HL. Mucoepidermoid carcinoma of the salivary glands: a study of 69 cases with special attention to histologic grading. Am J Clin Pathol 1984;81:696–701.

157. Evans HL. We have met that enemy, but its another neoplasm [Letter]. Am J Clin Pathol 1984; 82:512–3.

158. Fujino K, Ito J, Kanaji M, Shiomi Y, Saiga T. Adenosquamous carcinoma of the larynx. Am J Otolaryngol 1995;16:115–8.

159. Gerughty RM, Hennigar GR, Brown FM. Adenosquamous carcinoma of the nasal, oral and laryngeal cavities. A clinicopathologic study of ten cases. Cancer 1968;22:1140–55.

160. Martinez-Madrigal F, Baden E, Casiraghi O, Micheau C. Oral and pharyngeal adenosquamous carcinoma. A report of four cases with immunohistochemical studies. Eur Arch Otorhinolaryngol 1991;248:255–8.

161. Napier SS, Gormley JS, Newlands C, Ramsay-Baggs P. Adensquamous carcinoma. A rare neoplasm with an aggressive course. Oral Surg Oral Med Oral Pathol Oral Radiol Endod 1995;79:607–11.

162. Siar CH, Ng KH. Adenosquamous carcinoma of the floor of the mouth and lower alveolus: a radiation-induced lesion? Oral Surg Oral Med Oral Pathol 1987;63:216–20.

6
ADENOCARCINOMA (NONSALIVARY SUBTYPES)

Most adenocarcinomas affecting the head and neck region arise from major or minor salivary glands, or closely related seromucinous glands. Tumors of this type are discussed in the third series Fascicle, Tumors of the Salivary Glands (9). This section will discuss two broad categories of adenocarcinoma arising in the head and neck region that appear to be unrelated to salivary gland neoplasia.

SINONASAL INTESTINAL-TYPE ADENOCARCINOMA

Definition. This largest group of nonsalivary sinonasal adenocarcinomas consists of glandular or mucin-producing neoplasms composed of intestinal-type epithelial cells. Included in this group is a microscopic spectrum of neoplasia ranging from tumors resembling conventional colonic adenocarcinomas and mucinous adenocarcinomas to deceptively bland-appearing neoplasms resembling normal intestinal mucosa.

General Features. For more than half a century it has been known that tumors with an intestinal appearance occasionally arise in the sinonasal region (16). Renewed interest in these tumors was sparked in the early 1970s with the demonstration by Hadfield and colleagues (1,2,11,12) that these neoplasms were strongly associated with exposure to hardwood dust in the English furniture-making industry. This was subsequently confirmed in further studies from England, as well as other countries (3,8,14,15, 18). Exposure to softwood dusts in the logging and milling industries, as well as leather dust in the shoemaking industry, and possibly flour dust, have also been implicated as risk factors for the development of these neoplasms (4,8,15). In older studies, before the institution of dust control measures, the incidence of this tumor in long-time woodworkers approached 500 to 1000 times that of the general population (1). About 20 percent of these tumors have historically arisen in individuals with industrial wood dust exposure (2).

Clinical Features. Overall, 80 percent of reported intestinal-type sinonasal adenocarcinomas have occurred in men (4). Reported sites of origin have been as follows: ethmoid sinuses, 40 percent; nasal cavity, 28 percent; maxillary antrum, 23 percent; and indeterminate, 9 percent (4). Typical presenting symptoms include unilateral nasal obstruction, epistaxis, rhinorrhea, mass in the cheek, exophthalmos, or less commonly, symptoms relating to facial nerve involvement (4). Symptoms are typically present for less than a year, but may have been up to 5 years in duration. Often the initial clinical diagnosis is nasal polyps or chronic sinusitis rather than malignancy.

More recent studies have suggested some clinical differences between sinonasal intestinal-type tumors arising in occupationally dust-exposed individuals and those arising sporadically (4). Not surprisingly, tumors related to occupational exposure affect men in 85 to 95 percent of cases. In this setting the tumors show a strong tendency to arise in the ethmoid sinuses (11,12,18). Sporadic tumors frequently arise in women, and involve the maxillary antrum in 20 to 50 percent of cases (fig. 6-1) (4).

Gross Findings. The gross appearance of these tumors is similar to that of colonic adenocarcinomas, and occasionally may mimic the appearance of ulcerated or hemorrhagic inflammatory polyps. A fungating, grossly polypoid or papillary mass with a hemorrhagic to pink-white color is common. Areas of mucosal ulceration are typical and may have associated hemorrhage. Some tumors have a grossly mucoid or gelatinous appearance.

Microscopic Findings. As noted above, these tumors can recapitulate the entire spectrum of appearances assumed by normal, adenomatous, and overtly malignant small and large intestinal mucosae. At one extreme are neoplasms composed of multiple cell types native to the normal small intestine, including Paneth cells, goblet cells, resorptive cells, argentaffin cells, and even focally forming villi with an underlying muscularis mucosae (figs. 6-2–6-4) (16,20). More typical papillary tumors consist of elongated fronds lined by stratified, mitotically active, mildly dysplastic columnar and goblet cells, creating an appearance similar to that of an

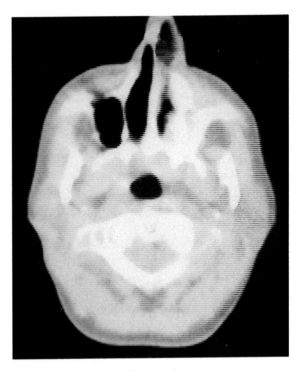

Figure 6-1
INTESTINAL-TYPE ADENOCARCINOMA
An intestinal-type adenocarcinoma involving the left maxillary antrum has produced opacification of the maxillary sinus and has encroached into the left nasal cavity.

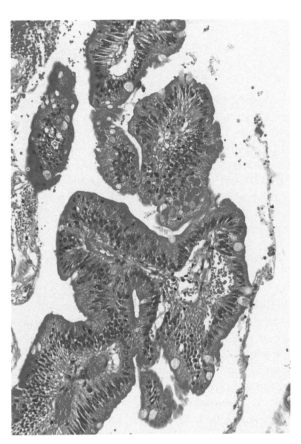

Figure 6-2
INTESTINAL-TYPE ADENOCARCINOMA
This papillary neoplasm consists of epithelial cells closely resembling those found in normal small intestine.

Figure 6-3
INTESTINAL-TYPE
ADENOCARCINOMA

A higher power magnification of the tumor seen in figure 6-2 shows goblet cells, resorptive cells, and Paneth cells. The latter are identified by their coarse eosinophilic cytoplasmic granularity.

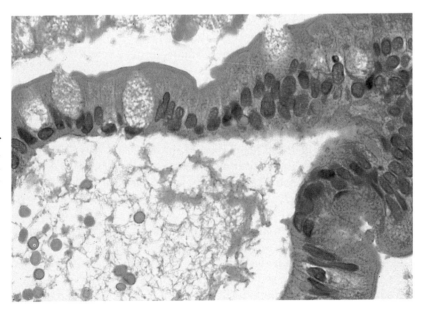

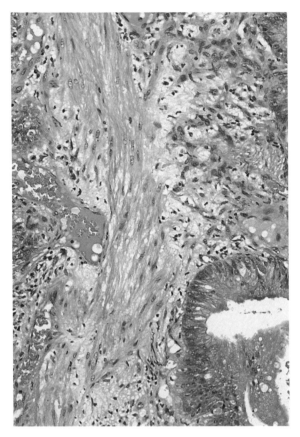

Figure 6-4
INTESTINAL-TYPE ADENOCARCINOMA
Smooth muscle resembling muscularis mucosae of the gastrointestinal tract is present just beneath the surface papillae of this very well-differentiated papillary neoplasm.

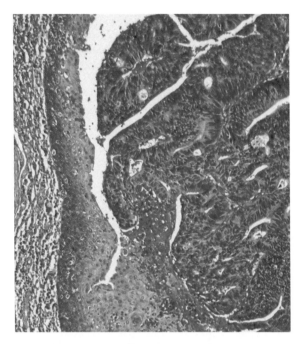

Figure 6-5
INTESTINAL-TYPE ADENOCARCINOMA
This intestinal-type adenocarcinoma grows as a partially exophytic mass adjacent to normal squamous mucosa.

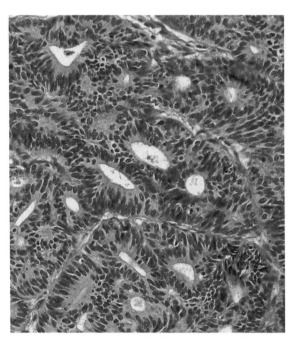

Figure 6-6
INTESTINAL-TYPE ADENOCARCINOMA
Higher magnification from an invasive portion of the tumor seen in figure 6-5 shows complex glandular arrays indistinguishable histologically or cytologically from an adenocarcinoma of the colon.

intestinal tubular or villous adenoma. The papillary neoplasms may be confined to the surface mucosa or be obviously invasive (fig. 6-5) (4,5).

The most common variant of intestinal-type adenocarcinoma resembles typical gland-forming colonic adenocarcinoma. In many instances, the biopsy specimens are completely indistinguishable from a primary colonic neoplasm (figs. 6-6, 6-7). Pleomorphic columnar cells line irregular, back-to-back glands. Mitotic figures, including apparently atypical forms, are easily identified in the glandular cells. Areas of "dirty necrosis" are common, with necrotic cellular debris partially filling glandular lumens. Intracellular and intraluminal mucin are present focally, but goblet cells are not a prominent component of the tumor. In poorly differentiated tumors,

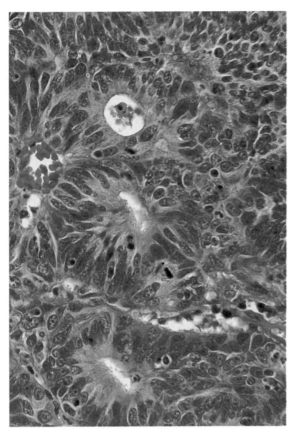

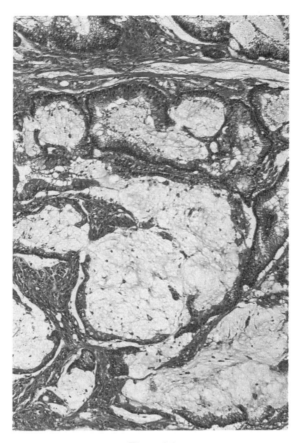

Figure 6-7
INTESTINAL-TYPE ADENOCARCINOMA
Glands in this sinonasal intestinal-type adenocarcinoma are comprised of pseudostratified, tall columnar cells with easily identified mitotic figures.

Figure 6-8
INTESTINAL-TYPE ADENOCARCINOMA
Sinonasal intestinal-type adenocarcinomas occasionally produce large pools of extracellular matrix and strikingly mimic "colloid carcinomas" of the gastrointestinal tract.

gland formation is less obvious and the tumors acquire more prominent "solid" components. Less frequently, sinonasal intestinal-type adenocarcinomas produce abundant mucin which may accumulate in large extracellular pools in a pattern identical to that of colonic colloid carcinoma (figs. 6-8, 6-9), or may be present predominantly intracellularly, forming prominent signet-ring cells (4,5).

Microscopic Grading/Subtyping. The grading of sinonasal intestinal-type adenocarcinoma has been the subject of several studies (4,5,10, 17). Batsakis et al. (5) divided these tumors into papillary, sessile, and alveolar-mucoid neoplasms. Papillary tumors were similar in appearance to colonic adenomas, often lacking clear-cut features of malignancy using criteria applied to analogous colonic lesions. Sessile carcinomas resembled con-

ventional colonic adenocarcinomas, and alveolar mucoid tumors were analogous to colloid or mucinous-type colonic neoplasms. Barnes (4), in an extensive review of the topic, recognized five variants of intestinal-type adenocarcinomas: papillary, colonic, solid, mucinous, and mixed. Papillary and colonic tumors were essentially equivalent to the papillary and sessile designations of Batsakis et al. Solid tumors were more poorly differentiated neoplasms with less obvious gland formation, and mucinous tumors included both extracellular mucinous (colloid) and intracellular mucinous (signet-ring) types. In a review of 79 sinonasal adenocarcinomas arising in woodworkers, Kleinsasser and Schroeder (17) recognized four primary tumor types, and a total of six tumor types and grades. These included papillary-tubular cylinder cell, grades I, II, III;

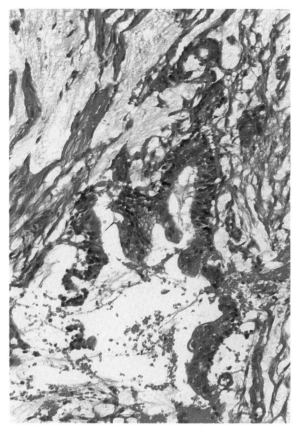

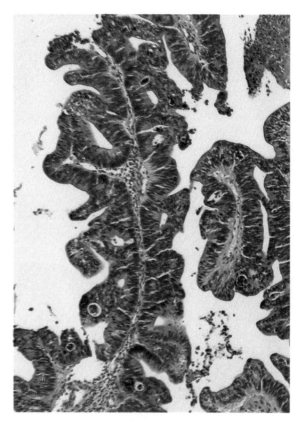

Figure 6-9
INTESTINAL-TYPE ADENOCARCINOMA
Higher magnification of figure 6-8 shows occasional strips of neoplastic columnar cells lining large pools of extracellular mucin.

Figure 6-10
INTESTINAL-TYPE ADENOCARCINOMA
This sinonasal intestinal-type adenocarcinoma shows focal cytoplasmic reactivity for carcinoembryonic antigen (CEA). Reactivity for CEA in these sinonasal tumors is usually negative, or less strongly positive than in analogous gastrointestinal tumors (anti-CEA, hematoxylin).

alveolar goblet cell; solid signet-ring cell; and transitional type neoplasms. The details of this grading system can be found in the literature (10,17). The grade I tumors closely resemble the papillary designation of Batsakis et al. grade II tumors are similar to their sessile designation, and the grade III tumors resemble the solid tumors of Barnes.

Immunohistochemical Findings. Initial immunohistochemical studies helped confirm the intestinal differentiation of these tumors by documenting the presence of intestinal-type hormones including gastrin, glucagon, serotonin, cholecystokinin, and leu-enkephalin in their cytoplasm (6). A subsequent study applied immunohistochemistry to these tumors to determine if diagnostically or prognostically significant profiles of reactivity could be documented (19).

These tumors commonly or uniformly express a spectrum of epithelial markers including cytokeratin, epithelial membrane antigen, B72.3, Ber-EP4, Leu M1, HMFG-2, and BRST-1 (19). Interestingly, although carcinoembryonic antigen is strongly expressed in virtually all colonic adenocarcinomas, only 2 of 12 sinonasal intestinal-type adenocarcinomas showed strong staining for this antigen, 6 showed focal positivity (fig. 6-10), and 4 were negative. In further distinction from colonic neoplasia, 9 of 12 sinonasal adenocarcinomas showed numerous chromogranin-positive cells (fig. 6-11), whereas only 3 of 12 colonic adenocarcinomas showed rare chromogranin positivity.

Ultrastructural Findings. The resemblance of the cells in these neoplasms to those of intestinal mucosa has been confirmed at the

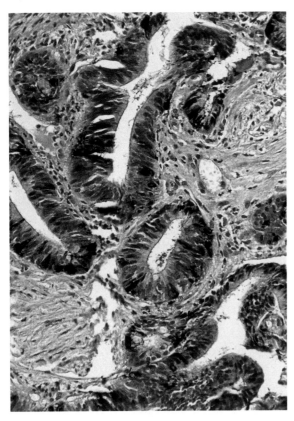

Figure 6-11
INTESTINAL-TYPE ADENOCARCINOMA
Many sinonasal intestinal-type adenocarcinomas show strong evidence of divergent neuroendocrine differentiation, as manifest by focally prominent reactivity for chromogranin (antichromogranin, hematoxylin).

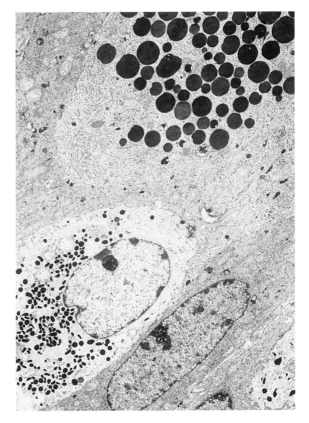

Figure 6-12
INTESTINAL-TYPE ADENOCARCINOMA
Ultrastructurally, this example of sinonasal intestinal-type adenocarcinoma shows Paneth cells with large zymogen-like granules (upper right) and neuroendocrine cells with much smaller dense-core granules (lower left).

ultrastructural level (6,20,22). Goblet cells, resorptive cells, Paneth cells, and argentaffin cells have all been present (fig. 6-12). In addition, several studies have documented muscularis mucosae-like smooth muscle (16,20,21).

Differential Diagnosis. When confronted with a histologically malignant-appearing intestinal-type adenocarcinoma in the sinonasal region, pathologists undoubtedly consider the possibility of metastatic disease, particularly if they have not previously encountered primary sinonasal tumors of this type. Gastrointestinal adenocarcinomas have been documented to metastasize to this region (7) and this concern is therefore reasonable. As noted above in the section on immunohistochemistry, strong staining for carcinoembryonic antigen supports the possibility of metastatic disease and, conversely,

strong staining for chromogranin is more typical of primary sinonasal tumors (19). This distinction is not a problem with the well-differentiated sinonasal intestinal-type tumors resembling colonic adenomas or even normal colonic mucosa.

Because of the presence of mucin-secreting cells, sinonasal intestinal-type adenocarcinomas occasionally may be confused with mucoepidermoid carcinoma. However, the former lacks the multiple, distinct cell types, including squamous cells, clear cells, intermediate cells, and mucinous cells, that typify mucoepidermoid carcinoma. Intestinal-type adenocarcinomas must also be distinguished from the low-grade adenocarcinomas of the sinonasal and nasopharyngeal regions described in detail in the next section (13,23). These tumors consist of well-formed glands lined by a single layer of cells without nuclear stratification. There is minimal mitotic activity. In our experience, the glands lack any resemblance to intestinal-type epithelium and may occasionally resemble papillary adenocarcinoma of the thyroid gland.

Spread and Metastasis. These neoplasms are characterized by one or more local recurrences in over half of patients (4). Regional lymph node and distant metastases are less common, seen in 8 percent and 13 percent of patients, respectively (4).

Treatment and Prognosis. The optimal treatment for sinonasal intestinal-type adenocarcinoma is complete surgical resection, with adjuvant radiation therapy to the region of the tumor. Given the low rate of regional lymph node metastasis, routine radical neck dissections are not recommended (4). Individual enlarged or suspicious lymph nodes may be initially evaluated by fine needle aspiration, followed by resection if necessary. Barnes (4) reviewed the clinical features of 213 cases, at least 19 percent of which occurred in woodworkers. Overall, 60 percent of patients were known to have died of disease, and 80 percent of these did so within 3 years of diagnosis. Survival up to 9 years before death from disease was noted. Some studies have shown a slight survival difference for patients with dust-related versus sporadic tumors: those with dust-related intestinal-type adenocarcinomas have an approximately 50 percent 5-year survival (18); sporadic tumors appear to have a poorer prognosis with a 20 to 40 percent survival at 5 years (4). Regardless of the pathogenesis, the clinical course for these tumors can be quite protracted and 5-year disease-free survival cannot be equated with cure.

Several studies have shown that grade and subtype correlate with patients' overall survival rate and duration of survival. Batsakis et al. (5) initially suggested a slightly better prognosis for patients with the papillary subtype, as opposed to those with the sessile and alveolar-mucoid variants. This was supported in a subsequent study (18). As described above, Barnes (4) recognized five variants of intestinal-type adenocarcinoma, and in his review, it was again noted that those with papillary tumors had a slightly better prognosis. In a review of 79 sinonasal adenocarcinomas arising in woodworkers by Kleinsasser and Schroeder (17), patients with grade 1 papillary-tubular tumors had the best 3-year survival

rate (82 percent); those with signet-ring cell tumors had the worse prognosis, with none of three patients alive at 3 years. We applied this grading approach to a series of 15 woodworking-related and sporadic intestinal-type adenocarcinomas (10). Although the number of cases was small, the 4 patients with grade 1 papillary tubular tumors had a median survival period of 9 years, whereas the median survival period for the 6 patients with grade 2 papillary tumors was 3 years.

Regardless of the degree of differentiation, all forms of intestinal-type adenocarcinoma should be considered to be locally aggressive. Even tumors deceptively resembling normal intestinal epithelial are known to be locally destructive, ultimately fatal neoplasms (16,20). Nonetheless, several studies have shown a somewhat better prognosis for the well-differentiated, papillary-tubular variant (10,17).

LOW-GRADE ADENOCARCINOMA

Definition. This is a microscopically somewhat heterogeneous group of well-differentiated, often papillary adenocarcinomas arising in the sinonasal and nasopharyngeal regions and lacking intestinal-like features. Tumors in this group will likely undergo additional definition and subdivision as more examples are studied.

General Features. Unlike intestinal-type sinonasal adenocarcinomas, risk factors have not been identified for these low-grade neoplasms. There is no apparent association with tobacco use or alcohol consumption, and no genetic, occupational, or environmental factors have been identified (26).

Clinical Features. In a review of 23 patients with low-grade lesions from the sinonasal region, age distribution ranged from 9 to 75 years, with most being in their fifth through seventh decades of life (24). There was no sex or racial predilection. Patients typically presented with nasal obstruction or epistaxis. Fewer than 10 percent complained of pain. Symptom duration averaged 5.5 months, but was 5 years in one case. Tumor location was as follows: ethmoid sinus, 30 percent; nasal cavity, 22 percent; nasal septum, 17.5 percent; multiple sinuses, 17.5 percent; and maxillary antrum, 13 percent. Similar clinical findings were seen in a study of nine microscopically analogous nasopharyngeal neoplasms (26).

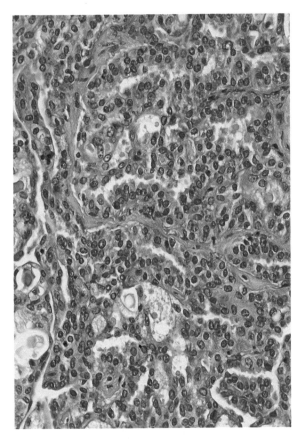

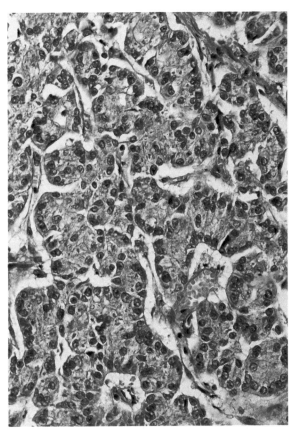

Figure 6-13
ADENOCARCINOMA
Some tumors classified as low-grade adenocarcinomas of the sinonasal region closely resemble acinic cell carcinomas and may derive from seromucinous glands.

Figure 6-14
ADENOCARCINOMA
The trabecular pattern of this well-differentiated adenocarcinoma and its basophilic cytoplasm suggest that it should be classified as an acinic cell carcinoma, rather than "low-grade" adenocarcinoma.

Gross Findings. The tumors have been described as often having a papillary or cauliflower-like gross appearance (26). The consistency is usually soft, but may be gritty if significant numbers of psammomatous calcifications are present. Tumors have ranged in size from 0.3 to 4.0 (median, 2.5) cm (26).

Microscopic Findings. Some lesions included under this rubric are comprised of cells with granular basophilic cytoplasm growing in acinar-like nests (fig. 6-13) (24). Tumors of the latter type are light microscopically indistinguishable from acinic cell carcinoma of salivary origin (fig. 6-14). In addition, we have personally encountered sinonasal and nasopharyngeal neoplasms resembling so-called oncocytoid adenocarcinomas and clear cell carcinomas with fea-

tures of epimyoepithelial carcinoma. In our opinion, these apparent salivary-type neoplasms should be segregated from other nonsalivary tumors in this group.

After elimination of apparent salivary-type neoplasms, one is left with a group of well-differentiated adenocarcinomas not resembling intestinal-type mucosa or neoplasia and characterized by papillary formations with well-formed glandular lumina. Some tumors in this category have a degree of morphologic and cytologic uniformity that is often confused with an adenoma or papilloma. There is considerable variation in cytologic appearance, suggesting that further subdivisions of this group may be forthcoming. Some tumors are composed of elongated cells with nonstratified, basally oriented nuclei and

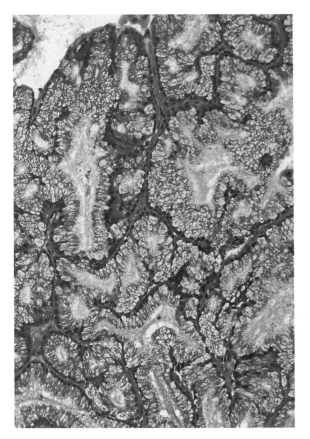

Figure 6-15
LOW-GRADE ADENOCARCINOMA
This well-differentiated sinonasal intestinal-type adenocarcinoma is comprised of columnar cells with nonstratified
basal nuclei and abundant intracytoplasmic mucin.

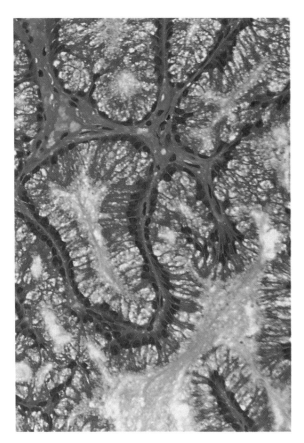

Figure 6-16
LOW-GRADE ADENOCARCINOMA
Higher magnification of the tumor seen in figure 6-15
shows glands lined by uniform cells resembling endocervical
cells. The basal uniform nuclei are unlike the stratified, more
pleomorphic nuclei seen in intestinal-type adenocarcinomas.

abundant intracytoplasmic mucin (figs. 6-15, 6-16). Neoplasms of this type somewhat resemble endocervical cells. Other tumors encompassed in this group have prominent papillations lined by cells with granular cytoplasm and overlapping, vesicular nuclei resembling the cells of papillary adenocarcinoma of the thyroid gland. Psammoma bodies have also been documented in tumors of this type. Importantly, immunohistochemistry for thyroglobulin has been nonreactive (26). Still other examples have large or cystically dilated glandular spaces with cell bridges producing a cribriform pattern somewhat evocative of cribriform intraductal carcinoma of the breast (24).

Immunohistochemical Findings. Only five examples of low-grade adenocarcinoma have been subjected to immunohistochemical study with a limited panel of antibodies (26). The neo-

plastic cells were strongly immunoreactive for cytokeratin and epithelial membrane antigen, focally reactive for carcinoembryonic antigen, and negative for glial fibrillary acidic protein, S-100 protein, and thyroglobulin.

Differential Diagnosis. Low-grade adenocarcinomas should be distinguished from intestinal-type neoplasms because of their considerably less aggressive clinical course and better survival rate (24,26). This is usually a straightforward determination. Low-grade adenocarcinomas, by definition, lack an "intestinal" microscopic appearance. Except for the rare intestinal-type tumor mimicking adenoma or even normal intestinal mucosa, the majority of intestinal-type neoplasms are considerably more pleomorphic than low-grade adenocarcinoma. As noted above, these tumors, in our opinion, should also be distinguished from neoplasms with features of salivary-type differentiation. Included in this group are acinic cell carcinomas, and, perhaps, oncocytic carcinomas with other features suggestive of minor salivary or seromucinous gland origin. As Heffner et al. (24) described, low-grade adenocarcinomas composed of cells with more granular, eosinophilic cytoplasm may be confused with oncocytic schneiderian papillomas. They considered the following criteria of value in making this distinction: 1) stratified epithelium in papillomas as opposed to the single layer of neoplastic cells in low-grade adenocarcinoma; 2) frequent, well-formed glandular lumina in adenocarcinoma; 3) often prominent myxoid stroma in papillomas.

As noted above, papillary low-grade adenocarcinomas may mimic thyroid neoplasia, a similarity enhanced by the presence of psammoma bodies and neoplastic cells with overlapping vesicular nuclei lining complex papillae. It seems prudent to assess thyroglobulin reactivity in all such cases in order to distinguish metastatic thyroid neoplasia (26).

Finally, low-grade adenocarcinomas should also be distinguished from epithelial adenomatoid hamartomas (25,27). These lesions grossly resemble inflammatory polyps, but microscopically contain often complex gland-like epithelial proliferations. The epithelial component often resembles normal respiratory mucosa, with a pseudostratified appearance composed of ciliated and scattered mucinous cells (25). The epithelial nests are often surrounded by prominent cuffs of stromal hyalinization (25). The overall appearance is easily distinguished from the uniform, nonstratified epithelium of low-grade adenocarcinoma. Uncommonly, epithelial adenomatoid hamartomas may contain seromucinous glands (25,27). The presence of multiple cell types, a prominent basal/myoepithelial cell layer, and the lack of a desmoplastic stromal reaction should allow distinction from low-grade adenocarcinoma.

Treatment and Prognosis. Treatment for these tumors has been surgical resection via an appropriate approach. Nasopharyngeal lesions have been removed by transpalatal resection (26). Sinonasal lesions may require a lateral rhinotomy, Caldwell-Luc procedure, and removal of the affected sinus or intranasal tumor (24). A few patients have received adjuvant radiation therapy, but given the overall good prognosis and limited number of cases, there is no evidence that this affects survival.

Of the 23 patients with low-grade adenocarcinoma in one study (24), a median follow-up interval of 6.3 years (range, 3.7 to 11.3 years) showed 18 patients (78 percent) had no evidence of disease; 3 patients were alive with locally recurrent disease, in 2 of whom recurrence was not extensive and potentially curable; and 2 patients (9 percent) died of disease, both following multiple local recurrences. One of the two latter patients developed apparent metastases to the oropharynx and larynx, and the other patient's tumor was said to have undergone anaplastic transformation.

REFERENCES

Adenocarcinoma (Nonsalivary Subtypes)

1. Acheson ED, Cowdell RH, Hadfield E, Macbeth RG. Nasal cancer in woodworkers in the furniture industry. Br Med J 1968;2:587–96.
2. Acheson ED, Cowdell RH, Jolles B. Nasal cancer in the Northhamptonshire boot and shoe industry. Br Med J 1970;1:385–93.
3. Andersen HC, Andersen I, Solgaard J. Nasal cancers, symptoms and upper airway function in woodworkers. Br J Ind Med 1977;34:201–7.
4. Barnes L. Intestinal-type adenocarcinoma of the nasal cavity and paranasal sinuses. Am J Surg Pathol 1986;10:192–202.
5. Batsakis JG, Holtz F, Sueper RH. Adenocarcinoma of the nasal and paranasal cavities. Arch Otolaryngol 1963;77:625–33.
6. Batsakis JG, Mackay B, Ordóñez NG. Enteric-type adenocarcinoma of the nasal cavity. An electron microscopic and immunocytochemical study. Cancer 1984;54:855–60.
7. Bernstein JM, Montgomery WW, Balogh K Jr. Metastatic tumors to the maxilla, nose, and paranasal sinuses. Laryngoscope 1966;76:621–50.
8. Cècchi F, Buiatti E, Kriebel D, Nastasi L, Santucci M. Adenocarcinoma of the nose and paranasal sinuses in shoemakers and woodworkers in the province of Florence, Italy (1963-77). Br J Med 1980;37:222–5.
9. Ellis GL, Auclair PL. Tumors of the salivary glands. Atlas of Tumor Pathology, 3rd Series, Fascicle 17. Washington, D.C.: Armed Forces Institute of Pathology, 1996.
10. Franquemont DW, Fechner RE, Mills SE. Histologic classification of sinonasal intestinal-type adenocarcinoma. Am J Surg Pathol 1991;15:368–75.
11. Hadfield EH. A study of adenocarcinoma of the paranasal sinuses in woodworkers in the furniture industry. Ann R Coll Surg Engl 1970;46:301–19.
12. Hadfield EH, Macbeth RG. Adenocarcinoma of ethmoids in furniture workers. Ann Otol Rhinol Laryngol 1971;80:699–703.
13. Heffner DK, Hyams VJ, Hauck KW, Lingeman C. Low-grade adenocarcinoma of the nasal cavity and paranasal sinuses. Cancer 1982;50:312–22.
14. Imbus HR, Dyson WL. A review of nasal cancer in furniture manufacturing and woodworking in North Carolina, the United States, and other countries. J Occup Med 1987;29:734–40.
15. Ironside P, Matthews J. Adenocarcinoma of the nose and paranasal sinuses in woodworkers in the state of Victoria, Australia. Cancer 1975;36:1115–24.
16. Jarvi O. Heterotopic tumors with an intestinal mucous membrane structure in the nasal cavity. Acta Otolaryngol 1945;33:471–85.
17. Kleinsasser O, Schroeder HG. Adenocarcinoma of the inner nose after exposure to wood dust. Morphological findings and relationships between histopathology and clinical behavior in 79 cases. Arch Otorhinolaryngol 1988;245:1–15.
18. Klintenberg C, Olofsson J, Hellquist H, Sokjer H. Adenocarcinoma of the ethmoid sinuses. A review of 28 cases with special reference to wood dust exposure. Cancer 1984;54:482–8.
19. McKinney CD, Mills SE, Franquemont DW. Sinonasal intestinal-type adenocarcinoma. Immunohistochemical profile and comparison with colonic adenocarcinoma. Mod Pathol 1995;8:421–6.
20. Mills SE, Fechner RE, Cantrell RW. Aggressive sinonasal lesion resembling normal intestinal mucosa. Am J Surg Pathol 1982;6:803–9.
21. Sanchez-Casis G, Devine KD, Weiland LH. Nasal adenocarcinomas that closely simulate colonic carcinomas. Cancer 1971;28:714–20.
22. Schmid KO, Aubock L, Albegger K. Endocrine-amphicrine enteric carcinoma of the nasal mucosa. Virchows Arch [A] 1979;383:329–43.
23. Wenig BM, Hyams VJ, Heffner DK. Nasopharyngeal papillary adenocarcinoma. A clinicopathologic study of a low-grade carcinoma. Am J Surg Pathol 1988;12:946–53.

Low-Grade Adenocarcinoma

24. Heffner DK, Hyams VJ, Hauck KW, Lingeman C. Low-grade adenocarcinoma of the nasal cavity and paranasal sinuses. Cancer 1982;50:312–22.
25. Wenig BM, Heffner DK. Respiratory epithelial adenomatoid hamartomas of the sinonasal tract and nasopharynx: a clinicopathologic study of 31 cases. Ann Otol Rhinol Laryngol 1995;104:639–45.
26. Wenig BM, Hyams VJ, Heffner DK. Nasopharyngeal papillary adenocarcinoma. A clinicopathologic study of a low-grade carcinoma. Am J Surg Pathol 1988;12:946–53.
27. Zarbo RJ, McClatchey KD. Nasopharyngeal hamartoma: report of a case and review of the literature. Laryngoscope 1983;93:494–7.

7
NEURAL, NEUROENDOCRINE, AND NEUROECTODERMAL NEOPLASIA

HETEROTOPIC GLIAL TISSUE (NASAL GLIOMA)

Definition. Glial heterotopia ("nasal glioma") is a congenital misplacement of central nervous system tissue in or about the nose. Glial heterotopias are thought to result from the failure of the developing frontal lobe to retract completely via the foramen cecum. Thus they represent sequestered encephaloceles, not true neoplasms (figs. 7-1, 7-2).

Clinical Findings. Virtually all are present at birth although rare lesions have been described in patients up to 50 years of age (11). Nasal gliomas are not familial and are not associated with other congenital anomalies. A 1.5–3.0 to 1 male predominance has been reported (1,5). About 25 percent of lesions occur posterior to the nasal bone and present as intranasal polypoid masses (1,4,5); 60 percent occur as subcutaneous lesions anterior to the nasal bone (fig.

7-3); and the remainder have combined features. Glial heterotopia at other locations in the upper aerodigestive tract is less common, with rare lesions reported in the nasopharynx, palate, paranasal sinuses, and tonsillar and pterygopalatine fossae (1,3,5,6,8,10).

Patients with intranasal lesions usually present within the first year of life. The lesions are often associated with respiratory distress, nasal obstruction, epistaxis, or cerebrospinal fluid rhinorrhea. The stalk or base of the lesion is frequently attached to the lateral nasal wall near the middle turbinate. Deviation of the septum, nasal bone, or both is common. Up to 25 percent of intranasal lesions are associated with an underlying bony defect, usually in the cribriform plate, and may be attached to the underlying dura by a fibrous stalk.

Subcutaneous lesions manifest as firm, rounded subcutaneous nodules on the bridge or side of the nose; patients present late in life with cosmetic concerns (11). Other subcutaneous sites

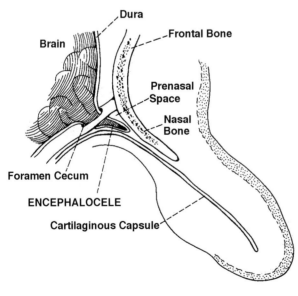

Figure 7-1
ENCEPHALOCELE

A sagittal section of the nose showing a developing encephalocele. (Fig. 2 from Katz A, Lewis JS. Nasal gliomas. Arch Otolaryngol 1971;94:351–5.)

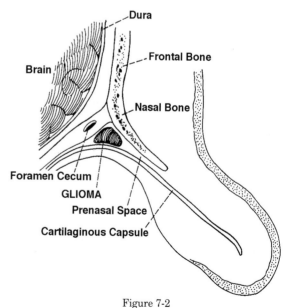

Figure 7-2
HETEROTOPIC GLIAL TISSUE/NASAL GLIOMA

Sagittal section of the nose: resultant glioma following closure of the foramen cecum. (Fig. 3 from Katz A, Lewis JS. Nasal gliomas. Arch Otolaryngol 1971;94:351–5.)

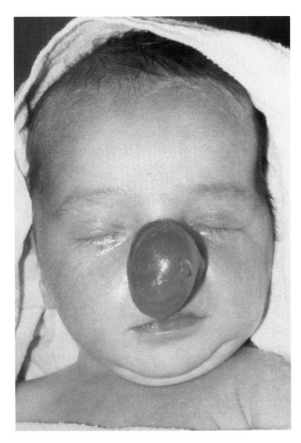

Figure 7-3
SUBCUTANEOUS GLIAL HETEROTOPIA
Sixty percent of nasal "gliomas" arise as subcutaneous lesions anterior to the nasal bone.

away from the bridge of the nose include the ethmoid bone, angle of the eye, and orbit

Glial heterotopias are benign and cured by simple excision, although rare local recurrences have been documented (1,5). About 25 percent retain communication with the central nervous system by a fibrous stalk and may be associated with postoperative cerebrospinal fluid leakage or meningitis. Magnetic resonance imaging (MRI) is superior to computed tomography (CT) for visualizing bony defects and intracranial extension (9). Unequivocal malignant transformation has not been described. Chan et al. (2) reported a bilateral intranasal glial lesion in continuity with a left frontal lobe astrocytoma. Whether this represented downward extension of the tumor or the coexistence of heterotopic glial tissue and an intracerebral astrocytoma is unclear.

Gross Findings. Glial tissue is never recognized on gross examination, thus macroscopic descriptions are rare. Intranasal lesions often appear as firm, lobulated fragments of gray-white, glistening tissue, either solid or partially cystic on cut section (8). Subcutaneous lesions appear as firm, white, circumscribed nodules within the deep dermis or subcutaneous fat.

Microscopic Findings. Histologically, glial heterotopias are circumscribed but unencapsulated proliferations of astrocytes and fibrillary glial processes (fig. 7-4). Most lesions consist of closely spaced lobules of glial tissue separated by

Figure 7-4
SUBCUTANEOUS
GLIAL HETEROTOPIA

A section of a subcutaneous heterotopic glial tissue presenting on the anterior bridge of the nose, showing a circumscribed but unencapsulated proliferation of central nervous system tissue and overlying squamous epithelium.

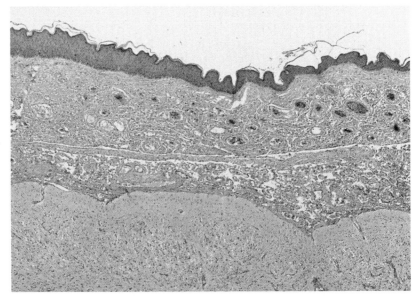

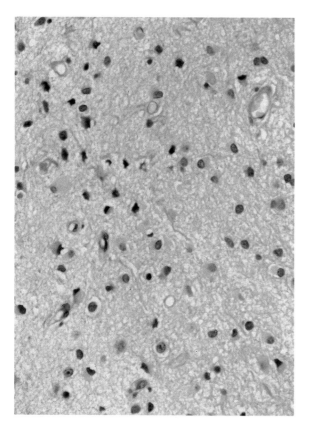

Figure 7-5
INTRANASAL GLIAL HETEROTOPIA
Intranasal heterotopic glial tissue showing a proliferation of astrocytes and fibrillary glial processes.

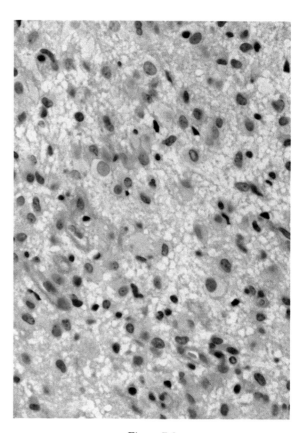

Figure 7-6
SUBCUTANEOUS GLIAL HETEROTOPIA
Occasional gliomas are composed of both bland, fusiform astrocytes as well as enlarged (gemistocytic) forms.

fibrovascular septa (fig. 7-5) (11). The astrocytes are usually fusiform, bland, and inconspicuous but may appear enlarged (gemistocytic), multinucleated, or mildly atypical (fig. 7-6) (2,11). Scattered neurons are present in a minority of cases (8). Rare cases with a prominent neuronal component have been reported (7). Choroid plexus and meningeal elements are not present. Typically there is no evidence of nuclear pleomorphism or mitotic activity. Intranasal lesions are often covered by nasal respiratory mucosa, whereas subcutaneous lesions are located deep to the reticular dermis (11).

Theaker et al. (11) described a sclerotic variant, composed of irregular, solid fibrous nodules with an inconspicuous or absent fibrillary background. Rare sclerotic lesions have small nests of astrocytes interspersed in a diffuse fibrous stroma.

Immunohistochemical Findings. The fibrillary matrix in nasal glioma is strongly pos-

itive for glial fibrillary acid protein and variably positive for neurofilament. The cellular (astrocyte/neuron) component is invariably positive for S-100 protein (fig. 7-7) (7,8,11). Epithelial and meningeal markers such as epithelial membrane antigen are absent (11).

Ultrastructural Findings. The few cases examined by electron microscopy have shown abundant collagen fibrils interspersed with astrocyte-like cells and glial processes (8,12). The cells are surrounded by a basal lamina and contain a moderate number of organelles with bundles of intermediate filaments. Apparent microglial cells with numerous mitochondria, lysozyomes, and microtubules have also been described (8).

Differential Diagnosis. It is important to distinguish glial heterotopias from true encephaloceles and meningoceles, as the latter lesions are in direct continuity with the intracranial space. True encephaloceles consist of mature glial

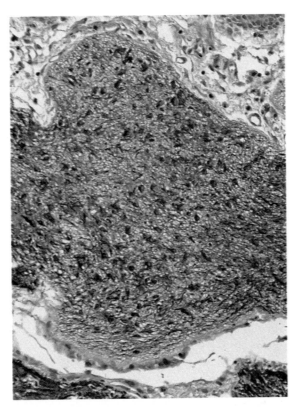 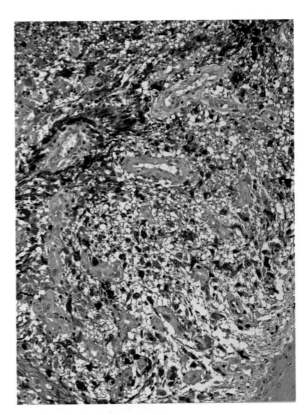

Figure 7-7
SUBCUTANEOUS GLIAL HETEROTOPIA
Glial heterotopias are typically immunohistochemically positive for glial fibrillary acid protein (left) and S-100 protein (right). The overlying epithelium is appropriately negative for both neural markers.

tissue, with the variable presence of dura and lepto-meninges. Encephaloceles without recognizable dura and leptomeninges can be distinguished from glial heterotopia only after clinicopathologic correlation. Clinically, intranasal and subcutaneous lesions may be confused with polyps and dermoid cysts, respectively. Immunostaining may be necessary for the diagnosis of sclerotic variants.

ECTOPIC PITUITARY TISSUE AND PITUITARY ADENOMA

General Features. Depending on the immuno-phenotype, 21 to 82 percent (mean: 35 percent estimated rate of gross invasion) of pituitary adenomas invade the dura and bones of the sella turcica (26). Most pituitary adenomas discovered in the upper aerodigestive tract extend from the floor of the sella turcica into the sphenoid sinus, nasopharynx, and, less commonly, the nasal cavity. Less often, pituitary adenomas arise from

ectopic tissue not in continuity with the intrasel-lar pituitary gland (13,16,17,23,27,28). Ectopic anterior lobe tissue may be found along the em-bryologic course of Rathke's pouch. Such tissue occurs within the sella turcica but outside the capsule of the pituitary gland; within the substance of the sphenoid bone or sinus; or, most commonly, in the soft tissues of the dorsal pharyngeal wall (13).

The pharyngeal pituitary lies deep within the midline of the pharyngeal mucosa or in the periosteum beneath or near the vomerosphenoidal articulation (22). Microscopic rests of ectopic pituitary tissue are found in the roof of the nasopharynx in almost 100 percent of people (22). In a study of 133 pharyngeal pituitaries, the maximum size was 9.6 mm long, 1.5 mm wide, and 1.0 mm deep (21). Embryologic remnants of Rathke's pouch may exhibit hormonal activity, and are occasionally important in hypophysectomized patients (23). They rarely give rise to adenomas. Of the 19 extracranial ectopic pituitary adenomas recorded in the literature, 68 percent arose in the sphenoid sinus (13); less often, they were found in the nasopharynx, nasal cavity, temporal bone, or clivus. Of 15 ectopic adenomas recently studied, the site of occurrence included the sphenoid sinus (8 cases), nasopharynx (5 cases), nasal cavity (1 case), and ethmoid sinus (1 case). Extrasellar pituitary adenoma may also occur in association with an intrasellar pituitary tumor; in this situation, the pathogenesis may be related to hematogenous or cerebrospinal fluid dissemination of the intrasellar neoplasm or to dislodgement of pituitary gland tumor cells at the time of a prior surgical procedure (23,27). Pituitary adenoma, ectopic or extending from the sella, may involve the clivus, clinically simulating a chordoma (29). Such lesions sometimes require immunohistochemistry or electron microscopy for diagnosis.

Clinical Features. The symptoms of an intracranial pituitary adenoma that extends to the upper aerodigestive tract are usually related to the intracranial portion of the neoplasm. These include headaches, visual field defects, and evidence of hormonal activity (16); nasal involvement may result in obstruction or epistaxis. For patients with ectopic adenomas, the age range is wide and symptoms are due to local mass effect or clinical evidence of hormonal secretion. Cushing's syndrome, acromegaly, hyperparathyroidism, and increased prolactin secretion have been described in these patients (13,16,17,27).

Microscopic Findings. Ectopic pituitary tissue, having a poorly defined capsule anteriorly, appears as irregular cords or islands of cells separated by vascularized connective tissue. These pituitary cells may intermingle with cells from the minor salivary glands. Acidophils, basophils, and chromophobe cells are often found in approximately the same proportion as in the normal anterior pituitary gland (24). In one autopsy study, 21 percent of tumors had collections of colloid and clumps of squamous cells (20); in 12 percent, the pharyngeal pituitary was reported to be composed exclusively of squamous cells. Mucinous acini are sometimes seen (14).

Ectopic pituitary adenomas are microscopically identical to their intrasellar counterparts, but because of their rarity and wide morphologic spectrum they may be misdiagnosed. They are submucosal and have a variety of growth patterns including solid, organoid, and trabecular (28). The tumor cells are set in a fibrovascular stroma and have round nuclei with dispersed chromatin and granular eosinophilic cytoplasm. Mitotic figures, necrosis, and marked pleomorphism are usually absent (figs. 7-8, 7-9) (28). The majority of ectopic adenomas consist of chromophobe cells (13). Correct classification of adenomas, however, is based upon the detection of hormones by immunohistochemical methods. Invasive adenomas show increased nuclear pleomorphism and mitotic figures compared to noninvasive tumors, but the features are sufficiently inconsistent and behavior cannot be predicted (15,19). Pituitary adenomas involving the clivus sometimes show nuclear pleomorphism and mitotic figures, raising other diagnostic possibilities (29).

Immunohistochemical Findings. The major hormones normally found in the anterior pituitary can be demonstrated immunohistochemically in ectopic pituitary tissue (20). In a study of eight adult pharyngeal pituitary glands, the percentage of the seven hormone-producing cell types varied from 1 to 30 percent. It may be important to ascertain the hormonal content of ectopic adenomas. Although immunostains for particular hormones may be applied depending upon the clinical setting, a full panel is usual, and includes antibodies to prolactin, adrenocorticotropic hormone (ACTH), growth hormone (GH), leutinizing hormone (LH), follicle-stimulating hormone (FSH), thyroid-stimulating hormone (TSH), and the alpha subunit (fig. 7-9) (26). In a study of 15 ectopic adenomas, 6 were immunoreactive with one pituitary hormone, 6 were positive for two or more hormones (plurihormonal), and one was negative (null cell) (28). Intrasellar pituitary adenomas are usually immunoreactive for cytokeratin (CAM5.2; 83 percent), chromogranin (70 percent), synaptophysin (100 percent) and neuron-specific enolase (100 percent) (18) and negative for S-100 protein, carcinoembryonic antigen, vimentin, epithelial membrane antigen, gastrin, calcitonin, insulin, glucagon, somatostatin, and CD34 (25). Occasional variations in the expected results may occur, however (25).

In a comparison study, 10 invasive pituitary adenomas involving the sphenoid sinus were more often immunohistochemically positive for IL-6 and heat shock protein 27 than the 10 noninvasive tumors (15). Antibodies to Ki-67 and PCNA failed

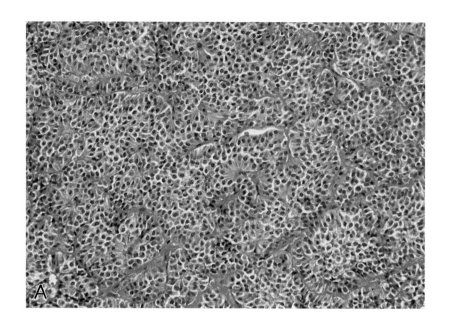

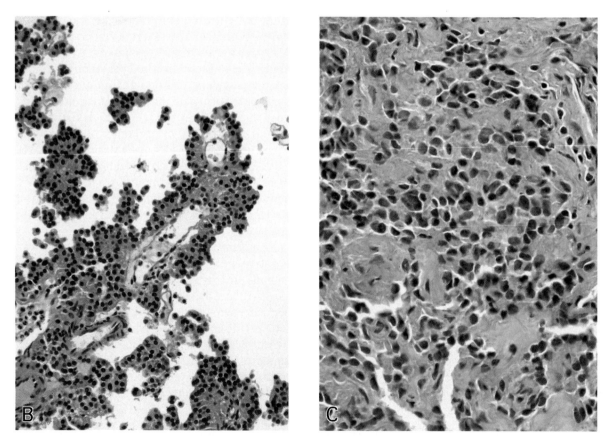

Figure 7-8
SINONASAL PITUITARY ADENOMA

Pituitary adenoma, whether it is intrasellar or ectopic, has a diffuse pattern of growth (A), forms papillae (B), or, uncommonly, consists of pleomorphic cells (C).

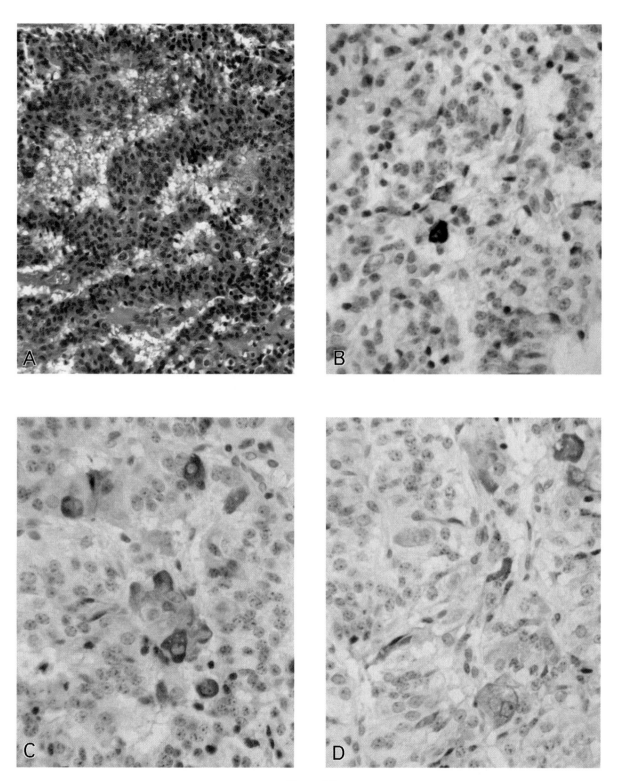

Figure 7-9
PITUITARY ADENOMA
This intrasellar adenoma that extended to the nasopharynx had a ribbon growth pattern focally (A). Immunohistochemistry, which may be important in separating pituitary adenoma from other neoplasms of the upper aerodigestive tract, was positive for ACTH (B), LH (C), and FSH (D). In addition, it was immunoreactive for prolactin (immunoperoxidase technique).

to predict biologic aggression. The biologic tendency to invade relates, in part, to the immunohistochemical characteristics (26). The lowest rate of invasion (21 percent) was found in adenomas containing FSH and LH cells, while the highest frequency of invasion (82 percent) was observed for adenomas with ACTH cells (26).

Differential Diagnosis. In the absence of pertinent clinical information, the diagnosis of ectopic pituitary adenoma may be problematic. Pituitary adenomas in biopsy specimens, particularly those that are small and distorted, may be difficult to distinguish from carcinoma, melanoma, paraganglioma, and olfactory neuroblastoma. An appropriate assortment of immunohistochemical stains, including those for pituitary hormones, is important for diagnosis. In lieu of immunohistochemistry, electron microscopy can help identify pituitary adenoma as well as classify it. Ultrastructural classification is based on the size of the cytoplasmic granules.

When involving the clivus the differential diagnosis includes chordoma, chondosarcoma, meningioma, astrocytoma, craniopharyngioma, germ cell tumor, lymphoma, melanoma, and metastatic carcinoma (29).

Treatment and Prognosis. Ectopic pituitary adenomas are usually managed surgically, which is typically curative (28). A combined sinonasal and anterior fossa approach may be necessary for the eradication of invasive examples (15). More aggressive surgery may be required for a more extensive neoplasm (13). If resection is incomplete, postoperative radiation therapy may be utilized.

NEUROFIBROMA

General Features. Neurofibroma of the upper aerodigestive tract may be solitary or multiple. Sometimes it represents a component of neurofibromatosis 1 (von Recklinghausen's disease) (30–32,35,38,39), an autosomal dominant disorder whose gene is located in the centromeric region of the long arm of chromosome 17 (17q11.2) (33,36). The neurofibromatosis 1 protein, neurofibromin, has a tumor suppressor function and has the ability to down-regulate p21-ras; uncontrolled cell growth or tumor formation would result from loss of neurofibromin (40).

In the oral cavity, neurofibroma is seen as a nontender solitary mass, as multiple nodules, or as diffuse tissue involvement. The tongue is the most frequent site affected, and there may be deep infiltration into the adjacent tissues of the neck. Neurofibroma arising in the nasal cavity or paranasal sinuses is rare (34,37,39), occurring less often than neurilemoma; a solitary sinonasal neurofibroma may involve more than one paranasal sinus. When located in the larynx, it usually occurs in the false cords or aryepiglottic folds (31,38). Neurofibroma, either solitary or in association with neurofibromatosis 1, rarely occurs in the nasopharynx or trachea (35). A few examples of malignant schwannoma arising within a neurofibroma have been documented in the upper aerodigestive tract.

Neurofibromas may be seen in patients with neurofibromatosis 2 as well. This clinically and genetically distinct disorder is described in the section on neurilemoma, as acoustic neurilemoma is really the hallmark of neurofibromatosis 2.

Clinical Features. The unilateral macroglossia seen in patients with neurofibromatosis 1 results from plexiform neurofibroma. Of 12 patients with neurofibromatosis macroglossia, almost all were less than 3 years old (30). Neurofibromas elsewhere in the oral cavity occur as asymptomatic submucosal masses in patients having a wide age range. Laryngeal involvement manifests as a fullness in the throat, cough, hoarseness, or dyspnea. Symptoms may be present for years. Although occurrence in the larynx may be seen at any age and may even be present at birth, young adults are most commonly affected (38). Symptoms from nasal or paranasal sinus neurofibroma include obstruction, swelling, and evidence of a mass.

Gross Findings. Solitary neurofibroma appears as an unencapsulated, tan to gray, submucosal nodule. The involved nerve may be seen entering and exiting the fusiform mass. The degenerative features typical of neurilemoma are lacking in neurofibroma. In patients with neurofibromatosis 1, neurofibromas are often multiple and there may be extensive infiltration into adjacent structures. Plexiform neurofibromas may have the characteristic "bag of worms" appearance.

Microscopic Findings. The solitary neurofibroma consists of an unencapsulated proliferation of interlacing bundles of spindle cells with

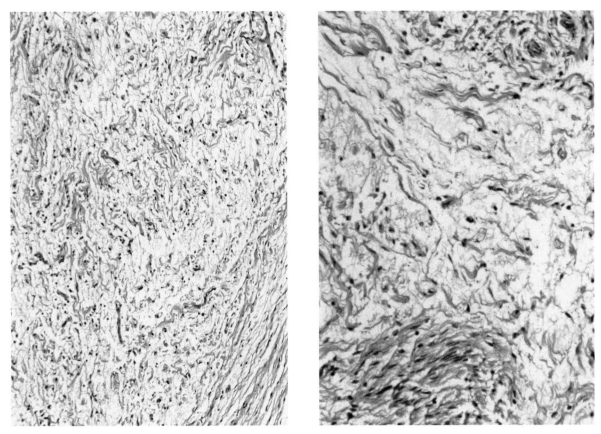

Figure 7-10
ORAL NEUROFIBROMA
Spindle cells with dark serpentine nuclei are surrounded by a myxoid matrix.

hyperchromatic serpentine nuclei. These cells are intermixed with foci of dense bundles of collagenous fibers, but there typically is a myxoid matrix separating the collagenous bands and the spindle-shaped cells (fig. 7-10). On occasion the matrix may be hyalinized (fig. 7-11). Neurofibromas lack the characteristic loose and dense foci seen in neurilemoma. In addition, Verocay bodies and blood vessels with dense, thickened walls are absent. Except for those that are plexiform, localized or multiple neurofibromas occurring in the setting of neurofibromatosis 1 are histologically identical to those that are solitary and not associated with this disorder. Neurofibromas of neurofibromatosis 1 may be more cellular, however, and malignant change may occur. Plexiform neurofibroma consists of a torturous mass of nerve branches, separated by increased endoneurial matrix material.

Immunohistochemical Findings. The Schwann cells of neurofibroma are immunoreactive for vimentin and S-100 protein; the axons for neurofilament protein. Epithelial membrane antigen helps distinguish plexiform neurofibroma from mucosal neuroma, as staining is absent in the former.

Treatment and Prognosis. The treatment for solitary neurofibroma is simple excision. This may be difficult when the lesion infiltrates adjacent structures. Complete surgical removal may not be possible when large numbers of lesions are present in neurofibromatosis 1. In such situations, surgery is indicated for lesions that are symptomatic or located in critical anatomic sites. Neurofibromas may recur if incompletely removed, and re-excision may be necessary. Malignant transformation, although quite rare in the upper aerodigestive tract, often leads to a poor prognosis (37).

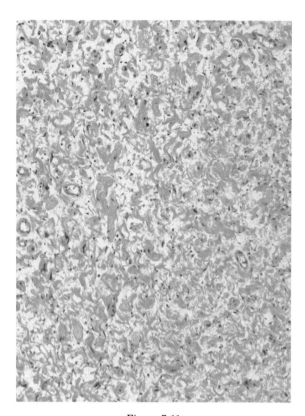

Figure 7-11
PARAPHARYNGEAL NEUROFIBROMA
This lesion shows a hyalinized matrix rather than a matrix with abundant mucosubstances.

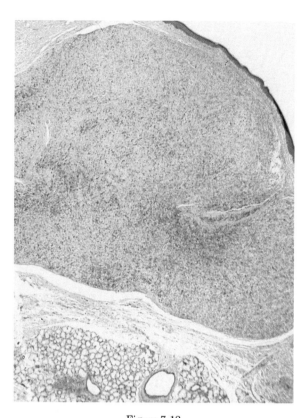

Figure 7-12
ORAL PALISADED ENCAPSULATED NEUROMA
This well-circumscribed lesion occurred as a 0.5 x 0.5 cm asymptomatic nodule on the hard palate.

NEUROMAS

Palisaded Encapsulated Neuroma (Solitary Circumscribed Neuroma)

General Features. Palisaded encapsulated neuroma, found typically on the facial skin of middle-aged adults (43), has been reported as a small solitary nodule of the oral mucosa. Chauvin et al. (42) described 13 cases, 9 of which were located on the hard palate. Other affected sites include soft palate, lower lip, upper lip, and maxillary alveolar ridge. The lesion occurs more often in men, and is not associated with neurofibromatosis or multiple endocrine neoplasia (MEN) type 2b. It accounted for 22 percent of intraoral neoplasms of peripheral nerve origin, exclusive of traumatic neuromas (42).

Gross Findings. The lesion appears usually as a 2- to 3-mm, firm, sessile, partly or completely encapsulated nodule (42). Ulceration of the mucosa is not characteristic.

Microscopic Findings. The moderately cellular, fascicular proliferation of spindle cells is partly or completely encapsulated (fig. 7-12). Nuclear palisading suggestive of neurilemoma may be seen (fig. 7-13), but Verocay bodies are absent (42). The fibrous capsule may be in continuity with the perineurium of an adjacent peripheral nerve bundle. The nodule consists of perineurial cells, Schwann cells, and variable numbers of peripheral nerve axons. Mucosal ulceration was seen in only one case (42). In cutaneous lesions, plexiform, multinodular, and fungating growth patterns have been described (41). In addition, fibrosis, myxoid change, and chronic inflammation have been noted (41).

Immunohistochemical Findings. Antibodies to S-100 protein label the Schwann cells. The variable number of peripheral nerve axons can be identified with antibodies to neurofilament protein. The perineurial cells in the capsule can be stained with an antibody to epithelial membrane antigen (41,42).

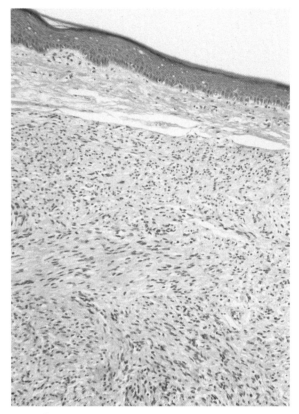

Figure 7-13
ORAL PALISADED ENCAPSULATED NEUROMA
The spindle cell proliferation is moderately cellular and has areas suggestive of neurilemoma. It lacks Verocay bodies and biphasic Antoni A and B foci, however.

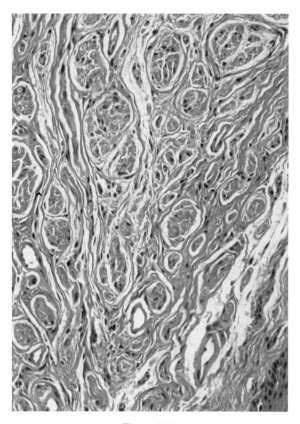

Figure 7-14
ORAL TRAUMATIC NEUROMA
The disorganized proliferation of nerve fascicles is embedded in a collagenous stroma in this example from the tongue.

Traumatic Neuroma

General Features. This non-neoplastic proliferation of nerve fascicles results from either amputation or injury to a nerve. It occurs when there is no distal nerve stump or when the severed ends of a nerve are not in close apposition (45). Traumatic neuromas are seldom encountered in biopsy specimens from the upper aerodigestive tract. This seems unusual given the number of surgical procedures that are performed in the head and neck area. It is likely that most traumatic neuromas in this anatomic area are subclinical. They receive clinical attention when they are painful or present as a mass. The oral and perioral regions (mental foramen, lower lip, tongue) are the most commonly affected sites. When present in the oral cavity they may be responsible for causing atypical facial pain or trigeminal neuralgia (46). Traumatic neuromas have also been reported in the larynx, where they have resulted in hoarseness, dysphagia, choking spells, intermittent aphonia, and cough (44).

Gross Findings. Traumatic neuromas are gray to white, firm nodules. They are usually small, rarely exceeding 2 cm, and are not encapsulated.

Microscopic Findings. The tangled, disorganized proliferation of nerve fascicles consists of axons, endoneurial and perineurial cells, and Schwann cells embedded in a collagenous stroma (fig. 7-14) (45). Occasionally, the stroma may be less collagenized and actually have a myxoid appearance.

Treatment and Prognosis. Simple removal is indicated when the neuroma is symptomatic or when it simulates recurrent cancer. Excision of the nodule with reimplantation of the proximal nerve stump in a location away from the scar tissue is effective therapy (45).

Mucosal Neuroma (Ganglioneuroma)

General Features. Mucosal neuroma is an important marker and also is the most constant component of MEN syndrome type 2b (48,49,52, 54). Only approximately 5 percent of patients with MEN 2 have the 2b type, an autosomal dominant disease consisting of gastrointestinal neuromas (ganglioneuromas); C-cell hyperplasia, medullary carcinoma of the thyroid, or both; pheochromocytoma, adrenal medullary hyperplasia, or both; and, rarely, parathyroid hyperplasia (50). Patients have a Marfan- like body appearance. The condition is typified by the characteristic facial appearance, mucosal neuromas, and constipation or diarrhea (due to ganglioneuromatosis of the gut) and usually manifests early in life (50).

Mutations in the *RET* gene located on chromosome 10q11.2 have been identified in 35 of 37 unrelated individuals with MEN 2b (51,53). A point mutation at codon 918 (exon 16) has been found in 95 percent of patients (50). It is likely that the majority of cases result from new mutations, since the reproductive rate of patients with MEN 2b is low (50). The RET protein belongs to the platelet-derived growth factor receptor subfamily of protein tyrosine kinases and is expressed in neural crest–derived tissues including those of patients with MEN 2, Hirschsprung's disease, medullary carcinoma of the thyroid, and pheochromocytoma (51). A codon 918 mutation activates the receptor tyrosine kinase, which may also bind and phosphorylate other substrates such as c-src and c-abl (50). If MEN 2b is suspected, then calcitonin levels should be measured after pentagastrin stimulation and RET mutations should be sought (50).

Usually multiple, neuromas manifest as fleshy and everted lips, and as nodules in the oral cavity, where they commonly arise on the tip and anterior edges of the tongue. They are also found in the buccal mucosa, gingiva, palate, nasal cavity, nasopharynx, and larynx. Mucosal neuromas are typically seen early in life as small mucosal nodules, and they may even be congenital (52). Diffuse ganglioneuromatosis may extend from the lips to the rectum (48).

Clinical Features. There is often diffuse enlargement of one or, more commonly, both lips, which have been described as "bumpy" or "blub-

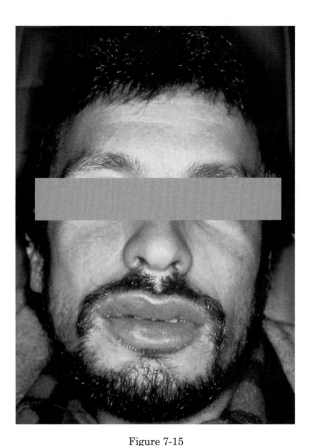

Figure 7-15
MUCOSAL NEUROMA
In MEN syndrome type 2b, both lips often appear fleshy and everted. (Courtesy of Dr. M. Bernstein, Louisville, KY.)

bery" (fig. 7-15) (52,54). The lesions appear on the anterior portion of the tongue as pink nodules (fig. 7-16). They range from 1 mm to several centimeters in size. Many symptoms of MEN 2b, particularly chronic constipation or those that are cosmetic, ocular, or neuromuscular are due to neuroma formation (49).

Microscopic Findings. Unencapsulated serpiginous bands of nerve tissue beneath the surface epithelium are surrounded by normal connective tissue (fig. 7-17) (47). The torturous axons are encased in a thickened perineurium. The nerve bundles vary in number and size. The stroma is sometimes loose and edematous or myxoid. Ganglion cells may be present, occasionally in large numbers (48). The trichrome stain highlights the increased amount of collagen around nerve bundles and within nerves; normal axons are highlighted by the Bodian stain. The appearance of disorganized neural fibers within

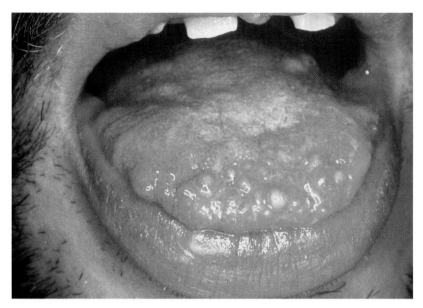

Figure 7-16
MUCOSAL NEUROMA
When present on the tongue, mucosal neuromas typically are seen as pink nodules on the anterior portion. (Courtesy of Dr. M. Bernstein, Louisville, KY.)

a thickened perineurium may lead to confusion with plexiform neurofibroma (47).

Immunohistochemical Findings. Schwann cells, endoneurial cells, and perineurial cells are immunoreactive with an antibody to vimentin (47). Schwann cells are also strongly positive for S-100 protein, while an antibody to epithelial membrane antigen labels the perineurial cells which surround the negative nerve fibers. Axons are labeled with antibodies to neurofilament protein. Epithelial membrane antigen may be useful in distinguishing mucosal neuroma from plexiform neurofibroma, as the latter lacks proliferating perineurial cells (47).

Treatment and Prognosis. It is important to identify mucosal neuroma since it clinically manifests before the development of thyroid and adrenal neoplasms. Patients' identified as having MEN type 2b should be examined periodically for medullary carcinoma of the thyroid and adrenal pheochromocytoma. Prophylactic thyroidectomy may be considered.

NEURILEMOMA (SCHWANNOMA)

General Features. Neurilemoma is found more often than neurofibroma in the upper aerodigestive tract (63,64). Sinonasal tumors arise chiefly from the ophthalmic or maxillary branches of the trigeminal nerve or branches of the autonomic nervous system. Schwann cells

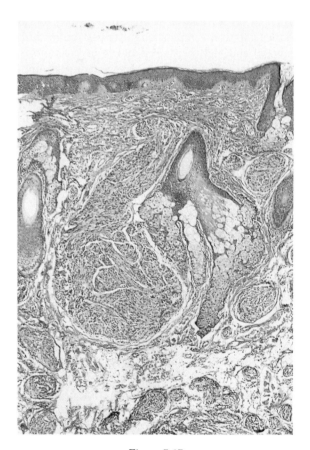

Figure 7-17
ORAL MUCOSAL NEUROMA
In this lip biopsy, tortuous bands of neural tissue surrounded by normal connective tissue lie beneath the surface squamous epithelium.

are normally absent from the olfactory nerve. Although there is occasional involvement of multiple sinuses, neurilemoma occurs more often in a solitary sinus, particularly the maxillary or ethmoid (63). Confinement to the sphenoid or frontal sinus is rare. Laryngeal tumors typically arise in the false cords or aryepiglottic folds. In a 1977 review of 152 schwannomas of the oral cavity (57), the tongue was the most common affected site (47 percent), followed by the buccal mucosa (12 percent), floor of mouth (9 percent), and palate (7 percent). Uncommon locations include mastoid, epiglottis, pharynx, soft palate, and trachea (60,61). Neurilemoma is among the most common neoplasms developing in the parapharyngeal space, arising from the vagus or cervical sympathetic nerve, and can be quite large in this location.

Acoustic neurilemoma (neuroma) accounts for almost 10 percent of all intracranial tumors. It is the most frequent neoplasm in the temporal bone. The tumor arises from the vestibular division of the eighth cranial nerve or, less often, from the cochlear division. Large tumors sometimes protrude from the internal auditory canal into the cerebellopontine angle, compressing the adjacent brain stem and cerebellum. Neurilemoma of the eighth cranial nerve is the only common neural neoplasm involving the external ear. Neurilemoma also occurs in the facial nerve, in its extratympanic (descending) portion.

In two series of acoustic neurilemomas, 228 lesions (94 percent) were unilateral and 15 (6 percent) were bilateral (56,59). The presence of bilateral neoplasms establishes the diagnosis of neurofibromatosis 2; bilateral tumors occur in more than 90 percent of these patients (55). Unilateral acoustic neurilemoma may be seen in neurofibromatosis 1. Neurofibromatosis 2, with an autosomal dominant inheritance pattern, is not associated with large numbers of cutaneous neurofibromas or café-au-lait spots. It occurs much less often (1 in 50,000 people) than neurofibromatosis type 1 (1 in 4,000 people) (62). In the absence of bilateral acoustic neurilemomas, neurofibromatosis 2 can be diagnosed when there is a first-degree relative with neurofibromatosis 2 and either a unilateral eighth nerve mass or two of the following: neurilemoma, neurofibroma, meningioma, glioma, and juvenile posterior subcapsular lenticular opacity (62). Neural

neoplasms in these patients frequently involve both the eighth nerve and other central nerves. There may be many small neurilemomas, neurofibromas, and meningiomas involving cranial nerves and the meninges near an acoustic neurilemoma. Small neural neoplasms may also be intermixed microscopically. Bilateral neurilemomas tend to be more invasive than single acoustic tumors, as they sometimes infiltrate the cochlea and vestibule. The gene for neurofibromatosis 2 has been mapped to the middle of the long arm of chromosome 22 (22q12) and, like the neurofibromatosis 1 gene, has a tumor suppressor function (65,66). Its protein, merlin, is homologous to other proteins that join cell membrane integral proteins to intracellular cytoskeletal constituents (65).

Clinical Features. Neurilemoma usually occurs as an asymptomatic mass, but it may cause a variety of symptoms depending upon its location. Symptoms include difficulties with eating, swallowing, phonation, breathing, and drainage; pain, tenderness, and paresthesia are seen uncommonly. Oral cavity tumors occur most often in patients in the second or third decade of life and vary from a few millimeters to several centimeters (57). Nasal or paranasal sinus neurilemomas are found in patients from 20 to 50 years of age (56,58). The neoplasm may mimic a nasal polyp or angiofibroma and may be bleed profusely on biopsy (56). In addition, there is sometimes local bony destruction and intracranial extension (58). Involvement of the larynx may result in fullness of the throat, hoarseness, cough, or dyspnea. Typically there is no vocal cord paralysis, but the size of the neoplasm may interfere with movement of the cords.

Unilateral acoustic neurilemoma occurs more often in women, three quarters of whom are over 40 years of age (56,59). Bilateral tumors are found in patients in the second or third decade of life (55,56). Acoustic neurilemoma may grow for many years without symptoms, and may even be initially diagnosed at autopsy. When symptoms are present, they include hearing loss, tinnitus, and vertigo.

Gross Findings. Neurilemomas are encapsulated, round or oval, firm masses that vary in size from a few millimeters to over 5 cm. The surface is smooth and sometimes lobulated, and on cut section they are tan, yellow, or pink. The tumor is typically solid, but may have soft,

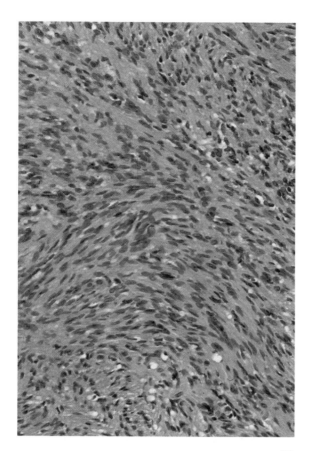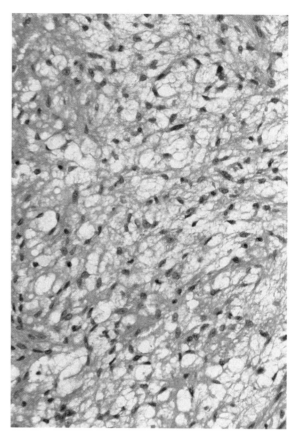

Figure 7-18
NASAL NEURILEMOMA
Cellular areas (Antoni A) (left) and loose, myxoid foci (Antoni B) (right) are usually both conspicuous.

myxoid, cystic, or calcified foci. When a large nerve is involved, it may be seen stretched over the surface of the neoplasm.

Microscopic Findings. Sinonasal tract and nasopharyngeal tumors are typically unencapsulated (58). The capsule of neurilemoma of other head and neck sites, when present, consists of epineurium with occasional residual nerve fibers. Characteristically, there are foci of cells with spindle-shaped nuclei and indistinct cytoplasmic margins (Antoni A cells; fig. 7-18, left) and other areas showing cells embedded in a loose, myxoid matrix (Antoni B cells; fig. 7-18, right). The amounts of Antoni A and Antoni B tissue may vary considerably. Typical of neurilemoma are Verocay bodies, which consist of spindle-shaped cells whose palisaded nuclei surround cellular eosinophilic processes and stroma (fig. 7-19). Mitotic figures are few or absent, but there may

be large, hyperchromatic and pleomorphic nuclei (fig. 7-20). Such nuclei are considered a degenerative phenomenon and should not be construed as evidence of malignancy. There may be focal granular cell change (58). Rarely, neurilemoma has a plexiform or multinodular pattern. The cellular variant has been reported in tumors of the sinonasal tract and nasopharynx (58).

Additional microscopic features seen in neurilemomas include occasional foci of necrosis, cystic degeneration, foam cells, hemosiderin, and calcification, as well as dense bands of hyalinized connective tissue. Prominent vessels with thick hyaline walls are usually present (fig. 7-21). Some vessels may be large and thin walled, and thrombi may also be observed.

Immunohistochemical Findings. Neurilemomas are uniformly immunopositive for S-100 protein. Vimentin is also characteristically present,

133

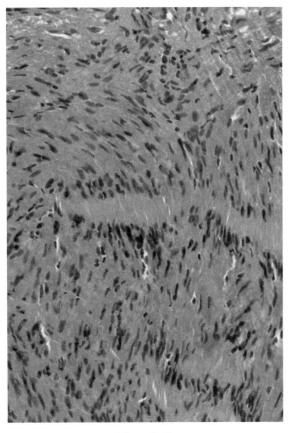

Figure 7-19
ACOUSTIC NEURILEMOMA
Verocay bodies consist of spindle-shaped cells whose nuclei surround an eosinophilic center.

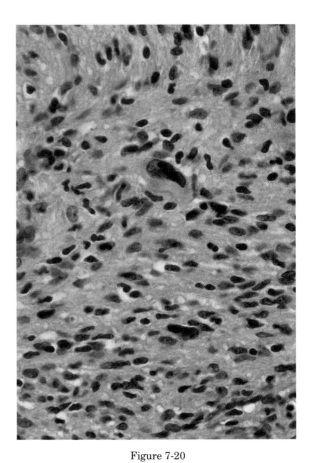

Figure 7-20
NASAL NEURILEMOMA
The finding of large, hyperchromatic nuclei in an otherwise typical neurilemoma is not indicative of aggressive behavior.

Figure 7-21
NASAL NEURILEMOMA
Vessels with thick hyaline walls are characteristically seen in neurilemoma.

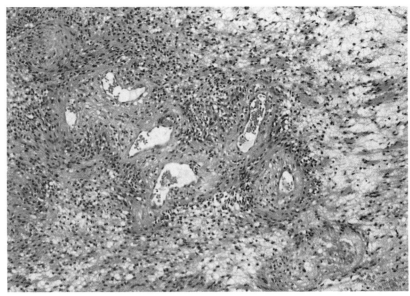

but cytokeratin is negative. Focal epithelial membrane antigen reactivity may be observed.

Ultrastructural Findings. Neurilemoma consists almost exclusively of a proliferation of Schwann cells. The thin, interdigitating processes are covered by a fine basal lamina. Giant fibers of collagen may also be seen.

Differential Diagnosis. Neurilemoma must be distinguished from any neoplasm of the upper aerodigestive tract consisting of spindle-shaped cells. Hence, neurofibroma, meningioma, melanoma, and leiomyoma, among others, are included in the differential diagnosis. Careful attention to the histologic findings and occasional immunohistochemical support is adequate to distinguish these neoplasms. Malignant neurilemomas show typical features of malignancy, but may be difficult to distinguish from other sarcomas. Benign neurilemoma is usually readily distinguishable from malignant schwannoma in resection specimens, but may be more problematic in small biopsy samples. Hypercellularity, lack of encapsulation, and locally destructive growth suggest malignancy in sinonasal and nasopharyngeal neoplasms; however, in an otherwise histologically typical neurilemoma, these findings are not indicative of malignant behavior (58).

Treatment and Prognosis. For most neurilemomas of the upper aerodigestive tract, complete removal leads to a cure. However, the tumor may be extensive and en bloc resection may be difficult or even impossible. Significant morbidity and even mortality may result from large acoustic neoplasms.

NERVE SHEATH MYXOMA (NEUROTHEKEOMA)

General Features. Nerve sheath myxoma was initially reported in 1969 as a cutaneous tumor (69). The lesion was later described in 1980 as neurothekeoma (67). Of 10 well-described intraoral nerve sheath myxomas, 4 occurred in the tongue (70–75). Other intraoral sites of neoplasm include buccal mucosa, retromolar area, and palate.

Clinical Features. The myxoma is a small, firm nodule which may be pedunculated. It occasionally is painful. The overlying mucosa is intact. The patient age range is 15 to 46 years.

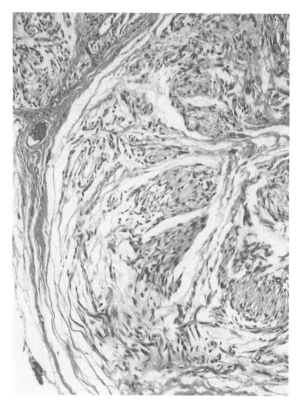

Figure 7-22
NERVE SHEATH MYXOMA
This lesion from the oral cavity contains spindle-shaped cells organized into lobules which are separated by thin fibrous septa.

Gross Findings. A small, submucosal, gray-white nodule is typical. The lesion is usually no larger than 1 cm. There may be myxoid or hemorrhagic foci.

Microscopic Findings. Myxomatous tissue is separated into lobules by fibrous septa (fig. 7-22). The connective tissue around myxomatous areas may be compressed. Spindle-shaped or stellate cells form net-like or syncytial patterns. Multinucleated giant cells may be present. Mitotic figures are sparse, if present. The myxomatous stroma is stained by alcian blue and is sensitive to hyaluronidase. Mast cells are sometimes numerous within the lesion.

Immunohistochemical Findings. Immunoreactivity for S-100 protein, vimentin, neuron-specific enolase, and glial fibrillary acid protein is frequent, but staining for cytokeratin is typically absent (68,71,72).

Treatment and Prognosis. Simple excision appears to be curative.

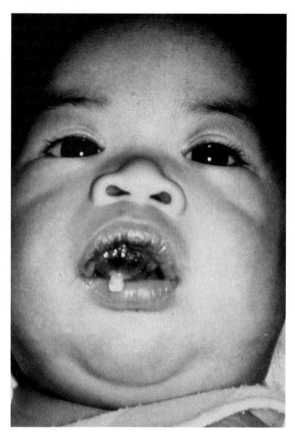

Figure 7-23
MELANOTIC NEUROECTODERMAL
TUMOR OF INFANCY
A clinical photograph of a melanotic neuroectodermal tumor of infancy involving the anterior maxilla.

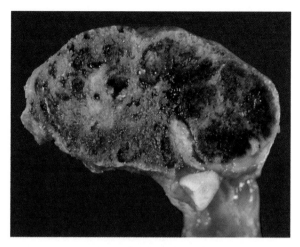

Figure 7-24
MELANOTIC NEUROECTODERMAL
TUMOR OF INFANCY
Expansile melanotic neuroectodermal tumor of infancy arising in the anterior maxilla has foci of blue-black pigmentation on cut surface. There is a tooth attached to the lower aspect of the specimen. (Courtesy of Dr. C. Manivel, Minneapolis, MN.)

MELANOTIC NEUROECTODERMAL TUMOR OF INFANCY

Definition. Melanotic neuroectodermal tumors of infancy (MNTI) are polyphenotypic neoplasms with evidence of epithelial, neural, mesenchymal, and neuroectodermal differentiation.

Clinical Features. Virtually all MNTIs arise in infants under 1 year of age. Gender distribution is approximately equal. Most tumors arise in the head and neck region, with nearly 70 percent in the anterior maxilla area (fig. 7-23) (78,85). Other commonly involved sites include in decreasing order, the skull, brain, mandible, and epididymis (76,78,82,85,86); rare cases involve the long bones, mediastinum, thigh, and skin (77,78,80, 82,84). Awareness of these uncommon anatomic locations is important for diagnosis. Purported

cases of MNTI arising in the ovary and uterus are poorly documented and probably do not represent bona fide examples (81,87). Intraosseous tumors are radiographically characterized by a central area of radiolucency with expansile margins displacing adjacent bone and teeth.

Following surgical excision with tumor-free margins, the clinical course is usually benign, with a 15 percent incidence of local recurrence (78). In a recent literature review of 195 cases, 13 patients (6.6 percent) developed metastases, usually to regional lymph nodes (85). The latter incidence, however, is probably an overestimation, since metastasizing tumors are more likely to be reported. Intracranial MNTIs tend to spread rapidly through the central nervous system to involve the meninges, brain, and spinal cord; adjunct chemotherapy following surgical extirpation has been advocated for these tumors (77).

Gross Findings. Tumors are usually firm, lobated, well-circumscribed, unencapsulated masses, ranging in size from 1.5 to 4.0 cm, although lesions up to 13 cm have been reported (85). The cut surface typically has a gray-white to dark brown variegated appearance with foci of blue-black pigmentation (fig. 7-24).

Microscopic Findings. Tumors are composed of a biphasic population of large and small

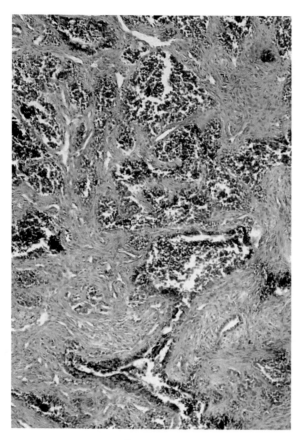

Figure 7-25
MELANOTIC NEUROECTODERMAL
TUMOR OF INFANCY

On low magnification, melanotic neuroectodermal tumors of infancy consist of strands, nests, tubules, and alveolar formations of neoplastic cells embedded in a densely collagenous stroma.

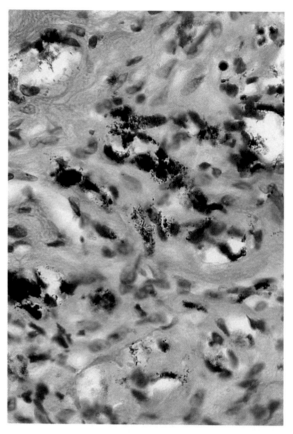

Figure 7-26
MELANOTIC NEUROECTODERMAL
TUMOR OF INFANCY

On high magnification, tumors are composed of two cell types: large cells with conspicuous melanin pigmentation accompanied by smaller cells with variable levels of pigmentation.

cells embedded in a dense collagenous stroma (fig. 7-25). Nests of small neuroblastic cells are often surrounded by larger, melanin-containing cells in an alveolar or tubular arrangement. The large tumor cells are polygonal, with abundant eosinophilic cytoplasm and vesicular nuclei with prominent nucleoli. A characteristic feature is that the large cells contain numerous, dark brown, elongated intracytoplasmic granules strongly positive with the Fontana-Masson melanin stain. The smaller cells show scant, pale cytoplasm and hyperchromatic nuclei (fig. 7-26). Melanin granules are rarely seen in the smaller cells. A neurofibrillary-type matrix is occasionally noted surrounding the smaller cells but rosettes are absent. Nuclear pleomorphism, mitoses, and necrosis are rarely noted. Occasional cases of MNTI may have a predominantly monophasic, poorly differentiated appearance similar to that of neuroblastoma (79,82).

Immunohistochemical Findings. Immunohistochemical findings vary according to the cell type examined. On fixed sections, the large cells are uniformly positive for cytokeratin, vimentin, and HMB-45. Both the small, neuroblastic cells and large cells are usually positive for neuron-specific enolase and occasionally reactive for Leu-7, desmin, and muscle-specific actin (fig. 7-27) (83, 85,86,88). Variable reactivity for epithelial membrane antigen (large cells only), as well as for synaptophysin, glial fibrillary acid protein, and microtubule-associated protein (small cells only) has also been reported (83,85,86).

Ultrastructural Findings. Three cell types can be distinguished by electron microscopic examination: undifferentiated cells, small cells

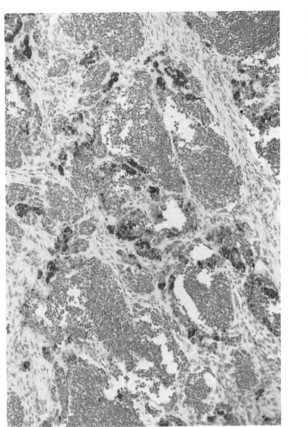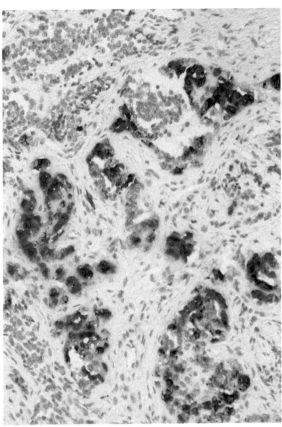

Figure 7-27

MELANOTIC NEUROECTODERMAL TUMOR OF INFANCY

Immunohistochemically, the large tumor cells are typically reactive for cytokeratin (left) and HMB-45 (right). (Courtesy of Dr. C. Manivel, Minneapolis, MN.)

with neuroblastic differentiation, and large, melanin-producing cells (78,79,85). The undifferentiated cells contain round nuclei with dense chromatin and scant cytoplasm with rare organelles. The small cells are characterized by ovoid nuclei with small marginal nucleoli, scant cytoplasm, and short, dendritic-like processes containing membrane-bound, neurosecretory-type granules. The larger cells are polygonal to dendritic, partially surrounded by a basement membrane and joined by poorly formed desmosomes. Nuclei are ovoid and irregular, with inconspicuous nucleoli. The large cell cytoplasm is typically abundant, with bundles of intermediate filaments and numerous organelles. Premelanosomes (stages I and II) and mature melanosomes (stages III and IV) are present in both cell types, but are much more numerous in the epithelioid cells (fig. 7-28). Occasionally, intermediate cells

containing both neurosecretory-type granules and melanosomes are seen.

Special Techniques. A total of 16 MNTIs have been studied by flow cytometric DNA analysis from tissue retrieved from paraffin blocks (83, 85). Of these, 5 were aneuploid and 11 were diploid. Follow-up was available on 4 aneuploid tumors, 3 of which recurred locally and 9 diploid tumors, 3 of which also recurred. Thus, DNA ploidy does not appear useful in predicting local recurrence.

Differential Diagnosis. The differential diagnosis of primitive craniofacial tumors in childhood includes metastatic neuroblastoma, malignant melanoma, primitive neuroectodermal tumor (PNET), and rhabdomyosarcoma. MNTI is distinguished from most of these tumors by its characteristic biphasic tumor cell population and pigmentation. Neuroblastomas may be pigmented and express both neural and neuroendocrine

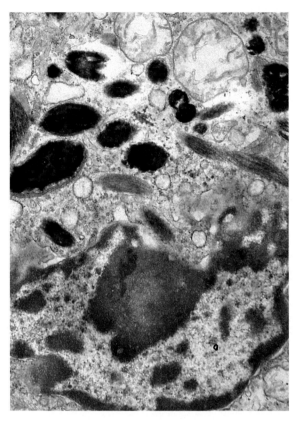

Figure 7-28
MELANOTIC NEUROECTODERMAL
TUMOR OF INFANCY
Ultrastructurally, both the large and, to a lesser extent,
the small tumor cells contain numerous premelanosomes
(stages I and II) and mature melanosomes (stages III and IV).

markers but are rarely positive for cytokeratin. Similarly, the tumor cells in melanoma are rarely reactive for cytokeratin and do not express neural or neuroendocrine markers such as neuron-specific enolase and synaptophysin. PNETs do not show evidence of epithelial or melanotic differentiation. Unusual desmin-reactive MNTIs may be confused with rhabdomyosarcoma, but the latter lesions are not pigmented and typically immunostain for myoglobin and muscle-specific actin.

GRANULAR CELL TUMOR/ CONGENITAL EPULIS

Definition. Granular cell tumors are relatively common benign neoplasms of possible neural differentiation. The light microscopically identical congenital epulis of the newborn is an uncommon benign tumor of uncertain differentiation.

Clinical Findings. Patients with granular cell tumors usually present in the fourth decade of life with an asymptomatic nodular mass (91, 102). The age range is wide, varying from 11 months to 68 years (102). Most studies report a 2 to 1 female predilection (98,99,102). Multiple primary lesions occur in about 10 percent of patients (102). Granular cell tumors have been reported in virtually every organ and tissue of the human body. The single most common anatomic site is the tongue, although relatively more tumors involve the skin or subcutaneous tissue. In a study of 118 tumors, Lack et al. (91) reported that 25 percent arose from the tongue, and 44 percent in the skin or subcutaneous tissues. In a review of 377 published cases, Peterson et al. (98) also found the most common site was the skin/subcutaneous tissue (33 percent of cases), followed by the oral cavity (28 percent), tongue (23 percent), and larynx (8 percent).

Biologically, most granular cell tumors are benign and cured by wide local excision. About 5 percent of benign tumors recur locally (91,102). Malignant versions occur but are rare, and comprise approximately 1 percent of all granular cell tumors (89,102). Distinguishing multifocal benign tumors, which may present synchronously or metachronously, from metastasizing lesions may be difficult. The presence of cellular pleomorphism and increased mitotic activity in the primary lesion, as well as a time course and anatomic distribution consistent with metastatic spread may be the only indicators. Metastases are usually to regional lymph nodes; other sites include the lung, subcutaneous fat, mediastinum, and heart (89,101–103).

Congenital epulides virtually always occur on the anterior alveolar ridge of newborn infants (90). The gingiva overlying future canine and lateral incisor teeth is most frequently involved, although the underlying bone or teeth are not affected. There is a strong predilection for newborn females (9 to 1). Multiple congenital epulides have been described but are rare. These lesions are always cured by local excision; even after incomplete excision, recurrence or metastatic behavior has not been reported (90).

Gross Findings. Granular cell tumors are usually firm, circumscribed nodular lesions with

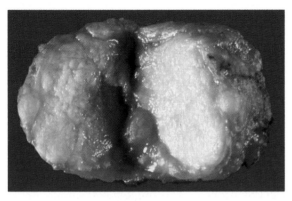

Figure 7-29
GRANULAR CELL TUMOR
Granular cell tumor excised from of a 65-year-old female.
The bisected tumor is circumscribed but unencapsulated,
with a tan-yellow, homogeneous cut surface.

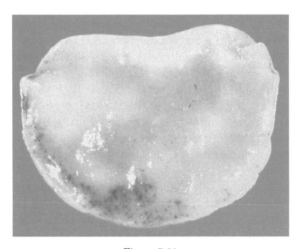

Figure 7-30
CONGENITAL EPULIS
Congenital epulis excised from the anterior alveolar
ridge of a newborn. The lesion is firm, pink-red, circumscribed, and focally hemorrhagic.

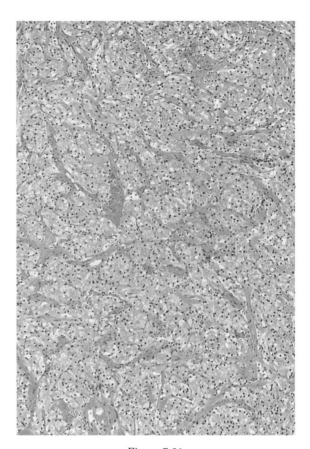

Figure 7-31
GRANULAR CELL TUMOR
On low magnification, granular cell tumors are composed
of sheets of polygonal granular cells supported by delicate,
fibrovascular septa.

a tan-yellow homogeneous cut surface (fig. 7-29).
Tumors are small and usually measure less than
4 cm in diameter (91,98,102).

Congenital epulides are fleshy, firm, pink-red
polypoid lesions with a broad-based attachment
to the alveolar ridge (fig. 7-30). Ulceration of the
overlying gingiva is unusual. Epulides are small,
with an average diameter of 1 cm (90).

Microscopic Findings. Granular cell tumors are composed of sheets, nests, and clusters
of tumor cells separated by a delicate, fibrovascular stroma (fig. 7-31). The tumor cells are
large, polygonal, and uniform, with distinct
cellular borders and abundant granular eosinophilic cytoplasm. The nuclei are small and
hyperchromatic, and may be either centrally or
eccentrically placed (fig. 7-32). Mitotic activity is
usually absent, although multinucleation and
mild nuclear pleomorphism are occasionally
noted (91). The coarsely granular cytoplasmic
material is periodic acid–Schiff positive and resistant to diastase. Large, inclusion-like granules surrounded by a distinct halo are commonly
seen (fig. 7-33). Older, sclerotic variants are occasionally encountered, with small nests of neoplastic cells embedded in a desmoplastic collagenous stroma (fig. 7-34) (95).

Marked pseudoepitheliomatous hyperplasia
of the overlying epithelium occurs in about 10
percent of cases, and may simulate squamous

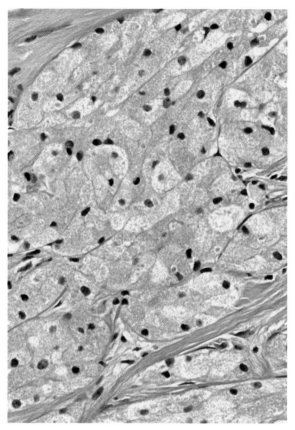

Figure 7-32
GRANULAR CELL TUMOR
The neoplastic cells have well-defined cytoplasmic borders, abundant eosinophilic granular cytoplasm, and small, hyperchromatic nuclei with little to no pleomorphism.

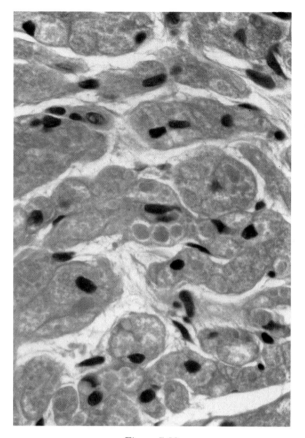

Figure 7-33
GRANULAR CELL TUMOR
Large, inclusion-like intracytoplasmic granules surrounded by a distinct halo are commonly seen in granular cell tumors.

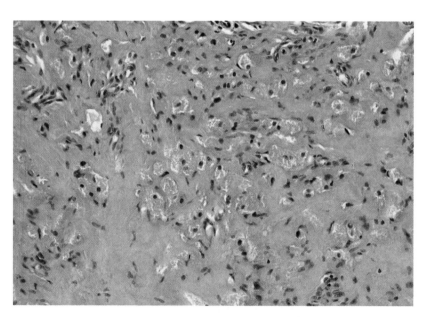

Figure 7-34
GRANULAR CELL TUMOR
Sclerotic granular cell tumor with nests and individual neoplastic cells embedded in a densely collagenous stroma.

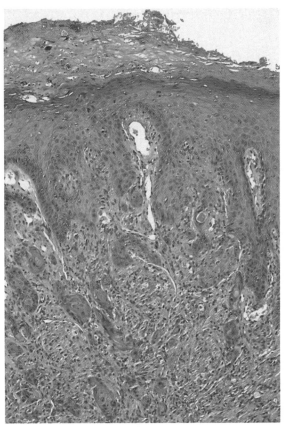

Figure 7-35
GRANULAR CELL TUMOR
A granular cell tumor of the tongue with prominent pseudoepitheliomatous hyperplasia of the overlying epithelium, simulating invasive squamous cell carcinoma.

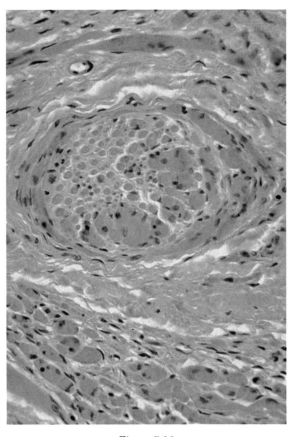

Figure 7-36
GRANULAR CELL TUMOR
A large myelinated nerve is surrounded by granular tumor cells. Neoplastic cells are also present within the perineural sheath. (Courtesy of Dr. E.E. Lack, Washington, DC.)

cell carcinoma (fig. 7-35) (91,102). Reports of granular cell tumors misdiagnosed as squamous cell carcinoma are common. A proportion of tumors are closely associated with myelinated peripheral nerve bundles (91,95,97). The granular cells may surround, involve, or nearly replace nerve fibers; residual neurites often require a silver preparation for recognition (fig. 7-36).

Malignant variants are histologically similar to benign tumors but often show increased mitotic activity and a greater degree of nuclear pleomorphism (89,93,103). Some metastasizing tumors are indistinguishable from benign lesions, however, even if examined in retrospect. To date there are no definitive histologic criteria that reliably separate benign from malignant (metastasizing) variants.

Congenital epulides of newborn infants are histologically identical to granular cell tumors but do not show pseudoepitheliomatous hyperplasia (91,92).

Immunohistochemical Findings. Granular cell tumors are virtually always immunoreactive for S-100 protein and vimentin (fig. 7-37) (92–94,96,97). Most tumors are positive for neuron-specific enolase, myelin-associated glycoprotein (antibody Leu-7), myelin-basic protein (93, 97,100) and peripheral nerve myelin proteins (96). Staining for keratin, neurofilament protein, glial fibrillary acid protein, desmin, muscle-specific actin, and myoglobin is uniformly negative (93,94, 96,97). Malignant variants have immunostaining profiles similar to benign tumors (93).

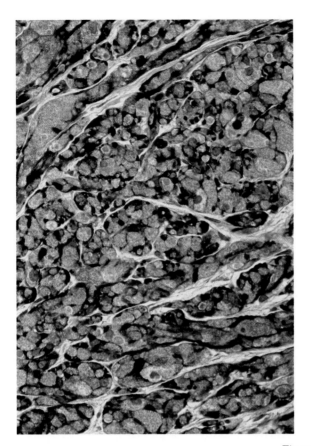
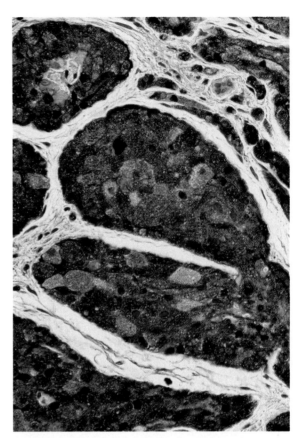

Figure 7-37
GRANULAR CELL TUMOR
Immunohistochemically, granular cell tumors are virtually always reactive for vimentin (left) and S-100 protein (right).

Unlike granular cell tumors, the few congenital epulides studied immunohistochemically do not stain for S-100 protein (92,97).

Ultrastructural Findings. Granular cell tumors are composed of large polyhedral cells, most of which are surrounded by basal lamina–like material and joined by intermediate-type cell junctions (91,94). A characteristic feature is the presence of abundant, intracytoplasmic membrane-bound granules containing fragments of electron-dense material resembling secondary lysozomes or phagolysosomal complexes (fig. 7-38) (91,94,99). Other organelles are inconspicuous. Membrane-bound, angular fibrillar aggregates composed of parallel arrays of microtubules, commonly referred to as angulate bodies, are infrequently encountered. The few malignant tumors studied have appeared ultrastructurally identical to their benign counterparts (89, 93,101,103).

The ultrastructure of the congenital epulis of the newborn is very similar to that of granular cell tumors, except that convincing angulate bodies are not found (91,92,99).

Differential Diagnosis. The histologic appearance of granular cell tumors is characteristic. The primary concern is differentiating benign from potentially malignant tumors. In general, large tumors and those with rapid growth, local recurrence, or histologic evidence of pleomorphism and mitotic activity are more likely to be malignant. However, there are no definitive criteria to prospectively identify malignant tumors in the absence of metastatic dissemination. Differentiation from other neoplasms in the upper aerodigestive tract is usually not difficult. The coarsely granular cytoplasm and absence of cross striations distinguish granular cell tumors from rhabdomyoma. The diastase-resistant periodic acid-Schiff–positive cytoplasm and diffuse

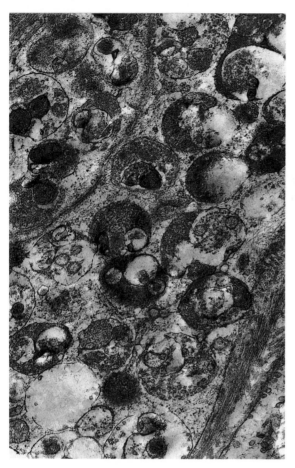

Figure 7-38
GRANULAR CELL TUMOR
Ultrastructural study of a granular cell tumor shows polygonal tumor cells containing abundant intracytoplasmic secondary lysosomes or phagolysosomal-like complexes. (Fig. 243, Fascicle 25, 2nd Series.)

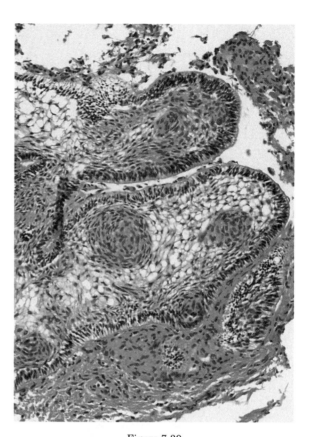

Figure 7-39
NASOPHARYNGEAL CRANIOPHARYNGIOMA
Basaloid squamous cells imparting an adamantinomatous appearance surround necrotic cystic contents.

expression of S-100 protein distinguishes problematic granular cell tumors from paragangliomas. Awareness of the frequent association of granular cell tumors with pseudoepitheliomatous hyperplasia should prevent a misdiagnosis of squamous cell carcinoma.

CRANIOPHARYNGIOMA

General Features. Craniopharyngioma occurs rarely in the infrasellar region. It most likely arises along the path of the craniopharyngeal duct. In a report of a case and review of the literature, Byme and Sessions (105) reported that all of nine extracranial craniopharyngiomas occupied the nasopharynx. Six of these neoplasms also were pres-

ent in the sella turcica and eight involved the sphenoid sinus. One tumor also involved the maxillary and ethmoid sinuses.

Clinical Features. In the above study (105), the patients with nasopharyngeal craniopharyngioma had symptoms that included headache, impaired vision, nasal obstruction, and epistaxis. Two thirds were in the first three decades of life. There was no sex predominance.

Gross Findings. Craniopharyngiomas vary in size, and typically have cystic components that contain brown (machine oil) fluid. Often, they adhere to adjacent structures.

Microscopic Findings. Nasopharyngeal neoplasms are identical to their suprasellar and intrasellar counterparts. Most have an adamantinomatous appearance consisting of cords of basaloid squamous cells plus foci of keratinized squamous cells (fig. 7-39). Keratin pearls may also be present. Such an appearance resembles that of ameloblastoma of the jaw. Craniopharyngioma even more closely resembles the keratinizing and calcifying odontogenic cyst, a lesion that contains proliferating ameloblastic epithelium, ghost keratin, calcifications, and cystic contents (104). A fibrous stroma, necrotic cystic contents, calcified foci, and cholesterol crystals are typically seen in craniopharyngioma, which in contrast to an epidermoid cyst, has a more complex pattern of epithelial proliferation. In small biopsy specimens, however, the lesions may be difficult to separate.

Treatment and Prognosis. Surgery is the mainstay of therapy. Incomplete resection is supplemented by radiation therapy. In the cases of nasopharyngeal craniopharyngioma reported in the literature, long-term follow-up was not available, but six patients whose tumors were excised had initial resolution of their symptoms (105). Progression of tumor was observed in one patient who had a biopsy only and another who received radiotherapy alone.

MENINGIOMA

General Features. Involvement of the upper aerodigestive tract by meningioma occurs in several ways: 1) an intracranial neoplasm directly extends extracranially; 2) extracranial growth from arachnoid cells accompanies cranial nerves (optic, oculomotor, facial, vagus, glossopharyngeal, spinal accessory, and hypoglossal) as they exit the skull foramina; 3) extracranial growth without any connection with foramina or cranial nerves arises from embryonic rests of arachnoid cells (ectopic); and 4) an intracranial source metastasizes (107). When a primary extracranial meningioma is suspected, it may be possible to demonstrate an intracranial origin. Hence, it is appropriate to search for an intracranial neoplasm prior to labeling a meningioma as a primary extracranial tumor. At times it may be impossible to exclude an intracranial origin for a meningioma believed to arise in an extracranial location. Both extracranial meningioma and those that are intracranial with extracranial extension may be found in the nasal cavity, paranasal sinuses, nasopharynx, pharyngeal space, middle ear, internal auditory meatus, and oral cavity (107–116). In one study, 20 percent of intracranial meningiomas extended beyond the cranial cavity and 3 percent secondarily involved

the nasal cavity, paranasal sinuses, or nasopharynx (106). When intracranial meningioma extends to the sinonasal area, it typically passes through the cribriform plate, orbital cavity, or medial portion of the sphenoidal ridge. It has been stated that the majority of meningiomas of the nasal cavity or paranasal sinuses represent true primary extracranial neoplasms (116). When located in the paranasal sinuses, the frontal, maxillary, sphenoid, and ethmoid sinuses are equally affected (116). Tumor may be present in more than one paranasal sinus.

Approximately 6 percent of all meningiomas arise from the anterior or posterior surface of the petrous bone, from which they may reach the middle ear (112). Nearly 70 percent of temporal bone meningiomas have both intracranial and intratemporal components; the remainder appear largely to be intratemporal neoplasms (114). There are numerous routes of extension into the temporal bone (114). When temporal bone involvement is extensive, the most frequent route of extratemporal extension is through the jugular foramen and foramen lacerum into the parapharyngeal space; the neoplasm often presents within the nasopharynx and lateral pharyngeal wall, and occasionally extends into the soft palate or tonsil. The origin for many intratemporal meningiomas is difficult to determine due to the size of the tumor, multiple areas of involvement, and extensive infiltration of bone (114). Extracranial meningiomas arise in various temporal bone sites, including the internal auditory meatus, jugular foramen, geniculate ganglion region, and roof of the eustachian tube. The most common temporal bone site for primary extracranial meningioma is the middle ear cleft. In one review, 45 percent of intratympanic meningiomas arose in the middle ear (they may actually have originated from the facial nerve or jugular bulb), 30 percent developed from the facial nerve, and a few arose within the internal auditory canal, eustachian tube, or jugular fossa (114). Meningioma may extend into the external auditory meatus, mastoid, or jugular fossa.

Clinical Features. Meningioma involving the upper aerodigestive tract has a variable presentation. Signs and symptoms are often related to a mass effect. Intracranial meningioma extending into the nasal cavity or paranasal sinuses occurs in patients of a broad age range but is found more often in women. Primary nasal cavity or paranasal sinus meningioma tends to be found in young patients who slightly more often are male (109). In young patients, primary meningioma has a predilection for the nasal cavity or paranasal sinuses (109). Symptoms are nonspecific but include nasal obstruction and epistaxis. Meningioma may present as a nasal polyp (111). Ear involvement is seen more often in women who present with otitis media, hearing loss, loss of equilibrium, headache, vertigo, otalgia, or tinnitus (114,115). Involvement of the chorda tympani and facial nerve result in disturbance of taste and facial nerve palsy, respectively.

Meningioma involving the upper aerodigestive tract may be found in patients with neurofibromatosis 2. In these patients, multiple small meningiomas may occur near the acoustic neurilemomas.

Gross Findings. The neoplasm appears as a tan, gray, or pink mass. It is firm and rubbery, and has a granular or gritty cut surface. When intracranial, it may be bulky or appear simply as a plaque. It sometimes spreads in bone along the canals of the haversian system, through neural foramina, or in bone marrow. Hyperostosis of adjacent bone may be seen, but necrosis, hemorrhage, and cyst formation are not typical.

Microscopic Findings. The microscopic appearance of meningioma is variable, reflecting the numerous subtypes: fibroblastic (fibrous), meningotheliomatous (syncytial), transitional (mixed) (fig. 7-40), psammomatous, and hemangioblastic, angioblastic, and angiomatous. Meningioma of the middle ear, nasal cavity, or paranasal sinus is most often meningotheliomatous or transitional; fibroblastic and psammomatous types are occasionally noted. Whorls of tumor cells, the presence of psammoma bodies (fig. 7-41), and the syncytial nature of the tumor cells are all diagnostic features. The cells have bland nuclear features and, often, intranuclear cytoplasmic inclusions, the presence of which may be a helpful diagnostic finding (fig. 7-42). Aggressive and malignant meningiomas (papillary and anaplastic) could potentially involve the upper aerodigestive tract. A neoplasm that has histologic features recognizable as meningioma, but that also has conspicuous mitotic figures and foci of tumor necrosis is probably malignant.

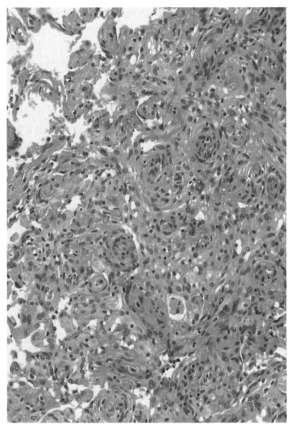

Figure 7-40
NASAL MENINGIOMA
Transitional cell meningiomas are composed of fibroblastic and syncytial components.

Immunohistochemical Findings. Meningiomas are characteristically immunoreactive for vimentin and epithelial membrane antigen (117). In one study of intracranial meningiomas, 12 percent were positive for cytokeratin, which was usually present only focally and was seen most often in the secretory variant of meningotheliomatous meningioma (117). In this same study, 15 percent of the neoplasms were positive for S-100 protein, but the reported frequency of staining for this antigen is quite variable. Meningiomas are characteristically negative for glial fibrillary acidic protein, factor VIII-reactive antigen, and Ulex agglutinin.

Ultrastructural Findings. Meningiomas have overlapping cell processes bound together by intracellular junctions or, occasionally, desmosomes. Intermediate filaments may insert at these junctions. Formation of basal lamina is variable.

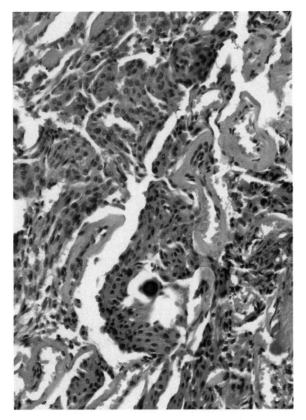

Figure 7-41
INNER EAR MENINGIOMA
The finding of one or more psammoma bodies in a neoplasm of the upper aerodigestive tract can be a helpful finding for the diagnosis of meningioma.

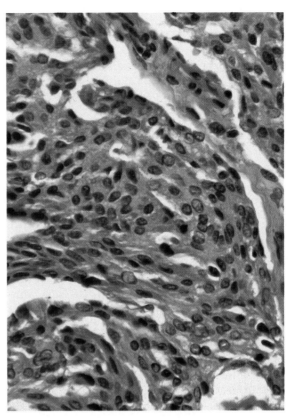

Figure 7-42
INNER EAR MENINGIOMA
The cells have nuclei that are typically bland and sometimes show intranuclear cytoplasmic inclusions. The finding of inclusions may be important in the differential diagnosis of neoplasms arising in the upper aerodigestive tract.

Differential Diagnosis. Because meningioma has a variable microscopic appearance, numerous other neoplasms are included in the differential diagnosis (113,116). When meningioma is found in the middle ear, a glomus tumor is often a diagnostic consideration. When present in the nasal cavity or paranasal sinus, melanoma, olfactory neuroblastoma, and carcinoma are tumors that need to be considered. Other diagnostic considerations include paraganglioma, neurofibroma, neurilemoma, fibrous histiocytoma, myoepithelioma of salivary gland origin, and cemento-ossifying fibroma.

Treatment and Prognosis. Surgery is the mainstay of therapy. The extent of the procedure depends upon the size of the neoplasm and its location. When the nasal cavity or paranasal sinus is involved, the prognosis is excellent for primary extracranial tumors. When an intracranial component is present, however, the neoplasm may be difficult to eradicate and radical surgery may be necessary. The prognosis is better for a meningioma that is limited to the middle ear than for a lesion invading from the petrous bone. In one review of middle ear neoplasms arising largely from the petrous surface of the temporal bone only 2 of 30 patients survived 5 years (112). Two patients with temporal bone meningioma had cervical lymph node metastases prior to surgery. The histologic appearance of the lymph node metastases was bland, and was identical to that seen in the primary temporal bone neoplasm. In general, meningiomas of the upper aerodigestive tract may be cured by radical surgery. There may be recurrences, however, which sometimes arise many years following the initial procedure.

PARAGANGLIOMA/CAROTID BODY TUMOR

Definition. Paragangliomas are neuroendocrine neoplasms derived from the extra-adrenal paraganglia of the autonomic nervous system.

General Findings. Paragangliomas can be subdivided into two groups, sympathetic and parasympathetic. Sympathetic paragangliomas originate from the adrenal medulla, extra-adrenal sympathetic paraganglia, and visceral autonomic paraganglia. Virtually all upper aerodigestive tract paragangliomas arise from the parasympathetic nervous system, including the carotid body, jugulotympanic (including the middle ear [glomus tympanicum] and jugular bulb [glomus jugulare]), laryngeal, and vagal paraganglia. Both paraganglioma types are composed of two separate cell populations: chief cells, which contain neurosecretory granules and may secrete catecholamines in the non-neoplastic and neoplastic state; and sustentacular cells, which convey unmyelinated nerve fibers into direct synapse with chief cells and lack neurosecretory granules (118–138).

Normally, carotid body and aorticopulmonary paraganglia function as chemoreceptors to modulate respiratory and cardiovascular function in response to changes in arterial oxygen tension and pH (122). The physiologic role of other paraganglia in the head and neck region is unknown, but their similar morphologic appearance suggests a similar function. Enlargement of the carotid body was reported by Arias-Stella (119) in Peruvian natives living in the Andes, 14,000 feet above sea level. An increased incidence of carotid body paragangliomas has been reported in other high altitude locations as well (132,133). Carotid body hyperplasia has also been observed in humans under hypoxic normobaric conditions, including those with chronic obstructive pulmonary disease, systemic hypertension, cystic fibrosis, and cyanotic congenital heart disease (127,128).

Clinical Findings. Paragangliomas usually occur in young or middle-aged adults, with a peak incidence in patients 40 to 60 years of age (mean, 50 years). Functional paragangliomas with signs and symptoms of excess catecholamine secretion are rare: Lack (129) noted no functional tumors in a review of 72 lesions. Paragangliomas have been reported to occur in famil-ial kindreds (126,129). Multiple paragangliomas, usually bilateral carotid body lesions, occur in about 10 percent of patients (126). Patients with multiple lesions or a family history of paragangliomas are usually younger as a group than those with solitary lesions (126).

Carotid body paragangliomas account for about 60 percent of head and neck paragangliomas, and typically present as painless, slow-growing masses near the angle of the jaw (129). Cranial nerve palsy with dysphonia or dysphagia may occur. Symptom duration ranges from 1 to 5 years prior to diagnosis. Most series show an equal sex predilection.

The middle ear is the next most common site of head and neck paragangliomas. Jugulotympanic paragangliomas may arise along the tympanic branch of the ninth cranial nerve, the auricular branch of the tenth cranial nerve, in the adventitia of the jugular bulb (glomus jugulare), the osseous canal connecting the jugular fossa to the middle ear, or within the middle ear itself (glomus tympanicum). These tumors occur significantly more often in females and usually present as a middle ear mass with loss of hearing, tinnitus, or cranial nerve palsies. Tumors may involve the temporal bone and extend intracranially, or occur at the base of the skull and erode the jugular foramen.

Less common sites of upper aerodigestive tract paragangliomas include the nodose ganglion of the vagus nerve (vagus body tumor), larynx, nasopharynx, nasal cavity, and paranasal sinuses. Patients with vagal body paragangliomas may present with a vagus nerve palsy and a lateral neck mass that may extend medially, displacing oropharyngeal structures, or superiorly into the base of the skull or nasopharynx. These tumors also have a predilection for women in the fourth and fifth decades of life. Laryngeal paragangliomas arise from two microscopic collections of paraganglia: a superior group near the aryepiglottic fold and an inferior group in the subglottic or tracheal area. Hoarseness and dysphagia are common complaints.

Gross Findings. Paragangliomas are firm, circumscribed tumors that appear red to light tan and focally hemorrhagic on cut section (fig. 7-43). Tumor size varies from 2 to 6 cm in most series.

Microscopic Findings. Paragangliomas are typically surrounded by a pseudocapsule of compressed fibrous tissue (fig. 7-44). Tumors appear

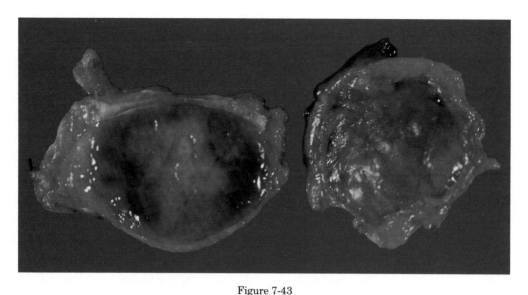

Figure 7-43
CAROTID BODY PARAGANGLIOMA
Irrespective of anatomic site, paragangliomas are grossly well-circumscribed lesions that often appear hemorrhagic on cut section.

as organoid nests (zellballen) of polygonal chief (type I) cells surrounded by sustentacular (type II) cells and a prominent capillary network (fig. 7-45). Less commonly, chief cells may form cords and irregular clusters without sustentacular support. The neoplastic chief cells are medium to large, and round to oval, with moderate amounts of eosinophilic granular cytoplasm and indistinct cell borders. Nuclei are usually small, centrally placed and vesicular with inconspicuous nucleoli. Sustentacular cells appear as spindled, attenuated cells encircling nests of chief cells, but are often difficult to identify in hematoxylin and eosin–stained sections (fig. 7-45). The mitotic rate is generally low, although nuclear hyperchromasia and pleomorphism have been observed in about 10 percent of tumors (fig. 7-46). Perineural and vascular invasion may be seen. "Oncocytic" tumors containing cells with deeply eosinophilic cytoplasm have been reported (129). Rare tumors may focally assume a spindled, or "sarcomatous" appearance without sustentacular cells, but typical organoid foci are usually present elsewhere in the tumor (129). Stromal edema, myxoid change, and diffuse stromal fibrosis (hyalinization) may occur, compressing and distorting the tumor nests.

Malignant tumors have been variably reported to show a higher incidence of necrosis, vascular invasion, and mitotic activity, and a lack

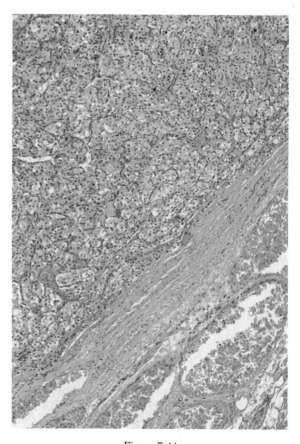

Figure 7-44
CAROTID BODY PARAGANGLIOMA
Tumors are usually separated from surrounding tissues by a pseudocapsule composed of compressed fibrous tissue.

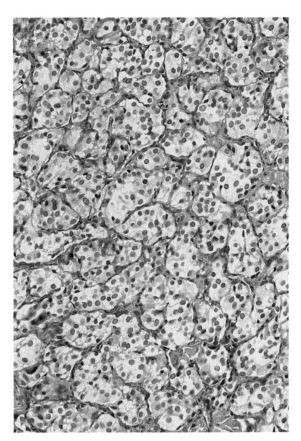

Figure 7-45
JUGULOTYMPANIC PARAGANGLIOMA
Histologically, paragangliomas invariably appear as organoid nests ("zellballen") of epithelioid neoplastic cells surrounded by sustentacular cells and a capillary network. Sustentacular cells are often difficult to distinguish on hematoxylin and eosin-stained sections.

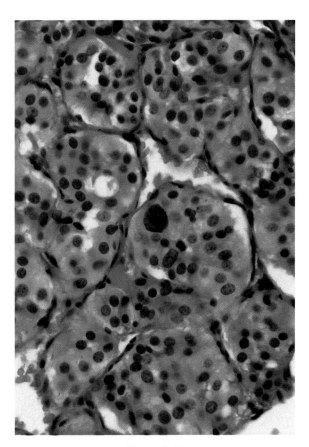

Figure 7-46
CAROTID BODY PARAGANGLIOMA
Paragangliomas often display mild nuclear pleomorphism.

of organoid architecture (126,129). Recent studies have suggested that a lack of sustentacular cells (demonstrated by S-100 protein or glial fibrillary acidic protein immunoreactivity) is associated with aggressive clinical behavior (118,126). One study identified type II sustentacular cells in 23 of 24 solitary, benign paragangliomas compared to 1 in 5 malignant paragangliomas (126). In general, however, sustentacular cells, as well as nuclear pleomorphism, necrosis, mitotic activity, and perineural, bony, and vascular invasion may be seen in both benign and malignant tumors.

Immunohistochemical Findings. The neoplastic chief cells in virtually all paragangliomas are immunohistochemically positive for at least one neuroendocrine marker: neuron-specific enolase, chromogranin, synaptophysin, or met-en-

kephalin (fig. 7-47) (125,126,135). Most tumors are also reactive for neuropeptides such as secretogranin II, serotonin, [Leu-5]-enkephalin, [Met-5]-enkephalin, and somatostatin (125,130,135). Vimentin is inconsistently present and rare tumors showing focal cytokeratin positivity have been reported (125). Overall, the single most sensitive chief cell marker is neuron-specific enolase (positive in 92 to 100 percent of cases), followed by synaptophysin (97 percent), chromogranin (84 to 89 percent), and met-enkephalin (73 percent) (125,126,130). The sustentacular cells are virtually always positive for S-100 protein and variably reactive for glial fibrillary acidic protein and vimentin (fig. 7-48) (125).

Ultrastructural Findings. The neoplastic chief cells are polygonal, with round to oval nuclei and variable numbers of mitochondria and other intracytoplasmic organelles. Ultrastructural examination of one tumor with oncocytic features

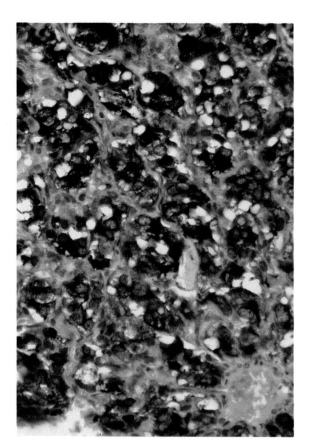
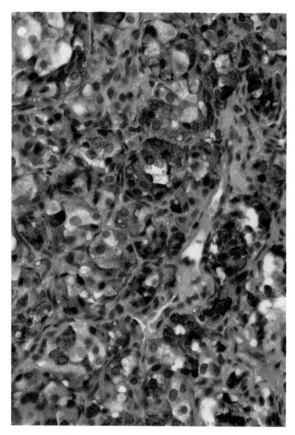

Figure 7-47
CAROTID BODY PARAGANGLIOMA
Immunohistochemical examination reveals the neoplastic cells positive for neuron-specific enolase (left) and chromogranin (right).

showed numerous mitochondria within the tumor cells (129). Occasional tumors contain abundant intracytoplasmic glycogen. Cells are joined by tight or, less commonly, desmosome-like junctions lacking tonofilaments. Electron-dense, membrane-bound neurosecretory granules are always present although variable in number; size ranges from 60 to 300 nm (fig. 7-49) (126). Sustentacular cells are occasionally identified as spindled to triangular cells with ovoid to fusiform nuclei and long cytoplasmic processes devoid of neurosecretory granules (129).

Special Studies/Techniques. DNA ploidy has been studied on several upper aerodigestive tract paragangliomas, primarily those of carotid body origin (121,123,134). In general, most paragangliomas are diploid. Of the few DNA abnormalities found, most were present in metastasizing or locally aggressive lesions. Ploidy anomalies have been reported in benign tumors as well, however,

thus DNA content cannot be used to definitively assess malignant potential in the individual case.

Differential Diagnosis. The differential diagnosis includes parathyroid and thyroid neoplasms, carcinoid tumors, alveolar soft-part sarcoma, granular cell tumor, melanoma, and metastatic renal cell carcinoma. Distinction from most of the latter lesions is usually enabled by recognition of the characteristic organoid (zellballen) cellular arrangement. Tumors with cells arranged in sheets or cords, however, may resemble medullary carcinoma of the thyroid or carcinoid tumor. In these and other problematic cases, immunopositivity for neuropeptides, the presence of S-100–positive sustentacular cells encircling tumor nests, and the absence of cytokeratin staining are virtually diagnostic of paraganglioma.

Treatment and Prognosis. The treatment of choice for paragangliomas, irrespective of anatomic site, is surgical excision. The incidence of

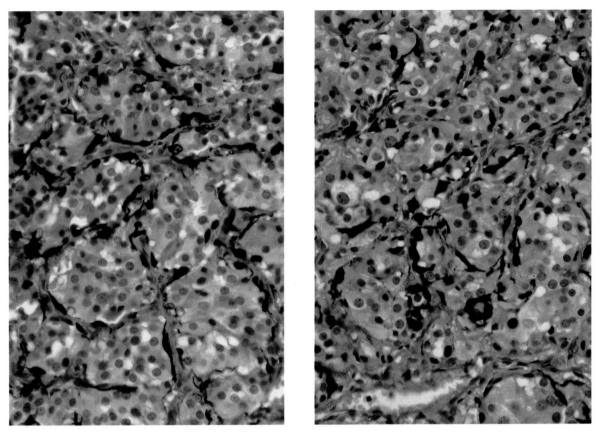

Figure 7-48
CAROTID BODY PARAGANGLIOMA
Sustentacular cells are often difficult to identify on routinely stained sections but are consistently immunoreactive for S-100 protein (left) and glial fibrillary acid protein (right).

Figure 7-49
CAROTID BODY
PARAGANGLIOMA
Ultrastructurally, paragangliomas contain numerous neurosecretory-type granules consistent with their neuroendocrine differentiation. (Fig. 22-8, Fascicle 19, 3rd Series.)

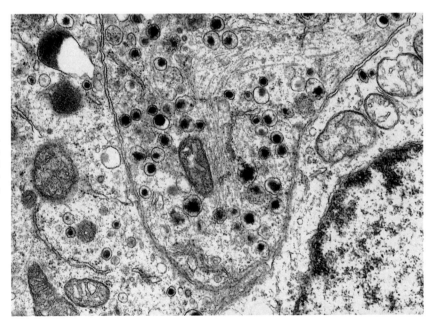

local recurrence and malignant behavior (regional or distant metastases) varies according to the anatomic site of origin. Combining the results of two large studies, 12 of 60 (20 percent) carotid body paragangliomas recurred following excision, as did 12 of 41 (29 percent) glomus jugulare/tympanicum tumors, 2 of 14 (14 percent) vagal body lesions, and 2 of 4 (50 percent) nasal paraganglioms (126,129). The prevalence of malignant behavior varies considerably from one series to another: 0 to 12 percent carotid body tumors are reportedly malignant (120,121,125,129,131,138), as are 0 to 25 percent of jugulotympanic paragangliomas (125,129) and 7 to 16 percent of vagal body tumors (124,129,137). Reliable prediction of biologic behavior on the basis of gross, histologic, or immunohistochemical features is notoriously difficult. In general, the only absolute criterion of malignancy is the presence of metastases; e.g., tumor in sites where paraganglionic tissue is not normally found. The more frequent sites of metastasis include regional lymph nodes, liver, lung, and bone, reflecting both lymphatic and hematogenous dissemination.

OLFACTORY NEUROBLASTOMA

Definition. Olfactory neuroblastoma is an uncommon malignant neuroendocrine neoplasm that arises from the olfactory mucosa (140,146,148, 159,162,168,173,181). A variety of other terms have been applied to these neoplasms, including *esthesioneuroblastoma, esthesioneurocytoma, esthesioneuroma, esthesioneuroepithelioma, intranasal neuroblastoma,* and *olfactory placode tumor.*

General Features. The availability of antibodies to olfactory marker protein has allowed for ready mapping of the normal olfactory mucosa (165,170). In the human fetus, the olfactory mucosa normally forms an irregular but continuous, sharply defined zone encompassing the superior one third to half of the nasal septum, the cribriform plate, and the superior-medial surface of the superior turbinate (169). In adults, this specialized mucosa undergoes progressive, multifocal degeneration with depletion of olfactory receptor cells and replacement by respiratory mucosa (169). This apparently normal phenomenon is usually asymptomatic. Evidence for the origin of olfactory neuroblastoma from the specialized olfactory epithelium is circumstantial, and based on the sharp

localization of these tumors to this region. The mitotically active reserve cell is the putative cell of origin, again on purely circumstantial grounds. During embryologic development, this cell gives rise to both neuronal and epithelial (sustentacular) cells; in adults, the reserve cells supply new sustentacular cells. It is unknown whether olfactory neuronal cells can regenerate in humans, although this has been suggested to occur in other mammalian species (169).

Causative factors have not been documented for human olfactory neuroblastoma. Tumors histologically identical to human olfactory neuroblastoma have been induced in the olfactory mucosa of Syrian hamsters by subcutaneous injection of diethylnitrosamine (156) and in rats with injection of N-nitrosopiperidine (184).

Clinical Features. Olfactory neuroblastomas occur in a broad patient age range with bimodal peaks at about 15 and 55 years of age (148). Males and females are equally affected (148). Presenting symptoms are usually related to nasal obstruction or hemorrhage (168). Less common complaints include headaches, anosmia, or visual disturbances. Physical examination typically demonstrates a polypoid mass high in the nasal cavity, often involving the ethmoid sinus. Although rare "ectopic" olfactory neuroblastomas probably do develop in the lower nasal cavity or maxillary antrum, this diagnosis should be viewed with great skepticism when the superior nasal cavity is not involved. Occasional olfactory neuroblastomas present as predominantly or exclusively intracranial masses that involve the superior aspect of the cribriform plate (141,154,171,176). Some have been documented to contain low levels of catecholamines without resulting in systemic symptoms (166), and to produce vasopressin with associated clinical findings of hypertension and hyponatremia (179).

Radiographic Appearance. Although the radiographic findings of olfactory neuroblastoma are nonspecific, they can be quite suggestive. In particular, the finding of a "dumbbell-shaped" lesion extending across the cribriform plate is highly supportive of this diagnosis (fig. 7-50). Involvement of the ethmoid sinuses with expansion into the roof of the orbit and the fronto-ethmoid complex is also typical (fig. 7-51) (187). The tumors typically show magnetic resonance imaging (MRI) changes indicative of a vascular lesion.

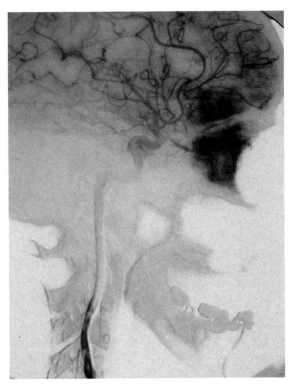

Figure 7-50
OLFACTORY NEUROBLASTOMA

As this subtraction angiogram indicates, olfactory neuroblastomas may have a significant intracranial component. The zone of extension through the cribriform plate is narrow, and gave the resected lesion a "dumbbell" appearance.

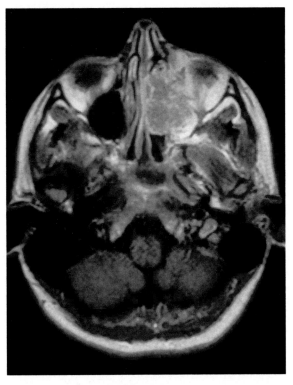

Figure 7-51
OLFACTORY NEUROBLASTOMA

This computerized tomography scan demonstrates a large olfactory neuroblastoma that filled the nasal cavity, extended into the maxillary antrum, and impinged on the orbit.

In particular, there is intense signal in precontrast T2-weighted images with marked enhancement of T1-weighted images following gadolinium injection (187). The latter technique is considered the optimum method for assessing extent of disease prior to craniofacial resection (187).

Gross Findings. Typically, olfactory neuroblastomas form a polypoid, vascular-appearing, red or tan mass located high in the nasal cavity (fig. 7-52). The overlying surface mucosa may be intact or focally ulcerated. Often the tumor is quite friable and bleeds easily on manipulation. The tumor may be as small as 1 cm or large enough to fill the nasal cavity and extend into adjacent paranasal sinuses. The epicenter of such larger lesions may be difficult to determine, but smaller tumors are more easily localized, and are often seen to attach to and invade the cribriform plate.

Microscopic Findings. At low magnification, olfactory neuroblastomas commonly display

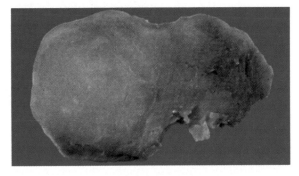

Figure 7-52
OLFACTORY NEUROBLASTOMA

Grossly, olfactory neuroblastomas vary from yellow tan, as seen, to more hemorrhagic in appearance.

one of two major growth patterns. Most often, they form sharply circumscribed nests of cells separated by stroma (fig. 7-53). Less commonly, the tumor grows as a diffuse sheet of neoplastic cells with a prominent background of capillaries but little intervening stroma (fig. 7-54) (168).

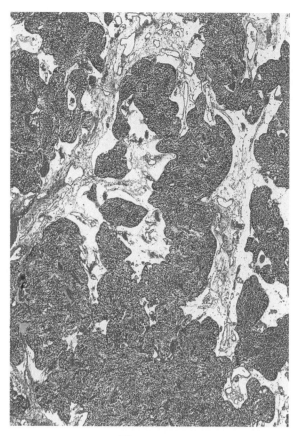

Figure 7-53
OLFACTORY NEUROBLASTOMA
Often, olfactory neuroblastomas grow as sharply demarcated nests of cells in an edematous stroma.

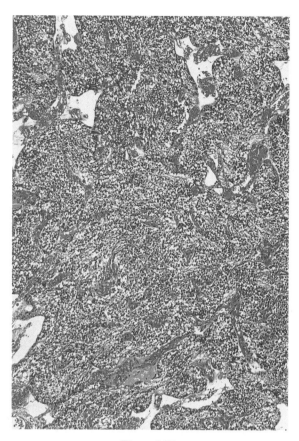

Figure 7-54
OLFACTORY NEUROBLASTOMA
Olfactory neuroblastomas may also grow as diffuse sheets of cells in a highly vascular stroma.

The neoplastic cells have small, round nuclei with coarse, punctate to fine chromatin and very little cytoplasm (fig. 7-55). Usually there is only mild to moderate nuclear pleomorphism. Numbers of mitotic figures are extremely variable and may be virtually absent or more than 10 per high-power field. Most often, mitotic activity is limited. Occasionally, the cells of olfactory neuroblastoma have more prominent, eosinophilic cytoplasm, and rare examples may have cells with clear cytoplasm (fig. 7-56), or cells containing melanin-like pigment (fig. 7-57) (145).

In our experience, as well as that of others (174), the key microscopic feature for a definitive diagnosis is the presence of a fibrillary cytoplasmic background (fig. 7-58). Such fibrils may be seen on hematoxylin and eosin–stained sections in about 86 percent of cases (168) and correspond to the neuronal cell processes seen

ultrastructurally. Another, less common diagnostic feature is the presence of Flexner-type (fig. 7-59) or Homer Wright–type (fig. 7-60) rosettes. The former are gland-like structures that are too infrequent to be of much diagnostic value, being encountered in about 5 percent or less of tumors. Homer Wright rosettes, also termed pseudorosettes, are annular arrays of cells surrounding central aggregates of cytoplasmic fibrils. They are most common in cases that contain a prominent fibrillary background (168). In our experience, about 28 percent of olfactory neuroblastomas contain well-formed Homer Wright rosettes, with equivocal structures encountered in an additional 43 percent (fig. 7-61) (168). Perivascular pseudorosettes (fig. 7-62), also encountered in these tumors as well as in many other tumor types, are of no diagnostic value. Ganglion cells are seen rarely in olfactory neuroblastoma (fig. 7-63), but

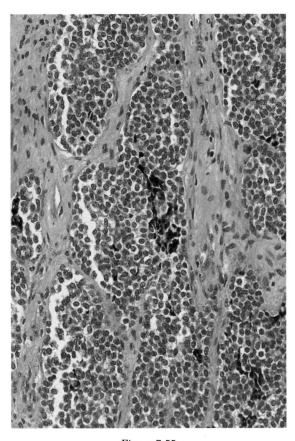

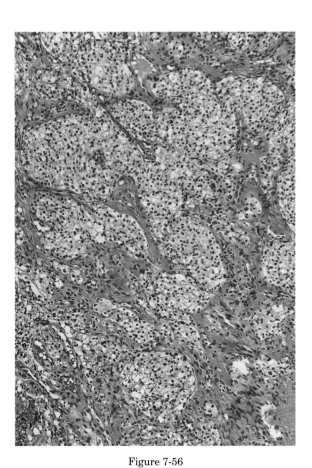

Figure 7-55
OLFACTORY NEUROBLASTOMA
Typically, olfactory neuroblastomas consist of "small blue cells" with little apparent cytoplasm.

Figure 7-56
OLFACTORY NEUROBLASTOMA
Rarely, olfactory neuroblastomas may have a "clear cell" appearance which may mimic a metastatic renal cell carcinoma.

Figure 7-57
OLFACTORY NEUROBLASTOMA
This olfactory neuroblastoma contains melanin-like pigment. This should not be confused with a malignant melanoma.

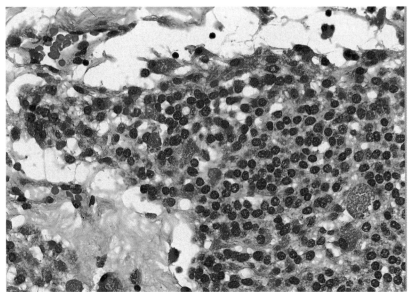

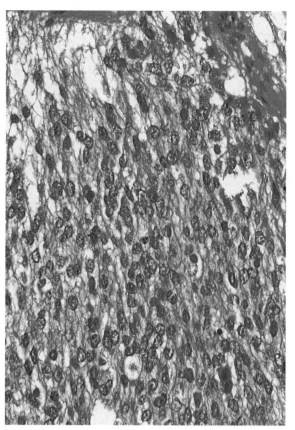

Figure 7-58
OLFACTORY NEUROBLASTOMA
The presence of a fibrillary cytoplasmic background, corresponding to neuronal cell processes, is a helpful diagnostic feature.

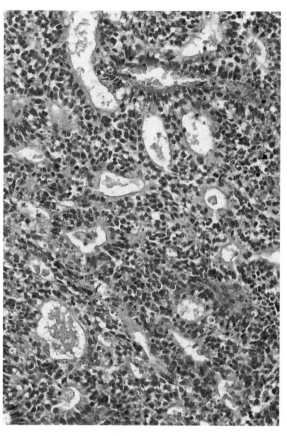

Figure 7-59
OLFACTORY NEUROBLASTOMA
The distinction between glandular spaces and Flexner-type rosettes may be arbitrary. These larger structures may represent areas of glandular differentiation in an otherwise typical olfactory neuroblastoma.

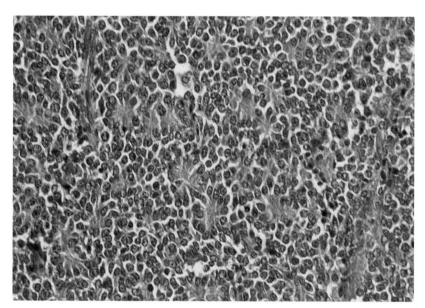

Figure 7-60
OLFACTORY NEUROBLASTOMA
Homer Wright-type rosettes may be encountered in olfactory neuroblastomas, although they are rarely this plentiful. Abundant rosette formation is invariably accompanied by a prominent fibrillary background.

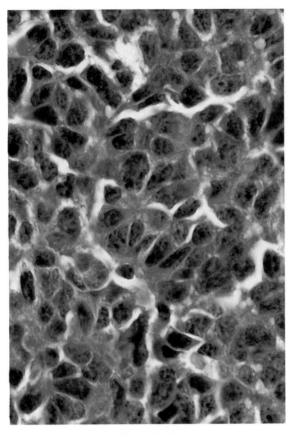

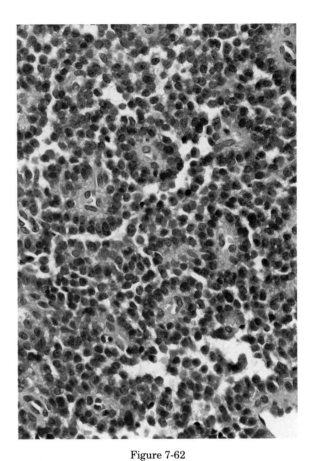

Figure 7-61
OLFACTORY NEUROBLASTOMA
More often, olfactory neuroblastomas contain equivocal rosette-like structures as seen in the center of this photograph.

Figure 7-62
OLFACTORY NEUROBLASTOMA
Perivascular pseudorosettes, as seen here, are of no diagnostic value and may be encountered in a wide variety of neoplasms.

Figure 7-63
OLFACTORY NEUROBLASTOMA
Ganglion cells, as seen in the center of this illustration, are rarely encountered in untreated olfactory neuroblastoma but, when present, are diagnostic. Olfactory neuroblastomas treated with chemotherapy or radiation may rarely show "maturation" with the presence of ganglion cells in post-treatment biopsies.

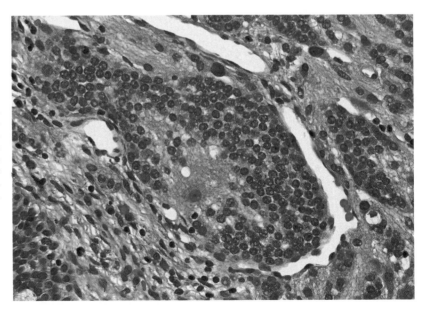

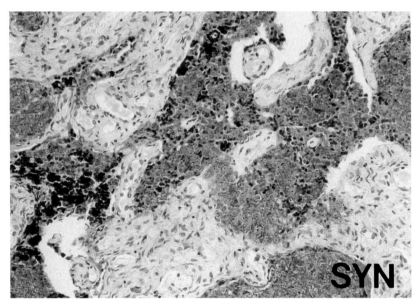

Figure 7-64
OLFACTORY NEUROBLASTOMA
Antibodies directed against synaptophysin are consistently strong markers for olfactory neuroblastoma.

when present, are also diagnostic (142,168). Rarely, olfactory neuroblastomas may show divergent differentiation in the form of adenocarcinoma-like areas (167,178), or even rhabdomyoblastic differentiation (180).

Microscopic Grading. The division of olfactory neuroblastomas into subtypes, based on morphologic features, particularly the degree of epithelial versus neuronal differentiation, has been of prognostic value in some studies (153,178), but most reports have been unable to correlate morphology and prognosis (140,146,162,173,181). In our own experience with 21 cases, necrosis was the only morphologic feature tending to show prognostic correlation (poorer survival if present) (168).

The experience of Hyams and colleagues (157) at the Armed Forces Institute of Pathology (AFIP) supported the use of a grading system for olfactory neuroblastoma. The features of this four-part grading approach are presented in Table 7-1. We would caution that the grade III and especially grade IV lesions in their system might, in some instances, be better classified as sinonasal undifferentiated carcinomas (see Differential Diagnosis section below).

Immunohistochemical Findings. Immunocytochemical staining is a valuable diagnostic adjunct. Between 75 and 100 percent of olfactory neuroblastoma are positive for neuron-specific enolase (139,151,163,181); synaptophysin is found in 64 to 100 percent (fig. 7-64) (151,186); neurofila-

Table 7-1

HYAMS GRADING SYSTEM FOR OLFACTORY NEUROBLASTOMA

Feature/Grade	I	II	III	IV
Lobular pattern	++	++	+/–	–/+
Uniform nuclei	++	+/–	–/+	–
Mitotic figures	–	+	++	++
Calcification	+/–	+/–	–	–
Necrosis	–	–	+/–	++
Fibrillary background	+++	++	+/–	–
Homer Wright rosettes	+/–	+/–	–	–
Flexner rosettes	–	–	++	–

ment protein (200 kD) in up to 73 percent (139, 151,181,183); and a similar number of cases contain scattered S-100–positive cells (139,144,151, 181). The latter are Schwann-like cells that are preferentially located at the periphery of neoplastic cell nests (fig. 7-65) (144,151,181). The scattered nature of the S-100–positive cells and their location should avoid confusion with the more diffuse S-100 staining in malignant melanoma. Most olfactory neuroblastomas also contain microtubule-associated protein-2 (MAP-2) and the class III beta-tubulin isotype (151). A few olfactory neuroblastomas stain for chromogranin (fig. 7-66), but

159

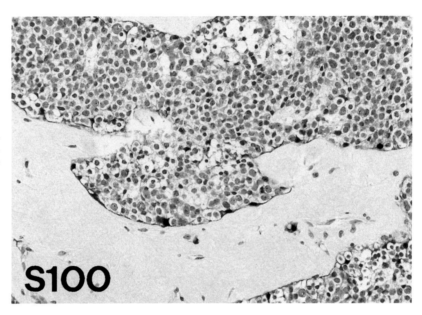

Figure 7-65
OLFACTORY NEUROBLASTOMA
When the cells of olfactory neuroblastoma grow as nests, the periphery of the cell nests often contains S-100 protein-positive cells.

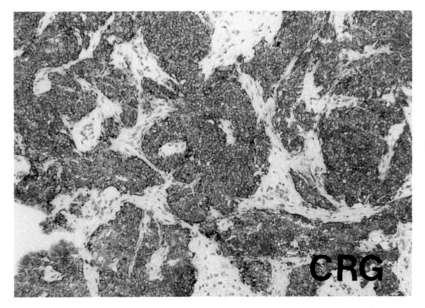

Figure 7-66
OLFACTORY NEUROBLASTOMA
Staining for chromogranin is less often positive than for synaptophysin, but some olfactory neuroblastomas are strongly positive for chromogranin.

this marker is not as useful as the other neuroendocrine antigens listed (139). Although some studies have noted negativity for cytokeratin (139, 186), up to 30 percent of olfactory neuroblastomas in other series have contained at least scattered cells that were positive for this marker (151,181). This is a potential source of confusion with nasopharyngeal-type carcinomas. Epithelial membrane antigen and carcinoembryonic antigen are typically absent (139,151). To add to the potential for confusion, rare olfactory neuroblastomas may stain focally with HMB-45, although the reported example was negative for vimentin or S-100 protein (186).

Ultrastructural Findings. In spite of the growing availability of neuroendocrine immunohistochemical markers, electron microscopy remains a useful ancillary technique for the diagnosis of olfactory neuroblastomas that lack fibrils, rosettes, or ganglion cells on hematoxylin and eosin–stained sections. Diagnostic ultrastructural features include moderate numbers of

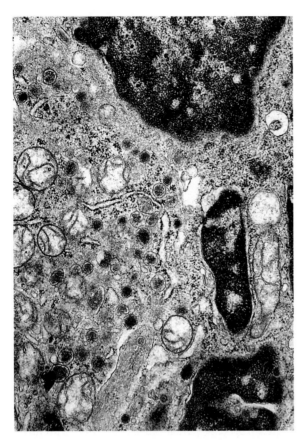

Figure 7-67
OLFACTORY NEUROBLASTOMA
Ultrastructurally, this olfactory neuroblastoma contains
neuronal cell processes, cut in cross section, which contain
multiple dense core granules.

dense core granules, usually measuring between 90 and 250 nm in diameter (fig. 7-67), and neurite-like cell processes containing neurofilaments or neurotubules (143,158,160,164,175,182). The dense core granules tend to cluster in the cell processes, in close approximation to the microtubules, and they also may be associated with smaller, clear vesicles. Fusion of vesicles with the cell membrane may be seen. Schwann-like cells with associated basal lamina can often be identified surrounding nests of neoplastic cells (175,182). Junctional complexes between neoplastic cells are rare (175, 182). It should be emphasized that the finding of scattered dense core granules alone is not sufficient for a diagnosis of olfactory neuroblastoma.

Other Special Techniques. Formaldehyde fume-induced fluorescence has been documented in olfactory neuroblastoma, but requires fresh tissue and experience with the technique

(158,166,178). Neuroblastomas arising from other sites have been noted on tissue culture assay to produce abundant neurite outgrowths, indicative of neuronal differentiation (177).

Differential Diagnosis. Olfactory neuroblastoma may be confused with a wide variety of tumors including malignant melanoma, lymphoma, embryonal rhabdomyosarcoma, small cell undifferentiated carcinoma, and other predominantly small cell neoplasms. In many instances, the diagnosis is relatively easy, given adequately processed tissue and, when necessary, the availability of specific immunohistochemical markers. This section will focus on several more problematic or potentially confusing diagnostic distinctions.

Malignant Melanoma. In our experience, confusion of olfactory neuroblastoma with malignant melanoma is very common. One should be particularly suspicious of diagnosing olfactory neuroblastoma when the tumor occurs low in the nasal cavity, beyond the realm of the normal olfactory mucosa. A number of factors conspire to further the confusion created by hematoxylin and eosin–based similarities. Rarely, sinonasal malignant melanoma may exhibit a distinctly fibrillar background, as well as forming structures resembling Homer Wright rosettes. Focal staining for neurofilament may also be encountered. However, the diffuse, strong S-100 positivity of malignant melanoma is not seen in olfactory neuroblastoma. In our experience, olfactory neuroblastoma does not stain with HMB-45 (149,186), although at least one example has been reported to stain focally with this marker (186). Interestingly, the reported example was negative for vimentin or S-100 protein.

Sinonasal Undifferentiated Carcinoma (SNUC). Olfactory neuroblastoma has a much better prognosis than SNUC and should be distinguished from the latter tumor. The cytologically more uniform cells and the frequently present fibrillary cytoplasmic background of the former are helpful differentiating features. The nuclei of olfactory neuroblastoma have punctate, "neural-like" chromatin, with small or absent nucleoli. In contrast, SNUC often has prominent eosinophilic nucleoli. Rosettes and ganglion cells are also diagnostic, when present. Individual cell necrosis and central necrosis of cell nests are common in SNUC and less often seen in olfactory neuroblastoma. Ultrastructurally, neuroblastoma contains cell processes and more numerous dense core granules than SNUC and S-100 positive cells often surround cell nests. Both tumors may label for cytokeratin, but SNUC is more frequently and strongly positive with this marker (150). The possible role of a deletion in the retinoblastoma gene with regard to the development of SNUC is under current investigation (155).

Pituitary Adenoma. As discussed elsewhere in this chapter, pituitary adenomas may present as nasopharyngeal or sinonasal masses either because of an ectopic origin or invasion from an adenoma originating in the sella turcica. Confusion with olfactory neuroblastoma is common, particularly when the biopsies are partially distorted. Location is a helpful distinguishing feature. Pituitary adenomas, whether ectopic or invasive, usually involve the sphenoid sinus or nasopharynx. Unlike olfactory neuroblastoma, nasal cavity lesions are rare. Adenomas are strongly positive for cytokeratin and chromogranin, positive for specific pituitary hormones, and negative for S-100 protein. Both tumors frequently express synaptophysin and neuron-specific enolase.

Peripheral Neuroectodermal Tumor (PNET). There have been recent reports of PNET-like tumors arising in the head and neck region, often in association with a prior retinoblastoma (152, 161). Several of these tumors have somewhat resembled SNUC and others have been composed of smaller, more primitive cells like those of other PNETs or Ewing's sarcoma. Both SNUC and PNET may be cytokeratin positive, although the former is more likely to be strongly so. "Divergent differentiation" may also be noted in the PNET-like tumors (152). Neuroendocrine markers are of no value in making this distinction.

Frozen Section. Experienced otolaryngologists often strongly suspect a diagnosis based on clinical and radiographic findings. Initial diagnosis of an olfactory neuroblastoma based on frozen section material is fraught with difficulty and should be avoided. Appropriate special stains not available at the time of frozen section are often required, such that definitive diagnosis almost always mandates evaluation of permanent section material. Furthermore, freezing artifact may hamper interpretation of the remaining tissue. If a frozen section is to be performed

for initial diagnosis, it should primarily confirm that neoplastic tissue has been obtained. Ideally, it should be first ascertained that adequate unfrozen tissue is available for further permanent section study. If sufficient material is available, a portion of the initial biopsy tissue should also be fixed in glutaraldehyde for possible electron microscopy. As with most small cell tumors, the cells are fragile and easily distorted by forceps biopsies. Incisional biopsies should be encouraged, with minimal tissue handling prior to fixation.

Spread and Metastasis. In one large literature review of patients with olfactory neuroblastoma who developed recurrences, 68 percent had local disease, 22 percent had nodal involvement, and 16 percent had distant spread (148). In a separate review of 40 patients from a single institution treated primarily with surgery followed by adjuvant radiation and, for high-stage disease, chemotherapy, 55 percent were initial treatment failures (147). Time to first recurrence ranged from 5 to 149 months (median, 21.5 months). Of these patients, 38 percent had locoregional disease, 10 percent had persistent local disease, and 8 percent developed distant metastases. Locoregional disease consisted of cervical lymph node involvement, recurrence in the nasal cavity and paranasal sinuses, or intracranial extension. Distant metastases may involve bone, lung, prostate, spinal cord, or other sites (147,148).

Staging. The Kadish staging system is applied to these tumors as follows (159): stage A, disease confined to the nasal cavity; stage B, disease confined to the nasal cavity and paranasal sinuses; and stage C, local or distant spread beyond the nasal cavity or sinuses. Stage B disease is most common and occurs in 40 to 50 percent of cases (148,168).

Treatment and Prognosis. Complete surgical excision, often supplemented by radiation therapy or chemotherapy, appears to offer the highest apparent cure rate of up to approximately 75 percent (30). In a review of all patients with olfactory neuroblastoma from a single institution, the overall 5-, 10-, and 15-year survival rates were 78 percent, 71 percent, and 68 percent, respectively (147). Long disease-free intervals do not indicate cure, as recurrence or metastases may develop after a decade or more. Prognosis has correlated with stage in some reports (148,159), with 5-year survival rates of 75 percent, 68 percent, and 41 percent for stages A, B, and C disease, respectively, in one large study (148). In another study, complete tumor resection was of more prognostic value than Kadish stage (168). Patients with advanced, unresectable disease benefit from chemotherapy: a 62 percent response rate was elicited with conventional chemotherapy protocols (185). Long-term survivors have been reported following high-dose chemotherapy and autologous bone marrow transplantation (147,172)

In the Armed Forces Institute of Pathology experience, grading of olfactory neuroblastoma correlated with survival (157). With a mean follow-up of 5 years, none of 6 patients with grade I disease had a recurrence; of 25 patients with grade II tumor, 19 were free of disease, 3 were living with disease, and 3 died of disease; of 11 patients with grade III tumors, 5 were free of disease and 6 died of disease; and finally, all 4 patients with grade IV tumors died of their disease. As noted above, the authors have some reservations regarding the nature of grade III and IV tumors.

SINONASAL UNDIFFERENTIATED CARCINOMA

Definition. Sinonasal undifferentiated carcinoma (SNUC) is a pathologically distinctive, clinically aggressive neoplasm composed of medium-sized, light microscopically undifferentiated cells. Ultrastructural and immunohistochemical studies demonstrate varying degrees of neuroendocrine differentiation. Other examples have been reported as anaplastic carcinoma.

General Features. SNUC is a rare but increasingly recognized neoplasm. In the past, these tumors were almost certainly lumped with poorly differentiated squamous cell carcinomas, malignant lymphomas, and, less often, with high-grade olfactory neuroblastomas. Although the tumors often show evidence of at least abortive neuroendocrine differentiation, they are composed of cells that are significantly larger than even the intermediate cells of small cell undifferentiated carcinoma. By definition, the tumors lack any light microscopic evidence of glandular or squamous differentiation. One study suggests an association with cigarette smoking, with 7 of 8 patients being smokers (190). One of the patients in our study (196) had long-term exposure to nickel refining fumes, a known head and

neck carcinogen. The possible role of Epstein-Barr virus (EBV) in the development SNUC is intriguing, given its known association with nasopharyngeal carcinoma. In one study, EBV RNA was identified in 7 of 11 Asian patients with SNUCs, but was not present in any of 11 Western patients with microscopically similar tumors (193). This suggests that there may be geographically variable factors associated with the development of these neoplasms. The possible role of the deletion of the retinoblastoma gene in the development of this tumor is also under study (191).

Clinical Features. The age range for affected patients has been broad, including both young adults and the elderly; the median age in our series was 53 years (190). The small number of reported cases suggests a slight female predominance (1.2–1.7 to 1) (190,192). Symptoms are nonspecific, of relatively short duration (median, 4 months), and indicative of an enlarging sinonasal mass. Common findings include nasal obstruction, proptosis, cranial nerve deficits, and periorbital swelling. Typically, multiple sinonasal structures are affected. Involvement of the nasal cavity, maxillary antrum, and ethmoid sinuses is most common. Extension into the sphenoid sinus, frontal sinus, orbit, and cranial cavity is also frequent. Radiographic studies almost invariably show marked destruction of sinus walls (fig. 7-68).

Gross Findings. The tumor typically presents as a large, grossly fungating mass obstructing a nasal cavity and freely invading multiple surrounding structures (fig. 7-69). Grossly obvious extension into the nasopharynx or, less commonly, the oral cavity may be present.

Microscopic Findings. SNUC consists of nests, trabeculae, ribbons, and sheets of medium-sized polygonal cells with an often "organoid" appearance (fig. 7-70). Nuclei are round to oval, slightly to moderately pleomorphic, and hyperchromatic. Chromatin varies from diffuse to coarsely granular. Nucleoli are typically large (fig. 7-71), but in some cases may be inconspicuous. Most cells have small to moderate amounts of eosinophilic cytoplasm with distinct cell borders. Mitotic figures are numerous (fig. 7-72), and vascular permeation is extensive. In some microscopic fields virtually all of the neoplasm is located within expanded vascular spaces (fig. 7-73). Individual cell necrosis and central necrosis of

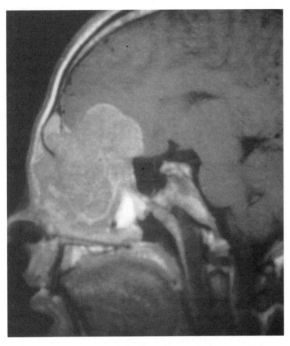

Figure 7-68
SINONASAL UNDIFFERENTIATED CARCINOMA
This large sinonasal undifferentiated carcinoma involves multiple paranasal sinuses and extends into the cranium.

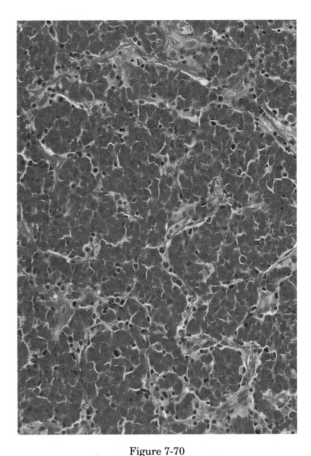

Figure 7-70
SINONASAL UNDIFFERENTIATED CARCINOMA
Sinonasal undifferentiated carcinoma often grows as cords, ribbons, and trabeculae of medium-sized cells.

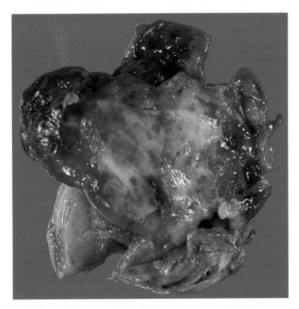

Figure 7-69
SINONASAL UNDIFFERENTIATED CARCINOMA
The large, composite resection of a sinonasal undifferentiated carcinoma includes a portion of the alveolar ridge and hard palate. The tumor completely filled the maxillary antrum.

cell nests are common (fig. 7-74). Homer Wright rosettes, cytoplasmic fibrils, and argyrophil granules are absent, as are features of squamous or glandular differentiation. Occasional SNUCs may be associated with severe dysplasia or carcinoma in situ of the surface mucosa.

Immunohistochemical Findings. Immunocytochemical stains for cytokeratin and epithelial membrane antigen are positive for one or both markers in virtually all cases (190). About 50 percent of cases are positive for neuron-specific enolase, but in our experience this is usually focal and of weak to moderate positivity (fig. 7-75). We have encountered a single SNUC with rare S-100 protein–positive neoplastic cells. Antibodies directed against more specific neuroendocrine markers such as synaptophysin, chromogranin, and neurofilament protein have been nonreactive in these neoplasms.

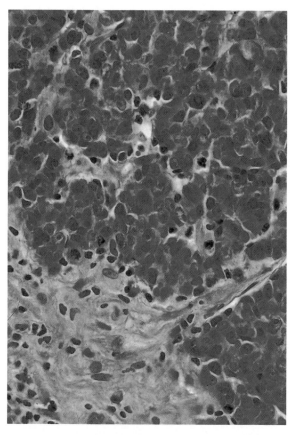

Figure 7-71
SINONASAL UNDIFFERENTIATED CARCINOMA
At higher magnification, the cells of sinonasal undifferentiated carcinoma have moderate amounts of amphophilic cytoplasm, with prominent nucleoli.

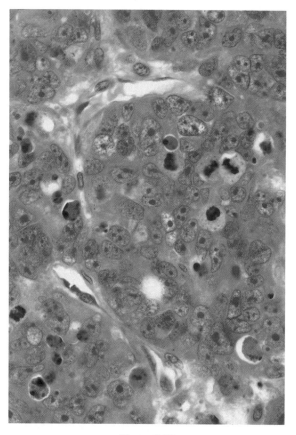

Figure 7-72
SINONASAL UNDIFFERENTIATED CARCINOMA
This example of sinonasal undifferentiated carcinoma has prominent nucleoli and an extremely high mitotic rate.

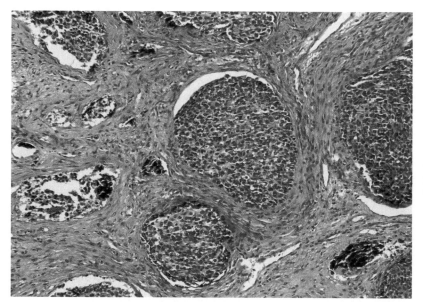

Figure 7-73
SINONASAL
UNDIFFERENTIATED
CARCINOMA
Intravascular growth with distended vascular spaces is a common pattern in sinonasal undifferentiated carcinoma.

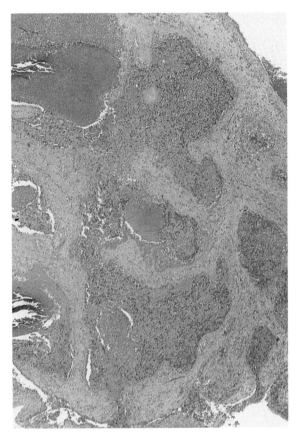

Figure 7-74
SINONASAL UNDIFFERENTIATED CARCINOMA
When sinonasal undifferentiated carcinoma forms larger cell nests, there is often central necrosis within these nests.

Ultrastructural Findings. At the ultrastructural level, the neoplastic cells have high nuclear to cytoplasmic ratios with scattered, poorly formed desmosomes that form intercellular connections (190). Well-formed cytoplasmic processes are absent, as are tonofilament bundles. Of five cases studied, each tumor contained a very few small, membrane-bound dense core granules compatible with neurosecretory-type granules (190). These were present in only rare cells and occurred singly, never in groups of granules.

Differential Diagnosis. *Nasopharyngeal Undifferentiated Carcinoma (Lymphoepithelioma).* SNUC is not simply a nasopharyngeal-type undifferentiated carcinoma (lymphoepithelioma) growing in the sinonasal region and should not be designated as such. Lymphoepithelioma-type undifferentiated carcinoma is composed of cells with more prominent cytoplasm and extremely chromatically uniform, vesicular nuclei. Nucleoli are usually small and less apparent than in SNUC. The cells grow singly or in syncytial-like sheets. In the latter growth pattern, cell borders are indistinct and nuclei appear to be "floating" in a syncytium of cytoplasm. Trabecular or "organoid" growth patterns, common in SNUC, are not seen in lymphoepithelioma-type undifferentiated carcinomas. Conversely, the prominent lymphoplasmacytic infiltrate of the latter is not a typical feature of SNUC. Patients from Western countries who have SNUC lack the association with EBV

Figure 7-75
SINONASAL
UNDIFFERENTIATED
CARCINOMA

Most sinonasal undifferentiated carcinomas show little or no staining for neuron-specific antigen, but occasional examples such as this one show uncharacteristically strong staining.

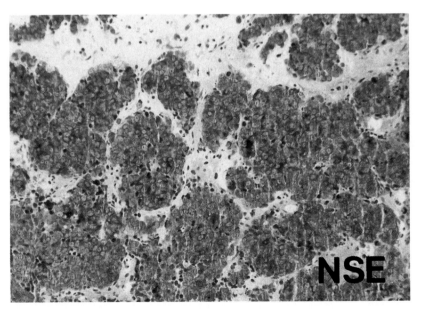

seen in patients with lymphoepithelioma-type undifferentiated carcinomas occurring at various head and neck sites (197). This suggests that these neoplasms have fundamental pathogenetic differences.

Small Cell Undifferentiated Carcinoma. True small cell undifferentiated carcinoma in the head and neck region, a tumor histologically identical to its pulmonary counterpart, is discussed in more detail elsewhere in this chapter, along with the features allowing its distinction from SNUC.

Olfactory Neuroblastoma. Because of the much worse prognosis of SNUC, it should be clearly distinguished from the less aggressive olfactory neuroblastoma. We believe that many "high-grade" olfactory neuroblastomas in the prior literature would be better interpreted as SNUC. Distinguishing features are discussed in the section on olfactory neuroblastoma.

Lymphoma. The light microscopic appearance of SNUC may closely mimic that of a large cell lymphoma. Prior to the advent of immunohistochemistry, misdiagnoses were undoubtedly made in both directions. The initial rapid response of SNUC to radiation therapy or chemotherapy is very "lymphoma-like" and may further the diagnostic confusion. The advent of immunohistochemistry and highly lineage-specific antibodies such as leukocyte common antigen and cytokeratin usually allow for straightforward distinction. A panel approach to immunohistochemistry should be utilized, rather than the application of single antibodies. Occasional large cell lymphomas are not immunoreactive for leukocyte common antigen and may be focally positive for epithelial membrane antigen (194). The use of additional lymphoid markers usually solves this dilemma. Rare lymphomas also express limited amounts of cytokeratin (189), but strong diffuse cytokeratin positivity, particularly with an antikeratin "cocktail" reactive to a variety of molecular weight cytokeratins typically allows distinction (188).

Spread and Metastasis. As noted above, local disease is invariably widespread at the time of diagnosis. In our experience, persistent, locally invasive disease is a major factor in the mortality associated with this tumor. Distant metastases to liver, bone, brain, and other sites may also occur.

Treatment and Prognosis. Surgical resection is almost never possible and radiation or chemotherapy have been of essentially no curative value, although there may be initial, clinically dramatic responses to both modalities. Median survival in one study was 4 months, with no disease-free patients. Occasional patients have been treated with high-dose chemotherapy and autologous bone marrow transplantation (195). We are aware of a single long-term survivor treated with the latter approach.

"CARCINOID TUMOR" AND "ATYPICAL CARCINOID TUMOR" (NEUROENDOCRINE CARCINOMA)

Definition. Typical carcinoid tumors arising in the head and neck are rare, low-grade neoplasms that are histologically indistinguishable from their more common intestinal or bronchial counterparts. Higher grade neoplasms exhibiting exclusively or predominantly neuroendocrine differentiation of greater degree than is encountered in so-called small cell undifferentiated (neuroendocrine) carcinoma are included under the designation of *neuroendocrine carcinoma*. There is considerable variation in the terminology applied to these neoplasms. For reasons discussed below, we use the above term rather than the World Health Organization terminology of *atypical carcinoid tumor* for higher grade tumors in this group (243).

General Features. In the head and neck region, carcinoid tumors and neuroendocrine carcinomas are virtually confined to the larynx. The first neuroendocrine neoplasm of the larynx was reported in 1969 by Goldman (221), who referred to the lesion as a "carcinoid tumor." Subsequently, a considerable number of such cases have been reported as carcinoids, atypical carcinoids, malignant carcinoids, aggressive carcinoids, and neuroendocrine carcinomas (198,200,204,206, 207,210,217,221–223,231,232,234,240,241,245, 249,252). In some of these earlier discussions, the cytologic and clinical features of the tumor were clearly malignant, yet the term carcinoid tumor was applied without further modification.

Most neuroendocrine carcinomas of the larynx seem to be tumors of intermediate differentiation, and are referred to by varying terms as discussed below. The relatively large number of

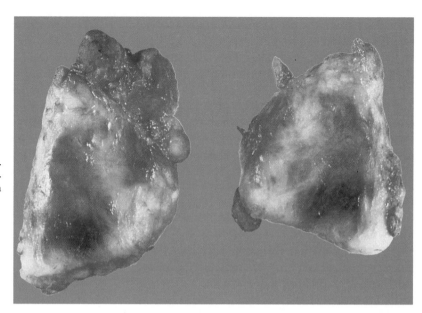

Figure 7-76
LARYNGEAL
NEUROENDOCRINE
CARCINOMA

This laryngeal neuroendocrine carcinoma formed a supraglottic, submucosal mass. The hemorrhagic region corresponds to an area of necrosis.

publications on this topic in recent times suggests that these are not rare neoplasms. Many have probably gone unrecognized and been interpreted as poorly differentiated carcinomas, without recognition of their neuroendocrine features. In their series from Memorial Sloan-Kettering, Woodruff and colleagues (258) indicated that such tumors accounted for 59 percent of nonsquamous laryngeal neoplasms.

Clinical Features. *Carcinoid Tumor.* A recent review by El-Naggar and Batsakis (211) indicated that slightly more than a dozen typical laryngeal carcinoid tumors have been adequately described. These predominantly involved the supraglottic larynx, often in the region of the arytenoid or aryepiglottic fold. There was a strong male predominance (11 to 1), with patients ranging in age from 45 to 80 years. Typical presenting complaints, often present for more than a year, included dysphagia, hoarseness, and a mass. There have been too few cases to assess the potential causative role of cigarette smoking. The percentage of patients with positive smoking histories appears lower than for neuroendocrine carcinomas (60 versus more than 70 percent), and the tumor has been documented in nonsmokers (211,255).

Neuroendocrine Carcinoma. There have been several series and literature reviews of moderately differentiated laryngeal neuroendocrine carcinomas/atypical carcinoid tumors (255,256,

259). There is a strong male predilection (2-3 to 1), and a high percentage of patients have been cigarette smokers (68 to 78 percent) (256,258). Patients range in age from 36 to 83 years (256); most are in their sixth or seventh decades of life. Most tumors involve the supraglottic larynx (96 percent), particularly the arytenoids or the epiglottis. Hoarseness and dysphagia are the most common complaints, with less common symptoms including hemoptysis, neck mass, or voice changes (255,256). About 10 percent of patients present with enlarged regional lymph nodes.

Gross Findings. The typical carcinoid tumors have ranged in size from 0.5 to 2 cm. A polypoid, submucosal mass in the supraglottic region is the usual gross appearance. Surface mucosal involvement or ulceration is absent (255). Similarly, neuroendocrine carcinomas tend to be submucosal, polypoid masses, although somewhat larger in size (up to 4 cm) (fig. 7-76) (255, 256). Unlike typical carcinoid tumors, surface ulceration is commonly present (255).

Microscopic Findings. *Carcinoid Tumor.* The hallmark of typical carcinoid tumor is a conspicuous low-power growth pattern consisting of cords, nests, and "glandular" or rosette-like structures, separated by a variably fibrotic stroma (fig. 7-77). The neoplastic cells have the classic features of carcinoid tumor, with small, uniform nuclei having finely stippled or "salt and pepper" chromatin (fig. 7-78). The cytoplasm may vary from clear

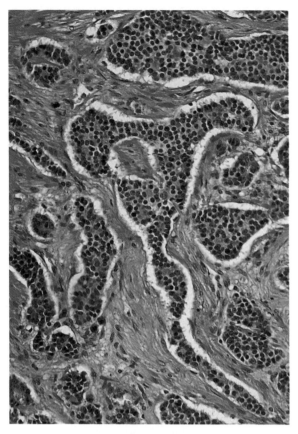

Figure 7-77
LARYNGEAL CARCINOID
The less common, "typical carcinoid tumors" of the larynx are composed of cords or nests of cytologically uniform cells.

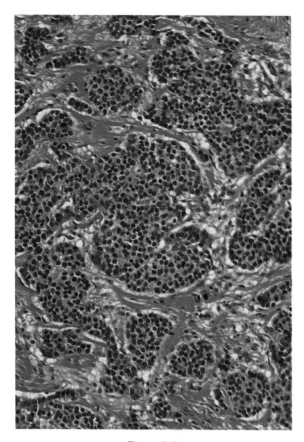

Figure 7-78
LARYNGEAL CARCINOID
This typical laryngeal carcinoid tumor is composed of uniform cells with punctate nuclear chromatin and moderate amounts of eosinophilic cytoplasm.

to eosinophilic. By definition, typical carcinoid tumors of the larynx lack cellular pleomorphism, necrosis, or more than rare, morphologically typical mitotic figures (211). Crush artifact, seen in tumors of higher grade neuroendocrine neoplasia is not present. Perineural and intravascular invasion are also absent (255). Argyrophil stains have been uniformly positive in a limited number of cases (211), and argentaffin stains are usually negative (255). Epithelial mucin may be present within the neoplastic cells (255).

Neuroendocrine Carcinoma. The tumor typically forms a submucosal mass which underlies at least partially intact, often focally ulcerated squamous mucosa (fig. 7-79) (255). The predominant growth pattern varies from one of nests, sheets, trabeculae, glandular structures, organoid formations, or acini (255). Combinations of patterns predominate and glandular formations are com-

mon. The nests vary considerably in size, from accumulations of only a few cells to large cell aggregates. Small to medium-sized cell nests may be present underlying the basal cell layer of the squamous mucosa and mimicking theques of melanocytic cells. Cytologically, the cells vary from larger cells with prominent eosinophilic cytoplasm to considerably smaller cells with scant amounts of similar-appearing cytoplasm. Even the latter cells, however, are two-fold larger than the cells of small cell undifferentiated carcinoma. There is mild to focally marked nuclear pleomorphism (fig. 7-80). In some areas, predominantly those composed of larger cells, the cells have more uniform nuclei, and in other areas, typically those with smaller cells, they exhibit tremendous nuclear variation. In general, nuclei have punctate chromatin with small or inapparent nucleoli. Multiple

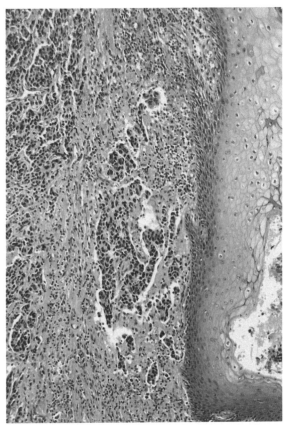

Figure 7-79
LARYNGEAL NEUROENDOCRINE CARCINOMA
Laryngeal neuroendocrine carcinomas often infiltrate beneath intact overlying squamous mucosa.

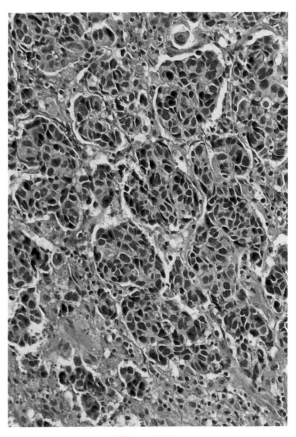

Figure 7-80
LARYNGEAL NEUROENDOCRINE CARCINOMA
At higher magnification the cells of this laryngeal neuroendocrine carcinoma exhibit moderate degrees of nuclear pleomorphism. Compare with figure 7-78.

eosinophilic nucleoli may be identified. In some foci the tumor cells may assume a spindled configuration (fig. 7-81), while maintaining their other cytologic and nuclear features. Occasional foci of squamous differentiation, complete with individual cell keratinization, may be present. Mitotic figures range from infrequent to prominent, and tend to be most apparent in areas with more striking nuclear pleomorphism. In some areas, particularly those with increased nuclear pleomorphism, there are often foci of necrosis, varying from more typical small aggregates of necrotic cells to less common prominent necrotic zones. Vascular, lymphatic, or perineural invasion may be present (255). Epithelial mucin stains are positive in over 90 percent of cases, argyrophilic stains are virtually always positive, but argentaffin stains are rarely reactive (6 percent) (255).

Microscopic Grading and Nomenclature.
The terminology surrounding neuroendocrine neoplasia at any anatomic site is currently in a state of flux. The lung is the prototypic location for this group of neoplasms. It is clear that neuroendocrine tumors in the lung, as well as the larynx and elsewhere, come in varying degrees of differentiation. In the larynx, the World Health Organization has divided these tumors into carcinoid, atypical carcinoid, and small cell carcinoma (214,243). This is certainly the oldest terminology applied to such lesions. There are, however, several problems with this approach. First, and most importantly, it requires that the clinician understand that an "atypical carcinoid" is an overtly malignant, usually high-grade neoplasm, meriting an aggressive clinical approach. This is counter intuitive to a name which seems

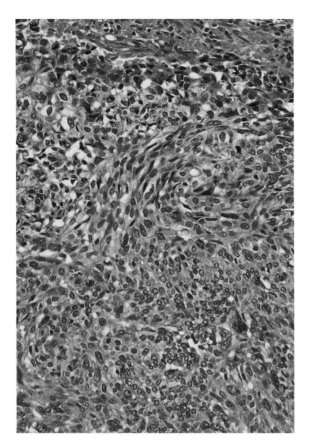

Figure 7-81
LARYNGEAL NEUROENDOCRINE CARCINOMA
Laryngeal neuroendocrine carcinomas may occasionally contain areas of spindled cells.

more closely allied to the indolent "typical" carcinoid tumor. Furthermore, although much is written about the spectrum of neuroendocrine tumors, it is unclear whether typical carcinoid tumor is a member of a blurred spectrum of neoplasms or an entity distinct from higher grades of neuroendocrine neoplasia. Typical carcinoid tumor of the lung, and possibly the larynx, is unrelated to smoking, whereas all other forms of neuroendocrine neoplasia show a striking association. Most "atypical carcinoid tumors" are highly malignant-appearing neoplasms, and there are many lesions for which the distinction between "atypical carcinoid" and small cell carcinoma is difficult, indicating a clear-cut morphologic "spectrum" between these lesions. In contrast, typical carcinoid tumor is almost never associated with areas of significant "atypia" and "atypical carcinoid tumors," in our experience, seldom if ever have areas so well

differentiated as to be confused with typical carcinoid tumor. Finally, "atypical carcinoids" and small cell carcinomas often show divergent differentiation in the form of foci of squamous or glandular cells. Such features are rare in typical carcinoid tumors. In other words, typical carcinoid tumor is a morphologically and clinically distinct lesion having little or no overlap with other, higher grade neuroendocrine proliferations. Therefore, we believe that such tumors should be distinguished by being the sole neoplasms to carry the "carcinoid" designation.

Several other systems of nomenclature have been advanced, but these also have problems, in our opinion (Table 7-2). Some authors have labeled typical carcinoid tumors as "very well-differentiated neuroendocrine carcinomas," and considered atypical carcinoids as "well-differentiated neuroendocrine carcinomas" (224,225). This approach, again, blurs the morphologically clear-cut and clinically important distinction between typical carcinoid tumor and higher grades of neuroendocrine neoplasia. Furthermore, there is nothing "well differentiated" about "well-differentiated neuroendocrine carcinomas" under their terminology. These are high-grade, aggressive neoplasms. Other authors have dealt with the latter problem by using the term "moderately differentiated neuroendocrine carcinoma" for the intermediate neoplasms (255,256), but then confused the issue by labeling typical carcinoid tumors as "well-differentiated neuroendocrine carcinomas."

We believe that the following nomenclatural approach best reflects the biology of these lesions (Table 7-2): true or typical carcinoid tumors should be designated as such to aid in their distinction from more aggressive neuroendocrine neoplasms and to emphasize their pathologic distinctness. Lesions formerly referred to as "atypical carcinoids" should be labeled as moderately differentiated neuroendocrine carcinomas. Small cell carcinomas may be referred to as such, or as poorly differentiated neuroendocrine carcinoma, small cell type. Does the entity of "well-differentiated neuroendocrine carcinoma" exist? In our experience, tumors with a histologic appearance only slightly more atypical than conventional carcinoid tumors are extremely rare, but such lesions would, theoretically, be in this category. Their

Table 7-2

NOMENCLATURE FOR NEUROENDOCRINE NEOPLASIA

Classic System	Gould Terminology	Wenig Terminology	Suggested Terminology
Carcinoid	Very well-differentiated neuroendocrine carcinoma	Well-differentiated neuroendocrine carcinoma	Carcinoid
Atypical carcinoid	Well-differentiated neuroendocrine carcinoma	Moderately differentiated neuroendocrine carcinoma	Moderately differentiated neuroendocrine carcinoma
Small cell undifferentiated carcinoma	Intermediate/poorly differentiated neuro-endocrine carcinoma	Poorly differentiated neuroendocrine carcinoma	Small cell neuro-endocrine (undifferen-tiated) carcinoma

clinical and microscopic features have not been adequately defined.

Immunohistochemical Findings. Seven convincingly typical carcinoid tumors of the larynx have been studied to varying degrees immunohistochemically (200,215,223,240,245,248). Positive results were as follows: keratin, 2 of 2 tumors; chromogranin, 3 of 3; neuron-specific enolase, 2 of 2; serotonin, 1 of 2; calcitonin, 0 of 2; somatostatin, 1 of 1. Single cases were negative for carcinoembryonic antigen, S-100 protein, and bombesin. Of the neuroendocrine carcinomas studied, the neoplastic cells were variably positive for neuron-specific enolase (39 to 100 percent) (fig. 7-82), synaptophysin (100 percent) (fig. 7-83), cytokeratin (96 percent), chromogranin (89 to 94 percent), calcitonin (67 to 81 percent), carcinoembryonic antigen (CEA) (50 to 75 percent), somatostatin (35 percent), adrenocorticotropic hormone (ACTH) (21 percent), S-100 protein (20 percent), gastrin (16 percent), glucagon (11 percent), and serotonin (10 percent) (256, 258,259). The S-100 protein positivity was confined to scattered cells and included nuclear staining (256). Notably, the tumors have been negative with HMB-45 (melanoma-specific protein) and for thyroglobulin (256).

Ultrastructural Findings. Electron microscopy of typical laryngeal carcinoid tumors has shown abundant membrane-bound, electron-dense, neurosecretory granules, ranging in size from 100 to 400 mm (211). Complex intercellular

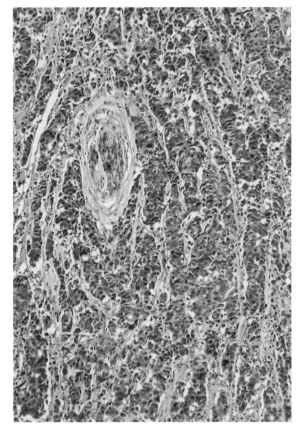

Figure 7-82

LARYNGEAL NEUROENDOCRINE CARCINOMA

This laryngeal neuroendocrine carcinoma exhibits strong cytoplasmic staining for neuron-specific enolase.

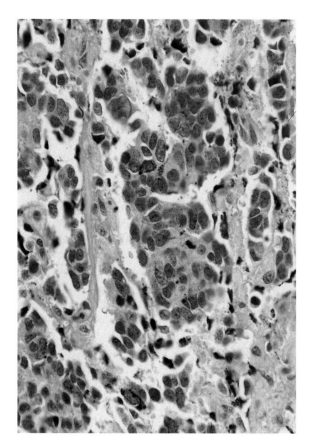

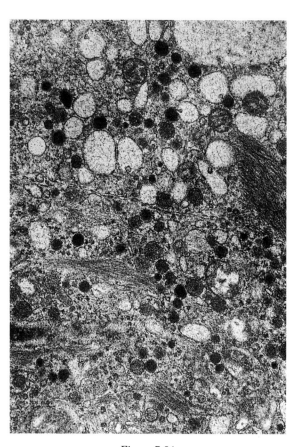

Figure 7-83
LARYNGEAL NEUROENDOCRINE CARCINOMA
Scattered cells in this laryngeal neuroendocrine carcinoma label for synaptophysin.

Figure 7-84
LARYNGEAL NEUROENDOCRINE CARCINOMA
Ultrastructurally, this laryngeal neuroendocrine carcinoma contained abundant, membrane-limited dense-core granules.

digitations with occasional intercellular junctions are variable features (211). Similar ultrastructural findings, with generally less abundant dense core granules and more prominent epithelial features have been described for neuroendocrine carcinomas (fig. 7-84) (256,258). The neoplastic cells are closely apposed, with variable numbers of junctional complexes (256). Intracellular and intercellular lumina with microvillous intraluminal projections may be present and, occasionally, bundles of intermediate filaments consistent with tonofilaments (256).

Differential Diagnosis. *Paraganglioma.* The larynx contains two matched sets of normal paraganglia (227,229,254). The superior paraganglia are located in the upper, anterior one third of the false vocal cords, in close approximation to the superior laryngeal artery and nerve (254). They measure approximately 0.1 to 0.3 cm

in diameter. The inferior paraganglia are slightly larger, measuring about 0.3 to 0.4 cm in diameter. They are located between the inferior horn of the thyroid cartilage and the cricoid cartilage, or between the cricoid cartilage and the first tracheal ring (227). These structures are, presumably, the site of origin for true laryngeal paragangliomas. Aberrant or ectopic laryngeal paraganglia have also been described (229).

Early studies of laryngeal "paragangliomas" indicated that such tumors appeared to be more frequently malignant than their counterparts occurring elsewhere in the body (198,232,244,253, 257). It has become apparent that many (most/all) such malignant tumors were, in fact, neuroendocrine carcinomas (247,256,258). Neuroendocrine carcinomas of the larynx can have a distinctly paraganglioma-like appearance with cell nests resembling "zellballen." In a large analysis of the literature regarding laryngeal "paragangli-omas," Barnes critically reviewed 78 purported cases (199). Of these, 34 were accepted as para-gangliomas, based on a characteristic photo-microscopic appearance. The remaining 44 cases were considered to be "unacceptable." In Barnes' review, true paragangliomas of the larynx oc-curred in a broad age range (14 to 80 years) and showed a 2.8 to 1 female predilection, in contrast to the striking male predilection of carcinoid tumor (255). The great majority (82 percent) occurred in the supraglottic larynx and appeared as highly vascular submucosal masses measur-ing approximately 2.5 cm in size. Hoarseness was the most common symptom, and pain was notably absent. Prior reports of painful laryn-geal paragangliomas appear to represent neuro-endocrine carcinomas (198,244). Only one of 34 laryngeal paragangliomas was potentially func-tional. Of the 30 patients with follow-up (mean age, 5.2 years), 5 developed local recurrences after limited local excisions. Only 1 of 30 patients (3 percent) developed a metastasis. This oc-curred in a lumbar vertebra 16 years after initial excision. This biologic behavior is quite analo-gous to that of paragangliomas arising at other locations and emphasizes the need for distin-guishing this lesion from the more aggressive neuroendocrine carcinoma.

Microscopically, true paragangliomas resem-ble their nonlaryngeal counterparts. They are highly vascular lesions with nests (zellballen) of chief cells having pink to clear cytoplasm and uniform to occasionally bizarrely atypical nuclei. Mitotic figures are absent or fewer than 2 to 3 per high-power field (199). Vascular invasion, necrosis, and perineural invasion are rare and do not predict a more aggressive clinical course (199).

Both paragangliomas and neuroendocrine carcinomas express neuroendocrine markers, including neuron-specific enolase, chromo-granin, and synaptophysin (235). However, the sustentacular cells of paragangliomas stain strongly for S-100 protein and glial fibrillary acidic protein (235). These cells are lacking in neuroendocrine carcinomas, although scattered S-100 protein–positive cells may be encountered (256). Most importantly, paragangliomas are cytokeratin negative, whereas this marker is almost invariably positive in moderately differ-entiated neuroendocrine carcinomas (235,256).

Interestingly, calcitonin has been demonstrated in laryngeal neuroendocrine carcinomas, adding to the potential confusion with metastatic med-ullary carcinoma, but has not been detected in true laryngeal paragangliomas (235).

Small Cell Neuroendocrine (Oat Cell) Carci-noma. With adequate material, this is unlikely to be a diagnostic problem. Small cell neuroendo-crine carcinomas of the larynx are uncommon but well-recognized neoplasms discussed in greater detail elsewhere in this text (201,203,205,208,213, 218–220,226,228,236–238,250,255). Microscopi-cally, the tumors are indistinguishable from their pulmonary counterparts. The sheet-like growth pattern, prominent necrosis, high nuclear to cytoplasmic ratio, prominent nuclear pleomor-phism, frequent crush artifact, and high mitotic rate of small cell carcinoma usually allow for distinction from better differentiated neuroen-docrine carcinomas (255). Because of the neuro-endocrine features of both tumors, immunohis-tochemical stains are of limited distinguishing value. Small cell carcinomas are at least occa-sionally positive for chromogranin, neuron-spe-cific enolase, calcitonin, ACTH, β-endorphin, gastrin-secreting polypeptide, and carcinoem-bryonic antigen (202,219,223,246,258).

Metastatic Medullary Carcinoma. The histo-logic similarity (identicality) of laryngeal neuro-endocrine carcinoma and medullary carcinoma of the thyroid gland has been well described (212, 256,258). Wenig (256) noted that the only defini-tive parameter separating the two lesions was the serum calcitonin level, which is almost in-variably elevated in patients with metastatic thy-roid carcinoma; only a single, somewhat contro-versial laryngeal neuroendocrine carcinoma has been associated with an elevated serum calcito-nin level (251). Woodruff et al. (258) reviewed the distinguishing microscopic features of the two lesions and noted that the presence of argyro-philia, epithelial mucin, epithelioid neoplastic cells, hyalinized stroma, cervical lymph node me-tastases, and ultrastructural features was of lit-tle or no distinguishing value. Amyloid was pres-ent in 27 percent of neuroendocrine carcinomas of the larynx versus 75 percent of medullary carcino-mas; tissue calcitonin staining was documented in 67 percent of neuroendocrine carcinomas versus 100 percent of medullary carcinomas, and tissue carcinoembryonic antigen staining was seen in

50 percent of neuroendocrine carcinomas versus 100 percent of medullary carcinomas (258)

Malignant Melanoma. The nesting pattern of laryngeal neuroendocrine carcinoma may be confused with the theques of malignant melanoma. The latter tumors do rarely arise in the larynx (209,216,230,239,242,256). Both tumors may be high-grade neoplasms, microscopically. Ultimately, immunohistochemistry may be necessary to resolve this differential possibility. Staining with HMB-45, a highly specific melanocytic marker, is not found in laryngeal neuroendocrine carcinomas (256). It should be noted that neuroendocrine carcinomas may contain occasional S-100 protein–positive cells (256).

Treatment and Prognosis. *Carcinoid Tumor.* In the review of 12 cases by El-Naggar and Batsakis (211), 3 patients were treated by local excision alone; 2 had local excision followed by laryngectomy; 1 had local excision followed by a laryngectomy 6 years later for recurrent disease; and 6 had at least laryngectomy as their initial therapy. Only 2 patients received adjuvant chemotherapy. Simple surgical excision, to the degree necessary to encompass the lesion, is considered accepted therapy for typical laryngeal carcinoid (211,215,223,255). Only 1 patient in the El-Naggar and Batsakis review died of disease. This individual developed liver and bone metastases and died 5 years after initial diagnosis. Nonetheless, 3 other patients in this study had metastases to liver (2 patients), bone (1 patient), lymph node (1 patient), and skin (1 patient), and 1 developed the carcinoid syndrome. In spite of this, these individuals were still alive 4 to 8 years after diagnosis. This biologic behavior (33 percent metastases) is significantly different from that of bronchial carcinoid tumor of typical type, and suggests that, with more adequate study, several of these tumors may be reclassified as more aggressive neoplasms. Overall, however, the behavior of this group of tumors is significantly better than that of laryngeal neuroendocrine carcinomas.

Neuroendocrine Carcinoma. Surgical resection is the primary mode of therapy for laryngeal neuroendocrine carcinoma. Of 127 patients with follow-up in Woodruff and Senie's review (259), 29 percent had regional lymph node metastases at the time of diagnosis and an additional 14 percent subsequently developed nodal involvement. At some point during the clinical course, 22 percent of tumors metastasized to skin or subcutaneous tissues, and 44 percent spread distally. The overall 5-year survival was 48 percent and 10-year survival was 30 percent. Radiation therapy did not significantly improve survival. The latter important fact emphasizes the need to distinguish these tumors from the more radiation-sensitive squamous cell carcinomas. Wenig and colleagues (256) noted an only slightly better prognosis in their review of 54 cases seen at the Armed Forces Institute of Pathology. About 22 percent of patients had documented regional lymph node metastases at the time of initial surgery. Sixteen of 48 patients (33 percent) with follow-up were alive and well from 2 to 16 years after diagnosis, 29 percent died without evidence of tumor, and 38 percent died with tumor. The mean survival of the latter group was 65 months (range, 3 months to 10 years).

SMALL CELL UNDIFFERENTIATED (NEUROENDOCRINE) CARCINOMA

Definition. This is a high-grade carcinoma composed of sheets of small to intermediate-sized cells that have a high nuclear to cytoplasmic ratio and a minimal amount of visible cytoplasm. Variable degrees of neuroendocrine differentiation may be demonstrable by electron microscopy or immunohistochemistry, but are not required for diagnosis.

General Features. Excluding Merkel cell carcinoma of the skin, in the head and neck region small cell undifferentiated carcinomas primarily arise from the major salivary glands, particularly the parotid gland; the larynx; and, rarely, the sinonasal region or hard palate. Small cell undifferentiated carcinomas of the parotid gland and other major salivary glands are described in another Fascicle. Whether tumors arising in the larynx, palate, and sinonasal structures are of seromucinous gland origin has been the subject of discussion (277). It has been noted that such tumors often occur in areas rich in seromucinous glands, are often centered in the submucosa, and may be covered by intact, uninvolved surface mucosal epithelium. However, direct origin from glandular structures has not been convincingly demonstrated.

Larynx. In the larynx, small cell undifferentiated carcinomas account for approximately 0.5

percent of all carcinomas (265,269) and about 4.5 percent of nonsquamous laryngeal malignancies (269,272). A review of laryngeal small cell carcinomas reported prior to 1991 documented approximately 125 cases (269).

Sinonasal. Approximately 30 small cell carcinoma-like neoplasms have been reported from the sinonasal region, under various designations (275,277,280). Some authors have considered these tumors to be equivalent to small cell undifferentiated carcinoma (261). However, on review, almost all of them lack the prototypical light microscopic appearance of small cell undifferentiated carcinoma (275,280,284). Their exact nosology is unclear, although some appear to be olfactory neuroblastomas or closely related neoplasms. The often protracted clinical course and relatively good prognosis of patients with such tumors provides further rationale for distinguishing these neoplasms from true small cell undifferentiated carcinomas (275,280,284). Acceptable examples of small cell undifferentiated carcinoma are quite rare in this location (277,282,283,289).

Clinical Features. *Larynx.* Small cell undifferentiated carcinoma of the larynx strongly predilects men (3 to 1) and tends to occur in patients in their sixth to seventh decades of life (269,270). The tumor is quite rare in patients under 40 years of age. There is a strong association with cigarette smoking (269,270) and a possible association with ethanol ingestion (270). Patients usually present with complaints of hoarseness, a neck mass, dysphagia, or cough (269,270). One patient had inappropriate antidiuretic hormone (ADH) secretion (270).

Sinonasal. There are too few well-documented cases of true small cell undifferentiated carcinoma at this location to allow for many generalizations regarding clinical features. Eight variably documented examples appearing to represent this tumor, rather than the variant lesions discussed above, have been reported (277,282,283,289). Five tumors involved the nasal cavity, two involved the ethmoid sinuses, and one the maxillary antrum (277,282,283, 289). In contrast to the larynx where these tumors show a striking male predominance, five of the eight sinonasal tumors occurred in women. Patients ranged in age from 26 to 77 years (median, 48 years), suggesting a younger age range than that for patients with laryngeal tumors

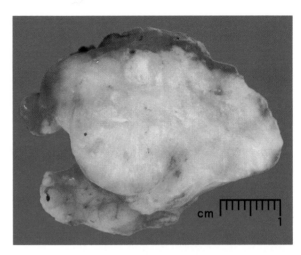

Figure 7-85
SMALL CELL UNDIFFERENTIATED CARCINOMA
This small cell undifferentiated carcinoma of the sinonasal region produced a large, polypoid mass.

(277,282,283,289). Complaints usually relate to a mass or hemoptysis.

Gross Findings. *Larynx.* The tumors may involve any portion of the larynx, but there is a strong predilection for the supraglottic region (269). The surface is typically ulcerated, but tumor epicenter in the submucosal region is common (269).

Sinonasal. A smooth polypoid mass or granular mucosal thickening has been described for nasal tumors of this type (fig. 7-85) (283,289).

Microscopic Findings. Regardless of their exact site of origin, small cell undifferentiated carcinomas arising in the head and neck are, by definition, histologically indistinguishable from their pulmonary counterparts. Typically, there are sheets, cords, and ribbons of small, light microscopically undifferentiated cells. The cells have little or no microscopically apparent cytoplasm and a correspondingly high nuclear to cytoplasmic ratio (figs. 7-86, 7-87). Nuclei are quite pleomorphic, ranging from densely hyperchromatic to more "open" nuclei with a delicate, punctate chromatin distribution (fig. 7-88) (269). Mitotic figures are numerous. Necrosis varies from scattered, individual cell death to irregular zones of infarct-like change (fig. 7-89). Adjacent to the latter areas are rare, smudged hematoxylin-staining deposits surrounding blood vessels (Azzopardi effect) (fig. 7-90). Intravascular and perineural

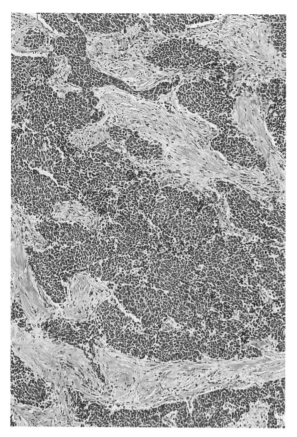

Figure 7-86
SMALL CELL UNDIFFERENTIATED CARCINOMA
Small cell undifferentiated carcinoma of the larynx infiltrates surrounding stroma as irregular nests of cells.

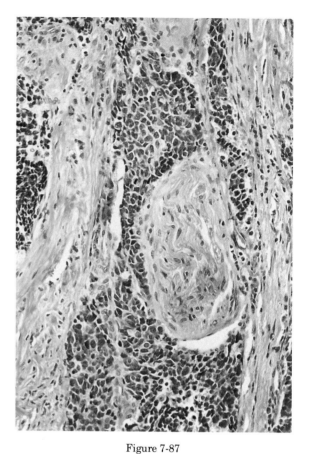

Figure 7-87
SMALL CELL UNDIFFERENTIATED CARCINOMA
At higher magnification, the small cell undifferentiated carcinoma seen in figure 7-86 is composed of small to intermediate-sized cells with little visible cytoplasm.

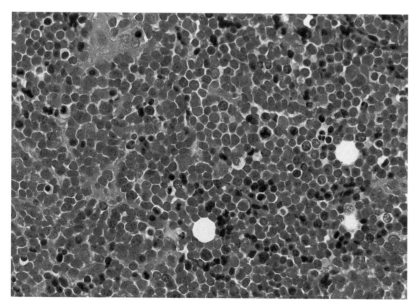

Figure 7-88
SMALL CELL UNDIFFERENTI-ATED CARCINOMA
This small cell undifferentiated carcinoma of the head and neck formed large, lymphoma-like sheets of light microscopically undifferentiated cells.

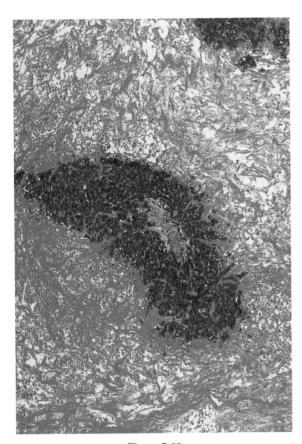

Figure 7-89
SMALL CELL UNDIFFERENTIATED CARCINOMA
Large areas of "geographic" necrosis are common in small cell undifferentiated carcinoma. In this example, the residual non-necrotic tumor forms a perivascular cuff.

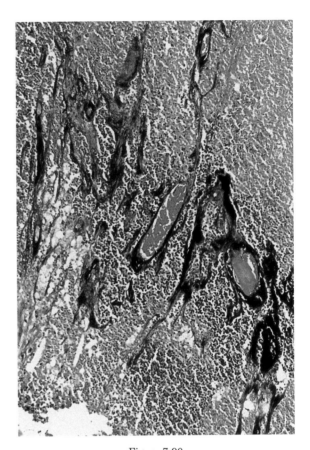

Figure 7-90
SMALL CELL UNDIFFERENTIATED CARCINOMA
Occasionally, small cell undifferentiated carcinoma of the head and neck, like its pulmonary counterpart, may be associated with smudged, hematoxylinophilic deposits in blood vessel walls ("Azzopardi effect").

invasion is common. As with their pulmonary counterparts, laryngeal small cell undifferentiated carcinomas may contain scattered "rosettes" (269). Continuing the pulmonary analogy, small cell undifferentiated carcinomas of the head and neck may contain areas of squamous cell carcinoma or, less commonly, adenocarcinoma. In the larynx, the presence of more than rare foci of squamous differentiation should strongly suggest the alternative diagnosis of basaloid squamous cell carcinoma (see Differential Diagnosis below). Even in areas without obvious glandular differentiation, scattered mucin-positive cells may be identified (269). Argyrophil stains are occasionally positive, but argentaffin stains are invariably negative (269,271,274,281,286).

Immunohistochemical Findings. Immunohistochemical stains are of less value for these lesions than for better differentiated forms of neuroendocrine carcinoma. Cytokeratin stains are typically positive, and may show the punctate perinuclear positivity typical of small cell carcinomas arising in other locations (fig. 7-91). Other markers documented to be at least occasionally positive include: chromogranin, neuron-specific enolase, calcitonin, ACTH, β-endorphin, gastrin-releasing polypeptide, carcinoembryonic antigen, serotonin, and bombesin (263,269,271,285,290).

Ultrastructural Findings. Electron microscopic study usually documents at least limited neuroendocrine differentiation in the form of scarce to rare membrane-bound, dense core neurosecretory granules ranging in size from 50 to 200 nm (261,262,269). Cell junctions are present to variable degree, ranging from absent to well-formed desmosomal attachments. Occasionally,

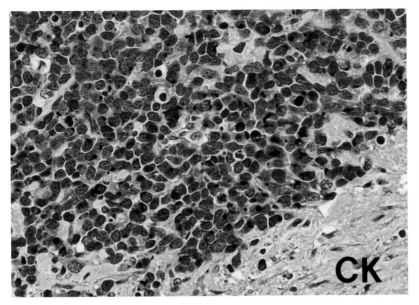

Figure 7-91
SMALL CELL
UNDIFFERENTIATED
CARCINOMA
Punctate, often perinuclear cytokeratin positivity is typical of small cell undifferentiated carcinomas arising in a wide variety of sites.

bundles of cytoplasmic intermediate filaments typical of tonofilaments are present.

Differential Diagnosis. *Moderately Differentiated Neuroendocrine Carcinoma.* The distinction between small cell undifferentiated carcinoma and better differentiated forms of neuroendocrine neoplasia is discussed under Carcinoid Tumor and Neuroendocrine Carcinoma, page 174.

Basaloid Squamous Cell Carcinoma. These tumors, when they involve the larynx, also show a marked predilection for the supraglottic region (260,276,278,279,288). Although they are aggressive neoplasms, primarily because of their advanced stage at presentation, stage for stage their behavior is analogous to that of more conventional squamous cell carcinomas. These tumors are often confused with small cell undifferentiated carcinoma due to the presence of a prominent, pleomorphic basaloid cell component. More conventional squamous cell carcinoma is invariably present in the basaloid variant. Because of this, the diagnosis of small cell undifferentiated carcinoma with focal squamous differentiation should be approached with caution in areas where basaloid squamous cell carcinoma frequently occurs. The presence of overlying squamous dysplasia is strongly supportive of the basaloid variant. Immunohistochemistry is of limited value in making this distinction; basaloid squamous cell carcinomas may contain scattered cells which label for neuron-specific enolase (260).

Sinonasal Undifferentiated Carcinoma. This microscopically distinctive variant of "anaplastic" carcinoma is described in detail on pages 163–167 (267,273). As discussed above, true small cell undifferentiated carcinomas are extremely rare in the sinonasal region. Most light microscopically "undifferentiated" tumors in this area are composed of distinctly larger cells with more prominent eosinophilic cytoplasm and large nuclei with often prominent eosinophilic nucleoli. These cells are obviously larger than the "intermediate cells" of small cell undifferentiated carcinoma. We apply the term sinonasal undifferentiated carcinoma to such lesions because of their considerably larger constituent cells (267). Unlike small cell undifferentiated carcinomas, sinonasal undifferentiated carcinomas originate from dysplastic surface mucosa (267). Having indicated these distinctions, however, it should be recognized that these two tumor types may be related. Sinonasal undifferentiated carcinomas may show at least abortive neuroendocrine differentiation (267). Moreover, both tumors have a highly aggressive clinical course with associated high mortality.

Malignant Lymphoma. Small cell undifferentiated carcinoma may mimic a high-grade lymphoma, at least on cursory examination. Given the well-developed radiation and chemotherapy protocols for the treatment of malignant lymphoma, this is an important distinction. If required, distinction can be easily made based on an immunohistochemical panel including broad spectrum lymphoid and epithelial markers.

Olfactory Neuroblastoma. Small cell undifferentiated carcinoma is less likely to be confused with olfactory neuroblastoma than the above entities if well-preserved tissue specimens are available. Olfactory neuroblastoma (see pages 153–163) is typically composed of minimally pleomorphic cells with punctate nuclear chromatin and an often prominent fibrillary background. Necrosis is usually absent or minimal. Immunohistochemical stains often demonstrate a prominent S-100 protein–positive cell at the periphery of cell nests, with strong positivity of the neoplastic cells for a variety of neuroendocrine markers including synaptophysin, MAP-2, β-tubulin, neurofilament (200 kD), neuron-specific enolase, and others (268,287). Cytokeratin is positive in a minority of cases (268,287). Small cell undifferentiated carcinomas show less obvious neuroendocrine differentiation and more frequent cytokeratin positivity.

Spread and Metastasis. Over 90 percent of patients with laryngeal small cell undifferentiated carcinoma eventually develop metastatic disease (269). The most common sites of spread from the larynx are cervical lymph nodes, liver, lung, and bone (270). The rare sinonasal small cell undifferentiated carcinomas seem to behave in a similarly aggressive fashion (277,289). Widespread metastases are common, as well as destructive local recurrences.

Treatment and Prognosis. Small cell undifferentiated carcinoma of the larynx is a highly lethal neoplasm. Because of the high rate of widespread dissemination, total laryngectomy is not considered appropriate therapy, at least by some authors (269). Selected lesions may be treated by conservative local excision, but the mainstay of treatment currently is radiation therapy combined with some mode of chemotherapy (269). This approach has been said to yield rare long-term survivors (264,266). In a review by Gnepp et al. (269,270), 73 percent of patients with laryngeal small cell undifferentiated carcinoma died of disease, with a mean survival time of 9.8 months (range, 1 to 26 months). The 2-year survival rate was 16 percent and the 5-year rate was only 5 percent. Interestingly, survival did not correlate with tumor size. This has been attributed to the prominent vascular invasion typically present in even small tumors (270).

Of five pathologically well-documented sinonasal small cell undifferentiated carcinomas, four patients died of disease from 8 months to 2.25 years after diagnosis. Of three patients with probable but inadequately illustrated disease, one died shortly after diagnosis (282), and two were disease free 12 months after diagnosis (283).

MALIGNANT MELANOMA

Definition. Malignant melanomas are neoplasms exhibiting melanocytic differentiation, based either on microscopically overt melanin pigment production, or immunohistochemical or ultrastructural evidence of such differentiation. Although most head and neck malignant melanomas arise from sun-exposed skin and, to a lesser degree, from the eye, this section deals only with the less common tumors arising from nonocular mucosal surfaces of the head and neck, particularly the sinonasal region.

General Features. Approximately 15 percent of all malignant melanomas arise in the head and neck, but over 80 percent of these develop on sun-exposed cutaneous surfaces. Of the remainder, about 80 percent are of ocular origin, with the rest arising from various mucosal surfaces. Of the head and neck mucosal sites, the mucosa lining the nasal cavity and paranasal sinuses is the most common, accounting for about 1 percent of all malignant melanomas (292,296,305,306,314, 315,318,324,325,328,336). Origin from other head and neck mucosal sites, including the oral cavity and larynx, is less common (300,303,309, 313,323,325,329,333). Melanocytes have been described in the sinonasal region, oral cavity, and larynx (299,302,310,342). Whether head and neck mucosal melanomas arise from these preexistent benign melanocytic precursors or represent "divergent differentiation" of a basal mucosal "stem cell" is controversial and, ultimately, of little or no clinical importance. Etiologic agents for head and neck mucosal malignant melanomas are unknown. Reuter and Woodruff (333) noted a 70 percent frequency of cigarette smoking in their series of 58 patients with head and neck mucosal melanomas with appropriate histories and suggested that further study of this known head and neck carcinogen was warranted.

Sinonasal Melanoma

Patients are typically adults, over 50 years of age, although occasional cases have been reported in children. Studies suggest either no male or female predilection or a slight male predominance. Presenting complaints are nonspecific and typical of a nasal mass, and include obstruction, epistaxis, and pain. Favored locations for sinonasal malignant melanoma, in decreasing order of frequency, include the nasal cavity, maxillary antrum, ethmoid sinuses, and sphenoid sinuses. Within the nasal cavity, melanoma predilects the anterior nasal septum, as well as the middle and lower turbinates. Malignant melanomas rarely, if ever, arise in the nasopharynx or the olfactory mucosa lining the superior portion of the nasal cavity. There have been rare descriptions of sinonasal malignant melanomas arising in schneiderian papillomas, and we have also encountered this phenomenon (311).

Oral Cavity

Oral cavity malignant melanomas, although less common than sinonasal lesions, have been well described (293,325,326,339). They may arise from virtually any mucosal surface (295, 326). The maxillary gingiva and hard palate are common locations of origin (326); the mandibular gingiva and soft palate are less common; and origin from the tongue, floor of mouth, and buccal mucosa are rare (326). It has been suggested that this tumor shows a female predilection and is more common in Japanese than Caucasians (320,338). Other studies have not noted a female predilection (326). The peak incidence is in the sixth decade of life, although patients in one study ranged in age from 32 to 92 years (326). About 75 percent of oral cavity malignant melanomas have a pigmented macule (radial phase) surrounding the tumor; the remaining one fourth of tumors have a purely nodular appearance, which is unpigmented in about 14 percent of all cases (326). Patients often present with advanced disease and a correspondingly poor prognosis (326).

Larynx

Rare examples of apparently primary malignant melanomas have been reported in the larynx (300,303,324,329,330,333,334). As with melanomas involving other unusual sites, it is difficult to exclude metastases for many of these cases. In a review, Reuter and Woodruff (333) noted only six laryngeal melanomas with associated melanoma in situ, presumably indicating primary disease. Conversely, primary lesions may lack an in situ component due to mucosal ulceration. Reports of primary laryngeal melanomas, although rare, outnumber reports of metastases to the larynx, but the latter do occur and undoubtedly are under-reported. In one study of laryngeal metastases, malignant melanomas were the most common, followed by renal cell carcinoma (340). Sites of involvement by purported primary laryngeal melanomas have included the ventricles, epiglottis, vocal cords, aryepiglottic fold, and arytenoid region (329, 333). Primary subglottic laryngeal malignant melanomas have not been convincingly documented. Melanomas of the larynx seem to predilect older males (333), but a 16-year-old with this neoplasm has been reported (324). As with other mucosal sites, tumors are typically polypoid, often pigmented masses; up to one third may be non-pigmented, however (333).

Head and Neck Mucosal Melanomas: General Findings

Gross Findings. Mucosal malignant melanomas, regardless of their origin, often have a grossly polypoid configuration (fig. 7-92). Alternately, the tumor may appear as a friable or partially necrotic, hemorrhagic mass. On cut section, areas of grossly visible pigment may be present, although many microscopically pigmented examples lack such gross pigmentation; in one series, over one third of head and neck mucosal melanomas lacked pigmentation (318).

Microscopic Findings. Malignant melanomas of mucosal origin may exhibit a bewildering array of light microscopic appearances, many of which are uncommon in their cutaneous counterparts. Common microscopic patterns include: small blue cell (fig. 7-93), spindle cell (fig. 7-94), epithelioid (fig. 7-95), and pleomorphic (305). Other patterns are less common, including one in which dissociated cells have prominent, refractile eosinophilic cytoplasm and eccentrically placed nuclei. The resultant image mimics the appearance of rhabdoid tumor or epithelioid sarcoma, and has been described in melanomas

181

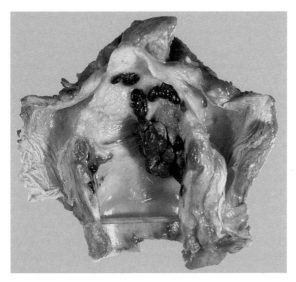

Figure 7-92
MALIGNANT MELANOMA OF THE LARYNX
This primary, polypoid malignant melanoma of the larynx is associated with several intramucosal metastases. (Slide 99 from Mills SE, Fechner RE. Pathology of the larynx. Chicago: ASCP 1985:81.)

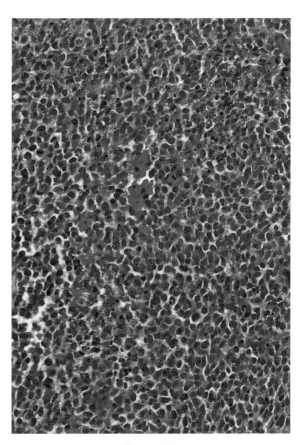

Figure 7-93
SINONASAL MALIGNANT MELANOMA
This sinonasal malignant melanoma has a "small blue cell" appearance, which may be confused with a lymphoma, olfactory neuroblastoma, or other small cell neoplasm.

arising from other sites (294,297). Each of these patterns is associated with specific differential diagnoses (see below).

About 30 percent of mucosal melanomas are microscopically weakly pigmented or nonpigmented, causing considerable diagnostic difficulty (see below) (305,318). In the sinonasal region, junctional change, a helpful diagnostic feature, is present in only about one third of cases, due to frequent surface ulceration (305). Reuter and Woodruff (333) noted, similarly, that only 6 of 22 reported laryngeal malignant melanomas showed adjacent in situ change. In the absence of intact surface mucosa, junctional change should be sought surrounding the underlying seromucinous glands (fig. 7-96). A nesting or theque-like growth pattern is also suggestive (fig. 7-97), but is, again, seen in only about one third of sinonasal cases (305). Oral cavity malignant melanomas often show an "acral lentiginous" pattern with combined radial and nodular growth phases (320,326,338). Between 8 and 23 percent of oral cavity melanomas present as de novo nodular lesions (320,326,338). The purely nodular lesions may lack gross or microscopic pigmentation, leading to the potential for diagnostic difficulty.

Immunohistochemical Findings. Strong immunohistochemical staining for S-100 protein, vimentin, and with HMB-45 is of diagnostic value (301,304,305,308,312,316,317,327,341). It has been suggested that HMB-45 may be superior to antibodies directed against S-100 protein in this group of tumors, particularly in archival material with prolonged storage (316). Additional melanoma-specific markers such as the melanoma-associated antigen, detected by monoclonal antibody NK1/C-3, have also been utilized (316). Rare mucosal malignant melanomas may contain scattered cells positive for cytokeratin and epithelial membrane antigen, but diffuse staining, as seen in carcinomas, is absent (305,321,343). Both olfactory neuroblastomas and occasional carcinomas may contain scattered S-100 protein–positive cells

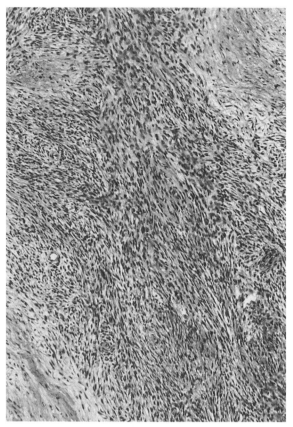

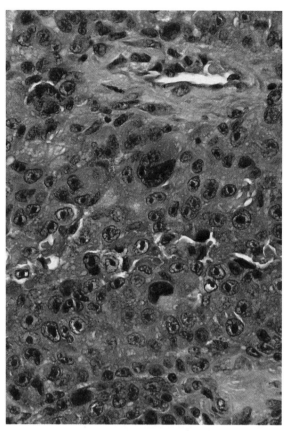

Figure 7-94
SINONASAL MALIGNANT MELANOMA
This sinonasal malignant melanoma has a spindle cell appearance and strikingly resembles a spindle cell sarcoma such as fibrosarcoma or malignant fibrous histiocytoma.

Figure 7-95
SINONASAL MALIGNANT MELANOMA
Sinonasal malignant melanomas may display considerable nuclear pleomorphism.

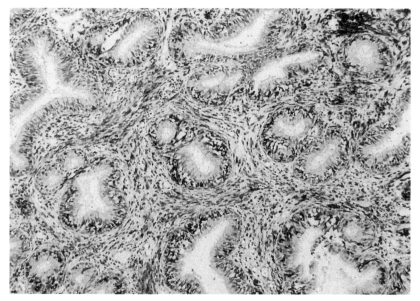

Figure 7-96
SINONASAL
MALIGNANT MELANOMA
This spindle cell sinonasal malignant melanoma has a "junctional" component involving seromucinous glands, as well as an invasive component. Both the junctional and invasive components stain strongly with HMB-45 (HMB-45 and hematoxylin).

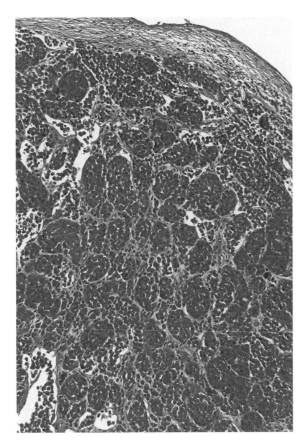

Figure 7-97
SINONASAL MALIGNANT MELANOMA

A nesting or "theque-like" growth pattern may be encountered in sinonasal malignant melanoma. Although somewhat suggestive of the diagnosis, this pattern may be encountered in a number of other tumors.

(301,317), but the diffuse staining of malignant melanoma is lacking in these tumors (see below).

Differential Diagnosis. The small cell pattern of mucosal malignant melanoma may be confused, depending on anatomic site, with olfactory neuroblastoma, lymphoma, rhabdomyosarcoma, small cell undifferentiated carcinoma, and other small cell neoplasms. The spindle cell pattern may be confused with a sarcoma or spindle cell (sarcomatoid) carcinoma. The epithelioid and pleomorphic variants are most often confused with carcinomas. Distinction is often possible based purely on the hematoxylin and eosin (H&E)-stained microscopy; this may be aided in selected cases by the application of immunohistochemistry, electron microscopy; or both. Specific diagnostic problems are discussed below.

Olfactory Neuroblastoma. In our experience, confusion of sinonasal malignant melanoma with olfactory neuroblastoma is a relatively common problem. One should be particularly suspicious of the latter diagnosis in tumors occurring low in the nasal cavity, beyond the realm of normal olfactory mucosa. Rarely, mucosal malignant melanomas may exhibit a distinctly fibrillar background, as well as forming structures resembling Homer Wright rosettes. A number of factors conspire to further the confusion created by H&E-based similarities. Focal staining for neurofilament may also be seen in malignant melanomas. Conversely, olfactory neuroblastomas frequently contain S-100 protein–positive cells (291,298,307). However, the diffuse, strong S-100 protein positivity of malignant melanoma is not seen in olfactory neuroblastoma, and the latter tumor lacks any staining with HMB-45, in our experience (305,341).

Undifferentiated Carcinoma. The epithelioid pattern of malignant melanoma may be confused with carcinoma, particularly lymphoepithelioma-like neoplasms. The syncytial growth of malignant melanoma, often coupled with a prominent inflammatory stroma, can closely mimic a lymphoepithelioma-type undifferentiated carcinoma. Location of the tumor is of value. Malignant melanoma predilects the paranasal sinuses and nasal cavity, whereas lymphoepithelioma-type undifferentiated carcinoma almost invariably arises in the nasopharynx or tonsil. As noted above, malignant melanoma may rarely show weak cytokeratin positivity and, conversely undifferentiated carcinomas may show patchy S-100 protein staining (305). Diffuse S-100 protein positivity and HMB-45 staining are diagnostic of malignant melanoma. This distinction is of considerable clinical importance, given the relative radiosensitivity of lymphoepithelioma-type undifferentiated carcinoma.

Sarcoma. The spindle cell pattern of malignant melanoma may be confused with a sarcoma such as malignant fibrous histiocytoma. Typically, consideration of the correct diagnosis, coupled with immunohistochemistry, allows for straightforward distinction.

Melanotic Neuroectodermal Tumor of Infancy. This very rare, almost invariably benign, partially melanocytic tumor shows a striking predilection for the bones of the head and neck in children under 1 year of age. The intraosseous origin and occurrence in the first year of life are clear-cut clinical distinctions from malignant melanoma. Nonetheless, we have encountered sinonasal malignant melanomas erroneously interpreted as melanotic neuroectodermal tumor. Microscopically, melanotic neuroectodermal tumors have a stereotypical tubular/alveolar pattern with a biphasic population of small, neuroblastoma-like cells and larger pigmented cells. Immunohistochemically, the tumors show a highly specific staining pattern with strong positivity for cytokeratin and HMB-45 in the larger cells; synaptophysin, neuron-specific enolase, and other neural markers stain primarily the smaller cell population (319,331). S-100 protein is rarely positive and mainly confined to the smaller cells (319,331).

Spread and Metastasis. Overall, about 40 percent of patients with head and neck mucosal melanomas have nonlocalized disease at the time of presentation (313). Of those receiving "curative" resection and developing recurrent disease, 44 percent have local recurrences, and the remainder have regional or distant recurrent disease (313). Local recurrence appears to be less of a problem for the subgroup of patients with laryngeal disease treated initially with complete surgical excision (321). Death from mucosal melanoma of the head and neck is due to either widespread metastases; persistent or recurrent local disease, often with intracranial extension; or both. In one study of patients dying of disease, 36 percent had both local and distant disease, 32 percent had distant disease only, and 32 percent had local disease only (309). In our smaller series of 14 patients with sinonasal tumors, all patients dying of disease had metastases at the time of death (305).

Treatment and Prognosis. Regardless of anatomic site in the head and neck region, complete excision is the treatment of choice, as radiation and chemotherapy have little or no value. For sinonasal lesions, the 5-year survival rate is approximately 10 to 21 percent (305,313), and median survival period is approximately 2 years (305). Five-year survival should not be equated with cure, as a significant number of tumor-related deaths occur after that time (306,315,324,328,335, 336). Patients with laryngeal melanomas have a similarly poor prognosis, with a reported 5-year survival rate of less than 20 percent and a median survival period of 3 to 3.5 years (333).

Oral cavity melanomas have been evaluated using the prognostic features applied to analogous cutaneous neoplasms (320,326,337,338). Most studies have shown a dismal overall prognosis, with 5-year survival rates of 10 to 20 percent, strikingly similar to those for other head and neck mucosal sites (322,326,332,339). In one review of 35 patients, lesions showing a radial growth phase (77 percent) were associated with a longer median survival time than purely nodular lesions (23.5 months versus 7.5 months) (326). Depth of invasion did not correlate with prognosis, although clinical stage I versus stage II did show prognostic significance (326). One recent study reported a good response to a combination of surgical excision, therapeutic neck dissection, and adjuvant immunochemotherapy (338). The 5-year survival rate for a group of five patients treated in this fashion was 65 percent.

PERIPHERAL NEUROECTODERMAL TUMOR/EXTRAOSSEOUS EWING'S SARCOMA

Definition. This is a primitive neuroectodermal round cell tumor with variable evidence of neural differentiation. Extraosseous Ewing's sarcoma (EOE) and peripheral neuroectodermal tumor (PNET) are closely related primitive neural neoplasms, with undifferentiated EOE at one end of the spectrum and PNET with neural features at the other. For the purposes of this section, no distinction will be made between them since they likely represent a single tumor type.

Clinical Findings. PNET/EOE are tumors of childhood and adolescence, with a mean peak incidence at 18 years of age (range, birth to 81 years) (346). Most series report a slight (1.2 to 1) male predilection (346,350,358). The predominant anatomic site of involvement is the thoracopulmonary region (so-called Askin tumors), followed by the extremities, abdominal/pelvic region, and the head and neck area (345,349,358). The combined results of four large studies reported 18 of 192 (9 percent) PNET/EOEs arising in the upper aerodigestive tract (head and neck) area, although the precise sites of origin were not further specified (345,349,358,362). Despite variable evidence of neural differentiation, most tumors are anatomically unassociated with nerves, ganglia, or other neural structures.

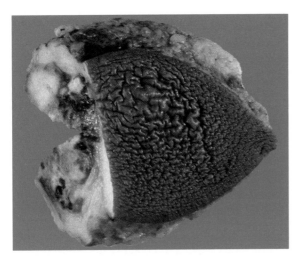

Figure 7-98
PERIPHERAL NEUROECTODERMAL TUMOR
Subcutaneous peripheral neuroectodermal tumor from
the posterior neck of a 25 year-old male. The tumor is poorly
defined and partially necrotic on cut surface.

Biologically, PNET/EOEs are highly aggressive tumors that often result in death within 2 years of diagnosis. If PNET and EOE are separated according to strictly defined criteria, some studies suggest differences in clinical outcome, with an overall survival rate of 30 percent for patients with PNET compared to 70 percent for those with EOE (352,357,358). Most patients present with localized disease, but local recurrence and metastasis to the lungs and bone generally occur within 1 to 2 years of diagnosis (349). Effective therapy to date has been principally limited to aggressive surgical resection. In general, adjuvant radiation or chemotherapy has no apparent effect on outcome.

Gross Findings. Tumors typically appear as ovoid, multinodular or lobulated masses with a granular, gray-white appearance on cut surface (344). Hemorrhage and necrosis are occasionally seen (fig. 7-98). Most tumors are circumscribed but unencapsulated.

Microscopic Findings. PNET/EOEs are characterized by sheets, lobules, or nests of homogeneous, closely packed, small round cells with an intervening fibrovascular stroma (fig. 7-99). The peripheral margins of the tumor often push, rather than infiltrate, into adjacent tissues. The neoplastic cells are round to elongated and invariably small; individual cells measure 10 to 4 µm in diameter (344). Cytoplasm is scant, and most cells appear to be composed almost entirely of a round, dense, hyperchromatic nucleus with inconspicuous nucleoli (fig. 7-100). Nuclei are usually compressed, but not molded, by adjacent tumor cells. Mitotic activity is high, in the range of 5 to 10 mitoses per 10 high-power fields. Homer Wright rosettes with centrally located fibrillary material are present in the majority of cases (345,348,350, 351,358,359). Structures resembling Flexner-Wintersteiner rosettes, with a sharply demarcated central lumen, have also been noted (345). Diastase-sensitive periodic acid–Schiff positivity is common, due to the presence of intracytoplasmic glycogen (fig. 7-101) (345,348,350,358). There are no histologic parameters predictive of clinical outcome (345).

Immunohistochemical Findings. Recent studies have identified the *MIC*-2 gene as a consistent and reliable marker of PNET/EOE. Monoclonal antibodies HBA-71, 12E7, and 013 directed against the MIC-2 protein product label more than 90 percent of PNET/EOEs on fixed sections in a diffuse, membranous pattern (fig. 7-102) (354,355,365). Virtually all tumors are reactive for neuron-specific enolase (345,351). A proportion of cases label with vimentin, synaptophysin, and S-100 protein, and occasional lesions stain for neurofilament (345,351,353). Rare cases are focally positive for low molecular weight keratins and desmin (345,353,355,359). In general, with the exception of the MIC-2 protein product, results of fixed section immunostaining are inconsistent and of limited diagnostic usefulness.

Ultrastructural Findings. Small, closely packed tumor cells extend short, neuritic cytoplasmic processes which are joined by poorly defined desmosomes and tight junctions (350,358). Cytoplasmic organelles, such as mitochondria, rough endoplasmic reticulum, and Golgi apparatti, are present in reduced numbers. Most tumors contain intracytoplasmic glycogen (7-103) (345, 350,358). The neuritic processes contain intermediate filaments, microtubules, and infrequent dense core neurosecretory-type granules that are 150 to 200 nm in diameter (344,358).

Special Techniques. Cytogenetic analysis of PNET/EOE has demonstrated a specific, reciprocal translocation between band q24 on chromosome 11 and band q12 on chromosome 22 (360,361, 364). Approximately 90 percent of PNET/ EOEs

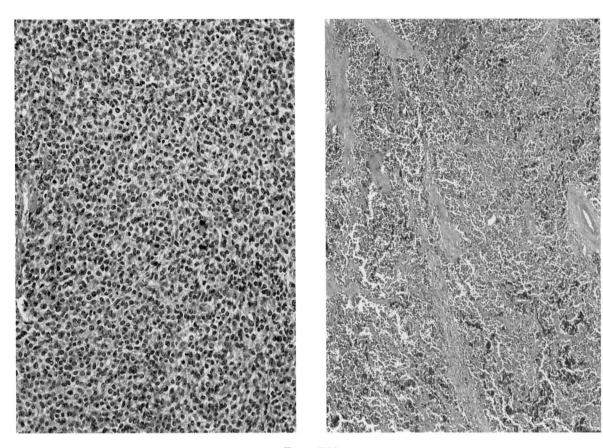

Figure 7-99
PERIPHERAL NEUROECTODERMAL TUMOR
Left: Peripheral neuroectodermal tumors are characterized by sheets of closely packed, small round cells resting on an almost inapparent fibrovascular stroma.
Right: Occasional tumors are composed of nests of neoplastic cells intersected by prominent bands of fibrous tissue.

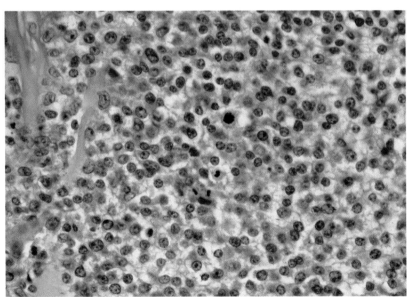

Figure 7-100
PERIPHERAL
NEUROECTODERMAL TUMOR
The neoplastic cells are small, and often appear to be composed almost entirely of a vesicular or hyperchromatic nucleus with inconspicuous nucleoli. Mitotic figures are easily identified.

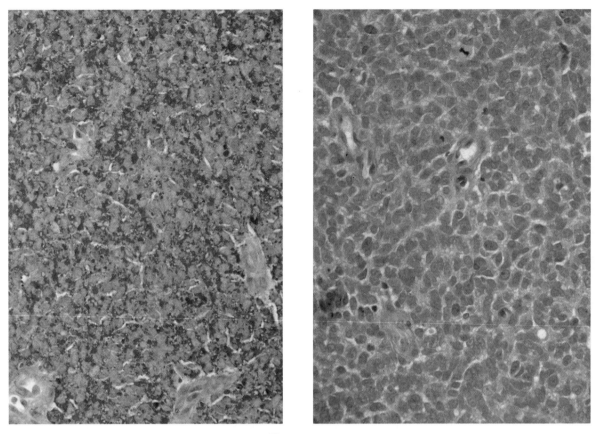

Figure 7-101
PERIPHERAL NEUROECTODERMAL TUMOR
Left: A proportion of tumors contain intracytoplasmic periodic acid-Schiff–positive material (periodic acid-Schiff stain, X400).
Right: The tumor is sensitive to diastase predigestion, consistent with the presence of glycogen (periodic acid-Schiff stain with diastase predigestion, X400).

Figure 7-102
PERIPHERAL
NEUROECTODERMAL TUMOR
Typical membrane-pattern immunoreactivity of a peripheral neuroectodermal tumor with monoclonal antibody HBA-71, directed against the MIC-2 protein product.

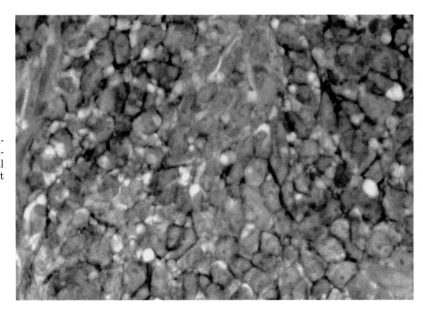

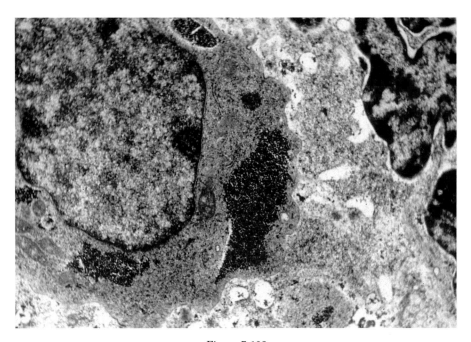

Figure 7-103
PERIPHERAL NEUROECTODERMAL TUMOR
Ultrastructural study shows poorly differentiated cells with few organelles and abundant intracytoplasmic particulate glycogen.

have either the standard t(11;22)(q24;q12) translocation (about 78 percent of cases), a variant translocation in which chromosome 22 and one or more chromosomes other than chromosome 11 are involved (7 percent), or a complex translocation involving a third chromosome in addition to chromosomes 11 and 12 (5 percent). The chromosome 22 breakpoint q12 is involved in over 90 percent of cases and may be the crucial event leading to malignant transformation.

The breakpoints of chromosomes 22 and 11 involve the *EWS* and *FLI*-1 genes, respectively. Most standard, variant, or complex translocations result in the fusion of these genes, with the production of a novel chimeric EWS/FLI-1 message. Unfortunately, successful karyotypes are obtained in PNET/EOE in less than half of the cases (347). However, the chimeric transcript may be detected by other means, including fluorescent in situ hybridization (363), the reverse transcriptase polymerase chain reaction (RT-PCR) (360), or Southern blot hybridization (360) in more than 90 percent of cases.

Differential Diagnosis. Included are all other small blue round cell tumors in the upper aerodigestive tract, such as rhabdomyosarcoma, small cell osteosarcoma, neuroblastoma, and non-Hodgkin's lymphoma. Distinction from small cell osteosarcoma, alveolar rhabdomyosarcoma, and neuroblastoma is usually possible on histologic grounds alone. Distinction from a proportion of neuroblastomas, embryonal rhabdomyosarcomas, the solid variant of alveolar rhabdomyosarcoma, and non-Hodgkin's lymphoma, however, often requires immunohistochemical examination. Virtually all neuroblastomas are nonreactive for vimentin, while MIC-2 is expressed in over 90 percent of PNET/EOEs compared to 0 percent of neuroblastomas (354,365). Distinction from lymphoma is potentially hazardous, since MIC-2 is expressed in most lymphoblastic lymphomas and related leukemias of T-cell derivation (356,365). Thus, immunostaining for B- and T- cell markers should be included in the evaluation of a suspected PNET/EOE. Finally, separation from embryonal and alveolar rhabdomyocarcoma is also problematic, since rare PNET/EOEs are focally immunopositive for desmin (345,359). Rhabdomyosarcomas, however, are usually diffusely desmin positive and negative for neural markers. Cytogenetic examination may be necessary to resolve equivocal cases.

REFERENCES

Heterotopic Glial Tissue (Nasal Glioma)

1. Black BK, Smith DE. Nasal glioma: two cases with recurrence. Arch Neurol Psychiatr 195;64:614–30.
2. Chan JK, Lau WH. Nasal astrocytoma or nasal glial heterotopia? Arch Pathol Lab Med 1989;113:943–5.
3. Feldman BA, Schwartz RH, Chandra R, Anderson K. Heterotopic brain tissue simulating a neonatal tonsil. Clin Pediatr 1982;21:428–30.
4. Gorenstein A, Kern EB, Facer GW, Laws ER. Nasal gliomas. Arch Otolaryngol 1980;106:536–40.
5. Karma P, Rasanen O, Karja J. Nasal gliomas. A review and report of two cases. Laryngoscope 1977;87:1169–79.
6. Katz A, Lewis JS. Nasal gliomas. Arch Otolaryngol 1971;94:351–5.
7. Mirra SS, Pearl GS, Hoffman JC, Campbell WG Jr. Nasal "glioma" with prominent neuronal component. Report of a case. Arch Pathol Lab Med 1981;105:540–1.
8. Patterson K, Kapur S, Chandra RS. "Nasal gliomas" and related brain heterotopias: a pathologist's perspective. Pediatr Pathol 1986;5:353–62.
9. Puppala B, Mangurten HH, McFadden J, Lygizos N, Taxy J, Pellettiere E. Nasal glioma. Presenting as neonatal respiratory distress. Definition of the tumor mass by MRI. Clin Pediatr 1990;29:49–52.
10. Shapiro MJ, Mix BS. Heterotopic brain tissue of the palate. A report of two cases. Arch Otolaryngol 1968;87:522–6.
11. Theaker JM, Fletcher CD. Heterotopic glial nodules: a light microscopic and immunohistochemical study. Histopathology 1991;18:255–60.
12. Whitaker SR, Sprinkle PM, Chou SM. Nasal glioma. Arch Otolaryngol 1981;107:550–4.

Ectopic Pituitary Tissue and Pituitary Adenoma

13. Anand VK, Osborne CM, Harkey HL III. Infiltrative clival pituitary adenoma of ectopic origin. Otolaryngol Head Neck Surg 1993;108:178–83.
14. Ciocca DR, Puy LA, Stati AO. Identification of seven hormone-producing cell types in the human pharyngeal hypophysis. J Clin Endocrinol Metab 1985;60:212–6.
15. Gandour-Edwards R, Kapadia SB, Janecka IP, Martinez AJ, Barnes L. Biologic markers of invasive pituitary adenomas involving the sphenoid sinus. Mod Pathol 1995;8:160–4.
16. Gillespie CA, Walker JS, Burch WM, Kenan PD, Kramer RS. Cushing's syndrome secondary to ectopic pituitary adenoma in the sphenoid sinus. Otolaryngol Head Neck Surg 1987;96:569–72.
17. Lloyd RV, Chandler WF, Kovacs K, Ryan N. Ectopic pituitary adenomas with normal anterior pituitary glands. Am J Surg Pathol 1986;10:546-52.
18. Lloyd RV, Scheithauer BW, Kovacs K. The immunophenotype of pituitary adenoma [Abstract]. Mod Pathol 1995;8:55A.
19. Luk IS, Chan JK, Chow SM, Leung S. Pituitary adenoma presenting as sinonasal tumor: pitfalls in diagnosis. Hum Pathol 1996;27:605–9.
20. McGrath P. Volume and histology of the human pharyngeal hypophysis. Aust NZ J Surg 1967;37:16–26.
21. McGrath P. Cysts of sellar and pharyngeal hypophysis. Pathology 1971;3:123–31.
22. Melchionna RH, Moore RA. The pharyngeal pituitary gland. Am J Pathol 1938;14:763–71.
23. Rasmussen P, Lindholm J. Ectopic pituitary adenomas. Clin Endocrinol 1979;11:69–74.
24. Richards SH, Evans IT. The pharyngeal hypophysis and its surgical significance. J Laryngol Otol 1974;88: 937–46.
25. Scheithauer BW. The pituitary and sellar region. In: Sternberg SS, ed. Diagnostic surgical pathology, 2nd ed. New York: Raven Press, 1994:493–522.
26. Scheithauer BW, Kovacs KT, Laws ER Jr, Randall RV. Pathology of invasive pituitary tumors with special reference to functional classification. J Neurosurg 1986;65:733–44.
27. Tovi F, Hirsch M, Sacks M, Leiberman A. Ectopic pituitary adenoma of the sphenoid sinus: report of a case and review of the literature. Head Neck 1990;12:264–8.
28. Wenig B, Heffess C, Adair C, Thompson L, Heffner D. Ectopic pituitary adenomas: a clinicopathologic study of 15 cases [Abstract]. Mod Pathol 1995;8:56A.
29. Wong K, Raisanen J, Taylor SL, McDermott MW, Wilson CB, Gutin PH. Pituitary adenoma as an unsuspected clival tumor. Am J Surg Pathol 1995;19:900–3.

Neurofibroma

30. Ayres WW, Delaney AJ, Backer MH. Congenital neurofibromatous macroglossia associated in some cases with von Recklinghausen's disease. A case report and review of the literature. Cancer 1952:5:721–6.
31. Chango-Lo M. Laryngeal involvement in von Recklinghausen's disease: a case report and review of the literature. Laryngoscope 1977;87:435–42.
32. Cummings CW, Montgomery WW, Balogh K Jr. Neurogenic tumors of the larynx. Ann Otol Rhinol Laryngol 1969;78:76–95.
33. Fountain JW, Wallace MR, Bruce MA, et al. Physical mapping of a translocation breakpoint in neurofibromatosis. Science 1989;244:1085–7.
34. Hillstrom RP, Zarbo RJ, Jacobs JJ. Nerve sheath tumors of the paranasal sinuses: electron microscopy and histopathologic diagnosis. Otolaryngol Head Neck Surg 1990:102:257–63.
35. Lossos IS, Breuer R, Lafair JS. Endotracheal neurofibroma in a patient with von Recklinghausen's disease. Eur Respir J 1988;1:464–5.

36. O'Connell P, Leach R, Cawthon RM, et al. Two NFI translocations map within a 600-kilobase segment of 17ql 1.2. Science 1989:244:1087–8.

37. Perzin KH, Panyu H, Wechter S. Nonepithelial tumors of the nasal cavity, paranasal sinuses, and nasopharynx. A clinicopathologic study. XII: Schwann cell tumors (neurilemoma, neurofibroma, malignant schwannoma). Cancer 1982:50:2193–202.

38. Pleasure J, Geller SA. Neurofibromatosis in infancy presenting with congenital stridor. Am J Dis Child 1967;113:390–3.

39. Robitaille Y, Seemayer TA, El Deiry A. Peripheral nerve tumors involving paranasal sinuses: a case report and review of the literature. Cancer 1975;35:1254–8.

40. Xu G, O'Connell P, Viskochil D, et al. The neurofibromatosis type 1 gene encodes a protein related to GAP. Cell 1990;62:599–608.

Palisaded Encapsulated Neuroma

41. Argenyi ZB, Cooper PH, Santa Cruz D. Plexiform and other unusual variants of palisaded encapsulated neuroma. J Cutan Pathol 1993;20:34–9.

42. Chauvin PJ, Wysocki GP, Daley TD, Pringle GA. Palisaded encapsulated neuroma of oral mucosa. Oral Surg Oral Med Oral Pathol 1992;73:71–4.

43. Fletcher CD. Solitary circumscribed neuroma of the skin (so-called palisaded, encapsulated neuroma). A clinicopathologic and immunohistochemical study. Am J Surg Pathol 1989;13:574–80.

Traumatic Neuroma

44. Daneshuar A. Pharyngeal traumatic neuromas and traumatic neuromas with mature ganglion cells (pseudoganglioneuromas). Am J Surg Pathol 1990:14:565–70.

45. Enzinger FM, Weiss SW. Soft tissue tumors. 2nd ed. St. Louis: CV Mosby, 1988:722.

46. Sist TC Jr, Greene GW. Traumatic neuroma of the oral cavity. Report of thirty-one new cases and review of the literature. Oral Surg Oral Med Oral Pathol 1981: 51:394–402.

Mucosal Neuroma (Ganglioneuroma)

47. Cangiarella J, Jagirdar J, Adelman H, Budzilovich G, Greco MA. Mucosal neuromas and plexiform neurofibromas: an immunocytochemical study. Pediatr Pathol 1993;13:281–8.

48. Carney JA, Go VL, Sizemore GW, Hayles AB. Alimentary-tract ganglioneuromatosis. A major component of the syndrome of multiple endocrine neoplasia, type 2b. N Engl J Med 1976;295:1287–91.

49. Dyck PJ, Carney JA, Sizemore GW, Okazaki H, Brimijoin WS, Lambert EH. Multiple endocrine neoplasia, type 2b: phenotype recognition; neurological features and their pathological basis. Ann Neurol 1979;6:302–14.

50. Eng C. The RET proto-oncogene in multiple endocrine neoplasia type 2 and Hirschspring's disease. N Engl J Med 1996;335:943–51.

51. Eng C, Smith DP, Mulligan LM, et al. Point mutation within the tyrosine kinase domain of the RET proto-oncogene in multiple endocrine neoplasia type 2B and related sporadic tumours. Hum Mol Genet 1994;3:237–41.

52. Gorlin RJ, Sedano HO, Vickers RA, Cervenka J. Multiple mucosal neuromas, pheochromocytoma and medullary carcinoma of the thyroid—a syndrome. Cancer 1968;22:293–9.

53. Hofstra RM, Landsvater RM, Ceccherini I, et al. A mutation in the RET proto-oncogene associated with multiple endocrine neoplasia type 2B and sporadic medullary thyroid carcinoma. Nature 1994;367:375–6.

54. Khairi MR, Dexter RN, Burzynski NJ, Johnston CC Jr. Mucosal neuroma, pheochromocytoma and medullary thyroid carcinoma: multiple endocrine neoplasia type 3. Medicine 1975;54:89–112.

Neurilemoma (Schwannoma)

55. Costantino PD, Friedman CD, Pelzer HJ. Neurofibromatosis type II of the head and neck. Arch Otolaryngol Head Neck Surg 1989;115:380–3.

56. Erickson LS, Sorenson GD, McGavran MH. A review of 140 acoustic neuromas (neurilemoma). Laryngoscope 1965;75:601–27.

57. Gallo WJ, Moss M, Shapiro DN, Gaul JV. Neurilemoma: review of the literature and report of five cases. J Oral Surg 1977;35:235-6.

58. Hasegawa SL, Mentzel T, Fletcher CD. Schwannomas of the sinonasal tract and nasopharynx. Mod Pathol 1997;10:777–84.

59. Kasantikul V, Netsky MG, Glasscock ME III, Hays JW. Acoustic neurilemoma. Clinicoanatomical study of 103 patients. J Neurosurg 1980;52:28–35.

60. Ma CK, Raju U, Fine G, Lewis JW Jr. Primary tracheal neurilemoma. Report of a case with ultrastructural examination. Arch Pathol Lab Med 1981;105:187–9.

61. Nass RL, Cohen NL. Neurilemoma of the trachea. Arch Otolaryngol 1979;105:220–1.

62. National Institutes of Health Consensus Development Conference Statement. Neurofibromatosis 1987;6:1–7.

63. Perzin KH, Panyu H, Wechter S. Nonepithelial tumors of the nasal cavity, paranasal sinuses, and nasopharynx. A clinicopathologic study. XII: Schwann cell tumors (neurilemoma, neurofibroma, malignant schwannoma). Cancer 1982;50:2193–202.

64. Robitaille Y, Seemayer TA, El Diery A. Peripheral nerve tumors involving paranasal sinuses: a case report and review of the literature. Cancer 1975;35:1254–8.

65. Trofatter JA, MacCollin MM, Rutter JL, et al. A novel moesin-, ezrin-, radixin-like gene is a candidate for the neurofibromatosis 2 tumor suppressor. Cell 1993;72:791–800.

66. Wertelecki W, Rouleau GA, Superneau DW, et al. Neurofibromatosis 2: clinical and DNA linkage studies of a large kindred. N Engl J Med 1988;319:278–83.

Nerve Sheath Myxoma (Neurothekeoma)

67. Gallager RL, Helwig EB. Neurothekeoma—a benign cutaneous tumor of neural origin. Am J Clin Pathol 1980;74:759–64.

68. Green TL, Leighty SM, Walters R. Immunohistochemical evaluation of oral myxoid lesions. Oral Surg Oral Med Oral Pathol 1992;73:469–71.

69. Harkin JC, Reed RJ. Tumors of the peripheral nervous system. The Atlas of Tumor Pathology, 2nd Series, Fascicle 3. Washington, DC: Armed Forces Institute of Pathology, 1969:60–4.

70. Mincer HH, Spears KD. Nerve sheath myxoma in the tongue. Oral Surg Oral Med Oral Pathol 1974;37:428–30.

71. Rodriguez-Peralto JL, el-Naggar AK. Neurothekeoma of the oral cavity: case report and review of the literature. J Oral Maxillofac Surg 1992;50:1224–6.

72. Smith BC, Ellis GL, Meis-Kindblom JM, Williams SB. Ectomesenchymal chondromyxoid tumor of the anterior tongue. Nineteen cases of a new clinicopathologic entity. Am J Surg Pathol 1995;19:519–30.

73. Tomich CE. Oral focal mucinosis: a clinicopathologic and histochemical study of eight cases. Oral Surg Oral Med Oral Pathol 1974;38:714–24.

74. Wright BA, Jackson D. Neural tumors of the oral cavity. A review of the spectrum of benign and malignant oral tumors of the oral cavity and jaws. Oral Surg Oral Med Oral Pathol 1980;49:509–22.

75. Yamamoto H, Kawana T. Oral nerve sheath myxoma: report of a case with findings of ultrastructural and immunohistochemical studies. Acta Pathol Jpn 1988; 38:121–7.

Melanotic Neuroectodermal Tumor of Infancy

76. Carpenter BF, Jimenez C, Robb IA. Melanotic neuroectodermal tumor of infancy. Pediatr Pathol 1985;3:227–44.

77. Cohen BH, Handler MS, DeVivo DC, Garvin JH, Hays AP, Carmel P. Central nervous system melanotic neuroectodermal tumor of infancy: value of chemotherapy in management. Neurology 1988;38:163–4.

78. Cutler LS, Chaudhry AP, Topazian R. Melanotic neuroectodermal tumor of infancy: an ultrastructural study, literature review, and reevaluation. Cancer 1981;48:257–70.

79. Dehner LP, Sibley RK, Sauk JJ Jr, et al. Malignant melanotic neuroectodermal tumor of infancy: a clinical, pathologic, ultrastructural and tissue culture study. Cancer 1979;43:1389–410.

80. Fowler M, Simpson DA. A malignant melanin-forming tumor of the cerebellum. J Pathol Bacteriol 1962;84:307–11.

81. Hameed K, Burslem MR. A melanotic ovarian neoplasm resembling the "retinal anlage" tumor. Cancer 1970;25:564–7.

82. Johnson RE, Scheithauer BW, Dahlin DC. Melanotic neuroectodermal tumor of infancy. A review of seven cases. Cancer 1983;52:661–6.

83. Kapadia SB, Frisman DM, Hitchcock CL, Ellis GL, Popek EJ. Melanotic neuroectodermal tumor of infancy. Clinicopathological, immunohistochemical, and flow cytometric study. Am J Surg Pathol 1993;17:566–73.

84. Misugi K, Okajima H, Newton WA Jr, Kmetz DR, DeLorimer AA. Mediastinal origin of a melanotic progonoma or retinal anlage tumor: ultrastructural evidence for a neural crest origin. Cancer 1965;18:477–84.

85. Pettinato G, Manivel JC, d'Amore ES, Jaszcz W, Gorlin RJ. Melanotic neuroectodermal tumor of infancy. A reexamination of a histogenetic problem based on immunohistochemical, flow cytometric, and ultrastructural study of 100 cases. Am J Surg Pathol 1991;15:233–45.

86. Raju U, Zarbo RJ, Regezi JA, Krutchkoff DJ, Perrin EV. Melanotic neuroectodermal tumors of infancy: intermediate filament-, neuroendocrine-, and melanoma-associated antigen profiles. Appl Immunohistochem 1993;1:69–76.

87. Schulz DM. A malignant melanotic neoplasm of the uterus, resembling the "retinal anlage" tumors: report of a case. Am J Clin Pathol 1957;28:524–32.

88. Stirling RW, Powell G, Fletcher CD. Pigmented neuroectodermal tumor of infancy: an immunohistochemical study. Histopathology 1988;12:425–35.

Granular Cell Tumor/Congenital Epulis

89. Klima M, Peters J. Malignant granular cell tumor. Arch Pathol Lab Med 1987;111:1070–3.

90. Lack EE, Perez-Atayde AR, McGill TJ, Vawter GF. Gingival granular cell tumor of the newborn (congenital "epulis"): ultrastructural observations relating to histogenesis. Hum Pathol 1982;13:686–9.

91. Lack EE, Worsham GF, Callihan MD, et al. Granular cell tumor: a clinicopathologic study of 110 patients. J Surg Oncol 1980;13:301–16.

92. Lifshitz MS, Flotte TJ, Greco MA. Congenital granular cell epulis. Immunohistochemical and ultrastructural observations. Cancer 1984;53:1845–8.

93. Mazur MT, Shultz JJ, Myers JL. Granular cell tumor: immunohistochemical analysis of 21 benign tumors and one malignant tumor. Arch Pathol Lab Med 1990;114:692–6.

94. Miettinen M, Lehtonen E, Lehtola H, Ekblom P, Lehto VP, Virtanen I. Histogenesis of granular cell tumor—an immunohistochemical and ultrastructural study. J Pathol 1984;142:221–9.

95. Morrison JG, Gray GF, Dao AH, Adkins RB. Granular cell tumors. Am Surg 1987;53:156–60.

96. Mukai M. Immunohistochemical localization of S-100 protein and peripheral nerve myelin proteins (P2 protein, P0 protein) in granular cell tumors. Am J Pathol 1983;112:139–46.

97. Nathratha WB, Remberger K. Immunohistochemical study of granular cell tumors. Demonstration of neurone specific enolase, S100 protein, lamin and alpha-1 antichymotrypsin. Virchows Arch [A] 1986;408:421–34.

98. Peterson LJ. Granular cell tumor. Review of the literature and report of a case. Oral Surg 1974;37:728–35.

99. Regezi JA, Batsakis JG, Courtney RM. Granular cell tumors of the head and neck. J Oral Surg 1979;37:402–6.

100. Smolle J, Konrad K, Kerl H. Granular cell tumors contain myelin-associated glycoprotein. An immunohistochemical study using Leu 7 monoclonal antibody. Virchows Arch [A] 1985;406:1–5.

101. Steffelaar JW, Nap M, Haelst UJ. Malignant granular cell tumor. Report of a case with special reference to carcinoembryonic antigen. Am J Surg Pathol 1982;6:665–72.

102. Strong EW, McDivitt RW, Brasfield RD. Granular cell myoblastoma. Cancer 1970;25:415–22.

103. Usui M, Ishii S, Yamawaki S, Sasaki T, Minami A, Hizawa K. Malignant granular cell tumor of the radial nerve: an autopsy observation with electron microscopic and tissue culture studies. Cancer 1977;39:1547–55.

Craniopharyngioma

104. Bernstein ML, Buchino JJ. The histologic similarity between craniopharyngioma and odontogenic lesions: a reappraisal. Oral Surg Oral Med Oral Pathol 1983;56:502–11.

105. Byme MN, Sessions DG. Nasopharyngeal craniopharyngioma. Case report and literature review. Ann Otol Rhinol Laryngol 1990;99:633–9.

Meningioma

106. Farr HW, Gray GF Jr, Vrana M, Panio M. Extracranial meningioma. J Surg Oncol 1973;5:411–20.

107. Friedman CD, Costantino PD, Teitelbaum B, Berktold RE, Sisson GA. Primary extracranial meningiomas of the head and neck. Laryngoscope 1990;100:41–8.

108. Granich MS, Pilch BZ, Goodman ML. Meningiomas presenting in the paranasal sinuses and temporal bone. Head Neck 1983;5:319–28.

109. Ho KL. Primary meningioma of the nasal cavity and paranasal sinuses. Cancer 1980:46:1442–7.

110. Kershishik M, Callender DL, Batsakis JG. Extracranial, extraspinal meningiomas of the head and neck. Ann Otol Rhinol Laryngol 1993;102:967–70.

111. Kjeldsberg CR, Minckler J. Meningiomas presenting as nasal polyps. Cancer 1972;29:153–6.

112. Nager GT. Meningiomas involving the temporal bone. Springfield, IL: Charles C. Thomas, 1964.

113. Perzin KH, Pushparaj N. Nonepithelial tumors of the nasal cavity, paranasal sinuses, and nasopharynx. A clinicopathologic study. XIII: Meningiomas. Cancer 1984;54:1860–9.

114. Rietz DR, Ford CN, Brandenburg JH, Kurtycz DF, Hafez GR. Significance of apparent intratympanic meningiomas. Laryngoscope 1983;93:1397–404.

115. Salama N, Stafford N. Meningiomas presenting in the middle ear. Laryngoscope 1982;92:92–7.

116. Taxy JB. Meningioma of the paranasal sinuses. A report of two cases. Am J Surg Pathol 1990;14:82–6.

117. Winek RR, Scheithauer BW, Wick MR. Meningioma, meningeal hemangiopericytoma (angioblastic meningioma), peripheral hemangiopericytoma, and acoustic schwannoma. A comparative immunohistochemical study. Am J Surg Pathol 1989;13:251–61.

Paraganglioma/Carotid Body Tumor

118. Achilles E, Padberg BC, Holl K, Kloppel G, Schroder S. Immunocytochemistry of paragangliomas—value of staining for S-100 protein and glial fibrillary acid protein in diagnosis and prognosis. Histopathology 1991;18:453–8.

119. Arias-Stella J, Valcarcel J. Chief cell hyperplasias in the human carotid body at high altitudes: physiologic and pathologic significance. Hum Pathol 1976;7:361–73.

120. Barnes L. Paraganglioma of the larynx. A critical review of the literature. ORL J Otorhinolaryngol Relat Spec 1991;53:220–34.

121. Barnes L, Taylor SR. Carotid body paragangliomas. A clinicopathologic and DNA analysis of 13 tumors. Arch Otolaryngol Head Neck Surg 1990;116:447–53.

122. Comroe JH Jr. The location and function of the chemoreceptors of the aorta. Am J Physiol 1939;127:176–91.

123. Granger JK, Hooun HY. Head and neck paragangliomas: a clinicopathologic study with DNA flow cytometric analysis. South Med J 1990;83:1407–12.

124. Heinrich MC, Harris AE, Bell WR. Metastatic intravagal paraganglioma. Case report and review of the literature. Am J Med 1985;78:1017–24.

125. Johnson TL, Zarbo RJ, Lloyd RV, Crissman JD. Paragangliomas of the head and neck: immunohistochemical neuroendocrine and intermediate filament typing. Mod Pathol 1988;1:216–23.

126. Kliewer KE, Wen DR, Cancilla PA, Cochran AJ. Paragangliomas: assessment of prognosis by histologic, immunohistochemical, and ultrastructural techniques. Hum Pathol 1989;20:29–39.

127. Lack EE. Carotid body hypertrophy in patients with cystic fibrosis and cyanotic congenital heart disease. Hum Pathol 1977;8:39–51.

128. Lack EE. Hyperplasia of vagal and carotid body paraganglia in patients with chronic hypoxemia. Am J Pathol 1978;91:497–516.

129. Lack EE, Cubilla AL, Woodruff JM. Paragangliomas of the head and neck region. A pathologic study of tumors from 71 patients. Hum Pathol 1979;10:191–218.

130. Linnoila RI, Lack EE, Steinberg SM, Keiser HR. Decreased expression of neuropeptides in malignant paragangliomas: an immunohistochemical study. Hum Pathol 1988;19:41–50.

131. Nora JD, Hallett JW Jr, O'Brien PC, Naessens JM, Cherry KJ Jr, Pairolero PC. Surgical resection of carotid body tumors: long-term survival, recurrence, and metastasis. Mayo Clin Proc 1988;63:348–52.

132. Pacheco-Ojeda L, Durango E, Rodriquez C, Vivar N. Carotid body tumors at high altitudes: Quito, Ecuador, 1987. World J Surg 1988;12:856–60.

133. Rodriquez-Cuevas H, Lau I, Rodriquez HP. High altitude paragangliomas: diagnostic and therapeutic considerations. Cancer 1986;57:672–6.

134. Sauter ER, Hollier LH, Bolton JS, Ochsner JL, Sardi A. Prognostic value of DNA flow cytometry in paragangliomas of the carotid body. J Surg Oncol 1991;46:151–3.

135. Schmid KW, Schroder S, Dockhorn-Dworniczak B, et al. Immunohistochemical demonstration of chromogranin A, chromogranin B, and secretogranin II in extra-adrenal paragangliomas. Mod Pathol 1994;7:347–52.

136. Schroder HD, Johannsen L. Demonstration of S-100 protein in sustentacular cells of phaeochromocytomas and paragangliomas. Histopathology 1986;10:1023–33.

137. Someren A, Karcioglu Z. Malignant vagal paraganglioma: report of a case and review of the literature. Am J Clin Pathol 1977;68:400–8.

138. Zbaren P, Lehmann W. Carotid body paraganglioma with metastases. Laryngoscope 1985;95:450–4.

Olfactory Neuroblastoma

139. Axe S, Kuhajda FP. Esthesioneuroblastoma. Intermediate filaments, neuroendocrine, and tissue-specific antigens. Am J Clin Pathol 1987;88:139–45.

140. Bailey BJ, Barton S. Olfactory neuroblastoma. Management and prognosis. Arch Otolaryngol 1975;101:1–5.

141. Banerjee AK, Sharma BS, Vashista RK, Kak VK. Intracranial olfactory neuroblastoma: evidence for olfactory epithelial origin. J Clin Pathol 1992;45:299–302.

142. Chan JK, Lau WH, Yuen RW. Ganglioneuroblastic transformation of olfactory neuroblastoma. Histopathology 1989;14:425–8.

143. Chaudhry AP, Haar JG, Koul A, Nickerson PA. Olfactory neuroblastoma (esthesioneuroblastoma): a light microscopic and ultrastructural study of two cases. Cancer 1979;44:564–79.

144. Choi HS, Anderson PJ. Olfactory neuroblastoma: an immuno-electron microscopic study of S-100 protein-positive cells. J Neuropathol Exp Neurol 1986;45:576–87.

145. Curtis JL, Rubinstein LJ. Pigmented olfactory neuroblastoma. A new example of melanotic neuroepithelial neoplasm. Cancer 1982;49:2136–43.

146. Djalilian M, Zujko RD, Weiland LH, Devine KD. Olfactory neuroblastoma. Surg Clin North Am 1977;57:751–62.

147. Eden BV, Debo RF, Larner JM, et al. Esthesioneuroblastoma. Long term outcome and patterns of failure—the University of Virginia experience. Cancer 1994;73:2556–62.

148. Elkon D, Hightower SI, Lim ML, Cantrell RW, Constable WC. Esthesioneuroblastoma. Cancer 1979;44:1087–94.

149. Franquemont DW, Mills SE. Sinonasal malignant melanoma. A clinicopathologic and immunohistochemical study of 14 cases. Am J Clin Pathol 1991;96:689–97.

150. Frierson HF Jr, Mills SE, Fechner RE, Taxy JB, Levine PA. Sinonasal undifferentiated carcinoma. An aggressive neoplasm derived from schneiderian epithelium and distinct from olfactory neuroblastoma. Am J Surg Pathol 1986;10:771–9.

151. Frierson HF Jr, Ross GW, Mills SE, Frankfurter A. Olfactory neuroblastoma. Additional immunohistochemical characterization. Am J Clin Pathol 1990;94:547–53.

152. Frierson HF Jr, Ross GW, Stewart FM, Newman SA, Kelly MD. Unusual sinonasal small-cell neoplasms following radiotherapy for bilateral retinoblastomas. Am J Surg Pathol 1989;13:947–54.

153. Gerard-Marchant R, Micheau C. Microscopical diagnosis of olfactory esthesioneuromas: general review and report of five cases. JNCI 1965;35:75–82.

154. Goldhammer Y, Sadeh M, Tadmor R, Leventon G. Intracranial esthesioneuroblastoma associated with unilateral visual loss. Case report. J Neurosurg 1980;53:836–40.

155. Greger V, Schirmacher P, Bohl J, et al. Possible involvement of the retinoblastoma gene in undifferentiated sinonasal carcinoma. Cancer 1990;66:1954–9.

156. Herrold KM. Induction of olfactory neuroepithelial tumors in Syrian hamsters by diethylnitrosamine. Cancer 1964;17:114–21.

157. Hyams VJ, Batsakis JG, Michaels L. Tumors of the upper respiratory tract and ear. Atlas of Tumor Pathology, 2nd series, Fascicle 25. Washington, D.C.: Armed Forces Institute of Pathology, 1988:240–8.

158. Judge DM, McGavran MH, Trapukdi S. Fume-induced fluorescence in diagnosis of nasal neuroblastoma. Arch Otolaryngol 1976;102:97–8.

159. Kadish S, Goodman M, Wang CC. Olfactory neuroblastoma. A clinical analysis of 17 cases. Cancer 1976;37:1571–6.

160. Kahn LB. Esthesioneuroblastoma. A light and electron microscopic study. Hum Pathol 1974;5:364–71.

161. Klein EA, Anzil AP, Mezzacappa P, Borderon M, Ho V. Sinonasal primitive neuroectodermal tumor arising in a long-term survivor of heritable unilateral retinoblastoma. Cancer 1992;70:423–31.

162. Lewis JS, Hutter RV, Tollefsen HR, Foote FW Jr. Nasal tumors of olfactory origin. Arch Otolaryngol 1965;81:169–74.

163. Lund VJ, Milroy C. Olfactory neuroblastoma: clinical and pathological aspects. Rhinology 1993;31:1–6.

164. Mackay B, Luna MA, Butler JJ. Adult neuroblastoma. Electron microscopic observations in nine cases. Cancer 1976;37:1334–51.

165. Margolis FL. Olfactory marker protein (OMP). Scand J Immunol 1982;15:181–99.

166. Micheau C, Guerinot F, Bohuon C, Brugere J. Dopamine-ß-hydroxylase and catecholamines in an olfactory esthesioneuroma. Cancer 1975;35:1309–12.

167. Miller DC, Goodman ML, Pilch BZ, et al. Mixed olfactory neuroblastoma and carcinoma. A report of two cases. Cancer 1984;54:2019–28.

168. Mills SE, Frierson HF Jr. Olfactory neuroblastoma. A clinicopathologic study of 21 cases. Am J Surg Pathol 1985;9:317–27.

169. Nakashima T, Kimmelman CP, Snow JB Jr. Structure of human fetal and adult olfactory neuroepithelium. Arch Otolaryngol 1984;110:641–6.

170 Nakashima T, Kimmelman CP, Snow JB Jr. Olfactory marker protein in the human olfactory pathway. Arch Otolaryngol 1985;111:294–7.

171. Ng HK, Poon WS, Poon CY, South JR. Intracranial olfactory neuroblastoma mimicking carcinoma: report of two cases. Histopathology 1988;12:393–403.

172. O'Conor GT Jr, Drake CR, Johns ME, Cail WS, Winn HR, Niskanen E. Treatment of advanced esthesioneuroblastoma with high-dose chemotherapy and autologous bone marrow transplantation. A case report. Cancer 1985;55:347–9.

173. Oberman HA, Rice DH. Olfactory neuroblastomas: a clinicopathologic study. Cancer 1976;38:2494–502.

174. Obert GJ, Devine KD, McDonald JR. Olfactory neuroblastomas. Cancer 1960;13:205–15.

175. Osamura RY, Fine G. Ultrastructure of esthesioneuroblastoma. Cancer 1976;38:173–9.

176. Pope TL Jr, Morris JL, Cail WS, Elkon D. Esthesioneuroblastoma presenting as an intracranial mass. South Med J 1994;73:643–5.

177. Reynolds CP, Smith RG, Frenkel EP. The diagnostic dilemma of the "small round cell neoplasm": catecholamine fluorescence and tissue culture morphology as markers for neuroblastoma. Cancer 1981;48:2088–94.

178. Silva EG, Butler JJ, Mackay B, Goepfert H. Neuroblastomas and neuroendocrine carcinomas of the nasal cavity. A proposed new classification. Cancer 1982;50:2388–405.

179. Singh W, Ramage C, Best P, Angus B. Nasal neuroblastoma secreting vasopressin. A case report. Cancer 1980;45:961–6.

180. Slootweg PJ, Lubsen H. Rhabdomyoblasts in olfactory neuroblastoma. Histopathology 1991;19:182–4.

181. Taxy JB, Bharani NK, Mills SE, Frierson HF Jr, Gould VE. The spectrum of olfactory neural tumors. A light-microscopic, immunohistochemical and ultrastructural analysis. Am J Surg Pathol 1986;10:687–95.

182. Taxy JB, Hidvegi DF. Olfactory neuroblastoma: an ultrastructural study. Cancer 1977;39:131–8.

183. Trojanowski JQ, Lee V, Pillsbury N, Lee S. Neuronal origin of human esthesioneuroblastoma demonstrated with anti-neurofilament monoclonal antibodies. N Engl J Med 1982;307:159–61.

184. Vollrath M, Altmannsberger M, Weber K, Osborn M. Chemically induced tumors of rat olfactory epithelium: a model for human esthesioneuroepithelioma. JNCI 1986;76:1205–16.

185. Wade PM Jr, Smith RE, Johns ME. Response of esthesioneuroblastoma to chemotherapy. Report of five cases and review of the literature. Cancer 1984;53:1036–41.

186. Wick MR, Stanley SJ, Swanson PE. Immunohistochemical diagnosis of sinonasal melanoma, carcinoma, and neuroblastoma with monoclonal antibodies HMB-45 and anti-synaptophysin. Arch Pathol Lab Med 1988;112:616–20.

187. Woodhead P, Lloyd GA. Olfactory neuroblastoma: imaging by magnetic resonance, CT and conventional techniques. Clin Otolaryngol 1988;13:387–94.

Sinonasal Undifferentiated Carcinoma

188. Battifora H. Clinical applications of the immunohistochemistry of filamentous proteins. Am J Surg Pathol 198;12(Suppl 1):24–42.

189. Frierson HF Jr, Bellafiore FJ, Gaffey MJ, McCary WS, Innes DJ Jr, Williams ME. Cytokeratin in anaplastic large cell lymphoma. Mod Pathol 1994;7:317–21.

190. Frierson HF Jr, Mills SE, Fechner RE, Taxy JB, Levine PA. Sinonasal undifferentiated carcinoma. An aggressive neoplasm derived from Schneiderian epithelium and distinct from olfactory neuroblastoma. Am J Surg Pathol 1986;10:771–9.

191. Greger V, Schirmacher P, Bohl J, et al. Possible involvement of the retinoblastoma gene in undifferentiated sinonasal carcinoma. Cancer 1990;66:1954–9.

192. Helliwell TR, Yeoh LH, Stell PM. Anaplastic carcinoma of the nose and paranasal sinuses. Light microcopy, immunohistochemistry, and clinical correlation. Cancer 1986;58:2038–45.

193. Lopategui JR, Gaffey MJ, Frierson HF Jr, et al. Detection of Epstein-Barr viral RNA in sinonasal undiffer-

entiated carcinoma from Western and Asian patients. Am J Surg Pathol 1994;18:391–8.

194. Pinkus GS, Kurtin PJ. Epithelial membrane antigen—a diagnostic discriminant in surgical pathology: immunohistochemical profile in epithelial, mesenchymal, and hematopoietic neoplasms using paraffin sections and monoclonal antibodies. Hum Pathol 1985;16:929–40.

195. Stewart FM, Laxarus HM, Levine PA, Stewart KA, Tabbara IA, Spaulding CA. High-dose chemotherapy and autologous marrow transplantation for esthesioneuroblastoma and sinonasal undifferentiated carcinoma. Am J Clin Oncol 1989;12:217–21.

196. Torjussen W, Solberg LA, Hogetveit AC. Histopathologic changes of the nasal mucosa in nickel workers. A pilot study. Cancer 1979;44:963–74.

197. Weiss LM, Movahed LA, Butler AE, et al. Analysis of lymphoepithelioma and lymphoepithelioma-like carcinomas for Epstein-Barr viral genomes by in-situ hybridization. Am J Surg Pathol 1989;13:625–31.

"Carcinoid Tumor" and "Atypical Carcinoid Tumor" (Neuroendocrine Carcinoma)

198. Ali S, Aird DW, Bihari J. Pain-inducing laryngeal paragangliomas (non-chromaffin). J Laryngol Otol 1983;97:181–8.

199. Barnes L. Paraganglioma of the larynx. A critical review of the literature. ORL J Otorhinolaryngol Relat Spec 1991;53:220–34.

200. Baugh RF, Wolf GT, Lloyd RV, McClatchey KD, Evans D. Carcinoid (neuroendocrine carcinoma) of the larynx. Ann Otol Rhinol Laryngol 1987;96:315–21.

201. Benisch BM, Tawfik B, Breitenbach EE. Primary oat cell carcinoma of the larynx: an ultrastructural study. Cancer 1975;36:145–8.

202. Bishop JW, Osamura RY, Tsutsumi Y. Multiple hormone production in an oat cell carcinoma of the larynx. Acta Pathol Jpn 1985;35:915–23.

203. Bitran JD, Toledo-Pereyra LH, Matz G. Oat cell carcinoma of the larynx: response to combined modality therapy. Cancer 1978;42:85–7.

204. Blok PH, Manni JJ, van den Brock P, van Haelst UJ, Slooff JL. Carcinoid of the larynx: a report of three cases and a review of the literature. Laryngoscope 1985;95:715–9.

205. Bone RC, Deer D. Oat cell carcinoma of the larynx. Laryngoscope 1978;88:1190–5.

206. Capper JW, Michaels L, Gregor RT. A malignant carcinoid tumor of the supraglottic larynx. J Laryngol Otol 1981;95:963–71.

207. Cefis F, Cattaneo M, Carnevale Ricci PM, Frigerio B, Usellini L, Capella C. Primary polypeptide hormones and mucin producing malignant carcinoid of the larynx. Ultrastruct Pathol 1983;5:45–53.

208. Chen DA, Mandell-Brown M, Moore SF, Johnson JT. "Composite" tumor-mixed squamous cell carcinoma and small cell anaplastic carcinoma of the larynx. Otolaryngol Head Neck Surg 1986;95:99–103.

209. Curtiss C, Kosinski AA. Primary malignant melanoma of the larynx: report of a case and review of the literature. Cancer 1955;8:961–3.

210. Dictor M, Tennvall J, Åkerman M. Moderately differentiated neuroendocrine carcinoma (atypical carcinoid) of the supraglottic larynx. A report of two cases including immunohistochemistry and aspiration cytology. Arch Pathol Lab Med 1992;116:253–7.

211. El-Naggar AK, Batsakis JG. Carcinoid tumor of the larynx. A critical review of the literature. ORL J Otorhinolaryngol Relat Spec 1991;53:188–93.

212. El-Naggar AK, Batsakis JG, Vasilopoulou-Sellin R, Ordóñez NG, Luna MA. Medullary (thyroid) carcinoma-like carcinoids of the larynx. J Laryngol Otol 1991;105:683–6.

213. Ferlito A. Oat cell carcinoma of the larynx. Ann Otol 1974;83:254–6.

214. Ferlito A. The World Health Organization's revised classification of tumours of the larynx, hypopharynx, and trachea. Ann Otol Rhinol Laryngol 1993;102:666–9.

215. Ferlito A, Friedmann I, Goldman NC. Primary carcinoid tumor of the larynx. ORL J Otohinolaryngol Relat Spec 1988;50:129–49.

216. Fisher GE, Odess JS. Metastatic malignant melanoma of the larynx. Arch Otolaryngol 1951;54:639–42.

217. Gapany-Gapanavicius B, Kenan S. Carcinoid tumor of the larynx. Ann Otol 1981;90:42–7.

218. Gelot R, Rhee TR, Lapidot A. Primary oat-cell carcinoma of head and neck. Ann Otol 1975;84:238–44.

219. Gnepp DR. Small cell neuroendocrine carcinoma of the larynx. A critical review of the literature. ORL J Otorhinolaryngol Relat Spec 1991;53:210–9.

220. Gnepp DR, Ferlito A, Hyams V. Primary anaplastic small cell (oat cell) carcinoma of the larynx. Review of the literature and report of 18 cases. Cancer 1983;51:1731–45.

221. Goldman NC, Hood CI, Singleton GT. Carcinoid of the larynx. Arch Otolaryngol 1969;90:90–3.

222. Goldman NC, Katibah GM, Medina J. Carcinoid tumors of the larynx. Ear Nose Throat J 1985;64:130–4.

223. Googe PB, Ferry JA, Bhan AK, Dickersin GR, Pilch BZ, Goodman M. A comparison of paraganglioma, carcinoid tumor, and small-cell carcinoma of the larynx. Arch Pathol Lab Med 1988;112:809–15.

224. Gould VE, Linnoila RI, Memoli VA, Warren WH. Neuroendocrine cells and neuroendocrine neoplasms of the lung. Pathol Ann 1983;18(1):287–330.

225. Gould VE, Linnoila RI, Memoli VA, Warren WH. Neuroendocrine components of the bronchopulmonary tract: hyperplasias, dysplasias, and neoplasms. Lab Invest 1983;49:519–37.

226. Johnson GD, Mahataphongse VP, Abt AB, Conner GH. Small cell undifferentiated carcinoma of the larynx. Ann Otol 1979;88:774–8.

227. Kleinsasser O. Das Glomus laryngicum inferior. Arch Ohrenheilk 1964;184:214–24.

228. Kyriakos M, Berlin BP, DeSchryver-Kecskemeti K. Oat-cell carcinoma of the larynx. Arch Otolaryngol 1978;104:168–76.

229. Lawson W, Zak FG. The glomus bodies ("paraganglia") of the human larynx. Laryngoscope 1974;84:98–111.

230. Loughead JR. Malignant melanoma of the larynx. Ann Otol Rhinol Laryngol 1952;61:154–8.

231. Markel SF, Magielski JE, Beals TF. Carcinoid tumor of the larynx. Arch Otolaryngol 1980;106:777–8.

232. Marks PV, Brookes GB. Malignant paraganglioma of the larynx. J Laryngol Otol 1983;97:1183–8.

233. Mills SE, Cooper PH, Garland TA, Johns ME. Small cell undifferentiated carcinoma of the larynx. Report of two patients and review of 13 additional cases. Cancer 1983;51:116–20.

234. Mills SE, Johns ME. Atypical carcinoid tumor of the larynx: a light microscopic and ultrastructural study. Arch Otolaryngol 1984;110:58–62.

235. Milroy CM, Rode J, Moss E. Laryngeal paragangliomas and neuroendocrine carcinomas. Histopathology 1991;18:201–9.

236. Mullins JD, Newman RK, Coltman CA. Primary oat cell carcinoma of the larynx. A case report and review of the literature. Cancer 1979;43:711–7.

237. Myerowitz RL, Barnes EL, Myers E. Small cell anaplastic (oat cell) carcinoma of the larynx: report of a case and review of the literature. Laryngoscope 1978;88:1697–702.

238. Olofsson J, van Nostrand AW. Anaplastic small cell carcinoma of larynx. Case report. Ann Otol 1972;81:284–7.

239. Pantazopoulos PE. Primary malignant melanoma of the larynx. Laryngoscope 1964;74:95–102.

240. Patterson SD, Yarrington CT. Carcinoid tumor of the larynx: the role of conservative therapy. Ann Otol Rhinol Laryngol 1987;96:12–4.

241. Porto DP, Wick MR, Ewing SL, Adams GL. Neuroendocrine carcinoma of the larynx. Am J Otolaryngol 1987;9:97–104.

242. Reuter VE, Woodruff JM. Melanoma of the larynx. Laryngoscope 1986;94:389–93.

243. Shanmugaratnam K, Sobin LH. The World Health Organization histological classification of tumours of the upper respiratory tract and ear. A commentary on the second edition. Cancer 1993;71:2689–97.

244. Sneige N, Mackay B, Ordóñez NG, Batsakis JG. Laryngeal paraganglioma. Report of two tumors with immunohistochemical and ultrastructural analysis. Arch Otolaryngol 1983;109:113–7.

245. Snyderman C, Johnson JT, Barnes L. Carcinoid tumor of the larynx: case report and review of the world literature. Otolaryngol Head Neck Surg 1986;95:158–64.

246. Soussi AC, Benghiat A, Holgate CS, Majumdar B. Neuroendocrine tumors of the head and neck. J Laryngol Otol 1990;104:504–7.

247. Spagnolo DV, Paradinas FJ. Laryngeal neuroendocrine tumour with features of a paraganglioma, intracytoplasmic lumina and acinar formation. Histopathology 1985;9:117–31.

248. Stanley RJ, DeSanto LW, Weiland LH. Oncocytic and oncocytoid carcinoid tumors (well-differentiated neuroendocrine carcinomas) of the larynx. Arch Otolaryngol Head Neck Surg 1986;112:529–35.

249. Stanley RJ, Weiland LH, Neel B. Pain-inducing laryngeal paraganglioma: report of the ninth case and review of the literature. Otolaryngol Head Neck Surg 1986;95:107–12.

250. Sun CJ, Hall-Craggs M, Adler B. Oat cell carcinoma of larynx. Arch Otolaryngol 1981;107:506–9.

251. Sweeney EC, McDonnell L, O'Brien C. Medullary carcinoma of the thyroid presenting as tumors of the pharynx and larynx. Histopathology 1981;5:263–75.

252. Tamai S, Iri H, Maruyama T, et al. Laryngeal carcinoid tumor. Light and electron microscopic studies. Cancer 1981;48:2256–9.

253. Vetters JM, Toner PG. Chemodectoma of larynx. J Pathol 1970;101:259–65.

254. Watska MA. Uber die Paraganglien in der Plica ventricularis des menschlichen Kehlkopfes. Dtsch Med Forsch 1963;1:19–20.

255. Wenig BM, Gnepp DR. The spectrum of neuroendocrine carcinomas of the larynx. Sem Diagn Pathol 1989; 6:329–50.

256. Wenig BM, Hyams VJ, Heffner DK. Moderately differentiated neuroendocrine carcinoma of the larynx. A clinicopathologic study of 54 cases. Cancer 1988;62:2658–76.

257. Wetmore RF, Tronzo RD, Lane RJ, Lowry LD. Nonfunctional paraganglioma of the larynx: clinical and pathological considerations. Cancer 1981;48:2717–23.

258. Woodruff JM, Huvos AG, Erlandson RA, Shah JP, Gerold FP. Neuroendocrine carcinomas of the larynx. A study of two types, one of which mimics thyroid medullary carcinoma. Am J Surg Pathol 1985;9:771–90.

259. Woodruff JM, Senie RT. Atypical carcinoid tumor of the larynx. A critical review of the literature. ORL J Otorhinolaryngol Relat Spec 1991;53:194–209.

Small Cell Undifferentiated (Neuroendocrine) Carcinoma

260. Banks ER, Frierson HF Jr, Mills SE, George E, Zarbo RJ, Swanson PE. Basaloid squamous cell carcinoma of the head and neck. A clinicopathologic and immunohistochemical study of 40 cases. Am J Surg Pathol 1992;16:939–46.

261. Baugh RF, Wolf GT, McClatchey KD. Small cell carcinoma of the head and neck. Head Neck Surg 1986;8:343–54.

262. Benisch BM, Tawfik B, Breitenbach EE. Primary oat cell carcinoma of the larynx: an ultrastructural study. Cancer 1975;36:145–8.

263. Bishop JW, Osamura RY, Tsutsumi Y. Multiple hormone production in an oat cell carcinoma of the larynx. Acta Pathol Jpn 1985;35:915–23.

264. Ferlito A. Diagnosis and treatment of small cell carcinoma of the larynx: a critical review. Ann Otol Rhinol Laryngol 1986;95:590–600.

265. Ferlito A, Friedmann I. Review of neuroendocrine carcinomas of the larynx. Ann Otol Rhinol Laryngol 1989;98:780–90.

266. Ferlito A, Pesavento G, Recher G, et al. Long-term survival in response to combined chemotherapy and radiotherapy in laryngeal small cell carcinoma. Auris Nasus Larynx 1986;13:113–23.

267. Frierson HF Jr, Mills SE, Fechner RE, Taxy JB, Levine PA. Sinonasal undifferentiated carcinoma. An aggressive neoplasm derived from schneiderian epithelium and distinct from olfactory neuroblastoma. Am J Surg Pathol 1986;10:771–9.

268. Frierson HF Jr, Ross GW, Mills SE, Frankfurter A. Olfactory neuroblastoma. Additional immunohistochemical characterization [see comments]. Am J Clin Pathol 1990;94:547–53.

269. Gnepp DR. Small cell neuroendocrine carcinoma of the larynx. A critical review of the literature. ORL J Otorhinolaryngol Relat Spec 1991;53:210–9.

270. Gnepp DR, Ferlito A, Hyams V. Primary anaplastic small cell (oat cell) carcinoma of the larynx. Review of the literature and report of 18 cases. Cancer 1983;51:1731–45.

271. Googe PB, Ferry JA, Bhan AK, Dickersin GR, Pilch BZ, Goodman M. A comparison of paraganglioma, carcinoid tumor, and small-cell carcinoma of the larynx. Arch Pathol Lab Med 1988;112:809–15.

272. Hamlyn PJ, O'Brien CJ, Shaw HJ. Uncommon malignant tumors of the larynx. A 35 year review. J Laryngol Otol 1986;100:1163–8.

273. Helliwell TR, Yeoh LH, Stell PM. Anaplastic carcinoma of the nose and paranasal sinuses. Light microscopy, immunohistochemistry, and clinical correlation. Cancer 1986;58:2038–45.

274. Johnson GD, Mahataphongse VP, Abt AB, Conner GH. Small cell undifferentiated carcinoma of the larynx. Ann Otol 1979;88:774–8.

275. Kameya T, Shimosato Y, Adachi I, Abe K, Ebihara S, Ono I. Neuroendocrine carcinoma of the paranasal sinus. A morphological and endocrinological study. Cancer 1980;45:330–9.

276. Klijanienko J, El-Naggar A, Ponzio-Prion A, Marandas P, Micheau C, Caillaud JM. Basaloid squamous carcinoma of the head and neck. Immunohistochemical comparison with adenoid cystic carcinoma and squamous cell carcinoma. Arch Otolaryngol Head Neck Surg 1993;119:887–90.

277. Koss LG, Spiro RH, Hajdu S. Small cell (oat cell) carcinoma of minor salivary gland origin. Cancer 1972;30:737–41.

278. Luna MA, El-Naggar A, Parichatikanond P, Weber RS, Batsakis JG. Basaloid squamous carcinoma of the upper aerodigestive tract. Clinicopathologic and DNA flow cytometric analysis. Cancer 1990;66:537–42.

279. Mills SE, Cooper PH, Garland TA, Johns ME. Small cell undifferentiated carcinoma of the larynx. Report of two patients and review of 13 additional cases. Cancer 1983;51:116–20.

280. Ordóñez NG, Mackay B. Neuroendocrine tumors of the nasal cavity. Pathol Annu 1993;28(2):77–111.

281. Pardo Mindan FJ, Algarra SM, Lozano BR, Tapia RG. Oat cell carcinoma of the larynx. A study of six new cases. Histopathology 1989;14:75–80.

282. Raychowdhuri RN. Oat cell carcinoma and paranasal sinuses. J Laryngol Otol 1965;79:253–5.

283. Rejowski JE, Campanella RS, Block LJ. Small cell carcinoma of the nose and paranasal sinuses. Otolaryngol Head Neck Surg 1982;90:516–7.

284. Silva EG, Butler JJ, Mackay B, Goepfert H. Neuroblastomas and neuroendocrine carcinomas of the nasal cavity. A proposed new classification. Cancer 1982;50:2388–405.

285. Soussi AC, Benghiat A, Holgate CS, Majumdar B. Neuroendocrine tumors of the head and neck. J Laryngol Otol 1990;104:504–7.

286. Sun CJ, Hall-Craggs M, Adler B. Oat cell carcinoma of larynx. Arch Otolaryngol 1981;107:506–9.

287. Taxy JB, Bharani NK, Mills SE, Frierson HF Jr, Gould VE. The spectrum of olfactory neural tumors. A light-microscopic, immunohistochemical and ultrastructural analysis. Am J Surg Pathol 1986;10:687–95.

288. Wain SL, Kier R, Vollmer RT, Bossen EH. Basaloid-squamous carcinoma of the tongue, hypopharynx, and larynx: report of 10 cases. Hum Pathol 1986;17:1158–66.

289. Weiss MD, deFies HO, Taxy JB, Braine H. Primary small cell carcinoma of the paranasal sinuses. Arch Otolaryngol 1983;109:341–3.

290. Woodruff JM, Huvos AG, Erlandson RA, Shah JP, Gerold FP. Neuroendocrine carcinomas of the larynx. A study of two types, one of which mimics thyroid medullary carcinoma. Am J Surg Pathol 1985;9:771–90.

Malignant Melanoma

291. Banerjee AK, Sharma BS, Vashista RK, Kak VK. Intracranial olfactory neuroblastoma: evidence for olfactory epithelial origin. J Clin Pathol 1992;45:299–302.

292. Barton RT. Mucosal melanomas of the head and neck. Laryngoscope 1975;85:93–9.

293. Berthelsen A, Andersen AP, Jensen S, Hansen HS. Melanomas of the mucosa in the oral cavity and the upper respiratory passages. Cancer 1984;54:907–12.

294. Bittesini L, Dei Tos AP, Fletcher CD. Metastatic melanoma showing a rhabdoid phenotype: further evidence of a nonspecific histological pattern. Histopathology 1992;20:167–70.

295. Calabrese V, Cifola M, Pareschi R, Parma A, Sonzogni A. Primary malignant melanoma of the oral cavity. J Laryngol Otol 1989;103:887–9.

296. Catlin D. Mucosal melanomas of the head and neck. Am J Roentgenol 1967;99:809–16.

297. Chang ES, Wick MR, Swanson PE, Dehner LP. Metastatic malignant melanoma with rhabdoid features. Am J Clin Pathol 1994;102:426–31.

298. Choi HS, Anderson PJ. Olfactory neuroblastoma: an immuno-electron microscopic study of S-100 protein-positive cells. J Neuropathol Exp Neurol 1986;45:576–87.

299. Cove H. Melanosis, melanocytic hyperplasia, and primary malignant melanoma of the nasal cavity. Cancer 1994;44:1424–33.

300. Curtiss C, Kosinski AA. Primary malignant melanoma of the larynx: report of a case and review of the literature. Cancer 1955;8:961–3.

301. Drier JK, Swanson PE, Cherwitz DL, Wick MR. S100 protein immunoreactivity in poorly differentiated carcinomas. Immunohistochemical comparison with malignant melanoma. Arch Pathol Lab Med 1987;111:447–52.

302. Eisen D, Voorhees JJ. Oral melanoma and other pigmented lesions of the oral cavity. J Am Acad Dermatol 1991;24:527–37.

303. Fisher GE, Odess JS. Metastatic malignant melanoma of the larynx. Arch Otolaryngol 1951;54:639–42.

304. Fitzgibbons PL, Chaurushiya PS, Nichols PW, Chandrasoma PT, Martin SE. Primary mucosal malignant melanoma: an immunohistochemical study of 12 cases with comparison to cutaneous and metastatic melanomas. Hum Pathol 1989;20:269–72.

305. Franquemont DW, Mills SE. Sinonasal malignant melanoma. A clinicopathologic and immunohistochemical study of 14 cases. Am J Clin Pathol 1991;96:689–97.

306. Freedman HM, DeSanto LW, Devine KD, Weiland LH. Malignant melanoma of the nasal cavity and paranasal sinuses. Arch Otolaryngol 1973;97:322–5.

307. Frierson HF Jr, Ross GW, Mills SE, Frankfurter A. Olfactory neuroblastoma. Additional immunohistochemical characterization [see comments]. Am J Clin Pathol 1990;94:547–53.

308. Gatter KC, Ralfkiaer E, Skinner J, et al. An immunocytochemical study of malignant melanoma and its differential diagnosis from other malignant tumors. J Clin Pathol 1985;38:1353–7.

309. Gaze MN, Kerr GR, Smyth JF. Mucosal melanomas of the head and neck: the Scottish experience. The Scottish Melanoma Group. Clin Oncol (R Coll Radiol) 1990;2:277–83.

310. Goldman JL, Lawson W, Zak FG, Roffman JD. The presence of melanocytes in the human larynx. Laryngoscope 1972;82:824–35.

311. Gouldesbrough DR, Martin-Hirsch DP, Lannigan F. Intranasal malignant melanoma arising in an inverted papilloma. Histopathology 1992;20:523–6.

312. Gown AM, Vogel AM, Hoak D, Gough F, McNutt MA. Monoclonal antibodies specific for melanocytic tumors distinguish subpopulations of melanocytes. Am J Pathol 1986;123:195–203.

313. Guzzo M, Grandi C, Licitra L, Podrecca S, Cascinelli N, Molinari R. Mucosal malignant melanoma of head and neck: forty-eight cases treated at Istituto Nazionale Tumori of Milan. Eur J Surg Oncol 1993;19:316–9.

314. Harrison DF. Malignant melanomata of the nasal cavity. Proc Royal Soc Med 1968;61:13–8.

315. Harrison DF. Malignant melanomata arising in the nasal mucous membrane. J Laryngol Otol 1976;90:993–1005.

316. Henzen-Logmans SC, Meijer CJ, Ruiter DJ, Mullink H, Balm AJ, Snow GB. Diagnostic application of panels of antibodies in mucosal melanomas of the head and neck. Cancer 1988;61:702–11.

317. Herrera GA, Turbat-Herrera EA, Lott RL. S100 protein expression by primary and metastatic adenocarcinomas. Am J Clin Pathol 1988;89:168–76.

318. Holdcraft J, Gallagher JC. Malignant melanomas of the nasal and paranasal sinus mucosa. Ann Otol Rhinol Laryngol 1969;78:5–16.

319. Kapadia SB, Frisman DM, Hitchcock CL, Ellis GL, Popek EJ. Melanotic neuroectodermal tumor of infancy. Clinicopathologic, immunohistochemical, and flow cytometric study. Am J Surg Pathol 1993;17:566–73.

320. Kato T, Takematsu H, Tomita Y, Takahashi M, Abe R. Malignant melanoma of mucous membranes. A clinicopathologic study of 13 cases in Japanese patients. Arch Dermatol 1987;123:216–20.

321. Lambe CD, Cartun RW, Knibb DR, Ricci AJ. Immunocytochemical reactivity with cytokeratin monoclonal antibodies in malignant melanoma. Further evidence dictating cautious interpretation of immuno-staining results [Abstract]. Mod Pathol 1989;2:50A.

322. Liversedge RL. Oral malignant melanoma. Br J Oral Surg 1975;13:40–55.

323. Loughead JR. Malignant melanoma of the larynx. Ann Otol Rhinol Laryngol 1952;61:154–8.

324. Lund V. Malignant melanoma of the nasal cavity and paranasal sinuses. J Laryngol Otol 1982;96:347–55.

325. Moore ES, Martin H. Melanoma of the upper respiratory tract and oral cavity. Cancer 1955;8:1167–76.

326. Ohashi K, Kasuga T, Tanaka N, Enomoto S, Horiuchi J, Okada N. Malignant melanomas of the oral cavity: heterogeneity of pathological and clinical features. Virchows Arch [A] 1992;420:43–50.

327. Ordóñez NG, Ji XL, Hickey RC. Comparison of HMB-45 monoclonal antibody and S100 protein in the immunohistochemical diagnosis of melanoma. Am J Clin Pathol 1988;90:385–90.

328. Panje WR, Moran WJ. Melanoma of the upper aerodigestive tract: a review of 21 cases. Head Neck Surg 1986;8:309–12.

329. Pantazopoulos PE. Primary malignant melanoma of the larynx. Laryngoscope 1964;74:95–102.

330. Pesce C, Toncini C. Melanin pigmentation of the larynx. Acta Otolaryngol 1983;90:189–92.

331. Pettinato G, Manivel JC, d'Amore ES, Jaszcz W, Gorlin RJ. Melanotic neuroectodermal tumor of infancy. A reexamination of a histogenetic problem based on immuno-

histochemical, flow cytometric, and ultrastructural study of 10 cases. Am J Surg Pathol 1991;15:233–45.

332. Rapini RP, Golitz LE, Greer RO, Krekorian EA, Poulson T. Primary malignant melanoma of the oral cavity. A review of 177 cases. Cancer 1985;55:1543–51.

333. Reuter VE, Woodruff JM. Melanoma of the larynx. Laryngoscope 1986;94:389–93.

334. Shanon E, Covo J, Loeventhal M. Melanoma of the epiglottis. A case treated by supraglottic laryngectomy. Arch Otolaryngol 1970;91:304–5.

335. Snow GB, Van der Esch EP, Van Slooten EA. Mucosal melanomas of the head and neck. Head Neck Surg 1978;1:24–30.

336. Trapp TK, Fu YS, Calcaterra TC. Melanoma of the nasal and paranasal sinus mucosa. Arch Otolaryngol Head Neck Surg 1987;113:1086–9.

337. Umeda M, Mishima Y, Teranobu O, Nakanishi K, Shimada K. Heterogeneity of primary malignant melanomas in oral mucosa: an analysis of 43 cases in Japan. Pathology 1988;20:234–41.

338. Umeda M, Shimada K. Primary malignant melanoma of the oral cavity—its histological classification and treatment. Br J Oral Maxillofac Surg 1994;32:39–47.

339. van der Waal RI, Snow GB, Karim AB, van der Waal I. Primary malignant melanoma of the oral cavity: a review of eight cases. Br Dent J 1994;176:185–8.

340. Whicker JH, Carder GA, Devine KA. Metastasis to the larynx. Report of a case and review of the literature. Arch Otolaryngol 1972;96:182–4.

341. Wick MR, Stanley SJ, Swanson PE. Immunohistochemical diagnosis of sinonasal melanoma, carcinoma, and neuroblastoma with monoclonal antibodies HMB-45 and antisynaptophysin. Arch Pathol Lab Med 1988;112:616–20.

342. Zak FG, Lawson W. The presence of melanocytes in the nasal cavity. Ann Otol Rhinol Laryngol 1974;83:515–9.

343. Zarbo RJ, Gown AM, Nagle RB, Visscher DW, Crissman JD. Anomalous cytokeratin expression in malignant melanoma: one- and two-dimensional western blot analysis and immunohistochemical survey of 100 melanomas. Mod Pathol 1990;3:494–501.

Peripheral Neuroectodermal Tumor/Extraosseous Ewing's Sarcoma

344. Askin FB, Rosai J, Sibley RK, Dehner LP, McAlister WH. Malignant small cell tumor of the thoracopulmonary region in childhood. Cancer 1979;43:2438–51.

345. Cavazzana AO, Ninfo V, Roberts J, Triche TJ. Peripheral neuroepithelioma: a light microscopic, immunocytochemical, and ultrastructural study. Mod Pathol 1992;5:71–8.

346. Dehner LP. Primitive neuroectodermal tumor and Ewing's sarcoma. Am J Surg Pathol 1993;17:1–13.

347. Douglass EC. Chromosomal rearrangements in Ewing's sarcoma and peripheral neuroectodermal tumor (PNET). Semin Devel Biol 1990;1:393–6.

348. Gonzalez-Crussi F, Wolfson SL, Misugi K, Nakajima T. Peripheral neuroectodermal tumors of the chest wall in childhood. Cancer 1984;54:2519–27.

349. Jurgens H, Bier V, Harms D, et al. Malignant peripheral neuroectodermal tumors: a retrospective analysis of 42 patients. Cancer 1988;61:349–57.

350. Llnnoila RI, Tsokos M, Triche TJ, Marangos PJ, Chandra RS. Evidence for neural origin and PAS-pos-

itive variants of the malignant small cell tumor of thoracopulmonary region ("Askin tumor"). Am J Surg Pathol 1986;10:124–33.

351. Liombart-Bosch A, Terrier-Lacombe J, Peydro-Olaya A, Contesso G. Peripheral neuroectodermal sarcoma of soft tissue (peripheral neuroepithelioma): a pathologic study of ten cases with differential diagnosis regarding other small, round-cell sarcomas. Hum Pathol 1989;20:273–80.

352. Marina NM, Etcubanas E, Parham DM, Bowman LC, Green A. Peripheral neuroectodermal tumor (peripheral neuroepithelioma) in children. A review of the St. Jude experience and controversies in diagnosis and management. Cancer 1989;64:1952–60.

353. Moll R, Lee I, Gould VE, Berndt R, Roessner A, Franke WW. Immunocytochemical analysis of Ewing's tumors. Patterns of expression of intermediate filaments and desmosomal proteins indicate cell type heterogeneity and pluripotential differentiation. Am J Pathol 1987;127:288–304.

354. Pappo AS, Douglass EC, Meyer WH, Marina N, Parham DM. Use of HBA 71 and anti-(beta)-microglobulin to distinguish peripheral neuroepithelioma from neuroblastoma. Hum Pathol 1993;24:880–5.

355. Parham DM, Dias P, Kelly DR, Rutledge JC, Houghton P. Desmin positivity in primitive neuroectodermal tumors of childhood. Am J Surg Pathol 1992;16:483–92.

356. Riopel M, Dickman PS, Link MP, Perlman EJ. MIC2 analysis in pediatric lymphomas and leukemias. Hum Pathol 1994;25:396–9.

357. Schmidt D, Herrmann C, Jurgens H, Harms D. Malignant peripheral neuroectodermal tumor and its necessary distinction from Ewing's sarcoma. A report from the Kiel pedatric tumor registry. Cancer 1991;68:2251–9.

358. Shimada H, Newton WA, Soule EH, Qualman SJ, Aoyama C, Maurer HM. Pathologic features of extraosseous Ewing's sarcoma: a report from the intergroup rhabdomyosarcoma study. Hum Pathol 1988;19:442–53.

359. Shinoda M, Tsutsumi Y, Hata JI, Yokoyama S. Peripheral neuroepithelioma in childhood: immunohistochemical demonstration of epithelial differentiation. Arch Pathol Lab Med 1988;112:1155–8.

360. Sorensen PH, Liu XF, Delattre O, et al. Reverse transcriptase PCR amplification of EWS/FLI-1 fusion transcripts as a diagnostic test for peripheral primitive neuroectodermal tumors of childhood. Diagn Mol Pathol 1993;2:147–57.

361. Stephenson CF, Bridge JA, Sandberg AA. Cytogenetic and pathologic aspects of Ewing's sarcoma and neuroectodermal tumors. Hum Pathol 1992;23:1270–7.

362. Swanson PE, Humphrey PA, Dehner LP. Immunoreactivity for bcl-2 protein in peripheral primitive neuroectodermal tumors. Appl Immunohistochem 1993;1:182–7.

363. Taylor C, Patel K, Jones T, Kiely F, DeStavola BL, Sheer D. Diagnosis of Ewing's sarcoma and peripheral neuroectodermal tumor based on the detection of t(11;22) using fluorescence in situ hybridization. Br J Cancer 1993;67:128–33.

364. Turc-Carel C, Aurias A, Mugneret F, et al. Chromosomes in Ewing's sarcoma. I. An evaluation of 85 cases of remarkable consistency of t(11;22)(q24;q12). Cancer Genet Cytogenet 1988;32:229–38.

365. Weidner N, Tjoe J. Immunohistochemical profile of monoclonal antibody 013: antibody that recognizes glycoprotein p30/32mic2 and is useful in diagnosing Ewing's sarcoma and peripheral neuroepithelioma. Am J Surg Pathol 1994;18:486–94.

8

LYMPHOID LESIONS

HYPERPLASIA OF WALDEYER'S RING IN HUMAN IMMUNODEFICIENCY VIRUS INFECTION

The function of the tonsils and adenoid is to protect the upper aerodigestive tract from external antigens. The adenoid is lined by ciliated or squamous epithelium and nonciliated flat epithelium composed of cells with multiple microfolds (M cells) (fig. 8-1) (5). These M cells form compartments (intraepithelial channels) for lymphocytes. This lymphoepithelium probably transplants antigen via the M cells to the lymphoid follicles lying below. In addition to M cells, immunophenotypic examination has shown that the crypt epithelium overlying the lymphoid follicles in the tonsils and adenoid resembles Peyer's patch mucosa, as it contains intraepithelial B lymphocytes, some clusters of CD4-positive T lymphocytes, and some Leu-8–positive cells (fig. 8-2) (2). Clusters of CD19-, CD20-, and CD22-positive B cells are accompanied by fewer CD3- and CD4-positive T lymphocytes, which are often present in small groups. Some intraepithelial lymphocytes are also positive for

CD5, CD8, and CD7. There are more α/β T lymphocytes than γ/δ T cells in crypt epithelium and in the superficial lamina propria. The squamous epithelium contains CD1a-positive Langerhans cells and CD1a-negative dendritic mononuclear cells. The germinal centers within follicles have the expected number of B cells, which are positive for CD19, CD20, CD21, and CD22. Tingible body macrophages and follicle dendritic cells are also conspicuous. The interfollicular zone contains predominately T lymphocytes with larger numbers of CD4- than CD8-positive T cells.

General Features. Lymphoid hyperplasia of the tonsils and adenoid is commonly observed in young children and adolescents. This condition typically poses no clinical or pathologic diagnostic dilemma. In adults, however, enlargement of Waldeyer's ring (adenoid, tonsils, and base of the tongue) may be due to neoplasm or to specific infections; hyperplasia of the tonsils and adenoid is sometimes observed in patients infected with the human immunodeficiency virus 1 (HIV-1) (1,3,4).

Clinical Features. Most patients with HIV infection and hyperplasia of the lymphoid tissue of Waldeyer's ring are men in the third to fifth

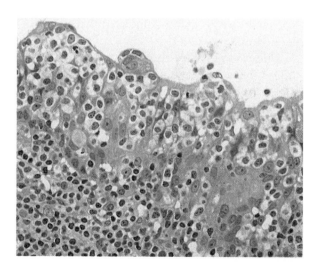 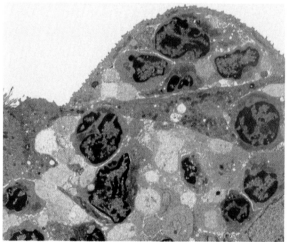

Figure 8-1
NORMAL ADENOID
M cells, which are nonciliated and flat epithelial cells, form compartments for lymphocytes that are important for recognition and response to external antigens. (Courtesy of Dr. D.J. Innes, Jr., Charlottesville, VA.)

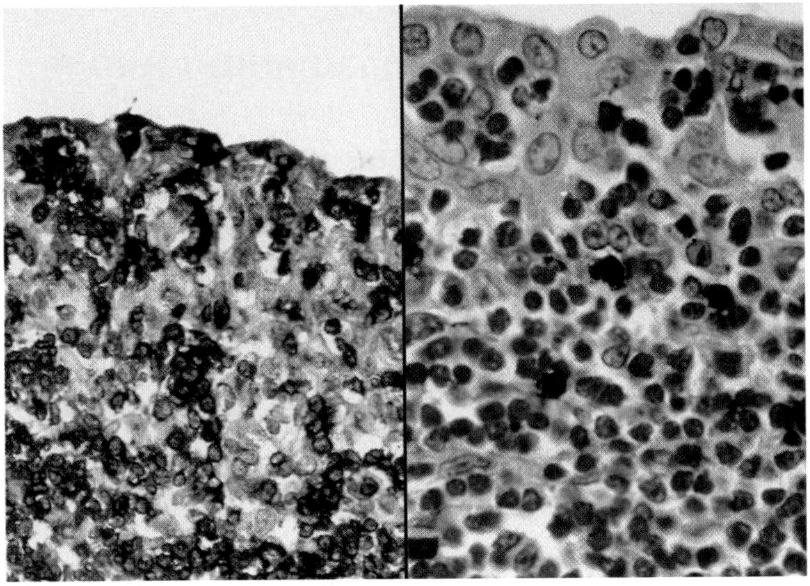

Figure 8-2
NORMAL ADENOID
Intraepithelial and subepithelial B cells (CD22 positive) outnumber T cells (CD3 positive). (Courtesy of Dr. D.J. Innes, Jr., Charlottesville, VA.)

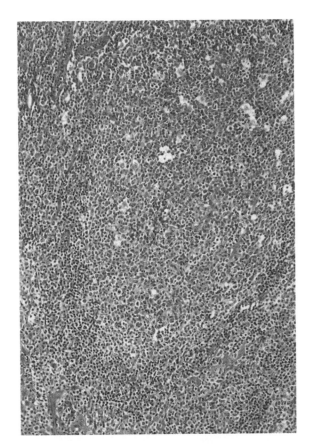

Figure 8-3
HYPERPLASIA OF WALDEYER'S RING IN
HUMAN IMMUNODEFICIENCY VIRUS INFECTION
Lymphoid tissue of the tonsil shows follicular hyperplasia with attenuated mantle zones.

decade of life (3,4). Many have no symptoms of HIV infection, but some are known to be HIV positive or to have acquired immunodeficiency syndrome (AIDS). Symptoms include a nasopharyngeal mass, nasal stuffiness, pharyngitis, epistaxis, hearing loss, otalgia, serous otitis media, and fever. Sometimes cervical lymphadenopathy is observed. The diffuse enlargement of tonsils is usually symmetrical, but may be quite bulky, simulating neoplasia. Enlargement of Waldeyer's ring lymphoid tissue may then prompt surgery.

Gross Findings. Hyperplastic lymphoid tissue is tan-white, soft to somewhat firm, and may be nodular.

Microscopic Findings. The histologic features (florid follicular hyperplasia with or without follicle lysis and the presence of multinucleated giant cells) are highly suspicious for HIV infection even when they are seen in asymptomatic young men (4). The florid follicular hyperplasia with enlarged follicles and irregularly shaped germinal centers is similar to that seen in lymph nodes of patients with early HIV infection (fig. 8-3) (3,4). The germinal centers typically contain prominent tingible body macrophages and mitotic figures. The mantle zones may be attenuated or virtually absent. Follicle lysis, the apparent invagination of mantle zone lymphocytes into follicular centers, is commonly observed. In addition there is monocytoid B-cell hyperplasia and interfollicular expansion of immunoblasts, plasma cells, small lymphocytes,

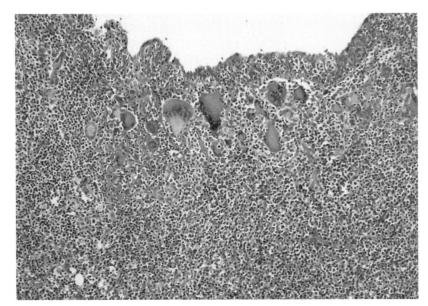

Figure 8-4
HYPERPLASIA OF WALDEYER'S
RING IN HUMAN
IMMUNODEFICIENCY
VIRUS INFECTION
Multinucleated giant cells are often located just beneath the tonsillar epithelium.

and histiocytes. Foci of hemorrhage may be present in the interfollicular areas. Multinucleated giant cells were observed in 10 of 12 patients in one study (4). When present, they tend to be located adjacent to the surface or tonsillar crypt squamous epithelium (fig. 8-4). They may also be scattered randomly within the lymphoid tissue and occasionally are present within germinal centers. The nuclei of the giant cells are usually seen along the periphery of the cytoplasm, but occasionally they are clustered in the center (fig. 8-5). Giant cells are seen more often in patients with early HIV infection, and can be absent in advanced disease. They may play an important role as reservoirs of HIV and in transmission of the virus within cells of extranodal lymphoid tissue (4). Histochemical stains for fungi and acid fast bacteria are typically negative in these cells.

In late stage HIV infection, lymphoid tissue within Waldeyer's ring may involute or even atrophy. Germinal centers are few or absent, and the interfollicular areas consist of modest numbers of immunoblasts and plasma cells, and stromal vascular proliferation.

Immunohistochemical Findings. The germinal centers show a dense and intact meshwork of CD21-positive dendritic reticulum cells. HIV p24 core protein has been localized to the follicular dendritic cells, scattered interfollicular lymphoid cells, dendritic cells within the surface and crypt squamous epithelium, and within the

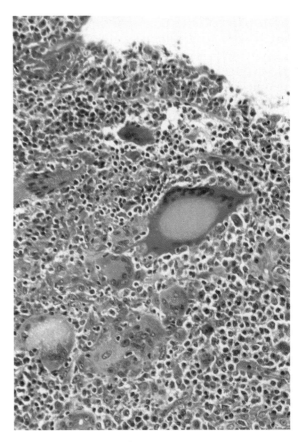

Figure 8-5
HYPERPLASIA OF WALDEYER'S RING IN
HUMAN IMMUNODEFICIENCY VIRUS INFECTION
Multinucleated giant cells in the tonsil are likely important in the transmission of the virus.

multinucleated giant cells (1,4). The multinucleated giant cells are S-100 and CD68 positive, but lack the immunoreactivity typical of B or T cells (4). In the late stages of HIV infection when lymphoid depletion is apparent, there is a relative lack of CD3-positive cells and an increase in polyclonal plasma cells.

Differential Diagnosis. The finding of florid follicular hyperplasia (with or without follicle lysis) and multinucleated giant cells in the tonsils or adenoid of young men should suggest the possibility of HIV infection. Malignant lymphoma is typically not a consideration in resected tonsils or adenoid with these microscopic features (4). Patients with HIV infection may develop lymphoma in the upper aerodigestive tract, however; such lymphomas typically are high grade (6).

Treatment and Prognosis. Excision of tonsils, adenoid, or both may be necessary if symptoms related to enlargement do not subside. For instance, adenoidectomy may be required for hearing loss. Overall, the long-term prognosis for patients with Waldeyer's ring lymphoid hyperplasia due to HIV infection is not different from that for patients with HIV infection in general.

INFECTIOUS MONONUCLEOSIS

General Features. When primary infection with the Epstein-Barr virus (EBV) is delayed until adolescence or young adulthood, infectious mononucleosis develops in approximately 50 percent of infected patients (11). Viral entry is likely into B lymphocytes located in Waldeyer's ring (15,19,20). The diagnosis of infectious mononucleosis is based on typical clinical, hematologic, and serologic findings. Cervical lymph nodes or tonsils are not biopsied in usual cases, but may be sampled when the diagnosis has not been established or when there are atypical clinical findings. Biopsy may be obtained when lymphoma is a clinical possibility, which may be suspected in a patient more than 30 years old who has generalized lymphadenopathy or isolated adenopathy in an unusual site, tonsillar enlargement producing obstruction, or a negative heterophil antibody test (18). When infectious mononucleosis is not suspected clinically, the microscopic findings in tonsillar specimens can pose difficult diagnostic problems for the surgical pathologist, and may lead to a misdiagnosis of malignant lymphoma.

Clinical Features. Infectious mononucleosis occurs in patients of all ages, but most often presents in adolescents or young adults. There is no sex predilection. The usual clinical features are sore throat, fever, malaise, cervical lymphadenopathy, and occasional splenomegaly. There is also lymphocytosis in the peripheral blood with atypical lymphocytes observed. The diagnosis is usually based upon these clinical findings as well as positive serology (positive Mono-Spot test or positive Paul-Bunnell heterophile antibody test). Other serologic tests that may be required include those for EBV viral capsid antigen, nuclear antigen, or early antigen.

Gross Findings. The tonsils are enlarged, swollen, and may show a tan-gray surface exudate.

Microscopic Findings. Changes range from obviously benign findings to those highly suggestive of malignant lymphoma (9). Importantly, there is some distortion but not complete effacement of the lymphoid tissue (10,16,18). Reactive follicular hyperplasia, which is often moderate or marked, is a typical microscopic feature (fig. 8-6). The follicles may be bizarre shaped and fused. Within the follicles, tingible body macrophages are quite conspicuous. The interfollicular areas are expanded by immunoblasts, small lymphocytes, plasma cells, and histiocytes. Immunoblasts are present in clusters and sheets, and mitotic figures are usually readily seen. Immunoblasts may cluster around necrotic foci (fig. 8-7). Apoptotic cells are also observed. Necrosis of surface epithelium may be striking. Although the proliferation of immunoblasts may simulate malignant lymphoma, there is a merging of the immunoblasts with the cells in the reactive follicles and paracortex. Reed-Sternberg–like cells may be present, particularly beneath the crypt epithelium and adjacent to areas of necrosis (fig. 8-8) (9,13,18). These cells have single or multiple, basophilic nuclei which, in most cases, lack the inclusion-like large eosinophilic nucleoli of Reed-Sternberg cells. The cytoplasm of these mimics of Reed-Sternberg cells is basophilic, and there is often a juxtanuclear clear zone. Such cells are not numerous.

Immunohistochemical and In Situ Hybridization Findings. The lymphoid proliferation consists predominantly of activated T lymphocytes (1). There may be a predominance of CD8- over CD4-positive T cells. The immunoblasts may be of B cell

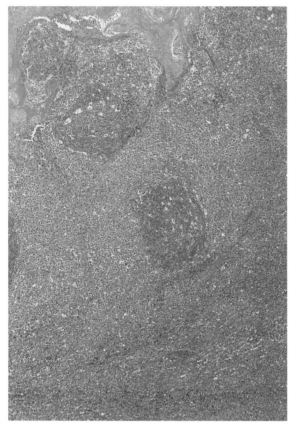

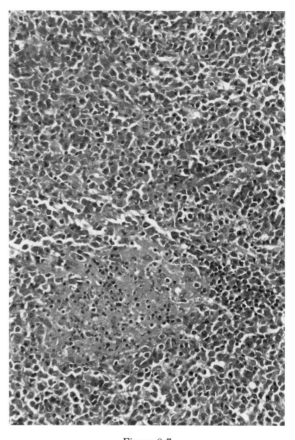

Figure 8-6
INFECTIOUS MONONUCLEOSIS
Tonsillar involvement is manifest by follicular hyperplasia and marked interfollicular expansion by immunoblasts, plasma cells, and plasmacytoid lymphocytes.

Figure 8-7
INFECTIOUS MONONUCLEOSIS
Sheets of immunoblasts and plasma cells surround foci of necrosis.

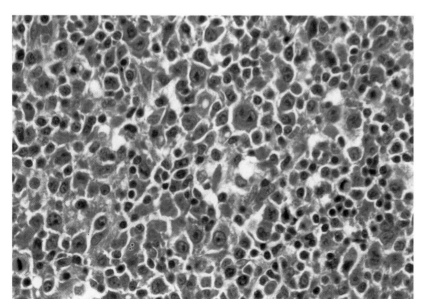

Figure 8-8
INFECTIOUS MONONUCLEOSIS
Although a few cells somewhat resemble Reed-Sternberg cells, their cytoplasm is basophilic and there may be a juxtanuclear clear zone (hof), which is not well formed in these cells.

(CD20 positive) or T cell (CD3 positive) type. They are sometimes CD30 positive (7), but are characteristically CD15 negative (19). The B cells are polyclonal. Reed-Sternberg–like cells are usually B cells that are CD30 positive and contain polytypic immunoglobulin light chains (13). Like true Reed-Sternberg cells, some may be negative for CD45 and CD20 (13). Infected cells are immunoreactive for EBV nuclear antigen (EBNA) 2 and latent membrane protein (LMP) 1 (8).

EBV-encoded RNA (EBER) transcripts are most abundant in latently infected cells. In patients with previous asymptomatic EBV infection, a few EBER-positive small lymphocytes can be detected in the lymphoid tissue of Waldeyer's ring (19,20). Since infectious mononucleosis consists of a mixture of lytic and latently infected cells (12), EBER-positive cells can be demonstrated by in situ hybridization in the transformed immunoblastic cells, which are CD20 positive, usually CD30 positive, and CD3 negative (8). The number of EBER-positive cells can be quite variable and, at times, are numerous (14). EBV DNA can also be demonstrated in B-cell immunoblasts and Reed-Sternberg–like cells in interfollicular and perifollicular areas by in situ hybridization (15,18). Infected cells that are EBER negative can be identified by probing reiterated EBV DNA sequences by in situ hybridization, a technique that targets cells producing abundant EBV DNA (12).

Southern blot hybridization can be used for the detection of EBV DNA (12). The linear viral DNA is identified as a ladder array of terminal restriction fragments. This is different than that seen in EBV-infected neoplasms where a single clone predominates and produces a unique band representing an intracellular fused terminal fragment. The polymerase chain reaction technique can also be used to detect EBV (12).

Differential Diagnosis. The most important considerations include non-Hodgkin's lymphoma, especially the large cell type with immunoblastic or anaplastic features, and Hodgkin's disease. It is quite important to be aware of the clinical setting such as the presence of tonsillar enlargement or cervical lymphadenopathy in adolescents or young adults. Unlike non-Hodgkin's lymphoma, the histologic findings in infectious mononucleosis include clearly reactive foci, transformed lymphocytes without severe nu-

clear irregularities, relative preservation of lymphoid architecture, and nonuniform interfollicular expansion (9). Immunoglobulin and T-cell receptor gene rearrangements are lacking in infectious mononucleosis. In situ hybridization for EBV DNA and immunoglobulin light chain mRNA have been used to establish the diagnosis of infectious mononucleosis in an 80-year-old man whose tonsil contained CD20- and CD45-positive lymphoid cells suggestive of diffuse large cell lymphoma (17). Although anaplastic large cell lymphoma may occur in children and, like infectious mononucleosis, contains CD30-positive cells (7), the cells are characteristically much more pleomorphic and numerous than those in infectious mononucleosis.

Both Reed-Sternberg–like cells in infectious mononucleosis and true Reed-Sternberg cells in Hodgkin's disease are frequently immunoreactive for EBV latent membrane protein (LMP) (13). Some cells in both conditions may contain EBV DNA and EBER transcripts. The large cells in infectious mononucleosis are sometimes transformed T cells and, unlike most cells of Hodgkin's disease, are CD15 negative (9). In addition, the Reed-Sternberg–like cells usually do not closely simulate classic Reed-Sternberg cells. Reactive follicular hyperplasia is typically present in infectious mononucleosis while the mixed cellular background typical of Hodgkin's disease is absent.

Treatment and Prognosis. Only supportive therapy is indicated for patients with infectious mononucleosis, as the disease is acute and resolves without sequelae. Resolution is accomplished by virus-specific antibodies and T-cell–mediated response, eliminating all but a few latently infected lymphoid cells (11). Rare fatal cases occur in patients with X-linked lymphoproliferative syndrome (11). Once infected (either with asymptomatic disease or with overt infectious mononucleosis), EBV remains in the body for life. In asymptomatic primary infection, the virus persists in healthy seropositive carriers and chiefly resides in the upper aerodigestive tract, which is the site of replication. A few small EBER-positive lymphocytes can be detected in the stroma of normal nasopharyngeal mucosa in patients with previous asymptomatic primary infection (19,20). The small lymphocytes are usually B cells (19,20).

SINUS HISTIOCYTOSIS WITH MASSIVE LYMPHADENOPATHY

General Features. This condition is also referred to as *Rosai-Dorfman disease,* named for the individuals who originally described the entity in 1969 (26) and defined it further in 1972 (27). The disease is rare, idiopathic, and typically involves lymph nodes, especially those in the cervical chain. Of 423 patients catalogued in the Sinus Histiocytosis with Massive Lymphadenopathy Registry (23), 43 percent had involvement of at least one extranodal site. The most common extranodal locations included skin, nasal cavity and paranasal sinuses, soft tissue, and bone; other sites of involvement included the genitourinary tract, lower respiratory system, and oral cavity. Forty-eight patients in the registry had nasal/paranasal sinus disease; 10 of them did not have lymph node disease. About 70 percent of the patients with sinonasal disease had other extranodal sites of involvement such as the orbit/eyelid, skin, or oral cavity. Eleven patients had sinus histiocytosis of the oral cavity, most often affecting the palate; 90 percent of these patients had other sites of extranodal disease, especially the sinonasal tract. Each of these 11 patients had lymphadenopathy. Four patients had tonsillar involvement, while 6 had laryngeal disease. The trachea was rarely involved.

Clinical Features. Overall, there is a wide age range, from newborns to those in the eighth decade (23); the average age is approximately 20 years. Of 305 patients catalogued in the Sinus Histiocytosis with Massive Lymphadenopathy Registry (23), 44 percent were white and 44 percent were black; 58 percent were men. There was no predilection for a particular socioeconomic status. Cervical lymphadenopathy was seen in approximately 90 percent of patients at presentation.

Symptoms of involvement of the upper aerodigestive tract may occur at initial presentation (22) or may develop months or even years following the onset of the disease. Fever is the most common symptom, and sometimes there is pharyngitis. Patients occasionally have associated immune-mediated disorders, especially hematologic autoantibody disease and joint manifestations. Additional clinical manifestations include anemia, elevation of white count with neutrophilia, hypoalbuminemia, and elevated poly-

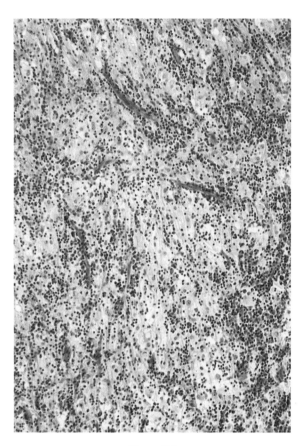

Figure 8-9
SINUS HISTIOCYTOSIS WITH
MASSIVE LYMPHADENOPATHY
In this specimen from the sinonasal tract, there is a predominance of plasma cells and histiocytes that contain abundant pale cytoplasm.

clonal gamma globulins (22). The sedimentation rate is commonly elevated. Patients may complain of nasal obstruction, discharge, polyps, or epistaxis (28). Other symptoms include dyspnea, stridor, and facial pain or tenderness.

Gross Findings. The mucosa appears thickened or polypoid. Resected tissue is rubbery and pink, tan-gray, or yellow.

Microscopic Findings. The infiltrate is polymorphous, consisting of mature small lymphocytes, plasma cells with some Russell bodies, and histiocytes in clusters or sheets (fig. 8-9). There are no well-formed granulomas. Lymphoid aggregates are common, but germinal center formation is not usually conspicuous. A few eosinophils may be noted, but they are rarely prominent. The polymorphous infiltrate is often separated by bands of fibrosis imparting a nodular appearance. The histiocytes have round or oval nuclei with single small nucleoli. On occasion, nucleoli may be more conspicuous. The cytoplasm is granular, clear, or vacuolated. Mitotic figures are usually few. The hallmark of sinus histiocytosis with massive lymphadenopathy is the presence of histiocytes with abundant eosinophilic cytoplasm containing phagocytized mononuclear cells (emperipolesis) (fig. 8-10) (26,27). These phagocytizing histiocytes range from few to many. Most of the phagocytized cells are small lymphocytes, but sometimes plasma cells, polymorphonuclear leukocytes, or red blood cells are ingested. In tonsillar tissue, the sinuses are packed with histiocytes producing an appearance identical to that of involved lymph nodes (22).

The overlying epithelium of the upper aerodigestive tract is typically not involved by the cellular infiltrate. The infiltrate greatly expands the submucosa and surrounds but does not destroy seromucous minor salivary glands. There may, however, be extension into bone, skeletal muscle, or other soft tissue structures. Special stains for microorganisms characteristically fail to reveal the presence of any type of infectious disease.

Immunohistochemical Findings. The histiocytes do not belong to the family of dendritic cells, but have immunophenotypic features of functionally activated macrophages (21). They are immunoreactive for pan-macrophage antigens as well as lysozyme, MAC 387, alpha-1-antitrypsin, alpha-1-antichymotrypsin, HAM56, and CD68. Staining for S-100 protein (using monoclonal or polyclonal antibodies) is virtually always seen. In at least half of the cases, there is immunoreactivity using antibodies for Ki-1, Leu-22, or LN-1. Staining for CD1a is typically absent (25). The histiocytes often are immunopositive for polyclonal immunoglobulins, while the plasma cells in the mixed infiltrate are polyclonal. Phagocytized lymphocytes include polytypic B cells and T cells.

Differential Diagnosis. Considerations include a variety of benign and malignant conditions (28). Like sinus histiocytosis with massive lymphadenopathy, rhinoscleroma consists of a mixed infiltrate of small lymphocytes, plasma cells, polymorphonuclear leukocytes, and histiocytes. In rhinoscleroma, however, the histiocytes contain abundant foamy cytoplasm, and bacteria can be demonstrated within the cells with

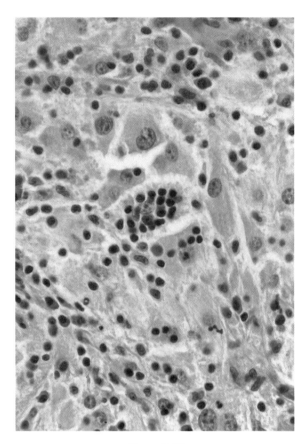

Figure 8-10
SINUS HISTIOCYTOSIS WITH
MASSIVE LYMPHADENOPATHY
Emperipolesis is a characteristic feature, and may be overt or less conspicuous.

Gram's stain or a Warthin-Starry silver stain. Phagocytosis of lymphocytes, plasma cells, and polymorphonuclear leukocytes is typically absent in rhinoscleroma.

Although there is a mixed cellular infiltrate in Wegener's granulomatosis, the finding of vasculitis, scattered giant cells without emperipolesis, and tissue necrosis are features not seen in sinus histiocytosis with massive lymphadenopathy. In addition, the cells in Wegener's granulomatosis are S-100 negative. Antineutrophil cytoplasmic autoantibodies are typically increased in Wegener's granulomatosis, and are absent in sinus histiocytosis with massive lymphadenopathy.

Langerhans' cell granulomatosis, extremely rare in the upper aerodigestive tract, consists of conspicuous numbers of eosinophils and Langerhans' cells, the latter having characteristic reniform nuclei and immunoreactivity for CD1a. Other diagnostic considerations include leprosy and T cell/natural killer (T/NK) cell lymphoma. The former condition reveals mycobacteria on an acid fast stain, while the latter consists of foci of lymphoid cells with overtly malignant cytologic features.

Treatment and Prognosis. In general, sinus histiocytosis with massive lymphadenopathy does not require therapy (24). Occasionally, surgery, radiation therapy, or chemotherapy is needed for severe disease (24,28). The most effective chemotherapeutic agents include vinca alkaloids, alkylating agents, and corticosteroids (24).

The disease is usually indolent and self-limited. The prognosis, however, does correlate with the number of involved nodal groups and the number of affected extranodal sites. Involvement of the nasal cavity, paranasal sinuses, or larynx does not affect the overall prognosis (23). Of patients with oral cavity disease, 9 percent died, but none directly from sinus histiocytosis with massive lymphadenopathy (23). Each of four patients with tonsillar disease had persistence of the disorder. Of 238 patients with a disease course of 1 year or longer, 49 were alive without evidence of disease, 36 were alive possibly with residual tumor, 129 were alive with disease, 3 had progressive disease, 4 died of disease, 13 died with disease, and 4 patients died without evidence of disease (23).

NON-HODGKIN'S LYMPHOMA

Oral Cavity

General Features. Non-Hodgkin's lymphoma of the oral cavity, exclusive of lymphomas of Waldeyer's ring and endemic Burkett's lymphoma of the jaw, is rare (29,35,37,40,44,46,47). In one Japanese series of 50 primary oral lymphomas, the palate and gingiva were the most common sites of origin followed by the tongue, buccal mucosa, floor of mouth, and lip (47). Although T/NK cell lymphomas may present in the oral cavity, these EBV-related lymphomas typically begin in the sinonasal tract and extend to palatal structures resulting in midline destruction (30–32,34,38,39,41,43,45,49). The destructive process may involve other oral structures including the tongue and lip (31).

One case of a low-grade mucosal T-cell lymphoproliferative disease of the digestive tract has been described in which multiple oral lesions and colonic ulcers arose and then regressed over a 17-year period (33). Rare examples of EBV-related oral T-cell lymphomas associated with HIV infection have been described; two patients had concurrent oral hairy leukoplakia (48).

Although biopsy of the lip has chiefly been used for the diagnosis of Sjogren's syndrome (36), this technique has recently been employed to detect the evolution of malignant lymphoma arising in the setting of Sjogren's syndrome (42). The polymerase chain reaction has been used to detect monoclonal immunoglobulin heavy chain gene rearrangements in labial salivary gland biopsies from patients under investigation for Sjogren's syndrome. Eleven such patients had monoclonal immunoglobulin heavy chain gene rearrangements; 4 of these subsequently were diagnosed with extrasalivary mucosa-associated lymphoid tissue (MALT) lymphoma. Many of these examples with immunoglobulin heavy chain gene rearrangements lacked histologic features of extranodal lymphoma, however.

Clinical Features. Patients with oral non-Hodgkin's lymphoma typically have no symptoms that would raise the clinical suspicion of lymphoma. Usually there is a painless swelling of the oral tissue (35). In the large study from Japan, the median age was 53 years, and almost twice as many patients were men as women (47). The growth appears exophytic or polypoid, and ulceration has been noted in approximately one third of the cases.

Gross Findings. Polypoid masses measure from 1 to 10 cm (mean, 3 cm) in greatest dimension (47). On cut section, they are gray-white with occasional foci of hemorrhage. At times, the surface is ulcerated.

Microscopic Findings. A wide spectrum of primary non-Hodgkin's lymphomas of the oral cavity has been described. Most are diffuse, as primary follicular lymphomas are quite unusual in this area. The majority have been diffuse large cell lymphomas (fig. 8-11). High-grade subtypes such as undifferentiated and lymphoblastic have also been reported. Low-grade lymphomas including a few examples of MALT lymphoma have also been described (47); MALT lymphomas typically consist of sheets of small centrocyte-like cells, some of which show intraepithelial infiltration of minor salivary glands.

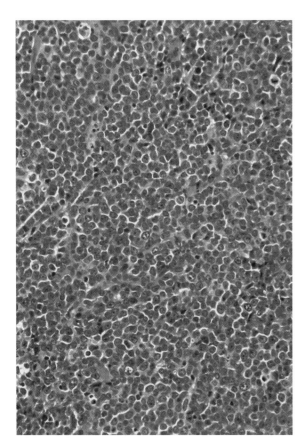 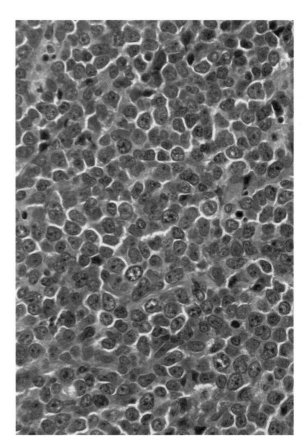

Figure 8-11
NON-HODGKIN'S LYMPHOMA
Diffuse large cell lymphoma is the most frequent subtype of primary lymphoma of the oral cavity.

The single example of a T-cell (CD3 positive, CD20 negative, CD56 negative, CD57 negative with T-cell gene rearrangements) lymphoproliferative disorder consisted of a diffuse monotonous proliferation of small lymphocytes with surface epithelial ulcerations.

The microscopic features of T/NK cell lymphoma are described in the section on sinonasal T/NK cell lymphoma.

Immunohistochemical Findings. In a study from the United States, 13 of 15 primary oral non-Hodgkin's lymphomas were B-cell neoplasms (44), while 39 of 45 from Japan were B-cell malignancies (fig. 8-12) (47).

Treatment and Prognosis. Treatment consists of radiation therapy with or without chemotherapy. Survival varies according to tumor grade and stage. The prognosis is typically poor for patients with sinonasal T/NK cell lymphoma that extends to oral cavity structures (31,34,38,43,45,49).

Waldeyer's Ring

Waldeyer's ring consists of the circle of nasopharyngeal (adenoid), oropharyngeal tonsillar, and base of tongue lymphoid tissue. This tissue is responsible for the recognition and processing of antigens presented to the upper aerodigestive tract. The immunophenotypic description of intraepithelial and subepithelial mononuclear cells of the upper aerodigestive tract appears in the section on hyperplasia of Waldeyer's ring in human immunodeficiency virus infection (57). The lymphoid tissues of Waldeyer's ring are not readily included among those of MALT (57), but they do possess some similarities. These include the absence of sinusoids, the introduction of antigen through crypt epithelium, and the presence of marginal zone-related B lymphocytes (61). Waldeyer's ring lymphoid tissue serves as an interface between gut-associated lymphoid tissue and systemic lymphoid tissue (72).

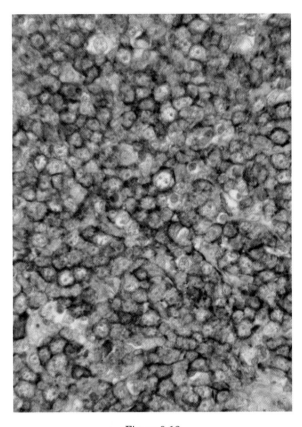

Figure 8-12
NON-HODGKIN'S LYMPHOMA
Most primary lymphomas of the oral cavity are B-cell neoplasms and are immunoreactive for CD20.

General Features. Approximately 5 to 10 percent of non-Hodgkin's lymphomas in patients living in the United States involve Waldeyer's ring (59,64). Of extranodal lymphomas, this is second in frequency only to those that arise in the gastrointestinal tract. In a study from Hong Kong, 15 percent of non-Hodgkin's lymphomas occurred in Waldeyer's ring (54). Lymphomas in this anatomic location constitute 10 to 20 percent of all lymphomas in Japan (73). Sixty to 70 percent of all extranodal lymphomas of the head and neck area occur in Waldeyer's ring (64) and the faucial tonsil is the most frequent location for its development. Of 68 lymphomas of Waldeyer's ring, 51 percent involved the tonsil, 35 percent the nasopharynx, 9 percent the base of the tongue, and 4 percent involved multiple sites (64).

The majority of lymphomas involving Waldeyer's ring occur as localized neoplasms (stage I or II). Waldeyer's ring may be involved by lym-phoma in patients with advanced disease, however. Blind biopsy of Waldeyer's ring as a staging procedure for patients with lymphoma lacks clinical value (50). In one study, a Waldeyer's ring biopsy positive for lymphoma was noted only in patients with stage IV disease; there was an absence of positive biopsies in patients who had positive cervical lymph nodes without clinical involvement of the nasopharynx (50). Synchronous or metachronous involvement of Waldeyer's ring has been noted in patients with lymphoma of the gastrointestinal tract (56,63,64); a proportion of Waldeyer's ring lymphomas also relapse in the gastrointestinal tract. The involvement of Waldeyer's ring lymphoid tissue and sites in the gastrointestinal tract by lymphoma may possibly represent a homing tendency of the malignant lymphoid cells.

Clinical Features. The age range for patients with Waldeyer's ring lymphoma is broad, from the first to the tenth decade. In most studies, the median age has ranged from 55 to 64 years (51, 54,59,60,62,64,65,69,70). In nine studies totaling 425 patients, 60 percent of the neoplasms occurred in males (51,54,59,60,62,64,65,69,70). Symptoms of lymphoma of the tonsil or tongue base include sore throat and dysphagia. Nasopharyngeal involvement leads to nasal, auditory, or cranial nerve symptoms.

Gross Findings. In one study, the clinical estimation of size ranged from 2.5 to 10 cm (mean, 4.6 cm) (51). Lymphoma has a gray-white appearance, and may feel rubbery. Ulceration and necrosis may be observed.

Microscopic Findings. Virtually all subtypes of non-Hodgkin's lymphoma have been described in Waldeyer's ring (Table 8-1) (68). Using the Revised European-American Classification of Lymphoid Neoplasms (REAL) (58), of 418 cases compiled from seven studies, 85 percent would be classified as diffuse lymphomas (51,59,64,65,68,73,74), over half of which are diffuse large cell lymphomas (fig. 8-13). High-grade lymphomas usually show a destructive pattern of growth, and surface ulceration is often observed. The surface epithelium is often intact in low-grade lymphomas, which may infiltrate crypt epithelium (60). Waldeyer's ring is a relatively frequent site for mantle cell lymphoma (52). In a study from the Kiel Lymph Node Registry (62), 12 of 329 cases of low-grade B-cell

Table 8-1

WALDEYER'S RING AS INITIAL EXTRANODAL SITE OF INVOLVEMENT BY LYMPHOMA IN THE NATIONAL CANCER INSTITUTE SPONSORED STUDY OF CLASSIFICATIONS OF NON-HODGKIN'S LYMPHOMAS

| Lymphoma Subtype | No. of Cases | | |
	Waldeyer's Ring	Total Extranodal Sites	(%)
Diffuse small cleaved cell	25	119	(21)
Diffuse mixed small and large cell	17	107	(16)
Diffuse large cell	38	326	(12)
Diffuse large cell immunoblastic	13	121	(11)
Follicular large cell	6	61	(10)
Small noncleaved cell	7	101	(7)
Lymphoblastic	6	81	(7)
Follicular mixed small and large cell	5	91	(5)
Small lymphocytic	3	73	(4)
Follicular small cleaved cell	11	344	(3)

lymphoma of Waldeyer's ring consisted of low-grade B-cell MALT lymphomas. These neoplasms demonstrated an extrafollicular pattern of growth and a marginal zone–like arrangement of cells with centrocyte-like morphology. Eleven of the 12 cases were located in the palatine tonsil. Two had a high-grade component. The cells of low-grade MALT lymphoma showed a tropism for the overlying epithelium, but this finding cannot be considered evidence for the presence of a true lymphoepithelial lesion, which involves glandular epithelium (60).

T/NK cell lymphoma may involve the nasopharynx, either arising in this location or, perhaps more commonly, extending from the sinonasal tract (53,67). This lymphoma is particularly manifest in Asian populations, in which it appears to be more frequent than in Western patients (53).

Immunohistochemical Findings. The proportion of B-cell (fig. 8-14) and T-cell lymphomas vary according to location in Waldeyer's ring and patient populations. In two studies from Europe, 93 of 98 lymphomas of Waldeyer's ring exhibited a B-cell immunophenotype (60,70). In Chinese populations, most Waldeyer's ring lymphomas, except for those involving the nasopharynx, are B-cell neoplasms (54); at least half of the nasopharyngeal

lymphomas exhibit a T/NK cell phenotype (53, 66,74). Of 100 non-Hodgkin's lymphomas of Waldeyer's ring from Japan, 72 percent exhibited a B-cell immunophenotype (65,69,73). Some examples of T-cell lymphoma in Japan represent tumors induced by human T-cell leukemia/lymphoma virus (69). The immunophenotypic characteristics of T/NK cell lymphoma are described in the section on sinonasal T/NK cell lymphoma.

Other Special Techniques. In a study from the United States, 2 of 10 B-cell lymphomas of Waldeyer's ring were positive for EBV DNA by in situ hybridization (71). One of the positive cases was a Burkitt's lymphoma, while the other was a diffuse large cell lymphoma. Using in situ hybridization and the polymerase chain reaction, Tomita and colleagues (69) found EBV in 3 of 40 B-cell lymphomas and 3 of 13 T-cell lymphomas in Japanese patients. Evidence for the presence of the human T-cell leukemia/lymphoma virus was observed in 11 of the 13 T-cell lymphomas. In a study from Hong Kong, each of 20 B-cell and one T-cell lymphoma from the tongue or tongue base lacked EBER mRNA by in situ hybridization (55). EBV has typically been associated, however, with T/NK cell lymphomas involving the nasopharynx.

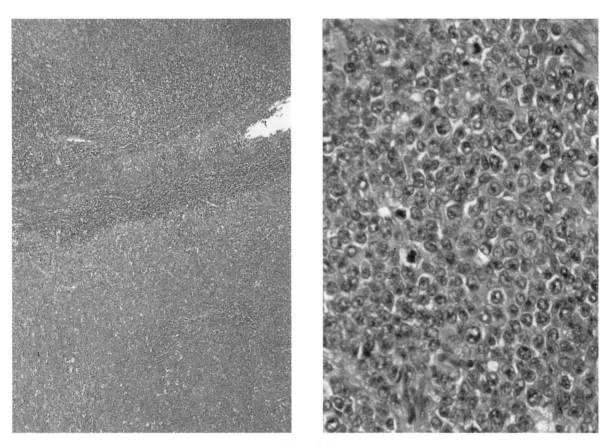

Figure 8-13
NON-HODGKIN'S LYMPHOMA
Diffuse large cell is the most common type of lymphoma of the tonsil.

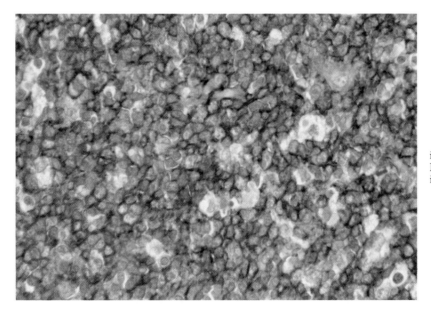

Figure 8-14
NON-HODGKIN'S LYMPHOMA
Most lymphomas of Waldeyer's ring in patients from the United States or Europe are B-cell neoplasms and are immunoreactive for CD20.

Differential Diagnosis. The distinction of non-Hodgkin's lymphoma from infectious mononucleosis has been described in the section on infectious mononucleosis. Non-Hodgkin's lymphomas of Waldeyer's ring must also be distinguished from undifferentiated carcinoma (lymphoepithelioma) which may arise in this anatomic site. Unlike non-Hodgkin's lymphoma, undifferentiated carcinoma shows a syncytial pattern of growth, is immunohistochemically positive for cytokeratin, and lacks immunoreactivity for leukocyte common antigen. The features of plasmacytoma and extramedullary myeloid cell tumor have been described in the specific sections on these two hematolymphoid neoplasms.

Treatment and Prognosis. Treatment for localized lymphoma of Waldeyer's ring consists of radiation therapy. Chemotherapy is used for higher stage lesions. The prognosis for patients depends upon tumor histologic grade and stage. Patients with low-grade and low-stage lymphomas have a better prognosis than those with higher grade and stage lesions. In a recent study of 77 patients with assorted lymphomas of Waldeyer's ring (70 percent stage I or II), the overall 5-year survival rate was 65 percent (60).

Larynx and Trachea

General Features. Localized laryngeal non-Hodgkin's lymphoma is rare (75–77,79,81,86,88, 90). It accounts for less than 1 percent of all laryngeal neoplasms (75). In one series from Japan, only 4 percent of extranodal non-Hodgkin's lymphomas of the head and neck involved the larynx (88). Lymphoma in the larynx may be localized or part of disseminated disease, or may extend from other upper aerodigestive tract sites such as the nasal cavity or nasopharynx. In a literature review of primary hematolymphoid neoplasms of the larynx, 90 were plasmacytomas, and 65 were non-Hodgkin's lymphomas (81). Most laryngeal lymphomas arise in the supraglottic area, especially the epiglottis or aryepiglottic folds; only a few arise in the glottic region or are subglottic.

Rare examples of primary non-Hodgkin's lymphoma of the trachea have been described; as of 1996, there were six documented in the literature (78,82,84,85,87,91). Otherwise, tracheal involvement by lymphoma usually occurs by displacement from adjacent lymph nodes, resulting in luminal narrowing or tracheal wall erosion (78).

Clinical Features. Of 65 cases of laryngeal lymphoma collected from the literature, the male to female ratio was 1.3 to 1 (56). The age range was 4 to 90 years, with a median age of 58 years; only four arose in children. Presenting symptoms included hoarseness, dysphonia, dysphagia, stridor, cough, and weight loss. The six patients with localized tracheal lymphoma initially presented with dyspnea, sometimes with wheezing or stridor (78,82,84,85,87,91). Their age range was 52 to 81 years.

Gross Findings. The endoscopic appearance of a submucosal, nonulcerated lesion in the supraglottis should arouse suspicion for the presence of a hematolymphoid malignancy. Occasionally the nodule appears polypoid, but usually is not pedunculated. Diffuse thickening of laryngeal structures is unusual. Lymphoma of the larynx typically measures 1 to 3 cm in greatest dimension and is tan and fleshy.

Microscopic Findings. The majority of laryngeal lymphomas reported in the literature are poorly documented, as there is often a lack of appropriate photomicrographs, and few have been studied immunohistochemically. The majority appear to be B-cell lymphomas, but there are some examples of T/NK cell lymphoma (80,83,89). Most are diffuse large cell lymphomas (fig. 8-15), but some are probably low-grade MALT lymphomas. Many of the cases formerly designated as diffuse poorly differentiated lymphocytic lymphoma may be examples of MALT lymphoma or mantle cell lymphoma. Nodular lymphomas are extremely rare in the larynx.

T/NK cell lymphoma may involve the larynx as an extension from the sinonasal tract or as a primary laryngeal lymphoma. The microscopic description of these EBV-related lymphomas can be found in the section on nasal and paranasal sinus T/NK cell lymphoma.

Of the six primary tracheal lymphomas, two were classified as lymphocytic, one was described as mixed small and large cell, one was an anaplastic large cell lymphoma, and two were MALT or probable MALT lymphomas (78,82,84,85,87,91). Hence, the majority of primary tracheal lymphomas are low grade. In MALT lymphoma, there is diffuse infiltration by small lymphocytes and centrocyte-like cells surrounding reactive follicles

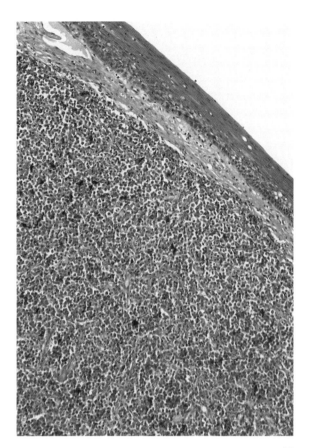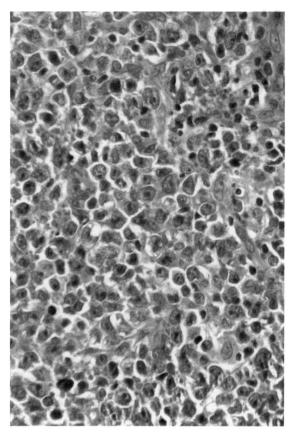

Figure 8-15
NON-HODGKIN'S LYMPHOMA
Most laryngeal lymphomas are diffuse large cell neoplasms.

(84). The vaguely nodular proliferation expands the submucosa, and surrounds and obliterates submucosal glands. Overlying invasion of the mucosa is present. Plasmacytoid differentiation is seen, as are lymphoepithelial lesions.

Immunohistochemical Findings. Well-characterized immunophenotypic cases of laryngeal or tracheal lymphoma are few (fig. 8-16). Some laryngeal lesions have immunophenotypic features of T/NK cell lymphoma (80,83,89). In one MALT lymphoma of the trachea, the monoclonal proliferation of cells was CD45RA positive, CD20 positive, CD22 positive, CD5 negative, CD10 negative, CD3 negative, CD5 negative, and CD45RO negative (84). The tracheal anaplastic large cell lymphoma was positive for CD15, CD30, and CD20 (78).

Differential Diagnosis. In small biopsy specimens, a variety of small blue cell neoplasms may enter into the differential diagnosis. Immu-

nohistochemical findings should separate those of hematolymphoid origin from other neoplasms. Lymphoma of the larynx must also be differentiated from plasmacytoma and leukemia. Examples of pseudolymphoma arising in the larynx that appear in the older literature are suspect, as they have been poorly characterized and lack convincing morphologic descriptions, immunophenotyping, and follow-up. It is likely that so-called laryngeal pseudolymphomas are examples of low-grade MALT lymphoma.

Treatment and Prognosis. Radiation therapy is standard treatment for localized non-Hodgkin's lymphoma of the trachea and larynx. Some patients have been treated with resection, however. Four of five patients with primary tracheal lymphomas responded well to radiation or surgery or both (one also received chemotherapy): complete remission was achieved at 12, 13, 22, and

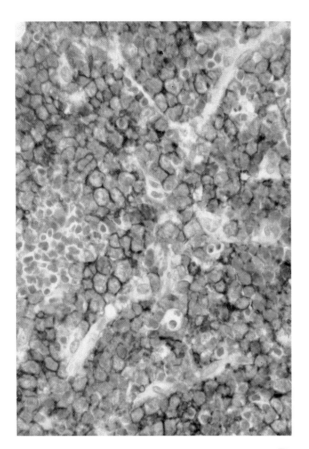
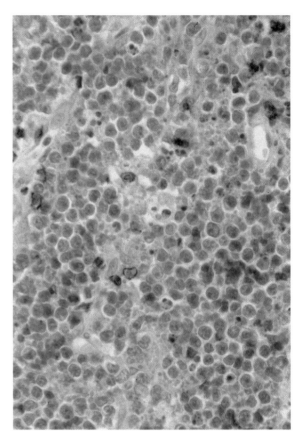

Figures 8-16
NON-HODGKIN'S LYMPHOMA
The majority of diffuse large cell lymphomas of the larynx are immunopositive for CD20 (left) and negative for CD45RO (right).

64 months after therapy (78,85,87,91). It has been suggested that for localized tracheal lymphoma, limited chemotherapy followed by radiation therapy is appropriate (78). Surgery should be employed for resistant disease or for tracheomalacia (78). Localized laryngeal neoplasms may respond completely to radiation therapy despite having an unfavorable histology. Survival is quite good for patients with localized laryngeal lymphoma, and long-term survival would be expected. Patients with laryngeal involvement as part of generalized lymphoma typically have a poor prognosis despite chemotherapy. Death may occur suddenly by acute laryngeal obstruction before therapy is instituted. Surgery may be necessary for patients who have acute obstruction or massive hemorrhage. Patients with T/NK cell lymphoma involving the larynx have a less favorable prognosis than those with other types of lymphoma.

Sinonasal B-Cell Lymphoma

General Features. Malignant lymphomas of the sinonasal tract are uncommon, comprising approximately 6 percent of all sinonasal malignant neoplasms (103). In our own patient population only 1.5 percent of all non-Hodgkin's lymphomas arose in the sinonasal tract (99). Of 33,402 cases of lymphoma in the Kiel Lymph Node Registry (96), only 0.17 percent arose in the sinonasal area, and only 0.44 percent of all extranodal lymphomas were sinonasal lesions. Sinonasal lymphomas appear to occur more frequently in Asian (Chinese) populations, where the majority are of T/NK cell type (94,102,105,110). B-cell lymphomas may be more frequent than T/NK cell lymphomas in Western patients, but the data to support this conclusion are not uniform (92,96,97, 98,106). In a study from Germany, 30 of 38 lymphomas were of B-cell immunophenotype (96). In the largest study of sinonasal lymphomas from the United States, 65 were of B-cell phenotype, while 55 showed T-cell immunophenotypic features (92). Although it is, at times, difficult to determine whether a lymphoma is strictly confined to the nasal cavity or, alternatively, to a paranasal sinus, 34 of 64 lymphomas that appeared to be confined to the nasal cavity were T-cell lymphomas; those that appeared to be confined to a paranasal sinus more often had a B-cell immunophenotype (30 of 39 cases) (92). Although B-cell lymphoma may be confined to the nasal cavity or a paranasal sinus, quite often multiple sinuses are affected, most commonly the maxillary antrum and ethmoid sinus (95,100). Spread to other sites in the upper aerodigestive tract and face may be observed, and it is not unusual for a sinonasal B-cell lymphoma to spread to the palate, nasopharynx, cheek, or orbit. Some cases of sinonasal B-cell lymphoma have been associated with EBV, but less frequently than that seen for T/NK cell lymphoma (93,108,109).

Clinical Features. In two studies from the United States totaling 91 cases, 56 patients were male and 35 female (92,99). The age range was 3 to 94 years; the median age was in the sixth decade of life.

Presenting symptoms of sinonasal B-cell lymphoma include nasal obstruction, nasal mass, discharge, and facial swelling. Less often there is facial numbness, epistaxis, pain, headache, proptosis, and vision disturbances. Fever, weight loss, malaise, and anorexia are uncommonly observed.

Gross Findings. Sinonasal B-cell lymphoma sometimes occurs as a polypoid mass. On cut section it is gray-tan and fleshy.

Microscopic Findings. Of 142 sinonasal B-cell lymphomas, 106 (75 percent) consisted of a diffuse proliferation with large cells (large cell, large cell with immunoblastic features, or diffuse mixed small and large cell) (fig. 8-17) (92,96, 98,101,104,108); 18 (12 percent) were classified as Burkitt's lymphoma; 1 as lymphoblastic lymphoma; 6 as small lymphocytic lymphoma; 7 as follicular center cell lymphoma; 2 had features of monocytoid B-cell lymphoma; and 2 were classified as lymphoplasmacytoid lymphoma. Low-grade B-cell lymphoma of MALT, in general, does not arise in the sinonasal tract.

Sinonasal B-cell lymphomas typically consist of sheets of malignant lymphoid cells that ex-

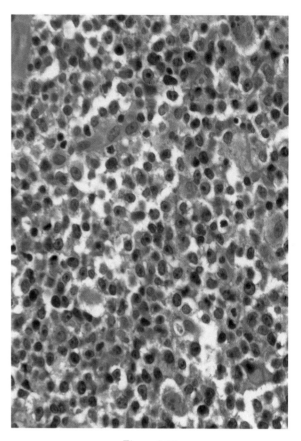

Figure 8-17
SINONASAL B-CELL LYMPHOMA
Most represent diffuse large cell neoplasms.

pand the subepithelial tissue. There may be infiltration of adjacent soft tissue and underlying bone. Unlike T/NK cell lymphomas, they lack a polymorphous cellular infiltrate, fibrosis, extensive necrosis, and angiocentricity.

Immunohistochemical Findings. Sinonasal B-cell lymphomas are usually positive for CD20 and CD45RA (fig. 8-18, left). They are characteristically negative for CD3, CD43, and CD45RO (fig. 8-18, right), although occasionally they may be CD43 or CD45RO positive. Kappa light chain restriction is seen more often than lambda light chain restriction. In a study from Japan, 13 of 22 sinonasal B-cell lymphomas were positive for EBV latent membrane protein (108).

Other Special Techniques. Thirty-one diffuse large cell lymphomas have been studied for EBV nucleic acids by in situ hybridization (93,104,108,109). Twelve were positive for either EBV DNA or RNA.

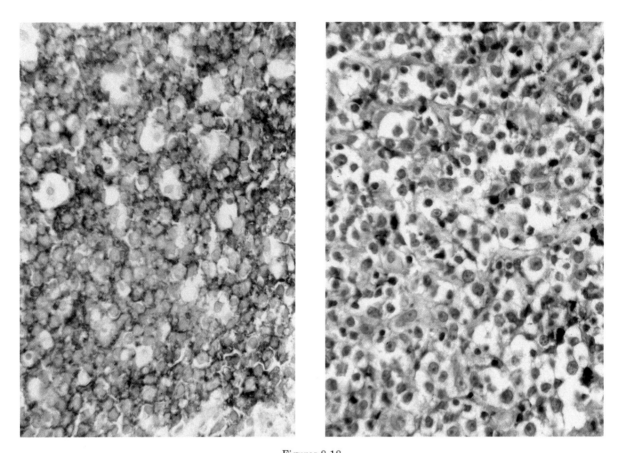

Figures 8-18
SINONASAL B-CELL LYMPHOMA
These neoplasms are typically immunoreactive for CD20 (left) and are negative for CD45RO (right).

Differential Diagnosis. Sinonasal B-cell lymphomas differ from T/NK cell lymphomas both morphologically and immunophenotypically. As mentioned above, the former lack angiocentricity, marked necrosis, and a polymorphous cellular infiltrate. The majority of sinonasal B-cell lymphomas are easily distinguished from plasmacytoma, but, on occasion, a large cell lymphoma with immunoblastic features may raise the possibility of anaplastic plasmacytoma. Sinonasal B-cell lymphoma should also be distinguished from extramedullary myeloid cell tumors; the immunophenotypic findings for the latter neoplasm have been described in the section on extramedullary myeloid and lymphoid cell tumors. Nonhematopoietic lesions included in the differential diagnosis are melanoma, sinonasal undifferentiated carcinoma, olfactory neuroblastoma, and rhabdomyosarcoma. In the

majority of cases, these nonhematolymphoid lesions have morphologic features sufficiently distinctive from lymphoma that immunohistochemistry is not required. However, in difficult diagnostic situations immunohistochemistry with antibodies to CD45, S-100 protein, HMB-45, cytokeratin, desmin, and muscle-specific actin readily distinguish them.

Treatment and Prognosis. Radiation therapy is the treatment of choice for almost all sinonasal B-cell lymphomas, and may be used alone for small localized neoplasms (107). For those patients with locally advanced tumors or disseminated neoplasm, chemotherapy is typically added. The prognosis largely depends on histologic type and tumor stage. Data regarding outcome for patients with sinonasal B-cell lymphoma are sparse, and they are difficult to evaluate due to differences in lymphoma classification, geographic distribution of patients, and difficulties in determining local extent of the neoplasm. In two studies from the United States comprising 57 patients, 29 either died of disease or were alive with tumor (92,99).

Sinonasal T/NK Cell Lymphoma

The intraepithelial lymphocyte component of the normal nasal mucosa differs from that of the tonsil and adenoid (132). Intraepithelial lymphocytes within the normal nasal lining epithelium consist of CD3-positive, CD8-positive, and Leu-8-negative T cells. These T cells are chiefly CD5 positive, but are often CD7 negative. In three fourths of specimens from one study, CD4-positive intraepithelial lymphocytes were absent or present only in sparse numbers (132). Eighty to 90 percent of intraepithelial T cells express the α/β T-cell receptor. Almost no B cells reside in the normal nasal epithelium, but intraepithelial dendritic cells (not Langerhans' cells) are observed.

In a study of frozen sections of normal nasal mucosae from 40 volunteers older than 18 years, the lymphocyte to monocyte/macrophage ratio of cells within the subepithelial tissue was 10 to 1 (176). T cells outnumbered B cells by 3 to 1, while T helper cells outnumbered T cytotoxic/suppressor cells 2.5 to 1. A relative increase in T cytotoxic/suppressor cells was observed around submucosal glands, while B lymphocytes resided in lymphoid aggregates in the lamina propria. Lymphoid aggregates, however, were seen in no more than one third of specimens. Within the subepithelial nasal tissue, the number of T and B lymphocytes equaled approximately $1000/mm^2$; in the interglandular area, $600/mm^2$; and in deeper vascular stroma, $300/mm^2$. No lymphocyte aggregates were noted in close contact with altered epithelium of the lymphoepithelial type. The above findings are not consistent with the presence of MALT in normal nasal tissues.

General Features. T/NK cell lymphoma is the most recent term used for an aggressive, destructive lymphoma of the upper aerodigestive tract or midline facial tissue (144). Former terms used to describe this malignancy include polymorphic reticulosis, malignant midline reticulosis, lethal midline granuloma, idiopathic midline destructive disease, midfacial necrotizing lesion, midfacial destructive lesion, midline

destructive granuloma, midline granuloma syndrome, nonhealing midline granuloma, and pseudolymphoma. We agree that these former terms should be considered archaic (137). T/NK cell lymphoma has also been encompassed under the category of angiocentric immunoproliferative lesions. Although the designation lymphomatoid granulomatosis has been used to describe a destructive lymphoreticular lesion of the aerodigestive tract, this term is currently best reserved for a T-cell–rich EBV-associated B-cell lymphoproliferative disorder, usually of pulmonary origin, but also often involving the skin, kidney, and central nervous system (133,144,150,175).

Evidence that T/NK cell lymphoma is a malignancy having T-cell immunophenotypic features began to appear in Asian populations in 1982 (141). Current evidence shows that this lymphoma is an EBV-associated angiocentric neoplasm with T-cell or NK cell phenotypic and genotypic features. This distinct lymphoma is included as an angiocentric lymphoma in the Revised European-American Classification of Lymphoid Neoplasms (136). Identical lymphomas may occur in extranasal sites such as the skin, subcutaneous tissue, and gastrointestinal tract, among others, and are referred to as nasal-type T/NK cell lymphomas (144,151,169). They typically arise in the absence of peripheral lymphadenopathy. There are also rare examples of leukemia that are morphologically, phenotypically, and genotypically similar to nasal T/NK cell lymphoma (144,160). A few of these patients have had nasal involvement (160).

T/NK cell lymphoma is often immunoreactive for CD56, an isoform of neural cell adhesion molecule (NCAM). This antigen is observed in NK cells, NK-like T cells (122), and neural/neuroendocrine tissues and neoplasms. Formerly, CD56 immunoreactivity could only be reliably determined on fresh or frozen tissues, but recently a paraffin section-reactive CD56 antibody (123C3) has been developed (168). T/NK cell lymphomas have been reported more often in Asian than Western patients (144), and therefore have not been particularly well studied with antibodies to CD56 or with Southern blot hybridization for T-cell receptor gene rearrangements in Western patients. Sinonasal T/NK cell lymphomas have been reported in patients from Peru and Mexico, likely indicating a racial predisposition (115,152). Tumor incidence is higher in Peru as well as Asia (113,130,138, 154): the incidence ranges from 6.7 to 7.2 percent in Asian countries (140,154) and 8 percent in a study of patients from Peru (147) compared to only 1.5 percent in the United States (129), and 0.17 percent in Germany (127). Although sinonasal B-cell lymphomas appear to be more frequent than those of T/NK cell type in Western populations, some of the data have been conflicting (128,159). In a study of 120 sinonasal non-Hodgkin's lymphomas collected at the Armed Forces Institute of Pathology (AFIP), 65 had a B-cell phenotype while 55 showed T-cell immunohistochemical features (111).

Clinical Features. T/NK cell lymphoma may occur at almost any age: patients range in age from the first through ninth decades (median, fifth or sixth decade). In one large series of 126 cases of "polymorphic reticulosis," the median age was 47, while the male to female ratio was 1.7 to 1 (113). A male predominance has been consistently reported. Patients present with midfacial destruction of the nasal cavity and paranasal sinuses; often, the palate and other oral and midfacial structures are involved. The entire upper aerodigestive tract to the larynx may be involved by T/NK cell lymphoma (144). Swelling, erythema, and, at times, pain are present. Epistaxis, nasal obstruction, and a nasal mass are also commonly observed. Ulceration, necrosis, septal perforation, collapse of the nasal bridge, and sinocutaneous fistulas have been described. The above findings may be accompanied by fever and weight loss. The duration of symptoms ranges from months to sometimes years. The neoplasm most commonly spreads to other extranodal sites such as the skin, subcutaneous tissue, gastrointestinal tract, and testis (144). Rarely, T/NK cell lymphoma may arise in the skin or soft tissue and relapse in the nasal cavity (144).

Gross Findings. Biopsy fragments consist of gray or tan, hemorrhagic or necrotic tissue.

Microscopic Findings. The ulceration, inflammatory exudate, and necrosis are often extensive (fig. 8-19). At the ulcer margins, the mucosal surface may show squamous metaplasia. It is likely that examples of T-cell lymphoma with florid pseudoepitheliomatous hyperplasia are examples of T/NK cell lymphoma (117,128). When the destructive process is marked, cartilage and bone may be involved. The cellular mixture consists of

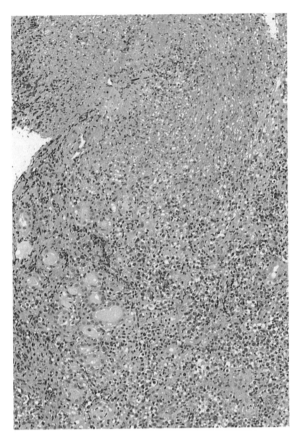

Figure 8-19
SINONASAL T/NK CELL LYMPHOMA
A diffuse population of malignant lymphoid cells infiltrates minor salivary glands. Areas of necrosis are almost always present. (Courtesy of Dr. J.K.C. Chan, Kowloon, Hong Kong.)

normal-appearing small lymphocytes, plasma cells, immunoblasts, and cytologically atypical lymphocytes; polymorphonuclear leukocytes, eosinophils, and histiocytes also are often present. The cellular infiltrate is invested by numerous capillaries, while foci of fibrosis may also be present. The cytologically malignant lymphoid cells sometimes invade the surface epithelium or minor salivary gland epithelium.

The angiocentric pattern of these cells results in angioinvasion (infiltration and destruction of vessel walls) (fig. 8-20) affecting muscular arteries, arterioles, and small veins. Thrombosis may also be observed. Angiocentricity does not include the concentration of malignant cells around blood vessels during the entrapment of these vessels in a massive infiltrate of lymphoma (144). Angiocentricity is seen in up to two thirds of cases of

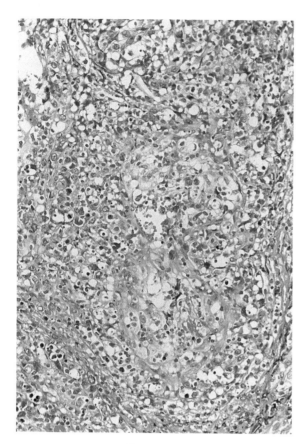

Figure 8-20
SINONASAL T/NK CELL LYMPHOMA
Angioinvasion by the lymphoma cells may nearly obliterate the affected vessel. (Courtesy of Dr. J.K.C. Chan, Kowloon, Hong Kong.)

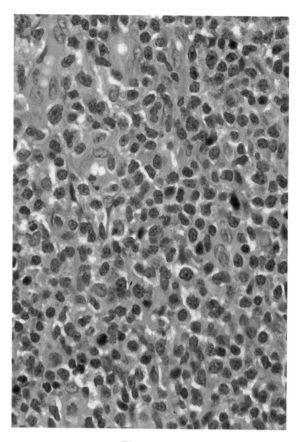

Figure 8-21
SINONASAL T/NK CELL LYMPHOMA
Sometimes the malignant cells consist entirely of small cleaved lymphocytes. (Courtesy of Dr. J.K.C. Chan, Kowloon, Hong Kong.)

T/NK cell lymphoma (144), and its absence may be related to sampling artifact, particularly in small biopsy specimens (143).

Necrosis of the lymphoma cells, normal tissues, or both is almost always seen (fig. 8-19) (133,144). This arises as a result of occlusion of vessels or the overexpression of tumor necrosis factor or other cytokines, possibly induced by EBV (144).

The cytologic spectrum of the malignant lymphoid cells is broad, ranging from small or medium-sized lymphocytes to large transformed cells. Quite often there is a mixture of malignant lymphoid cells of various size. Mitotic figures are common in the malignant cellular infiltrate. The cytologic spectrum is reflected in the fact that T/NK cell lymphomas have been formerly classified as diffuse small cleaved cell lymphoma (fig. 8-21), diffuse mixed small and large cell lym-

phoma (fig. 8-22), diffuse large cell lymphoma (fig. 8-23), and large cell immunoblastic lymphoma (117). In Giemsa-stained touch imprint specimens, the malignant cells often show azurophilic granules, likely representing cytotoxic granules (114,158,172).

Immunohistochemical Findings. T/NK cell lymphoma is typically immunoreactive for CD2, but immunoreactivity for CD5, CD7, CD4, and CD8 is variable (144). Most cases show cytoplasmic immunoreactivity for CD3 in paraffin-embedded sections (fig. 8-24), but lack surface staining for CD3 in frozen sections (112,118–120,149,156,162–165). In one study, 90 percent of cases that were negative for surface CD3 in frozen sections were positive for cytoplasmic CD3 in paraffin sections (120). The lack of surface CD3 immunostaining in fresh or frozen tissues and the presence of

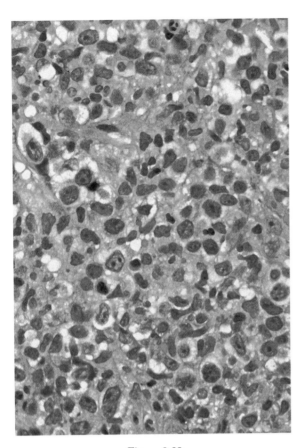

Figure 8-22
SINONASAL T/NK CELL LYMPHOMA
This lesion contains both small and large malignant lymphoid cells. (Courtesy of Dr. J.K.C. Chan, Kowloon, Hong Kong.)

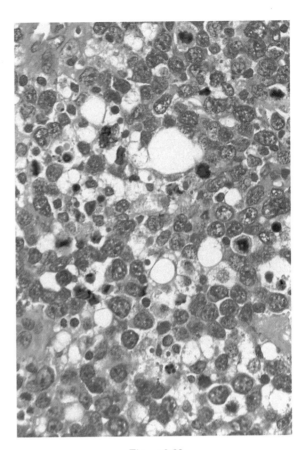

Figure 8-23
SINONASAL T/NK CELL LYMPHOMA
This large cell lymphoma contains numerous mitotic figures and shows prominent apoptosis. (Courtesy of Dr. J.K.C. Chan, Kowloon, Hong Kong.)

cytoplasmic CD3 immunostaining in paraffin sections is consistent with a NK cell phenotype. Immunostaining for T-cell receptor α/β chains (using βF1) and γ/δ T-cell receptor chains (using TCRδ1) is usually negative (144). The lymphoma in paraffin-embedded sections is also typically immunoreactive for CD45RO and CD43, while a few examples have been CD30 positive (145). Cytotoxic granules have been immunoreactive for granzyme B (172) and also for cytotoxic granule–associated protein TIA-1 (126,158). Neoplastic cells are positive for perforin, a specific marker of NK cells and cytotoxic T cells (149). They are negative for B-cell markers.

Nonneoplastic NK cells are typically positive for CD56, CD2, and CD7, and negative for CD5 and T-cell receptor proteins (126). T-cell receptor gene rearrangements also are absent in non-neoplastic NK cells. The majority of T/NK cell lymphomas have been immunoreactive for CD56 (fig. 8-25), an antigen also detected in a subset of T cells, neural and neuroendocrine tissues and neoplasms, and, occasionally, in lymphoblasts, myeloid leukemia, rhabdomyosarcoma, and multiple myeloma (170,172). In one study of 38 T/NK cell lymphomas, 71 percent were CD56 positive (173). The CD56 antibody 123C3 has been shown to be effective in paraffin sections after epitope retrieval. In one study of 32 cases of T/NK lymphoma, there was complete concordance between 123C3 and a CD56 antibody used on frozen sections (168). None of 24 CD56-negative T-cell lymphomas and none of 50 CD56-negative B-cell lymphomas stained with antibody 123C3. T/NK cell lymphomas typically lack immunoreactivity for CD57 and CD16 (other markers of NK cells) (144,149,155).

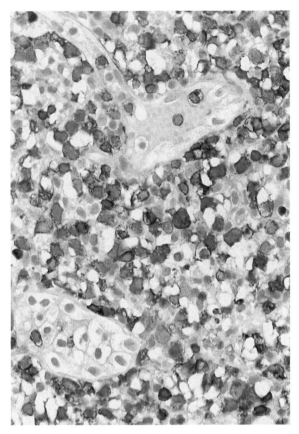

Figure 8-24
SINONASAL T/NK CELL LYMPHOMA
Cytoplasmic CD3 is observed with a polyclonal antibody in paraffin sections. (Courtesy of Dr. J.K.C. Chan, Kowloon, Hong Kong.)

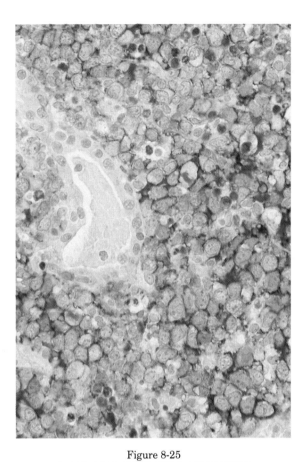

Figure 8-25
SINONASAL T/NK CELL LYMPHOMA
CD56 can be demonstrated in paraffin sections using the antibody 123C3 and epitope retrieval. (Courtesy of Dr. J.K.C. Chan, Kowloon, Hong Kong.)

Although most T/NK cell lymphomas are associated with EBV, staining for latent membrane protein 1 (LMP-1) has been variable in paraffin-embedded sections (124,144). This protein has often been observed in frozen sections, however, suggesting a low level of expression (145).

Other Special Techniques. Immunoglobulin heavy and light chain genes are typically not rearranged in T/NK cell lymphoma. Although most cases show T-cell receptor genes in the germline configuration, some have had T-cell receptor gene rearrangements (122,126,134,139,143,144). It is possible that cases of CD56-positive or -negative, EBV-positive sinonasal lymphomas with T-cell receptor gene rearrangements represent true T-cell lymphomas. In a recent study from Japan, 10 of 10 nasal T-cell lymphomas associated with EBV showed T-cell receptor gene rearrange-

ments (134). The discrepancy in the presence or absence of T-cell gene rearrangements in nasal T/NK cell lymphomas may have resulted from the different numbers of probes that were used in Southern blot analysis, problems of sampling small biopsy specimens, racial/geographic differences, or technical problems. Recently two cases with a CD2-positive, CD3 surface-negative, CD56-positive phenotype had truncated Tβ and multiple unrearranged Tδ transcripts with germline T-cell receptor β, γ, and δ genes consistent with NK cell lineage (122). Another nasal lymphoma, however, positive for CD2, CD3 surface, CD8, and CD56 expressed full-length Tα, Tβ, and Tγ transcripts with rearranged T-cell receptor β, γ, and deleted δ genes, consistent with T-cell lineage (122).

Most cases of nasal T/NK cell lymphoma have been associated with EBV, most often detected

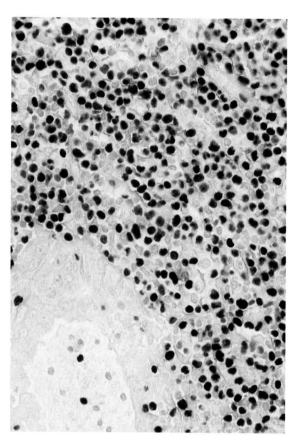

Figure 8-26
SINONASAL T/NK CELL LYMPHOMA
EBV-encoded small nuclear RNA (EBER) can be detected by in situ hybridization in most cases. (Courtesy of Dr. J.K.C. Chan, Kowloon, Hong Kong.)

by in situ hybridization for EBV-encoded small nuclear RNA1/2 (EBER1/2) (fig. 8-26). The finding of EBV in nasal T/NK cell lymphomas has been consistent in all populations, including those from Asia, South America, Europe, and the United States (115,116,121,124,125,134,135, 139,142–146,148,149,152,157,158,161,166,167, 171–173). In studies totaling 134 patients, 119 had evidence of EBV within the neoplastic cells (121,173). EBV has also been identified by Southern blot analysis and by the polymerase chain reaction. The clonality of EBV with terminal repeat probes has been demonstrated by Southern blot analysis (128,134,135,146). Using in situ hybridization and reverse transcriptase polymerase chain reaction (RTPCR), van Gorp and colleagues (173) found that T/NK cell lymphomas typically were EBER positive, BARF0 mRNA pos-

itive, EBNA1 mRNA positive, and LMP1 mRNA positive. A few cases showed LMP2A mRNA, LMP2B mRNA, and ZEBRA mRNA. EBNA2 mRNA was characteristically absent. The above mRNA findings are indicative of a type 2 EBV latency pattern which is similar to that observed in nasopharyngeal carcinoma, somewhat like that seen in Hodgkin's disease, but unlike that observed for African Burkett's lymphoma (type 1 latency) and B-cell lymphoma in immunocompromised patients (type 3 EBV latency). In one small study from Europe, half of the T/NK cell lymphomas contained EBV subtype A while the other half contained EBV subtype B (116). In a Japanese study, most nasal T/NK cell lymphomas had EBV subtype A (167).

Differential Diagnosis. A variety of non-neoplastic and neoplastic conditions may be confused with nasal T/NK cell lymphoma. Various fungi and bacteria may result in marked inflammation and necrosis of sinonasal structures. Similarly, Wegener's granulomatosis may clinically simulate sinonasal lymphoma. The finding of cytologic atypia and conspicuous mitotic features in the lymphoid cellular component are helpful in excluding non-neoplastic conditions. When biopsy specimens are small, in situ hybridization for EBV may be useful in distinguishing nasal T/NK cell lymphoma from benign or malignant sinonasal lesions (125). Immunostaining for CD56 using the antibody 123C3 in paraffin-embedded sections may also be useful: more than 20 percent of cells positive with 123C3 or the presence of multiple large clusters (more than 6 cells) of 123C3-positive cells is consistent with T/NK cell lymphoma (168).

Malignant hematolymphoid conditions that should be considered include blastic NK cell leukemia/lymphoma, extramedullary myeloid or lymphoid cell leukemia, and sinonasal B-cell lymphoma (142,144). Unlike nasal T/NK cell lymphoma, these lesions are typically not associated with EBV, although a few examples of EBV-associated sinonasal B-cell lymphoma have been described (174). It is important to note that myeloid leukemias may be CD56 positive (172), but unlike T/NK cell lymphoma, lack marked destruction and necrosis as well as the polymorphous cellular infiltrate. Like nasal T/NK cell lymphoma, lymphomatoid granulomatosis shows necrosis, angiocentricity, and association with EBV, but most examples arise in the lung, have B-cell immunophenotypic features, and have an exuberant T-cell reaction. Nasal T/NK cell lymphoma can readily be distinguished from various small blue cell neoplasms arising in the sinonasal tract. It should be remembered, however, that CD56 may be observed in neuroectodermal tumors, rhabdomyosarcoma, and plasmacytoma/myeloma (170,172).

Treatment and Prognosis. Optimal treatment includes radiation therapy with or without chemotherapy. Despite sensitivity to radiation therapy, relapses are common. In a compilation of nine studies (obviously varying in patient populations, treatment modalities, and follow-up) 87 of 143 patients (61 percent) either were alive with disease or died of disease (111,112,116,121, 134,138,161,162,172). Five-year survival rates have ranged from 46 to 63 percent. In one study, however, the 3-year survival rate was only 9 percent (134). Relapse may be detected from a few months after initial therapy up to many years later; recurrent tumor has been noted in patients as late as 18 and 24 years following initial treatment (145,161). The prognosis is quite poor after tumor dissemination; dissemination to extranodal sites such as the skin, subcutaneous tissue, gastrointestinal tract, and testis is typical (142), as well as to lymph nodes, liver, and spleen. Several examples of an associated hemophagocytic syndrome have been described (fig. 8-27) (111,128,131,153): it occurs at any time during the course of nasal T/NK cell lymphoma, is associated with EBV, and is typically fatal.

Malignant Lymphoma with Pseudoepitheliomatous Hyperplasia

General Features. Although malignant lymphoma with pseudoepitheliomatous hyperplasia is not a specific subtype of lymphoma, it is included here to delineate its histologic features which may be misinterpreted as squamous cell carcinoma, particularly in small biopsy specimens. Some if not all of these lesions represent examples of T/NK cell lymphoma (177).

General Features. Each of the six cases reported in detail has involved the nasal cavity, either primarily or as recurrent disease (178,179). Other additional sites of involvement included the nasopharynx, paranasal sinuses, palate, alveolar ridge, pterygopalatine fossa, and cheek. Chan and colleagues (177) observed pseudoepitheli-

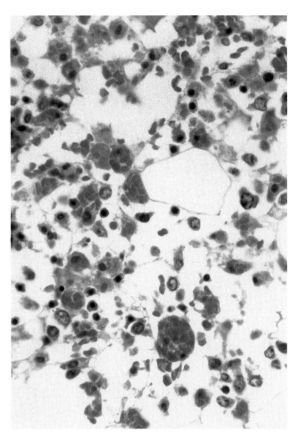

Figure 8-27
SINONASAL T/NK CELL LYMPHOMA
This case was associated with the hemophagocytic syndrome. There was striking hemophagocytosis in the bone marrow, but involvement by lymphoma was absent.

omatous hyperplasia in 3 of 11 nasal/nasopharyngeal T/NK cell lymphomas.

Clinical Features. The patients ranged in age from 27 to 78 years (178,179). Five of the six patients were women. Each neoplasm arose as a stage I lymphoma. Presenting sinonasal symptoms were nonspecific.

Microscopic Findings. Each case showed striking pseudoepitheliomatous hyperplasia (fig. 8-28), which in one case led to a misdiagnosis of squamous cell carcinoma. Located within and beneath the squamous proliferation were lymphoid cells with malignant cytologic features. Four cases showed angioinvasion by the tumor cells. In addition, necrosis was frequently observed. Two of the lymphomas were classified as diffuse mixed small and large cell lymphoma, while four were classified as diffuse large cell immunoblastic lymphoma with polymorphous features.

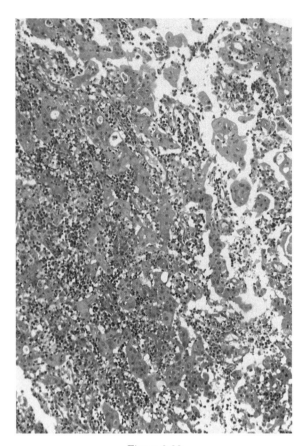

Figure 8-28
MALIGNANT LYMPHOMA WITH
PSEUDOEPITHELIOMATOUS HYPERPLASIA
Hyperplasia of squamous epithelium is surrounded by a
bulky lymphoid infiltrate in this nasal T-cell lymphoma.

Immunohistochemical Findings. Of the
five neoplasms that were immunophenotyped,
four had findings that were typical or suggestive
of T-cell differentiation (178,179). Although these
cases were not examined for CD56, it is possible
that some would have been immunoreactive.

Differential Diagnosis. The chief differential diagnostic consideration is squamous cell
carcinoma. Unlike squamous cell carcinoma, the
cells of pseudoepitheliomatous hyperplasia lack
marked nuclear pleomorphism and hyperchromatism. In addition, mitotic figures in pseudoepitheliomatous hyperplasia are present in modest numbers, typically along the basal layers of
the epithelium. Attention to the malignant cytologic features of the adjacent lymphocytes is, of
course, important for the proper diagnosis of
malignant lymphoma.

Treatment and Prognosis. Each patient
was treated initially with local radiation therapy
(178,179). Several of the patients also received
chemotherapy, chiefly for recurrent disease. At
follow-up, three of the six patients had no evidence of disease at 1 1/2, 2, and 10 years, respectively. One patient died of lymphoma at 11
months, while two are alive with tumor; one of
these latter two patients has disease 7 years
after initial diagnosis.

EXTRAMEDULLARY PLASMACYTOMA

General Features. Numerous studies and
literature reviews over the past 50 years have
catalogued examples of extramedullary plasmacytoma of the upper aerodigestive tract (181–184,186,
190–192,194,196,198), which is the most common
site for the occurrence of extraosseous disease. It
has been noted that 80 percent of extramedullary plasmacytomas arise in the head and neck
area (192). Plasmacytoma is usually solitary in
this anatomic location, but in some instances, it
is found in the setting of known multiple myeloma or precedes the development of multiple
myeloma. Of 299 cases of extramedullary plasmacytoma of the upper aerodigestive tract collected from the literature and from the files of the
AFIP, 52 percent arose in the sinonasal tract, 22
percent in the nasopharynx, 8 percent in the larynx, 7 percent in the tonsil, 6 percent in the pharynx, 2 percent in the soft palate, and 1 percent each
in the tongue, gingiva, and trachea (190,192,193).
Extramedullary plasmacytoma is the most frequent primary hematolymphoid neoplasm arising
in the larynx. A total of 90 cases had been reported
as of 1995 (189). Most involved the supraglottic
portion of the larynx, particularly the epiglottis,
while the subglottic portion was involved in less
than 10 percent of cases.

Clinical Features. There is a wide age
range, but most patients are in the fifth to seventh decades of life. Approximately 80 percent of
patients are men. Presenting symptoms include
a nasal mass, facial swelling, airway obstruction,
epistaxis, facial pain, nasal discharge, proptosis,
dysphagia, or hoarseness. Fever is typically absent. Although it is appropriate to evaluate the
patient for systemic disease, the bone marrow is
usually negative, and serum and urine proteins
are usually in the normal range. Extramedullary

plasmacytoma of the head and neck involves the draining cervical lymph nodes in 8 to 32 percent of cases (186).

Gross Findings. Plasmacytoma usually appears as an elevated, smooth-surfaced, subepithelial mass that bulges into the affected lumen. It may also be polypoid. The mass usually measures from 2 to 5 cm in greatest diameter. The soft or firm neoplasm is pink-tan, gray, or red. Ulceration of the overlying epithelium is unusual.

Microscopic Findings. There is a subepithelial monomorphous proliferation of plasma cells, whose cytologic features vary from case to case (fig. 8-29). The plasma cells may appear mature or pleomorphic (anaplastic) (fig. 8-30). Atypical cytologic features include large nuclei, an increased nuclear to cytoplasmic ratio, coarse nuclear chromatin, and prominent nucleoli. Mitotic figures range from 0 to 1 or 2 per high-power field. Local invasion of underlying tissues is common. In the AFIP series, 20 percent of the 53 cases had large deposits of amyloid (fig. 8-31) (190). There is no firm evidence that the degree of differentiation of the plasma cells correlates with long-term prognosis.

Immunohistochemical Findings. Immunohistochemical stains for kappa or lambda light chains show a monoclonal proliferation (fig. 8-32). Plasmacytomas characteristically are positive for cytoplasmic immunoglobulin and negative for surface immunoglobulin (8). Most of the B-cell associated antigens (CD19, CD20, CD22) are negative, but CD79a is positive in over 50 percent of cases (187). The pan-leukocyte marker CD45 is positive in less than half of the cases (fig. 8-33), while CD43 is present in more than half (187). On occasion, the T-cell antigens CD2, CD4, and CD9 may be observed (195). The NK antigen, CD56, is positive in over 50 percent of all plasmacytomas (187,195), CD38 is detected in over 90 percent (187,195), over half are immunoreactive for CD30, and positivity for epithelial membrane antigen may also be observed (187). The myelomonocytic antigens CD13, CD14, CD15, and CD33 may occasionally be found in plasmacytomas/myelomas (195).

Other Special Techniques. By in situ hybridization for kappa or lambda mRNA, 22 of 23 extramedullary plasmacytomas of the head and neck showed light chain mRNA restriction (177). Twenty-one of these 23 cases were monoclonal for either kappa or lambda by standard immu-

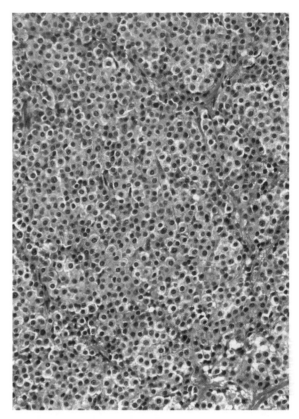

Figure 8-29
PLASMACYTOMA
Sheets of monotonous-appearing plasma cells were observed in this tumor from the nasopharynx.

nohistochemistry. Plasmacytomas/myelomas have immunoglobulin heavy and light chain gene rearrangements or deletions (187). EBV does not seem to be important in the pathogenesis of these tumors, as the majority of cases in one study lacked EBV DNA and RNA (177).

Differential Diagnosis. A variety of lesions arising in the upper aerodigestive tract enter into the differential diagnosis in small biopsy specimens. These include extramedullary myeloid cell tumor, undifferentiated carcinoma, olfactory neuroblastoma, melanoma, large cell lymphoma, and reactive plasmacytosis. Anaplastic plasmacytomas may be difficult to distinguish from other poorly differentiated round cell neoplasms. Large cell lymphoma with immunoblastic features may also be confused with poorly differentiated plasmacytoma, and, at times, the diagnosis is almost arbitrary. Obviously, cases with overt plasma cell cytologic features should be

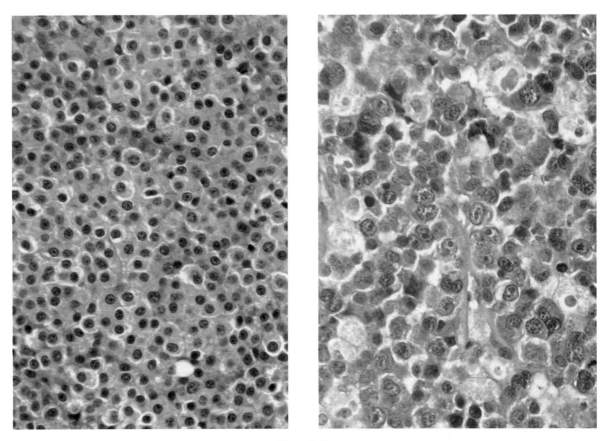

Figure 8-30
PLASMACYTOMA
The neoplastic cells may appear relatively mature, as seen in this nasopharyngeal example (left), or pleomorphic, as observed in this sinonasal neoplasm (right). For the latter neoplasm, the differential diagnosis would include a large cell lymphoma with immunoblastic features.

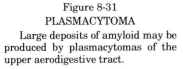

Figure 8-31
PLASMACYTOMA
Large deposits of amyloid may be produced by plasmacytomas of the upper aerodigestive tract.

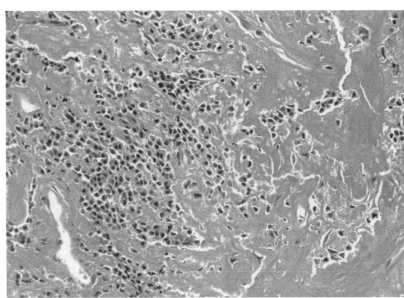

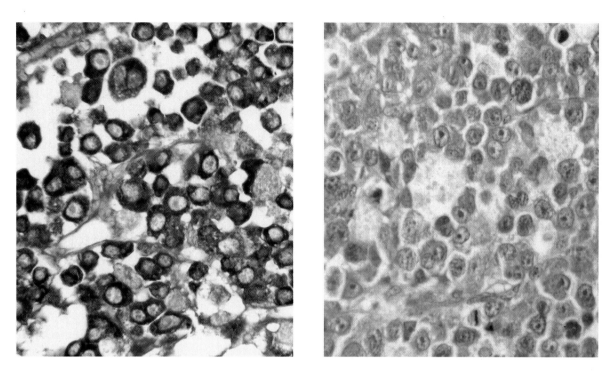

Figure 8-32
PLASMACYTOMA
Neoplastic plasma cells typically show light chain restriction. This neoplasm was immunoreactive for lambda light chain (left) and negative for kappa light chain (right).

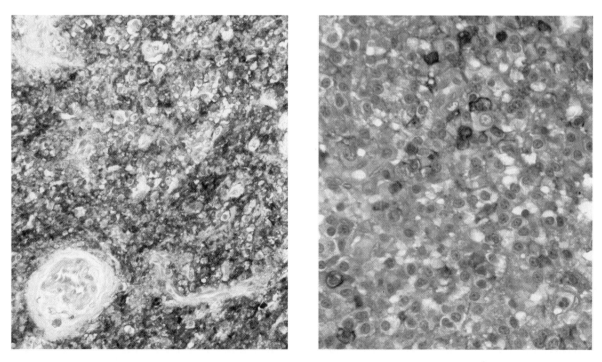

Figure 8-33
PLASMACYTOMA
Immunostaining for CD45 is variable. If positive, staining may be diffuse or focal.

classified as plasmacytoma. A panel of antibodies to B-cell antigens, CD45, and CD38, may help in the differential diagnosis. One study showed some differences in immunophenotype between plasmacytoma/multiple myeloma and large cell immunoblastic lymphoma in frozen sections (197).

Plasmacytoma should also be distinguished from mucous membrane plasmacytosis, which was described in the upper aerodigestive tract of nine patients in one study (185). Most of these patients had more than one site of involvement in the aerodigestive tract. In mucous membrane plasmacytosis the mucosa appears warty or cobblestone. This is reflected by psoriasiform epithelial hyperplasia with dyskeratosis, dense subepithelial plasmacytosis, and scattered polymorphonuclear leukocytes and lymphocytes. The plasma cells are characteristically mature and are polyclonal for kappa and lambda light chains. The etiology of mucous membrane plasmacytosis is unknown, and the lesion usually shows no regression. In two patients there was progression to airway obstruction requiring tracheostomy. There has been no progression to malignancy, but effective medical therapy has also not been reported.

Treatment and Prognosis. Radiation therapy is standard treatment for patients with extramedullary plasmacytoma of the upper aerodigestive tract (188). Radical surgery is usually not indicated, but may be appropriate for locally persistent or recurrent neoplasm. It has been shown that if amyloid is absent in a neoplasm, the plasmacytoma completely disappears within 3 months after completion of radiation therapy (188). Much slower tumor regression is observed in lesions that contain amyloid (188). Some plasmacytomas with amyloid show only a partial response to radiation therapy, and surgical resection is indicated for eradication of residual neoplasm. Patients with disseminated plasmacytoma/myeloma are treated best with chemotherapy.

Thirty-one to 75 percent of patients with primary plasmacytomas of the upper aerodigestive tract survive 5 years (189,191,192). Dissemination occurs in approximately 35 to 50 percent of patients, sometimes several decades later (191,192). Ten to 15 percent of patients have local persistence or recurrence, while 10 to 15 percent develop additional plasmacytomas at other sites (191). If there is multiple myeloma, the median survival is typically less than 2 years (191). The behavior of the

neoplasm cannot be predicted from its histologic features (192). Tumor site and the presence or absence of bone destruction are important factors to predict the development of multiple myeloma (188). Plasmacytomas of the tonsil, parapharyngeal space, nasal cavity, and nasopharynx proceed less often to multiple myeloma than those elsewhere in the head and neck area. Patients whose plasmacytomas show bone destruction are at increased risk for progression to multiple myeloma and death. The presence or absence of an M protein peak does not influence survival (188).

POST-TRANSPLANTATION LYMPHOPROLIFERATIVE DISORDER

General Features. Post-transplantation lymphoproliferative disorder (PTLD), arising in patients who have received a solid organ transplant, consists of a morphologically heterogeneous EBV-driven B-cell proliferation whose clonal status is variable (201). Most cases have been associated with latent EBV infection, although lytic activity may be important in initiating the process (204). PTLD has been reported in 1 to 5 percent of patients after transplant, and this rate depends in part upon the type of organ transplanted (201, 203,205); the type and severity of PTLD also varies according to the immunosuppressive regimen employed. PTLD may regress after reduction of immunosuppression, but may also progress despite therapy. In the evolution of pathologic classifications to predict the behavior of PTLD, the most recent system of Knowles et al. (201) appears to be quite useful. The three groups of PTLD in this scheme include: 1) plasmacytic hyperplasia; 2) polymorphic B-cell hyperplasia and polymorphic B-cell lymphoma; and 3) immunoblastic lymphoma and multiple myeloma.

The most common anatomic sites of occurrence of PTLD are cervical lymph nodes, the gastrointestinal system, liver, and Waldeyer's ring. In one series of 43 patients with PTLD, 28 percent involved Waldeyer's ring (205).

Clinical Features. Most patients with PTLD involving Waldeyer's ring are children or young adults. Children without previous exposure to EBV may develop PTLD localized to the tonsils and adenoid, and biopsy of these areas may permit early diagnosis and treatment (202). Of 14 patients with PTLD involving Waldeyer's ring, the onset after transplantation ranged from 2 to 162 months (median, 1 year) (202,205). Most patients had a mononucleosis-like syndrome with fever, lymphadenopathy, and tonsillitis (202,205). Other findings included hoarseness, otitis, and symptoms of upper respiratory tract infection. Upper respiratory tract obstruction by PTLD may be life threatening in children (205).

Gross Findings. PTLD appears as a solid tumor simulating lymphoma, a diffuse infiltrate of an organ, or enlargement of a native lymphoid organ. For tonsils and adenoid, there is enlargement, lobulation, and a gray-white color.

Microscopic Findings. A spectrum of histologic, phenotypic, and genotypic features ranges from a polymorphous, polyclonal lymphoid hyperplasia to a monomorphic, monoclonal proliferation with features of high grade lymphoma (201). Using the classification of Knowles et al. (201), group 1 (plasmacytic hyperplasia) consists of plasmacytoid lymphocytes with conspicuous plasma cells and sparse immunoblasts. Plasmacytic hyperplasia most often arises in the oropharynx or lymph nodes. It is almost always polyclonal, usually contains multiple EBV infection events or only a minor population of cells infected by a single form of EBV, and lacks oncogene and tumor suppressor gene alterations. The polymorphic B-cell hyperplasia of group 2 PTLD consists of a mixture of plasmacytoid lymphocytes, abundant plasma cells, and immunoblasts without atypia. There may be necrosis of single cells or a few small necrotic foci. Polymorphic B-cell lymphoma shows plasmacytic differentiation with prominent cytologic atypia of immunoblasts. There may be large foci of necrosis. Type 2 PTLD usually involves lymph nodes, lungs, or the gastrointestinal system. The proliferation is almost always monoclonal, usually contains a single form of EBV, and lacks oncogene and tumor suppressor gene alterations. Group 3 PTLD consists of large cell immunoblastic lymphoma and multiple myeloma. It is monoclonal, has a single form of EBV, and contains alterations of one or more oncogenes or tumor suppressor genes (N-*ras* mutation, p53 mutation, or c-*myc* gene rearrangement). Most patients with type 3 PTLD have widely disseminated disease.

Immunohistochemical Findings and Other Special Techniques. As mentioned above, most examples of PTLD of Waldeyer's ring consist of

plasmacytic hyperplasia. Immunophenotypically, plasmacytic hyperplasia does not show immunoglobulin light chain restriction, although a small clonal B-cell population may be observed uncommonly (201). EBV in PTLD can be detected by several techniques including the polymerase chain reaction for EBV DNA, in situ hybridization for EBV mRNA (EBER), and immunohistochemical methods for EBV latent membrane protein (202). EBV latent membrane protein is observed in the large lymphocytes and immunoblasts; EBV mRNA is detected in CD20-positive lymphocytes. Using immunohistochemistry and in situ hybridization, approximately 90 percent of specimens in one study showed evidence of at least one of the lytic EBV nucleic acids and proteins (204). The degree of lytic activity did not vary with the particular histopathologic findings.

Treatment and Prognosis. Patients with plasmacytic hyperplasia usually have regression of disease following reduction in immunosuppression (199,202). As PTLD of Waldeyer's ring typically consists of plasmacytic hyperplasia, the prognosis for patients with PTLD of the tonsils and adenoid is typically excellent. Of 13 patients with PTLD of head and neck sites in one study, 10 were alive from 7 to 64 months after diagnosis (205). There was recurrence in only 1 patient, while another died of laryngospasm after a clinical examination. Most of those with polymorphic B-cell hyperplasia and polymorphic B-cell lymphoma also regress following decrease in immunosuppression (199). Patients with large cell immunoblastic lymphoma or multiple myeloma, however, usually have advanced stage disease that cannot be halted. Despite reduction in immunosuppression, these patients usually die.

EXTRAMEDULLARY TUMORS OF MYELOID OR LYMPHOID BLASTS

General Features. Extramedullary myeloblastic or lymphoblastic proliferations appear as mass lesions or leukemic infiltrates. Extramedullary myeloid cell tumors occur in association with acute or chronic myeloid leukemia, myeloproliferative disorders, or without initial evidence of leukemia (212,213). They may arise in virtually any body site, although lymph nodes appear to be the most common location. Extramedullary myeloid cell tumors have been described in the nasopharynx, tonsil, pharynx, oral cavity, nasal cavity, and paranasal sinuses (210); tumors of the larynx are extremely rare (209).

Clinical Features. Overall, there is a wide age distribution, from very young children to very old adults (213). There is no sex predilection. The clinical appearance is usually that of a mass lesion, but oral cavity involvement, typically seen in monocytic or myelomonocytic leukemias, manifests as gingival hypertrophy, gingivitis, hemorrhage, petechiae, or ulceration (207). The gingival hypertrophy is usually generalized and varies in severity. The gingiva appear boggy, erythematous, and edematous; they often bleed easily. Loosening of the teeth may be observed.

Gross Findings. Extramedullary blastic cell tumors appear fleshy and tan-white. Those of myeloid differentiation (chloroma) may be pale green.

Microscopic Findings. The cells are lymphoblastic, myeloblastic, or monoblastic. Their growth is diffuse and infiltrative (fig. 8-34) and the neoplastic infiltrates may separate minor salivary glands. Large areas of necrosis are unusual, but single cell necrosis is common.

Lymphoblasts are slightly larger than normal small lymphocytes. Their nuclei are round or convoluted, and the chromatin is fine and homogeneous; nucleoli are inconspicuous. Mitotic figures are numerous, and a starry-sky low-power microscopic appearance may be obvious. There are no morphologic features that distinguish T-cell from B-cell lymphoblastic proliferations (208).

Myeloid or monocytic blasts are approximately the size of large lymphocytes, and contain nuclei that are round, oval, reniform, or multilobated. Their nuclear membranes appear delicate. Nucleoli are small or large, and the cytoplasm is scant to moderate. Mitotic figures are characteristically numerous. The myeloid cells show varying states of differentiation; eosinophilic myelocytes and mature eosinophils, when present, are important for the diagnosis. Touch imprint specimens may show granules within the cytoplasm, and the finding of Auer rods is diagnostic of myeloid differentiation. Extramedullary myeloid cell tumors have been classified as well differentiated, poorly differentiated, or blastic (215). Well-differentiated tumors show conspicuous numbers of mature myeloid cells including eosinophilic myelocytes, whereas poorly differentiated myeloid lesions have only occasional to rare eosinophilic

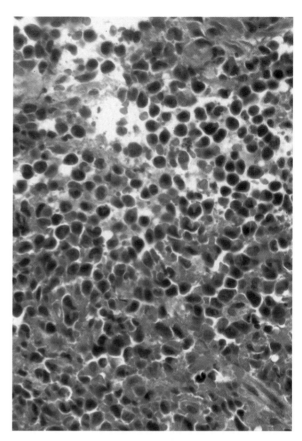

Figure 8-34
EXTRAMEDULLARY MYELOID CELL TUMOR
This nasopharyngeal neoplasm consists of sheets of noncohesive hematolymphoid cells having irregular nuclear outlines.

myelocytes. Blastic myeloid tumors show no morphologic evidence of myeloid differentiation; these neoplasms typically have round nuclei with fine nuclear chromatin, occasional small nucleoli, large numbers of mitotic figures, and a starry-sky pattern. Overall, eosinophilic myelocytes are absent in 50 to 70 percent of extramedullary myeloid cell tumors (207,211,213, 215). The Leder stain (naphthol AS-D chloroacetate esterase) is useful in diagnosing myeloid differentiation (fig. 8-35), but is absent in 25 to 33 percent of cases (207,213,215).

Immunohistochemical Findings. Immunohistochemical stains are often critical in determining lymphoid or myeloid differentiation. For frozen section specimens, stains for CD45, CD7, CD3, CD10, CD19, CD13, and CD33 are the most important (214). In paraffin-embedded sections,

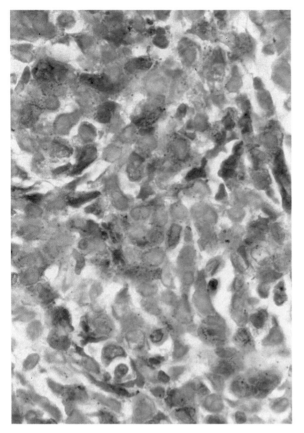

Figure 8-35
EXTRAMEDULLARY MYELOID CELL TUMOR
Positivity with the Leder stain (naphthol AS-D chloroacetate esterase) in the neoplastic cells confirms the presence of myeloid differentiation.

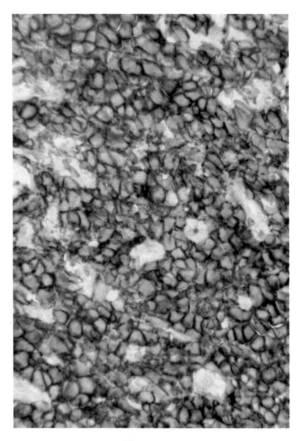

Figure 8-36
EXTRAMEDULLARY MYELOID CELL TUMOR
CD43 is present in virtually all extramedullary myeloid cell neoplasms and assists in confirming a hematolymphoid origin.

CD45 may be negative in both lymphoblastic and myeloblastic cells. CD43, while not lineage specific, may be helpful when positive (fig. 8-36) in identifying a CD45-negative tumor as having a hematolymphoid origin (214). CD45RA (4KB5) and CD45RO (UCHL1) although usually indicative of B-cell and T-cell differentiation, respectively, may stain myeloid cells (207). In series examining various markers for their use in the diagnosis of extramedullary myeloid cell tumors, CD45 was immunopositive in 81 percent, CD43 in 100 percent, CD20 in 4 percent, CD34 in 36 percent, myeloperoxidase in 93 percent, CD68 in 79 percent, MAC387 in 87 percent, lysozyme in 81 percent (fig. 8-37), CD15 in 44 percent, and elastase in 51 percent (207,213,215). In these studies, the Leder stain was positive in 71 percent of the cases. Hence, to determine lymphoblas-

tic or myeloblastic differentiation in paraffin-embedded sections, the most useful immunostains include antibodies to CD20, CD43, CD68, CD45RO, CD45, CD3, CD79a, and antimyeloperoxidase (214,215). MAC387 and lysozyme may also be of value.

Differential Diagnosis. A high index of suspicion is often required in order to avoid misdiagnosis. The diagnosis of extramedullary myeloid cell neoplasms may be exceptionally difficult in the absence of known leukemia. In such situations, it is important to recognize that the hematolymphoid (myeloid) proliferation does not easily fit into standard subtypes of lymphoma. Immunophenotypic results, as discussed above, are critical for the diagnosis of most cases. Additional diagnostic considerations include plasmacytoma, undifferentiated carcinoma, olfactory

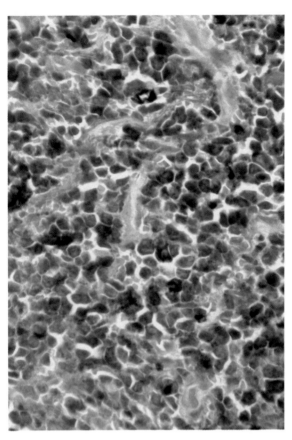

Figure 8-37
EXTRAMEDULLARY MYELOID CELL TUMOR
The majority of these neoplasms are immunoreactive for lysozyme.

neuroblastoma, rhabdomyosarcoma, and melanoma. For each of these, immunohistochemistry may be essential.

Treatment and Prognosis. Chemotherapy is the most important therapeutic modality, and the specific regimen depends upon whether differentiation is lymphoblastic or myeloblastic. Patients with extramedullary myeloid cell tumors and concurrent acute myeloid leukemia have no prognostic differences from those with acute myeloid leukemia alone (213). The finding of extramedullary myeloid cell tumor in a patient with a known myeloproliferative disorder is indicative of transformation to acute leukemia (213). Although the majority of patients who present with extramedullary myeloid cell tumor alone ultimately develop acute myeloid leukemia, a small subset appear to have localized disease that fails to progress (212).

HODGKIN'S DISEASE OF WALDEYER'S RING

General Features. Hodgkin's disease rarely occurs in Waldeyer's ring. Of 659 cases of Hodgkin's disease reviewed in one large series, only 6 involved Waldeyer's ring (217). Some of the purported examples of Hodgkin's disease of Waldeyer's ring are incompletely documented, and in only a few studies are the cases supported by immunohistochemical staining (216,218–220). Some of the older reports of Hodgkin's disease of Waldeyer's ring may be examples of non-Hodgkin's lymphoma, in particular Lennert's lymphoma (221).

Clinical Features. In the largest series of Waldeyer's ring Hodgkin's disease supported with immunohistochemical findings, Kapadia and colleagues (219) studied 16 patients whose ages ranged from 14 to 74 years (median, 41 years). There were 8 men and 7 women. The clinical presentation most often included symptoms of airway obstruction or unilateral tonsillar enlargement. Characteristically, there was no fever, night sweats, or weight loss. Of the 16 cases, 46 percent were stage I, 39 percent were stage II (involving cervical lymph nodes), and 15 percent were stage III (involving the spleen). The tonsil or nasopharyngeal lymphoid tissue was most often involved by Hodgkin's disease, while involvement of the base of tongue was unusual.

Microscopic Findings. Of the 16 cases reported by Kapadia et al. (219), 8 were of mixed cellularity Hodgkin's disease; 4 were nodular sclerosis; 1, nodular lymphocyte predominance; and 3, interfollicular Hodgkin's disease (fig. 8-38). The examples of interfollicular Hodgkin's disease showed prominent reactive secondary follicles with scattered interfollicular clusters of Hodgkin's cells and typical Reed-Sternberg cells; the normal lymphoid architecture was not effaced. Seven other well-documented examples of nodular lymphocyte predominance Hodgkin's disease have been reported in Waldeyer's ring tissue (216,220). In two studies of Hodgkin's disease involving extranodal sites, 6 of 29 cases involved Waldeyer's ring (216,220). The histologic appearance was similar to that of nodal nodular lymphocyte predominance Hodgkin's disease. In tonsillar tissue, the nodular proliferation distorted epithelial islands, but there was

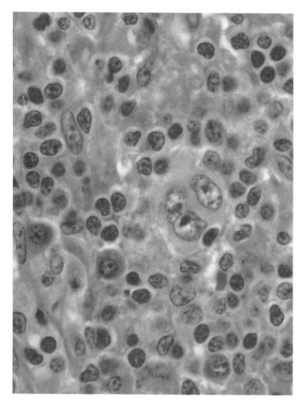

Figure 8-38
HODGKIN'S DISEASE
The finding of Reed-Sternberg cells in Waldeyer's ring is
diagnostic of Hodgkin's disease. (Courtesy of Dr. S.B. Kapadia, Pittsburgh, PA.)

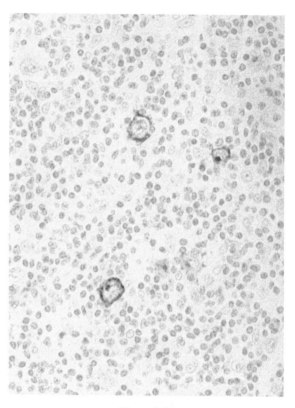

Figure 8-39
HODGKIN'S DISEASE
The malignant cells in Hodgkin's disease involving
Waldeyer's ring lymphoid tissue are typically immunoreactive
for CD15. (Courtesy of Dr. S.B. Kapadia, Pittsburgh, PA.)

no infiltration of the epithelium by lymphocytic
and histiocytic (L&H) cells (216).

Immunohistochemical Findings. The malignant cells in mixed cellularity, nodular sclerosis, and interfollicular Hodgkin's disease typically show an absence of immunostaining for
CD45, CD20, and CD45RO. They are immunoreactive, however, for CD15 (fig. 8-39), CD30, or
both. In nodular lymphocyte predominance
Hodgkin's disease, the neoplastic cells are usually immunoreactive for CD45 and CD20, but
lack staining for CD45RO, CD15, and CD30.

Other Special Techniques. Using in situ
hybridization, EBV EBER1 mRNA has been
demonstrated in the Reed-Sternberg cells of 8 of
12 cases of Waldeyer's ring Hodgkin's disease
(219). These EBER1 mRNA-positive cases were
examples of mixed cellularity or nodular sclerosis, while the one example of nodular lymphocyte
predominance Hodgkin's disease lacked evi-

dence of EBV. These results are an indication of
the greater prevalence of EBV-related Hodgkin's
disease in Waldeyer's ring lymphoid tissue than
in nodal Hodgkin's disease. This may be related
to the fact that Waldeyer's ring is a natural
reservoir for latent EBV infection (219).

Differential Diagnosis. Hodgkin's disease in
Waldeyer's ring should be distinguished from T-
cell lymphoma, T-cell–rich B-cell lymphoma, undifferentiated carcinoma, and infectious mononucleosis (219). T-cell lymphoma arising in Waldeyer's
ring consists of a spectrum of atypical lymphoid
cells that include small and large lymphocytes
which demonstrate a T-cell immunophenotype.
T-cell–rich B-cell lymphoma consists of CD20-pos-
itive, large B-cells that are CD15 and CD30 negative, occurring in a setting of numerous small T-lym-
phocytes. Unlike Hodgkin's disease, infectious
mononucleosis shows foci of follicular hyperplasia,
a spectrum of transformed lymphocytes typically

with nests and sheets of immunoblasts, and individual cell necrosis. The enlarged transformed cells in infectious mononucleosis, unlike the malignant cells in mixed cellularity Hodgkin's disease, are CD45 positive and CD15 negative, and show a B-cell or T-cell immunophenotype.

Nodular lymphocyte predominance Hodgkin's disease should be distinguished from follicular lymphoma and MALT lymphoma (220). MALT lymphoma may be simulated by the nodular pattern of growth and a polymorphous lymphoid background of Hodgkins disease. Unlike MALT lymphoma, however, there are typical L&H cells and an absence of sheets of "centrocyte-like" cells.

Nodular lymphocyte predominance Hodgkin's disease should also not be confused with peripheral T-cell lymphoma with abundant epithelioid histiocytes (Lennert's lymphoma), which has a predilection for tonsillar involvement (216).

Treatment and Prognosis. In the series of patients with Hodgkin's disease of Waldeyer's ring, treatment was with local radiation with or without chemotherapy (219). A complete response was noted in 14 of 16 patients. One patient had a local recurrence, while 3 others had distant spread of disease. One patient with stage II and 1 patient with stage III Hodgkin's disease died of widespread neoplasm.

REFERENCES

Hyperplasia of Waldeyer's Ring in Human Immunodeficiency Virus Infection

1. Carbone A, Gloghini A, Vaccher E, Barzan L, Tirelli U. Nasopharyngeal lymphoid tissue masses in patients with human immunodeficiency virus-1 [Letter]. Cancer 1995;76:527–8.
2. Graeme-Cook F, Bhan AK, Harris NL. Immunohistochemical characterization of intraepithelial and subepithelial mononuclear cells of the upper airways. Am J Pathol 1993;143:1416–22.
3. Shahab I, Osborne BM, Butler JJ. Nasopharyngeal lymphoid tissue masses in patients with human immunodeficiency virus-1. Histologic findings and clinical correlation. Cancer 1994;74:3083–8.
4. Wenig BM, Thompson LD, Frankel SS, et al. Lymphoid changes of the nasopharyngeal and palatine tonsils that are indicative of human immunodeficiency virus infection. A clinicopathologic study of 12 cases. Am J Surg Pathol 1996;20:572–87.
5. Winther B, Innes DJ. The human adenoid. A morphologic study. Arch Otolaryngol Head Neck Surg 1994;120:144–9.
6. Ziegler JL, Beckstead JA, Volberding PA, et al. Non-Hodgkin's lymphoma in 90 homosexual men. Relation to generalized lymphadenopathy and the acquired immunodeficiency syndrome. N Engl J Med 1984;311:565–70.

Infectious Mononucleosis

7. Abbondanzo SL, Sato N, Straus SE, Jaffe ES. Acute infectious mononucleosis. CD30 (Ki-1) antigen expression and histologic correlations. Am J Clin Pathol 1990;93:698–702.
8. Brousset P, Schlaifer D, Roda D, Mussip P, Marchou B, Delsol G. Characterization of Epstein-Barr virus-infected cells in benign lymphadenopathy of patients seropositive for human immunodeficiency virus. Hum Pathol 1996;27:263–8.
9. Childs CC, Parham DM, Berard CW. Infectious mononucleosis. The spectrum of morphologic changes simulating lymphoma in lymph nodes and tonsils. Am J Surg Pathol 1987;11:122–32.
10. Dorfman RF, Warnke R. Lymphadenopathy simulating the malignant lymphomas. Hum Pathol 1974;5:519–50.
11. Epstein MA, Achong BG. Pathogenesis of infectious mononucleosis. Lancet 1977;2:1270–2.
12. Gulley ML, Raab-Traub N. Detection of Epstein-Barr virus in human tissues by molecular genetic techniques. Arch Pathol Lab Med 1993;117:1115–20.
13. Isaacson PG, Schmid C, Pan L, Wotherspoon AC, Wright DH. Epstein-Barr virus latent membrane protein expression by Hodgkin and Reed-Sternberg-like cells in acute infectious mononucleosis. J Pathol 1992;167:267–71.
14. Lones MA, Mishalani S, Shintaku IP, Weiss LM, Nichols WS, Said JW. Changes in tonsils and adenoids in children with posttransplant lymphoproliferative disorders: report of three cases with early involvement of Waldeyer's ring. Hum Pathol 1995;26:525–30.
15. Niedobitek G, Hamilton-Dutoit SH, Herbst H, et al. Identification of Epstein-Barr virus infected cells in tonsils of acute infectious mononucleosis by in situ hybridization. Hum Pathol 1989;20:796–9.
16. Salvador AH, Harrison EG Jr, Kyle RA. Lymphadenopathy due to infectious mononucleosis: its confusion with malignant lymphoma. Cancer 1971;27:1029–40.
17. Shin SS, Berry GJ, Weiss LM. Infectious mononucleosis. Diagnosis by in situ hybridization in two cases with atypical features. Am J Surg Pathol 1991;15:625–31.
18. Strickler JG, Fedeli F, Horowitz CA, Copenhaver CM, Frizzera G. Infectious mononucleosis in lymphoid tissue. Histopathology, in situ hybridization, and differential diagnosis. Arch Pathol Lab Med 1993;117:269–78.
19. Tao Q, Srivastava G, Chan AC, Chung LP, Loke SL, Ho FC. Evidence for lytic infection by Epstein-Barr virus in mucosal lymphocytes instead of nasopharyngeal epithelial cells in normal individuals. J Med Virol 1995;45:71–7.
20. Tao Q, Srivastava G, Chan AC, Ho FC. Epstein-Barr-virus-infected nasopharyngeal intraepithelial lymphocytes [Letter]. Lancet 1995;345:1309–10.

Sinus Histiocytosis with Massive Lymphadenopathy

21. Eisen RN, Buckley PJ, Rosai J. Immunophenotypic characterization of sinus histiocytosis with massive lymphadenopathy (Rosai-Dorfman disease). Semin Diagn Pathol 1990;7:74–82.
22. Foucar E, Rosai J, Dorfman RF. Sinus histiocytosis with massive lymphadenopathy. Ear, nose, and throat manifestations. Arch Otolaryngol 1978;104:687–93.
23. Foucar E, Rosai J, Dorfman R. Sinus histiocytosis with massive lymphadenopathy (Rosai-Dorfman disease): review of the entity. Semin Diagn Pathol 1990;7:19–73.
24. Komp DM. The treatment of sinus histiocytosis with massive lymphadenopathy (Rosai-Dorfman disease). Semin Diagn Pathol 1990;7:83–6.
25. Paulli M, Rosso R, Kindl S, et al. Immunophenotypic characterization of the cell infiltrate in five cases of sinus histiocytosis with massive lymphadenopathy (Rosai-Dorfman disease). Hum Pathol 1992;23:647–54.
26. Rosai J, Dorfman RF. Sinus histiocytosis with massive lymphadenopathy. A newly recognized benign clinicopathological entity. Arch Pathol 1969;87:63–70.
27. Rosai J, Dorfman RF. Sinus histiocytosis with massive lymphadenopathy: a pseudolymphomatous benign disorder. Analysis of 34 cases. Cancer 1972;30:1174–88.
28. Wenig BM, Abbondanzo SL, Childers EL, Kapadia SB, Heffner DR. Extranodal sinus histiocytosis with massive lymphadenopathy (Rosai-Dorfman disease) of the head and neck. Hum Pathol 1993;24:483–92.

Non-Hodgkin's Lymphoma of Oral Cavity

29. Blok P, van Delden L, van der Waal I. Non-Hodgkin's lymphoma of the hard palate. Oral Surg 1979;47:445–52.
30. Borisch B, Hennig I, Laeng RH, Waelti ER, Kraft R, Laissue J. Association of the subtype 2 of the Epstein-Barr virus with T-cell non-Hodgkin's lymphoma of the midline granuloma type. Blood 1993;82;858–64.
31. Chott A, Rappersberger K, Schlossarek W, Radaszkiewicz T. Peripheral T-cell lymphoma presenting primarily as lethal midline granuloma. Hum Pathol 1988;19:1093–101.
32. Dictor M, Cervin A, Kalm O, Rambech E. Sinonasal T-cell lymphoma in the differential diagnosis of lethal midline granuloma using in situ hybridization for Epstein-Barr virus RNA. Mod Pathol 1996;9:7–14.
33. Egawa N, Fukayama M, Kawaguchi K, et al. Relapsing oral and colonic ulcers with monoclonal T-cell infiltration. A low grade mucosal T-lymphoproliferative disease of the digestive tract. Cancer 1995;75:1728–33.
34. Emile JF, Boulland ML, Haioun C, et al. CD5- CD56+ T-cell receptor silent peripheral T-cell lymphomas are natural killer cell lymphomas. Blood 1996;87:1466–73.
35. Fukada Y, Ishida T, Fujimoto M, Ueda T, Aozusa K. Malignant lymphoma of the oral cavity: clinicopathologic analysis of 20 cases. J Oral Pathol 1987;16:8–12.
36. Greenspan JS, Daniels TE, Talal N, Sylvester RA. The histopathology of Sjogren's syndrome in labial salivary gland biopsies. Oral Surg 1974;37:217–29.
37. Handlers JP, Howell RE, Abrams AM, Melrose RJ. Extranodal oral lymphoma. Part I. A morphologic and immunoperoxidase study of 34 cases. Oral Surg Oral Med Oral Pathol 1986;61:362–7.
38. Harabuchi Y, Imai S, Wakashima J, et al. Nasal T-cell lymphoma causally associated with Epstein-Barr virus. Clinicopathologic, phenotypic, and genotypic studies. Cancer 1996;77:2137–49.
39. Ho FC, Choy D, Loke SL, et al. Polymorphic reticulosis and conventional lymphomas of the nose and upper aerodigestive tract: a clinicopathologic study of 70 cases, and immunophenotypic studies of 16 cases. Hum Pathol 1990;21:1041–50.
40. Howell RE, Handlers JP, Abrams AM, Melrose RJ. Extranodal oral lymphoma. Part II. Relationships between clinical features and the Lukes-Collins classification of 34 cases. Oral Surg Oral Med Oral Pathol 1987;64:597–602.
41. Jaffe ES, Chan JK, Su IJ, et al. Report of the workshop on nasal and related extranodal angiocentric T/natural killer cell lymphomas. Definitions, differential diagnosis, and epidemiology. Am J Surg Pathol 1996;20:103–11.
42. Jordan R, Diss TC, Lench NJ, Isaacson PG, Speight PM. Immunoglobulin gene rearrangements in lymphoplasmacytic infiltrates of labial salivary glands in Sjogren's syndrome: a possible predictor of lymphoma development. Oral Surg Oral Med Oral Pathol Oral Radiol 1995;79:723–9.
43. Kanavaros BP, Lescs MC, Briere J, et al. Nasal T-cell lymphoma: a clinicopathologic entity associated with peculiar phenotype and with Epstein-Barr virus. Blood 1993;81:2688–95.
44. Launder TM, Weathers DR, Farhi DC. Hematolymphoid lesions of the oral cavity [Abstract]. Am J Clin Pathol 1995;104:351–2.
45. Petrella T, Delfau-Larue MH, Caillot D, et al. Nasopharyngeal lymphomas: further evidence for a natural killer cell origin. Hum Pathol 1996;27:827–33.
46. Ratech H, Burke JS, Blayney DW, Sheibani K, Rappaport H. A clinicopathologic study of malignant lymphomas of the nose, paranasal sinuses, and hard palate, including cases of lethal midline granuloma. Cancer 1989;64:2525–31.
47. Takahashi H, Fujita S, Okabe H, Tsuda N, Tezuka F. Immunophenotypic analysis of extranodal non-Hodgkin's lymphomas in the oral cavity. Pathol Res Pract 1993;189:300–11.
48. Thomas JA, Cotter F, Hanby AM, et al. Epstein-Barr virus-related oral T-cell lymphoma associated with human immunodeficiency virus immunosuppression. Blood 1993;81:3350–6.
49. van Gorp J, De Bruin PC, Sie-Go DM, et al. Nasal T-cell lymphoma: a clinicopathological and immunophenotypic analysis of 13 cases. Histopathology 1995;27:139–48.

Non-Hodgkin's Lymphoma of Waldeyer's Ring

50. Albada J, Hordijk GJ, van Unnik JA, Dekker AW. Non-Hodgkin's lymphoma of Waldeyer's ring. Cancer 1985;56:2911–3.
51. Barton JH, Osborne BM, Butler JJ, et al. Non-Hodgkin's lymphoma of the tonsil. A clinicopathologic study of 65 cases. Cancer 1984;53:86–95.

52. Campo E, Jaffe ES. Mantle cell lymphoma. Accurate diagnosis yields new clinical insights [Editorial]. Arch Pathol Lab Med 1996;120:12–4.

53. Chan JK, Ng CS, Lau WH, Lo ST. Most nasal/nasopharyngeal lymphomas are peripheral T-cell neoplasms. Am J Surg Pathol 1987;11:418–29.

54. Chan JK, Ng CS, Lo ST. Immunohistochemical characterization of malignant lymphomas of the Waldeyer's ring other than the nasopharynx. Histopathology 1987;11:885–99.

55. Chan JK, Yip TT, Tsang WY, et al. Detection of Epstein-Barr viral RNA in malignant lymphomas of the upper aerodigestive tract. Am J Surg Pathol 1994;18:938–46.

56. Gospodarowicz MK, Sutcliffe SB, Brown TC, Chua T, Bush RS. Patterns of disease in localized extranodal lymphomas. J Clin Oncol 1987;5:875–80.

57. Graeme-Cook F, Bhan AK, Harris NL. Immunohistochemical characterization of intraepithelial and subepithelial mononuclear cells of the upper airways. Am J Pathol 1993;143:1416–22.

58. Harris NL, Jaffe ES, Stein H, et al. A revised European-American classification of lymphoid neoplasms: a proposal from the International Lymphoma Study Group. Blood 1994;84:1361–92.

59. Hoppe RT, Burke JS, Glatstein E, Kaplan HS. Non-Hodgkin's lymphoma. Involvement of Waldeyer's ring. Cancer 1978;42:1096–104.

60. Menarguez J, Mollejo M, Carrion R, et al. Waldeyer ring lymphomas. A clinicopathologic study of 79 cases. Histopathology 1994;24:13–22.

61. Morente MA, Piris M, Orradre JL, Rivas C, Villuendas R. Human tonsil intraepithelial B-cells: a marginal zone related subpopulation. J Clin Pathol 1992;45:668–72.

62. Paulsen J, Lennert K. Low-grade B-cell lymphoma of mucosa-associated lymphoid tissue type in Waldeyer's ring. Histopathology 1994;24:1–11.

63. Ree HJ, Rege VB, Knisley RE, et al. Malignant lymphoma of Waldeyer's ring following gastrointestinal lymphoma. Cancer 1980;46:1528–35.

64. Saul SH, Kapadia SB. Primary lymphoma of Waldeyer's ring. Clinicopathologic study of 68 cases. Cancer 1985;56:157–66.

65. Shimm DS, Dosoretz DE, Harris NL, Pilch BZ, Linggood RM, Wang CC. Radiation therapy of Waldeyer's ring lymphoma. Cancer 1984;54:426–31.

66. Sugimoto T, Hashimoto H, Enjoji M. Nasopharyngeal carcinomas and malignant lymphomas: an immunohistochemical analysis of 74 cases. Laryngoscope 1990;100:742–8.

67. Suzumiya J, Takeshita M, Kimura N, et al. Expression of adult and fetal natural killer cell markers in sinonasal lymphomas. Blood 1994;83:2255–60.

68. The Non-Hodgkin's Lymphoma Pathologic Classification Project. National Cancer Institute sponsored study of classifications of non-Hodgkin's lymphomas. Summary and description of a working formulation for clinical usage. Cancer 1982;49:2112–35.

69. Tomita Y, Ohsawa M, Kojya S, Aozasa K. Non-Hodgkin's lymphoma of the Waldeyer's ring as a manifestation of human T-cell leukemia virus type 1-associated lymphoproliferative diseases in southwest Japan [Abstract]. Mod Pathol 1996;9:124a.

70. Watson MG, Crocker J. Non-Hodgkin's lymphoma involving the tonsil: an immunohistochemical study. J Laryngol Otol 1991;105:445–50.

71. Weiss LM, Gaffey MJ, Chen YY, Frierson HF Jr. Frequency of Epstein-Barr viral DNA in "Western" sinonasal and Waldeyer's ring non-Hodgkin's lymphomas. Am J Surg Pathol 1992;16:156–62.

72. Wright DH. Lymphomas of Waldeyer's ring. Commentary. Histopathology 1994;24:97–9.

73. Yamanaka N, Harabuchi Y, Sambe S, et al. Non-Hodgkin's lymphoma of Waldeyer's ring and nasal cavity. Clinical and immunologic aspects. Cancer 1985;56:768–76.

74. Ye YL, Zhou MH, Lu XY, Dai YR, Wu WX. Nasopharyngeal and nasal malignant lymphoma: a clinicopathological study of 54 cases. Histopathology 1992;20:511–6.

Non-Hodgkin's Lymphoma of Larynx and Trachea

75. Anderson HA, Maisel RH, Cantrell RW. Isolated laryngeal lymphoma. Laryngoscope 1976;86:1251–7.

76. DeSanto LW, Weiland LH. Malignant lymphoma of the larynx. Laryngoscope 1970;80:966–78.

77. Ferlito A, Carbone A, Volpe R. Diagnosis and assessment of non-Hodgkin's malignant lymphomas of the larynx. ORL J Otorhinlaryngol Relat Spec 1981;43:61–78.

78. Fidias P, Wright C, Harris NL, Urba W, Grossbard ML. Primary tracheal non-Hodgkin's lymphoma. A case report and review of the literature. Cancer 1996;77:2332–8.

79. Gregor RT. Laryngeal malignant lymphoma—an entity? J Laryngol Otol 1981;95:81–93.

80. Harabuchi Y, Imai S, Wakashima J, et al. Nasal T-cell lymphoma causally associated with Epstein-Barr virus. Clinicopathologic, phenotypic, and genotypic studies. Cancer 1996;77:2137–49.

81. Horny HP, Kaiserling E. Involvement of the larynx by hematopoietic neoplasms. An investigation of autopsy cases and review of the literature. Pathol Res Pract 1995;191:130–8.

82. Houston HE, Payne WS, Harrison EG, Olson AM. Primary cancer of the trachea. Arch Surg 1969;99:132–40.

83. Jaffe ES, Chan JK, Su IJ, et al. Report of the workshop on nasal and related extranodal angiocentric T/natural killer cell lymphomas. Definitions, differential diagnosis, and epidemiology. Am J Surg Pathol 1996;20:103–11.

84. Kaplan MA, Pettit CL, Zukerberg LR, Harris NL. Primary lymphoma of the trachea with morphologic and immunophenotypic characteristics of low-grade B-cell lymphoma of mucosa-associated lymphoid tissue. Am J Surg Pathol 1992;16:71–5.

85. Maeda M, Kotake Y, Monden Y, Nakahara K, Kawashima Y, Kitamura H. Primary malignant lymphoma of the trachea. Report of a case successfully treated by primary end to end anastomosis after circumferential resection of the trachea. J Thorac Cardiovasc Surg 1981;81:835–9.

86. Morgan K, MacLennan KA, Narula A, Bradley PJ, Morgan DA. Non-Hodgkin's lymphoma of the larynx (stage 1E). Cancer 1989;64:1123–7.

87. Pradham DJ, Rabuzzi D, Meyer JA. Primary solitary lymphoma of the trachea. J Thorac Cardiovasc Surg 1975;70:938–40.

88. Shima N, Kobashi Y, Tsutsui K, et al. Extranodal non-Hodgkin's lymphoma of the head and neck. A clinicopathologic study in the Kyoto-Nara area of Japan. Cancer 1990;66:1190–7.

89. Strickler JG, Meneses MF, Habermann TM, et al. Polymorphic reticulosis: a reappraisal. Hum Pathol 1994; 25:659–65.

90. Swerdlow JB, Merl SA, Davey FR, Gacek RR, Gottlieb AJ. Non-Hodgkin's lymphoma limited to the larynx. Cancer 1984;53:2546–9.

91. Wiggins J, Sheffield E, Green M. Primary B-cell malignant lymphoma of the trachea. Thorax 1988;43:497–8.

Sinonasal B-Cell Lymphoma

92. Abbondanzo SL, Wenig BM. Non-Hodgkin's lymphoma of the sinonasal tract. A clinicopathologic and immunophenotypic study of 120 cases. Cancer 1995;75:1281–91.

93. Arber DA, Weiss LM, Albujar PF, Chen YY, Jaffe ES. Nasal lymphomas in Peru. High incidence of T-cell immunophenotype and Epstein-Barr virus infection. Am J Surg Pathol 1993;17:392–9.

94. Chan JK, Ng CS, Lau WH, Lo ST. Most nasal/nasopharyngeal lymphomas are peripheral T-cell neoplasms. Am J Surg Pathol 1987;11:418–29.

95. Cleary KR, Batsakis JG. Sinonasal lymphomas. Ann Otol Rhinol Laryngol 1994;103:911–4.

96. Fellbaum C, Hansmann ML, Lennert K. Malignant lymphomas of the nasal cavity and paranasal sinuses. Virch Arch [A] 1989;414:399–405.

97. Ferry JA, Sklar J, Zukerberg LR, Harris NL. Nasal lymphoma. A clinicopathologic study with immunophenotypic and genotypic analysis. Am J Surg Pathol 1991;15:268–79.

98. Frierson HF Jr, Innes DJ Jr, Mills SE, Wick MR. Immunophenotypic analysis of sinonasal non-Hodgkin's lymphomas. Hum Pathol 1989;20:636–42.

99. Frierson HF Jr, Mills SE, Innes DJ Jr. Non-Hodgkin's lymphomas of the sinonasal region: histologic types and their clinicopathologic features. Am J Clin Pathol 1984;81:721–7.

100. Fu YS, Perzin KH. Nonepithelial tumors of the nasal cavity, paranasal sinuses and nasopharynx. A clinicopathologic study. X. Malignant lymphomas. Cancer 1979;43:611–21.

101. Harris NL, Jaffe ES, Stein H, et al. A revised European-American classification of lymphoid neoplasms: a proposal from the International Lymphoma Study Group. Blood 1994;84:1361–92.

102. Ishii Y, Yamanaka N, Ogawa K, et al. Nasal T-cell lymphoma as a type of so-called "lethal midline granuloma." Cancer 1982;50:2336–44.

103. Kapadia SB, Barnes L, Deutsch M. Non-Hodgkin's lymphoma of the nose and paranasal sinuses: a study of 17 cases. Head Neck Surg 1981;3:490–9.

104. O'Leary G, Kennedy SM. Association of Epstein-Barr virus with sinonasal angiocentric T cell lymphoma. J Clin Pathol 1995;48:946–9.

105. Ng CS, Chan JK, Lo ST. Expression of natural killer cell markers in non-Hodgkin's lymphomas. Hum Pathol 1987;18:1257–62.

106. Ratech H, Burke JS, Blayney DW, Sheibani K, Rappaport H. A clinicopathologic study of malignant lymphomas of the nose, paranasal sinuses, and hard palate, including cases of lethal midline granuloma. Cancer 1989;64:2525–31.

107. Robbins KT, Fuller LM, Vlasak M, et al. Primary lymphomas of the nasal cavity and paranasal sinuses. Cancer 1985;56:814–9.

108. Tomita Y, Ohsawa M, Mishiro Y, et al. The presence and subtype of Epstein-Barr virus in B and T cell lymphomas of the sino-nasal region from the Osaka and Okinawa districts of Japan. Lab Invest 1995;73:190–6.

109. Weiss LM, Gaffey MJ, Chen YY, Frierson HF Jr. Frequency of Epstein-Barr viral DNA in "Western" sinonasal and Waldeyer's ring non-Hodgkin's lymphomas. Am J Surg Pathol 1992;16:156–62.

110. Yamanaka N, Harabuchi Y, Sambe S, et al. Non-Hodgkin's lymphoma of Waldeyer's ring and nasal cavity. Clinical and immunologic aspects. Cancer 1985;56:768–76.

Sinonasal T/NK Cell Lymphoma

111. Abbondanzo SL, Wenig BM. Non-Hodgkin's lymphoma of the sinonasal tract. A clinicopathologic and immunophenotypic study of 120 cases. Cancer 1995;75:1281–91.

112. Aozasa K. Author reply [Letter]. Cancer 1995;76:538.

113. Aozasa K, Ohsawa M, Tomita Y, Tagawa S, Yamamura T. Polymorphic reticulosis is a neoplasm of large granular lymphocytes with CD3+ phenotype. Cancer 1995;75:894–901.

114. Aozasa K, Ohsawa M, Tajima K, et al. Nation-wide study of lethal mid-line granuloma in Japan: frequencies of Wegener's granulomatosis, polymorphic reticulosis, malignant lymphoma and other related conditions. Int J Cancer 1989;44:63–6.

115. Arber DA, Weiss LM, Albujar PF, Chen YY, Jaffe ES. Nasal lymphomas in Peru. High incidence of T-cell immunophenotype and Epstein-Barr virus infection. Am J Surg Pathol 1993;17:392–9.

116. Borisch B, Hennig I, Laeng RH, Waelti ER, Kraft R, Laissue J. Association of the subtype 2 of the Epstein-Barr virus with T-cell non-Hodgkin's lymphoma of the midline granuloma type. Blood 1993;82:858–64.

117. Chan JK, Ng CS, Lau WH, Lo ST. Most nasal/nasopharyngeal lymphomas are peripheral T-cell neoplasms. Am J Surg Pathol 1987;11:418–29.

118. Chan JK, Tsang WY. Polymorphic reticulosis is a neoplasm of large granular lymphocytes with CD3+ phenotype [Letter]. Cancer 1995;76:537.

119. Chan JK, Tsang WY, Ng CS. Clarification of CD3 immunoreactivity in nasal T/natural killer cell lymphomas: the neoplastic cells are often CD3+ [Letter]. Blood 1996;87:839–40.

120. Chan JK, Tsang WY, Ng CS, Pau MY. Discordant CD3 expression in lymphomas when studied on frozen and paraffin sections. Hum Pathol 1995;26:1139–43.

121. Chan JK, Yip TT, Tsang WY, et al. Detection of Epstein-Barr viral RNA in malignant lymphomas of the upper aerodigestive tract. Am J Surg Pathol 1994;18:938–46.

122. Chiang AK, Srivastava G, Lau PW, Ho FC. Differences in T-cell-receptor gene rearrangement and transcription in nasal lymphomas of natural killer and T-cell types: implications on cellular origin. Hum Pathol 1996;27:701-11.

239

123. Chott A, Rappersberger K, Schlossarek W, Radaszkiewicz T. Peripheral T cell lymphoma presenting primarily as lethal midline granuloma. Hum Pathol 1988;19:1093–101.

124. de Bruin PC, Jiwa M, Oudejans JJ, et al. Presence of Epstein-Barr virus in extranodal T-cell lymphomas: differences in relation to site. Blood 1994;83:1612–8.

125. Dictor M, Cervin A, Kalm O, Rambech E. Sinonasal T-cell lymphoma in the differential diagnosis of lethal midline granuloma using in situ hybridization for Epstein-Barr virus RNA. Mod Pathol 1996;9:7–14.

126. Emile JF, Boulland ML, Haioun C, et al. CD5- CD56+ T-cell receptor silent peripheral T-cell lymphomas are natural killer cell lymphomas. Blood 1996;87:1466–73.

127. Fellbaum C, Hansmann ML, Lennert K. Malignant lymphomas of the nasal cavity and paranasal sinuses. Virchows Arch [A] 1989;414:399–405.

128. Ferry JA, Sklar J, Zukerberg LR, Harris NL. Nasal lymphoma. A clinicopathologic study with immunophenotypic and genotypic analysis. Am J Surg Pathol 1991;15:268–79.

129. Frierson HF Jr, Mills SE, Innes DJ Jr. Non-Hodgkin's lymphomas of the sinonasal region: histologic types and their clinicopathologic features. Am J Clin Pathol 1984;81:721–7.

130. Fu YS, Perzin KH. Nonepithelial tumors of the nasal cavity, paranasal sinuses and nasopharynx. A clinicopathologic study. X. Malignant lymphomas. Cancer 1979;43:611–21.

231. Gaffey MJ, Frierson HF Jr, Medeiros LJ, Weiss LM. The relationship of Epstein-Barr virus to infection-related (sporadic) and familial hemophagocytic syndrome and secondary (lymphoma-related) hemophagocytosis: an in situ hybridization study. Hum Pathol 1993;24:657–67.

132. Graeme-Cook F, Bhan AK, Harris NL. Immunohistochemical characterization of intraepithelial and subepithelial mononuclear cells of the upper airways. Am J Pathol 1993;143:1416–22.

133. Guinee D Jr, Jaffe E, Kingma D, et al. Pulmonary lymphomatoid granulomatosis. Evidence of Epstein-Barr virus infected B-lymphocytes with a predominant T-cell component and vasculitis. Am J Surg Pathol 1994;18:753–64.

134. Harabuchi Y, Imai S, Wakashima J, et al. Nasal T-cell lymphoma causally associated with Epstein-Barr virus. Clinicopathologic, phenotypic, and genotypic studies. Cancer 1996;77:2137–49.

135. Harabuchi Y, Yamanaka N, Kataura A, et al. Epstein-Barr virus in nasal T-cell lymphomas in patients with lethal midline granuloma. Lancet 1990;335:128–30.

136. Harris NL, Jaffe ES, Stein H, et al. A revised European-American classification of lymphoid neoplasms: a proposal from the International Lymphoma Study Group. Blood 1994;84:1361–92.

137. Heffner DK. Idiopathic midline destructive disease [Letter]. Ann Otol Rhinol Laryngol 1995;104:258.

138. Ho FC, Choy D, Loke SL, et al. Polymorphic reticulosis and conventional lymphomas of the nose and upper aerodigestive tract: a clinicopathologic study of 70 cases, and immunophenotypic studies of 16 cases. Hum Pathol 1990;21:1041–50.

139. Ho FC, Srivastava G, Loke SL, et al. Presence of Epstein-Barr virus DNA in nasal lymphomas of B and T cell type. Hematol Oncol 1990;8:271–81.

140. Ho FC, Todd D, Loke SL, Ng RP, Khoor KK. Clinicopathological features of malignant lymphomas in 294 Hong Kong Chinese patients, a retrospective study covering an eight-year period. Int J Cancer 1984;34:143–8.

141. Ishii Y, Yamanaka N, Ogawa K, et al. Nasal T-cell lymphoma as a type of so-called "lethal midline granuloma." Cancer 1982;50:2336–44.

142. Jaffe ES. Classification of natural killer (NK) cell and NK-like T-cell malignancies [Editorial]. Blood 1996;87:1207–10.

143. Jaffe ES. Nasal and nasal-type T/NK cell lymphoma: a unique form of lymphoma associated with the Epstein-Barr virus. Histopathology 1995;27:581–3.

144. Jaffe ES, Chan JK, Su IJ, et al. Report of the workshop on nasal and related extranodal angiocentric T/natural killer cell lymphomas. Definitions, differential diagnosis, and epidemiology. Am J Surg Pathol 1996;20:103–11.

145. Kanavaros P, Lescs MC, Briere J, et al. Nasal T-cell lymphoma: a clinicopathologic entity associated with peculiar phenotype and with Epstein-Barr virus. Blood 1993;10:2688–95.

146. Medeiros LJ, Peiper SC, Elwood L, Yano T, Raffeld M, Jaffe ES. Angiocentric immunoproliferative lesions: a molecular analysis of eight cases. Hum Pathol 1991;22:1150–7.

147. Misad O, Solidoro A, Quiroz L, Olivares L. An overview of lymphoreticular malignancies in Peru. Prog Cancer Res Ther 1984;27:85–97.

148. Mishima K, Horiuchi K, Kojya S, Takahashi H, Ohsawa M, Aozasa K. Epstein-Barr virus in patients with polymorphic reticulosis (lethal midline granuloma) from China and Japan. Cancer 1994;73:3041–6.

149. Mori N, Yatabe Y, Oka K, et al. Expression of perforin in nasal lymphoma. Additional evidence of its natural killer cell derivation. Am J Pathol 1996;149:699–705.

150. Myers JL, Kurtin PJ, Katzenstein AL, et al. Lymphomatoid granulomatosis. Evidence of immunophenotypic diversity and relationship to Epstein-Barr virus infection. Am J Surg Pathol 1995;19:1300–12.

151. Nakamura S, Suchi T, Koshikawa T, et al. Clinicopathologic study of CD56 (NCAM)-positive angiocentric lymphoma occurring in sites other than the upper and lower respiratory tract. Am J Surg Pathol 1995;19:284–96.

152. Navarro-Roman L, Zarate-Osorno A, Meneses A, Kingma DW, Jaffe ES. High grade AIL and Epstein-Barr virus infection in 22 cases from Mexico [Abstract]. Mod Pathol 1994;7:117a.

153. Ng CS, Chan JK, Cheng PN, Szeto SC. Nasal T-cell lymphoma associated with hemophagocytic syndrome. Cancer 1986;58:67–71.

154. Ng CS, Chan JK, Lo ST, Poon YF. Immunophenotypic analysis of non-Hodgkin's lymphomas in Chinese. A study of 75 cases in Hong Kong. Pathology 1986;18:419–25.

155. Ng CS, Chan JK, Lo ST. Expression of natural killer cell markers in non-Hodgkin's lymphomas. Hum Pathol 1987;18:1257–62.

156. Ohno T, Yamaguchi M, Oka K, Miwa H, Kita K, Shirakawa S. Frequent expression of CD3 in CD3 (Leu 4)-negative nasal T-cell lymphomas. Leukemia 1995;9:44–52.

157. O'Leary G, Kennedy SM. Association of Epstein-Barr virus with sinonasal angiocentric T cell lymphoma. J Clin Pathol 1995;48:946–9.

158. Petrella T, Delfau-Larue MH, Caillot D, et al. Nasopharyngeal lymphomas: further evidence for a natural killer cell origin. Hum Pathol 1996;27:827–33.

159. Ratech H, Burke JS, Blayney DW, Sheibani K, Rappaport H. A clinicopathologic study of malignant lymphomas of the nose, paranasal sinuses, and hard palate, including cases of lethal midline granuloma. Cancer 1989;64:2525–31.

160. Soler J, Bordes R, Ortuno F, et al. Aggressive natural killer cell leukemia/lymphoma in two patients with lethal midline granuloma. Br J Haematol 1994;86:659–62.

161. Strickler JG, Meneses MF, Habermann TM, et al. Polymorphic reticulosis: a reappraisal. Hum Pathol 1994;25:659–65.

162. Suzumiya J, Takeshita M, Kimura N, et al. Expression of adult and fetal natural killer cell markers in sinonasal lymphomas. Blood 1994;83:2255–60.

163. Suzumiya J, Takeshita M, Kimura N, Kikuchi M. Response [Letter]. Blood 1994;83:2994–6.

164. Suzumiya J, Takeshita M, Kimura N, Kikuchi M. Response [Letter]. Blood 1996;86:841.

165. Tao Q, Chiang AK, Srivastava G, Ho FC. TCR- CD56+ CD2+ nasal lymphomas with membrane-localized CD3 positivity: are the CD3+ cells neoplastic or reactive? [Letter] Blood 1995;84:2993–4.

166. Tao Q, Ho FC, Loke SL, Srivastava G. Epstein-Barr virus is localized in the tumour cells of nasal lymphomas of NK, T or B cell type. Int J Cancer 1995;60:315–20.

167. Tomita Y, Ohsawa M, Mishiro Y, et al. The presence and subtype of Epstein-Barr virus in B and T cell lymphomas of the sino-nasal region from the Osaka and Okinawa districts of Japan. Lab Invest 1995;73:190–6.

168. Tsang WY, Chan JK, Ng CS, Pau MY. Utility of a paraffin section-reactive CD56 antibody (123C3) for characterization and diagnosis of lymphomas. Am J Surg Pathol 1996;20:202–10.

169. Tsang WY, Chan JK, Yip TT, et al. In situ localization of Epstein-Barr virus encoded RNA in non-nasal/nasopharyngeal CD56-positive and CD56-negative T-cell lymphomas. Hum Pathol 1994;25:758–65.

170. van Camp B, Durie BG, Spier C, et al. Plasma cells in multiple myeloma express a natural killer cell-associated antigen: CD56 (NKH1; Leu19). Blood 1990;76:377–82.

171. van Gorp J, Brink A, Oudejans JJ, et al. Expression of Epstein-Barr virus encoded latent genes in nasal T-cell lymphomas. J Clin Pathol 1996;49:72–6.

172. van Gorp J, de Bruin PC, Sie-Go DM, et al. Nasal T-cell lymphoma: a clinicopathological and immunophenotypic analysis of 13 cases. Histopathology 1995;27:139–48.

173. van Gorp J, Weiping L, Jacobse K, et al. Epstein-Barr virus in nasal T-cell lymphomas (polymorphic reticulosis/ midline malignant reticulosis) in western China. J Pathol 1994;173:81–7.

174. Weiss LM, Gaffey MJ, Chen YY, Frierson HF Jr. Frequency of Epstein-Barr viral DNA in "Western" sinonasal and Waldeyer's ring non-Hodgkin's lymphomas. Am J Surg Pathol 1992;16:156–62.

175. Wilson WH, Kingma DW, Raffeld M, Wittes RE, Jaffe ES. Association of lymphomatoid granulomatosis with Epstein-Barr viral infection of B lymphocytes and response to interferon-2b. Blood 1996;87:4531–7.

176. Winther B, Innes DJ Jr, Mills SE, Mygind N, Zito D, Hayden FG. Lymphocyte subsets in normal airway mucosa of the human nose. Arch Otolaryngol Head Neck Surg 1987;113:59–62.

Malignant Lymphoma with Pseudoepitheliomatous Hyperplasia

177. Chan JK, Ng CS, Lau WH, Lo ST. Most nasal/nasopharyngeal lymphomas are peripheral T-cell neoplasms. Am J Surg Pathol 1987;11:418–29.

178. Ferry JA, Sklar J, Zukerberg LR, Harris NL. Nasal lymphoma. A clinicopathologic study with immunophenotypic and genotypic analysis. Am J Surg Pathol 1991;15:268–79.

179. Krasne DL, Warnke RA, Weiss LM. Malignant lymphoma presenting as pseudoepitheliomatous hyperplasia. A report of two cases. Am J Surg Pathol 1988;12:835–42.

Extramedullary Plasmacytoma

180. Aguilera NS, Kapadia SB, Nalesnik MA, Swerdlow SH. Extramedullary plasmacytoma of the head and neck: use of paraffin sections to assess clonality with in situ hybridization, growth fraction, and the presence of Epstein-Barr virus. Mod Pathol 1995;8:503–8.

181. Batsakis JG, Fries GT, Goldman RT, Karlsberg RC. Upper respiratory tract plasmacytoma. Extramedullary myeloma. Arch Otolaryngol 1964;79:613–8.

182. Castro EB, Lewis JS, Strong EW. Plasmacytoma of paranasal sinuses and oral cavity. Arch Otolaryngol 1973;97:326–9.

183. Dolin S, Dewar JP. Extramedullary plasmacytoma. Am J Pathol 1956;32:83–103.

184. Ewing MR, Foote FW Jr. Plasma-cell tumors of the mouth and upper air passages. Cancer 1952;5:499–513.

185. Ferreiro JA, Egorshin EV, Olsen KD, Banks PM, Weiland LH. Mucous membrane plasmacytosis of the upper aerodigestive tract. A clinicopathologic study. Am J Surg Pathol 1994;18:1048–53.

186. Fu YS, Perzin KH. Nonepithelial tumors of the nasal cavity, paranasal sinuses and nasopharynx. A clinicopathologic study. IX. Plasmacytomas. Cancer 1978;42:2399–406.

187. Harris NL, Jaffe ES, Stein H, et al. A revised European-American classification of lymphoid neoplasms: a proposal from the International Lymphoma Study Group. Blood 1994;84:1361–92.

188. Harwood AR, Knowling MA, Bergsagel DE. Radiotherapy of extramedullary plasmacytoma of the head and neck. Clin Radiol 1981;32:31–6.

189. Horny HP, Kaiserling E. Involvement of the larynx by hemopoietic neoplasms. An investigation of autopsy cases and review of the literature. Pathol Res Pract 1995;191:130–8.

190. Hyams VJ, Batsakis JG, Michaels L. Lymphoreticular tissue neoplasia. In: Tumors of the upper respiratory tract and ear. Atlas of Tumor Pathology, 2nd Series, Fascicle 25. Washington DC: Armed Forces Institute of Pathology, 1988:207–25.

191. Kapadia SB. Hematologic diseases: malignant lymphomas, leukemias, plasma cell dyscrasias, histiocytosis X, and reactive lymph node lesions. In: Barnes L, ed. Surgical pathology of the head and neck, Vol 2. New York: Marcel Dekker, 1985:1045–209.

192. Kapadia SB, Desai U, Cheng VS. Extramedullary plasmacytoma of the head and neck. A clinicopathologic study of 20 cases. Medicine 1982;61:317–29.
193. Kober SJ. Solitary plasmacytoma of the carina. Thorax 1979;34:567–8.
194. Kotner LM, Wang CC. Plasmacytoma of the upper air and food passages. Cancer 1972;30:414–8.
195. Ruiz-Arguelles GJ, San Miguel JF. Cell surface markers in multiple myeloma. Mayo Clin Proc 1994;69:684–90.
196. Stout AP, Kenney FR. Primary plasma-cell tumors of the upper air passages and oral cavity. Cancer 1949;2:261–78.
197. Strickler JG, Audeh MW, Copenhaver CM, Warnke RA. Immunophenotypic differences between plasmacytoma/multiple myeloma and immunoblastic lymphoma. Cancer 1988;61:1782–6.
198. Wiltshaw E. The natural history of extramedullary plasmacytoma and its relation to solitary myeloma of bone and myelomatosis. Medicine 1976;55:217–38.

Post-transplantation Lymphoproliferative Disorder

199. Chadburn A, Frizzera G, Chen J, Cesarman E, Michler R, Knowles DM. Clinicopathologic analysis of 28 posttransplantation lymphoproliferative disorders (PTLPDs) [Abstract]. Mod Pathol 1994;7:104a.
200. Ho M, Jaffe R, Miller G, et al. The frequency of Epstein-Barr virus infection and associated lymphoproliferative syndrome after transplantation and its manifestations in children. Transplantation 1988;45:719–27.
201. Knowles DM, Cesarman E, Chadburn A, et al. Correlative morphologic and molecular genetic analysis demonstrates three distinct categories of posttransplantation lymphoproliferative disorders. Blood 1995;85:552–65.
202. Lones MA, Mishalani S, Shintaku IP, Weiss LM, Nichols WS, Said JW. Changes in tonsils and adenoids in children with posttransplant lymphoproliferative disorder: report of three cases with early involvement of Waldeyer's ring. Hum Pathol 1995;26:525–30.
203. Malatack JJ, Gartner JC Jr, Urbach AH, Zitelli BJ. Orthotopic liver transplantation, Epstein-Barr virus, cyclosporine, and lymphoproliferative disease: a growing concern. J Pediatr 1991;118:667–75.
204. Montone KT, Hodinka RL, Salhany KE, Lavi E, Rostami A, Tomaszewski JE. Identification of Epstein-Barr virus lytic activity in post-transplantation lymphoproliferative disease. Mod Pathol 1996;9:621–30.
205. Nalesnik MA, Jaffe R, Starzl TE, et al. The pathology of posttransplant lymphoproliferative disorders occurring in the setting of cyclosporine A-prednisone immunosuppression. Am J Pathol 1988;133:173–92.

Extramedullary Tumors of Myeloid or Lymphoid Blasts

206. Curtis AB. Childhood leukemias: initial oral manifestations. J Am Dent Asso 1971;83:159–64.
207. Davey FR, Olsen S, Kurec AS, Eastman-Abaya R, Gottlieb AJ, Mason DY. The immunophenotyping of extramedullary myeloid cell tumors in paraffin-embedded tissue sections. Am J Surg Pathol 1988;12:699–707.
208. Harris NL, Jaffe ES, Stein H, et al. A revised European-American classification of lymphoid neoplasms: a proposal from the International Lymphoma Study Group. Blood 1994;84:1361–92.
209. Horny HP, Kaiserling E. Involvement of the larynx by hemopoietic neoplasms. An investigation of autopsy cases and review of the literature. Pathol Res Pract 1995;191:130–8.
210. Kapadia SB. Hematologic diseases: malignant lymphomas, leukemias, plasma cell dyscrasias, histiocytosis X, and reactive lymph node lesions. In: Barnes L, ed. Surgical pathology of the head and neck, Vol 2. New York: Marcel Dekker, 1985:1045–209.
211. Kurec AS, Cruz VE, Barrett D, Mason DY, Davey FR. Immunophenotyping of acute leukemias using paraffin-embedded tissue sections. Am J Clin Pathol 1990;93:502–9.
212. Meis JM, Butler JJ, Osborne BM, Manning JT. Granulocytic sarcoma in nonleukemic patients. Cancer 1986;58:2697–709.
213. Neiman RS, Barcos M, Berard C, et al. Granulocytic sarcoma: a clinicopathologic study of 61 biopsied cases. Cancer 1981;48:1426–37.
214. Quintanilla-Martinez L, Zukerberg LR, Ferry JA, Harris NL. Extramedullary tumors of lymphoid or myeloid blasts. The role of immunohistology in diagnosis and classification. Am J Clin Pathol 1995;104:431–43.
215. Traweek ST, Arber DA, Rappaport H, Brynes RK. Extramedullary myeloid cell tumors. An immunohistochemical and morphologic study of 28 cases. Am J Surg Pathol 1993;17:1011–9.

Hodgkin's Disease of Waldeyer's Ring

216. Chang KL, Kamel OW, Arber DA, Horyd ID, Weiss LM. Pathologic features of nodular lymphocyte predominance Hodgkin's disease in extranodal sites. Am J Surg Pathol 1995;19:1313–24.
217. Colby TV, Hoppe RT, Warnke RA. Hodgkin's disease: a clinicopathologic study of 659 cases. Cancer 1981;49:1848–58.
218. Dunphy CH, Saravia O, Varvares MA. Hodgkin's disease primarily involving Waldeyer's ring. Case report and review of the literature. Arch Pathol Lab Med 1996;120:285–7.
219. Kapadia SB, Roman LN, Kingma DW, Jaffe ES, Frizzera G. Hodgkin's disease of Waldeyer's ring. Clinical and histoimmunophenotypic findings and association with Epstein-Barr virus in 16 cases. Am J Surg Pathol 1995;19:1431–9.
220. Siebert JD, Stuckey JH, Kurtin PJ, Banks PM. Extranodal lymphocyte predominance Hodgkin's disease. Clinical and pathologic features. Am J Clin Pathol 1995;103:485–91.
221. Todd GB, Michaels L. Hodgkin's disease involving Waldeyer's lymphoid ring. Cancer 1974;34:1769–78.

9

VASCULAR LESIONS PREDILECTING THE HEAD AND NECK REGION

LOBULAR CAPILLARY HEMANGIOMA

Definition. This is a benign capillary proliferation with a microscopically distinctive lobular architecture that predilects the skin and mucous membranes of the oral cavity and sinonasal region.

General Features. In 1904, Hartzell (6) described four vascular tumors occurring on the fingers and arms that he termed "granuloma pyogenicum" because he believed that they represented a nonspecific granulation tissue response to any pyogenic agent. Even though he did not describe a lobular capillary pattern, it is evident in his illustration. This unique lobular arrangement of capillaries is the key feature of his pyogenic granuloma. Because of this, the more accurate term, lobular capillary hemangioma (LCH) is the preferred designation for these tumors. LCHs have been documented as deep intradermal (3), subcutaneous (3), and even intravenous lesions (2), in addition to the more common cutaneous and mucous membrane growths.

Many authors have equated pyogenic granuloma with granulation tissue, and in their illustrations have focused on the superficial, acutely inflamed portions of these masses. Conversely, vascular proliferations that lack granulation tissue have been diagnosed by others as nonspecific capillary hemangiomas (5). The fact that the capillary lobules in these nonulcerated lesions are identical to those seen in the deeper portions of polypoid, ulcerated, pyogenic granuloma has often gone unappreciated.

Such problems in terminology are best illustrated by the pyogenic granulomas of the larynx and trachea. Our review of these reports, as well as the 68 laryngo-tracheal "granulomas" present in our review of vascular tumors from this region, failed to reveal a single lesion with the characteristic features of LCH (4).

The pathogenesis of LCH is not known. Trauma appears to be a factor in only a minority of cases. The marked variation in sexual distribution with age and the frequent occurrence of LCH in pregnant women suggest that hormonal factors may be involved. The regression of these lesions in pregnant women following delivery and the development of LCH in women using oral contraceptives further support a hormonal role. However, in our study of 21 LCHs, including 6 from pregnant patients, we were unable to identify estrogen or progesterone receptors by immunohistochemical analysis (9).

Clinical Features. Within the head and neck region, the oral cavity is the most common site for LCH, followed by the nasal mucous membranes. In our study, 29 percent of lesions involved the nasal cavity (7): 13 arose from the nasal septum, 4 from the turbinates, and 4 from the nasal vestibule (fig. 9-1); there were no nasopharyngeal LCHs. Lesions of the oral and nasal

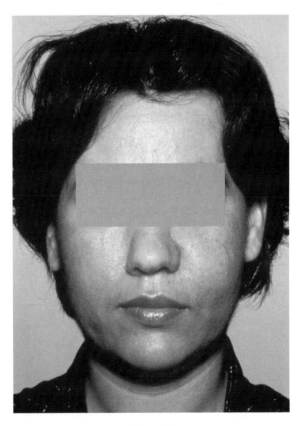

Figure 9-1
LOBULAR CAPILLARY HEMANGIOMA
A lobular capillary hemangioma of the nasal cavity has produced an external deformity of the left side of the nose in this young woman.

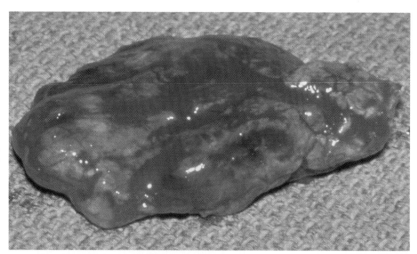

Figure 9-2
LOBULAR
CAPILLARY HEMANGIOMA
This large, resected lobular capillary hemangioma consists of a vascular appearing, noninvasive polypoid mass that was easily removed from the nasal cavity.

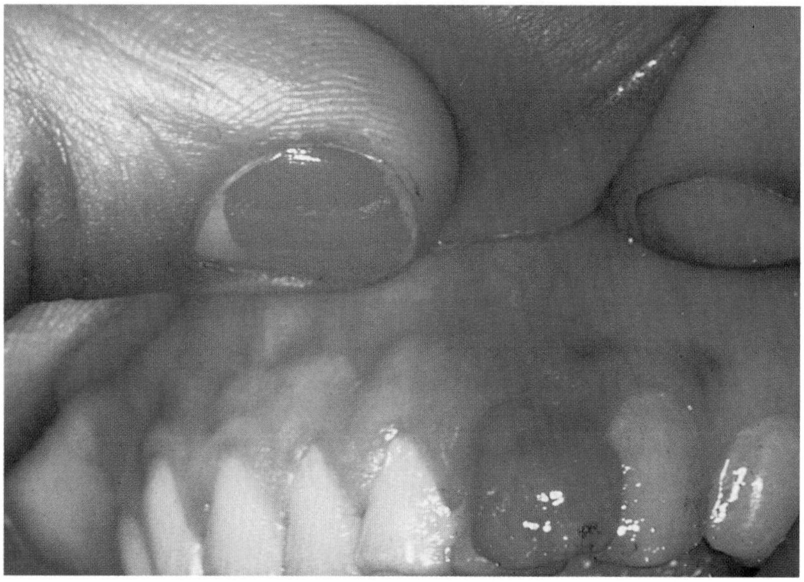

Figure 9-3
EPULIS OF PREGNANCY
The so-called "epulis of pregnancy," seen here as a highly vascular, "strawberry colored" mass involving the gingiva, has the microscopic features of a lobular capillary hemangioma.

mucous membrane show a marked sexual variation with age. Of the patients under 18 years of age, 82 percent were males; in contrast, 86 percent of patients 18 to 39 years of age were females. Eight of these women were pregnant and the histologic features of the LCH (pregnancy epulis) were indistinguishable from those of other patients in the series. Sexual predilection disappeared after the age of 39 years.

Clinically, patients with nasal LCH present with nasal obstruction and recurrent epistaxis. Excluding pain related to trauma to an existing lesion, LCH is nonpainful. They are typically described by clinicians as pedunculated, red or hemorrhagic masses, often with an ulcerated surface covered with a fibrinopurulent exudate. In 92 percent of cases, there is no history of trauma and the lesion appears to arise spontaneously.

Gross Findings. Grossly, LCHs are red, obviously vascular, polypoid masses attached to the gingiva, nasal septum, or other mucous membrane surfaces (fig. 9-2). Areas of secondary change including surface ulceration with hemorrhage, thrombosis, or both may be grossly visible. The nodules are usually less than 1.5 cm in greatest dimension and rarely exceed 2 cm. The so-called epulis of pregnancy is a polypoid, lobular capillary hemangioma, typically arising from the gingiva. It has a distinctive, often "strawberry colored" gross appearance (fig. 9-3).

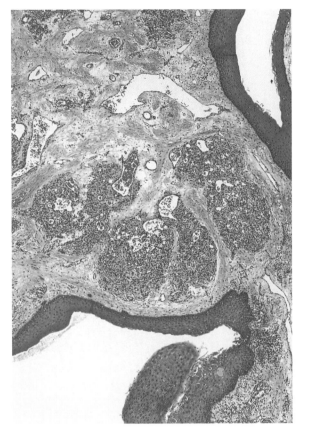

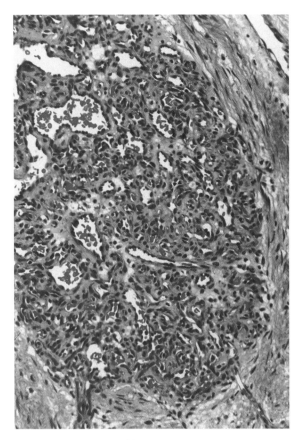

Figure 9-4
LOBULAR CAPILLARY HEMANGIOMA
At low-power magnification, the characteristic capillary lobules of lobular capillary hemangioma can be seen beneath intact nasal mucosa.

Figure 9-5
LOBULAR CAPILLARY HEMANGIOMA
A characteristic lobule of lobular capillary hemangioma is composed of tightly packed capillaries, as well as enlarged vascular spaces.

Microscopic Findings. The lesion contains lobules and anastomosing networks of capillaries in an edematous, fibroblastic stroma. In their most compact form, the capillary lobules consist of closely packed clusters of plump, cytologically bland endothelial cells with prominent mitotic figures and only scattered, indistinct capillary lumina (figs. 9-4, 9-5). In other areas, the capillaries form a more widely separated meshwork surrounded by a fibroblastic stroma. Large capillaries with angulated, branching lumina are present within and between the capillary lobules (figs. 9-6, 9-7).

Although LCH is a distinctive histologic entity, a number of secondary changes may occur. Marked stromal edema, often selectively located in the superficial areas, may distort the lobular pattern. Ulcerated lesions may show superficial inflammatory cell infiltrates and marked capillary dilation, as well as stromal edema. In some ulcerated lesions, the superficial capillaries may radiate to the surface in an acutely inflamed, edematous stroma, resulting in an appearance focally indistinguishable from that of granulation tissue, but with preservation of lobules in the deeper portions of the lesion (fig. 9-8).

Immunohistochemical Findings. The predominant endothelial cells of LCH stain strongly for factor VIII–related antigen and with *Ulex europaeus* lectin (9). More recent endothelial markers, CD34 and CD31, are also strongly positive in this cell population. A second, less prominent population of pericyte-like cells surrounds the luminal endothelial cells. This minor perivascular component can easily be overlooked on hematoxylin and eosin (H&E)-stained sections. It labels strongly for muscle-specific actin and collagen type IV (9). Stains for estrogen receptor and progesterone receptor have, thus far, been negative in (9).

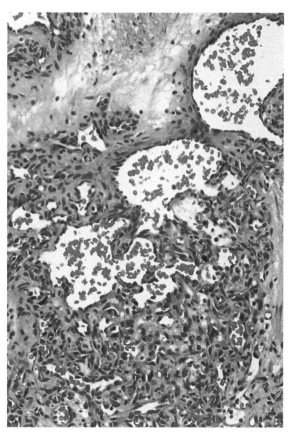

Figure 9-6
LOBULAR CAPILLARY HEMANGIOMA
Papillary tufts of endothelial cells may be present within the larger vascular spaces of lobular capillary hemangioma.

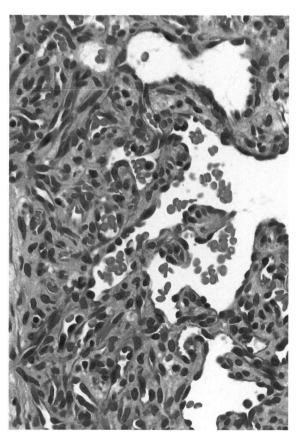

Figure 9-7
LOBULAR CAPILLARY HEMANGIOMA
Higher power magnification shows the papillary tufts in larger vascular spaces, as well as the surrounding zone of small capillaries. Mitotic figures may be extremely numerous in the endothelial cells forming these smaller capillaries.

Figure 9-8
LOBULAR
CAPILLARY HEMANGIOMA

This lobular capillary hemangioma has eroded through the mucosa and has a surface covered with nonspecific granulation tissue. In the deeper portions of the lesion, however, the characteristic lobules can be seen.

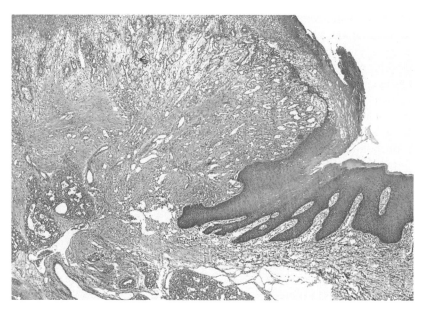

Differential Diagnosis. The following entities should be considered in the differential diagnosis of lobular capillary hemangioma.

Granulation Tissue. Masses of granulation tissue may assume a polypoid configuration that is grossly indistinguishable from that of LCH. The hallmark of granulation tissue is a radial arrangement of capillaries, often originating from a central fibrovascular stalk, and surrounded by an intensely inflamed, edematous stroma. Lesions of pure granulation tissue do not have an underlying, uninflamed LCH. In our experience, laryngotracheal "pyogenic granulomas" are invariably pure granulation tissue (4).

Angiofibroma. Nasal LCH often occurs in young males and may be confused clinically, as well as pathologically, with angiofibroma. Angiofibromas nearly invariably involve the nasopharynx and may extend to involve the paranasal sinuses. In a series of 120 angiofibromas, only 2 involved the nasal cavity alone (8). In our experience, LCH does not involve the nasopharynx and is confined to the nasal cavity, usually to the septal wall. Angiofibromas consist of angulated, branching, vascular channels of variable size that are uniformly distributed in fibrocollagenous stroma. Although the vascularity may vary considerably from case to case, it tends to be uniform within a given lesion. Angiofibromas do not have the distinctive lobules of closely packed capillaries that are characteristic of LCH.

Hemangiopericytoma. Sinonasal hemangiopericytomas are described in the next section (1). These neoplasms most commonly originate from the paranasal sinuses and involve the nasal cavity secondarily. They are commonly seen in adults in their sixth to seventh decades of life. Clinically, they resemble allergic polyps. Microscopically, the pattern is characteristic of a hemangiopericytoma and consists of ramifying vessels in a "deer antler" pattern, surrounded by delicate reticulin. The spaces between the capillaries are filled with spindle-shaped pericytes in a diffuse, nonorganoid arrangement. A multilobular organization of capillaries is not present. LCH lacks the distinctive spindle cell, pericytic component that is so characteristic of these lesions (7). Low-grade sinonasal hemangiopericytomas behave in a benign fashion and in one series only 2 of 22 cases recurred, regardless of treatment. Malignant sinonasal hemangiopericytomas with anaplastic spindle cells have also been described (1).

Nasal Polyps. LCH may resemble nasal polyps, clinically. Microscopically, nasal polyps may have areas of ulceration with a secondary granulation tissue response, but they do not have the lobular pattern of LCH. In areas of the polyp away from the ulceration, the more typical pattern of a nasal polyp may be appreciated.

Treatment and Prognosis. Recurrences of mucosal LCH are uncommon in completely excised lesions. Shave partial excisions or cauterizations result in a much higher recurrence rate.

SINONASAL HEMANGIOPERICYTOMA

Definition. This is a vascular, spindle cell neoplasm, with a distinct growth pattern composed of cells exhibiting at least minimal evidence of myogenous or pericytic differentiation at the ultrastructural level, but thus far lacking immunohistochemical features of myogenous differentiation. The light microscopic growth pattern is nonspecific and other, more specific directions of differentiation must be excluded.

General Features. When first described in the sinonasal region, there was some controversy regarding whether this neoplasm was fully analogous to soft tissue hemangiopericytoma. This uncertainty was reflected in the initial term of *hemangiopericytoma-like lesion* applied to these tumors (12,13). It is now generally, but not universally accepted that these neoplasms are part of the microscopic spectrum of hemangiopericytoma. In the Armed Forces Institute of Pathology (AFIP) series of cases from all anatomic sites, the head and neck region was the third most common location for hemangiopericytomas, following the lower extremity (most common site) and the retroperitoneum (15). Within the head and neck region, over half of the tumors occur within the sinonasal region, with the remainder involving a variety of structures including periorbital tissues, salivary glands, oral cavity, larynx, thyroid gland, and the bones of the skull.

Clinical Features. The features of hemangiopericytomas occurring in the upper aerodigestive tract, particularly in the nasal cavity and paranasal sinuses, have been summarized in several reviews (11,13,16–18,32). Most patients are middle-aged or older adults in their sixth or

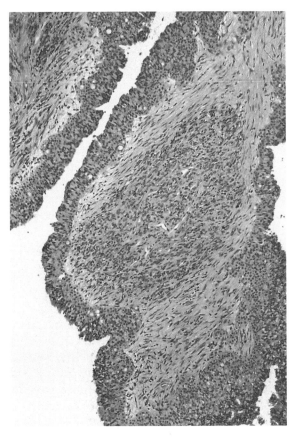

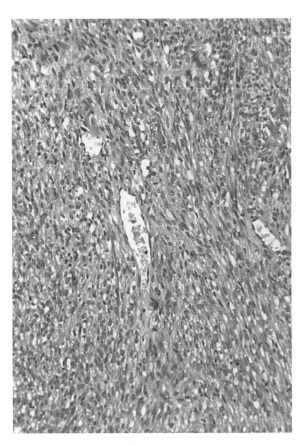

Figure 9-9
NASAL HEMANGIOPERICYTOMA
This nasal hemangiopericytoma has a low-power lobular pattern resembling that of lobular capillary hemangioma.

Figure 9-10
NASAL HEMANGIOPERICYTOMA
At higher magnification, nasal hemangiopericytoma is typified by a haphazard proliferation of spindle cells surrounding larger, often branching vascular channels.

seventh decades of life, with complaints of nasal obstruction or epistaxis. There is no sexual predilection. Radiographically, sinonasal hemangiopericytomas typically produce nasal cavity and paranasal sinus opacification with displacement of boundary structures or erosion of bone. Arteriograms may document a richly vascular stroma (15).

Gross Findings. Typically, the lesion forms a painless, polypoid mass that may be mistaken for an inflammatory polyp. Tumors up to 7 cm in size have been reported. The mass may have a gray-tan or more obviously vascular, red color. Some individuals have noted easy bleeding with manipulation and, as with angiofibroma, are cautioned against biopsy in an "uncontrolled" setting such as a physician's office.

Microscopic Findings. The histologic features of hemangiopericytomas will be covered in

greater detail in the upcoming Fascicle dealing with soft tissue neoplasms. The diagnosis remains to a large degree one of exclusion. A recent review noted that a hemangiopericytoma-like growth pattern may be seen in over a dozen distinct neoplasms (22). Many of these lesions are discussed in further detail under differential diagnosis.

In the head and neck region, these tumors are usually low grade and composed of uniform, ovoid or spindled cells forming tight aggregates, with little intervening stromal collagen (figs. 9-9–9-11). Only rare mitotic figures are seen, and there is no necrosis. The vascular pattern usually includes open, ramifying vascular spaces with the branching, prominent, vascular lumina often likened to "staghorns" (fig. 9-12). In other areas, the vessels may be smaller and less apparent (fig. 9-11). Typically, vessel walls lack an

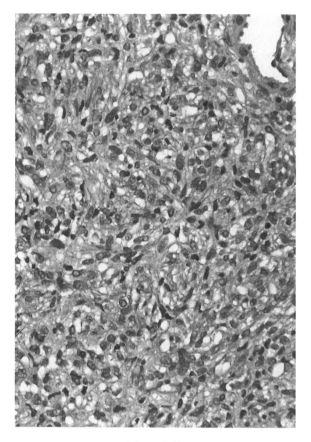

Figure 9-11
HEMANGIOPERICYTOMA
Higher magnification shows the uniform spindle cells of hemangiopericytoma. In this area, large vascular spaces are not as prominent.

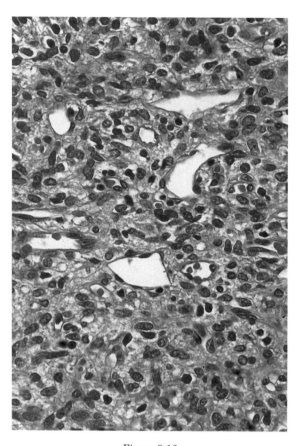

Figure 9-12
HEMANGIOPERICYTOMA
This low-grade hemangiopericytoma is composed of spindled to cuboidal stromal cells surrounding prominent capillaries.

obvious muscular coat. Higher grade hemangiopericytomas less commonly occur in this region, but should be distinguished from the low-grade forms because of their greater tendency for aggressive behavior, including metastasis.

Immunohistochemical Findings. Although normal pericytic cells "entrapped" within hemangiopericytomas stain strongly for smooth muscle actin and desmin, the neoplastic cells have failed, with one exception, to label for a variety of myogenous markers, notably muscle-specific actin and desmin, in multiple immunohistochemical studies (25,29). Of the actin and intermediate filaments, only vimentin is reproducibly present within these neoplasms. One study has noted the presence of myogenous markers in these tumors (20). This review of 28 cases reported that 65 percent expressed muscle-specific actin and 72 percent labeled for smooth

muscle actin. Staining for desmin was negative. Thus, the differential diagnostic value of immunohistochemical staining is not entirely clear. We view immunohistochemistry as primarily exclusionary, allowing elimination of other neoplasms exhibiting clear-cut myogenous, epithelial, or neural differentiation.

Ultrastructural Findings. Ultrastructurally, hemangiopericytomas have some features of pericytes, including pericellular basal lamina, pinocytotic vesicles, aggregates of thin cytoplasmic filaments, dense bodies, and, less frequently, membranous attachment plaques (10,14). These features support at least primitive myogenous differentiation.

Differential Diagnosis. The concept of hemangiopericytoma as a diagnostic entity continues to be associated with some uncertainty, more than 50 years after its initial description by Stout and Murray (31). Stout, himself, noted several years after his initial description that, "our general attitude in regard to hemangiopericytoma is to reject it as a diagnosis if we can think of any more reasonable explanation for the tumor" (30). Neoplasms with documented evidence of epithelial, melanocytic, myogenous, or neural differentiation, usually based on immunohistochemical studies, should be excluded from this diagnostic category (22). In a recent review by Nappi et al. (22), 14 distinct neoplasms were listed that were capable of assuming a "hemangiopericytoma-like" growth pattern. Neoplasms particularly prone to exhibit this growth pattern include: monophasic synovial sarcoma, mesenchymal chondrosarcoma, endometrial stromal sarcoma, infantile fibrosarcoma, and malignant fibrous histiocytoma.

Angiofibroma. There are obvious clinical differences between hemangiopericytoma and angiofibroma. The latter neoplasm virtually always arises in the nasopharynx, always occurs in males, and rarely occurs beyond or before the adolescent years. Although angiofibromas may have areas of increased stromal cellularity, they lack the uniformly hypercellular stroma of hemangiopericytoma. The vascular spaces in angiofibroma are smaller and less apparent at low-power magnification than the gaping, "staghorn" vascular spaces of hemangiopericytoma. Immunohistochemical stains are of limited discriminatory value. Angiofibromas may show limited staining for muscle-specific actin (22), but often the stromal cells, as in hemangiopericytoma, label only for vimentin.

Lobular Capillary Hemangioma. The distinction between LCH and hemangiopericytoma is discussed in the previous section.

Solitary Fibrous Tumor. It has recently been recognized that the upper respiratory tract may give rise to a benign fibrous proliferation that microscopically resembles so-called benign fibrous mesothelioma of the pleura. The term *solitary fibrous tumor* has been applied to these neoplasms (34,35). The clinical presentation of these lesions, as a solitary polypoid mass in the nasal cavity, may be identical to that of hemangiopericytoma. To further complicate the distinction, areas of prominent vascularity with a hemangiopericytoma-like pattern may be seen in solitary fibrous tumors (34). However, virtually by defi-

nition, the latter areas must be only a minor component of a solitary fibrous tumor. Solitary fibrous tumor has been know to label with CD34, but this marker may be encountered in hemangiopericytoma as well (22). The overlapping microscopic features of solitary fibrous tumor and well-differentiated hemangiopericytoma suggest closely related entities distinguished primarily by the degree of stromal vascularity.

Meningioma. Meningiomas may arise in the nasopharyngeal region, or secondarily invade the region (24,26). The generally vascular, spindle cell appearance may be confused with that of hemangiopericytoma. Positivity for epithelial membrane antigen may aid in the distinction as hemangiopericytomas are uniformly negative for this marker (33). We agree with others that so-called angioblastic meningioma is a meningeal hemangiopericytoma.

Synovial Sarcoma. This soft tissue sarcoma may rarely arise in the neck (27) and its monophasic form is noted to have a distinctly hemangiopericytoma-like light microscopic appearance. Staining for cytokeratin in monophasic, spindle cell synovial sarcoma allows ready distinction from cytokeratin-negative hemangiopericytoma.

Mesenchymal Chondrosarcoma. This soft tissue neoplasm commonly involves the head and neck region, including the periorbital tissues, meninges, and craniofacial bones (19,28). The hemangiopericytoma-like growth pattern is highly typical of the "undifferentiated" stromal component of these neoplasms. The diagnosis is based on the finding of sharply demarcated islands of cartilage within the tumor. In small biopsy specimens, the absence of these cartilaginous islands precludes a diagnosis and may easily lead to interpretation as hemangiopericytoma.

Treatment and Prognosis. Surgical resection is the mainstay of therapy. In general, predicting biologic behavior for hemangiopericytomas has been notoriously difficult. Considering all anatomic sites, approximately half of these lesions have been said to metastasize, although one wonders if this reflects a bias towards over-reporting malignant variants (21,23). Most hemangiopericytomas occurring in the head and neck are extremely well-differentiated lesions with a benign clinical course, regardless of therapy (12,13). Only rare tumors have behaved in a locally aggressive fashion or metastasized (16,32). Based on 42 patients from a series by Cantrell et al. (11), and Compagno and Hyams (12), 6 patients (14 percent) developed recurrences, and only 3 (7 percent) developed metastatic disease.

NASOPHARYNGEAL ANGIOFIBROMA

Definition. This is a clinicopathologically distinctive, locally destructive fibrovascular tumor arising in the region of the posterior nasal cavity and nasopharyngeal wall.

General Features. Nasopharyngeal angiofibromas are uncommon tumors that occur exclusively in the lateral nasopharynx and posterior portion of the nasal cavity (36,42,50,55,57, 61). The exclusive occurrence of nasopharyngeal angiofibromas in males (see below), particularly during adolescence, and the clinically observed reduction in size and vascularity of these masses following estrogen therapy suggests a hormonally sensitive lesion (53). This is further supported by anecdotal reports of tumor enlargement following testosterone administration. Estrogen receptors are lacking (52,53), but testosterone receptors have been found in these tumors, initially by cytosol preparations and, more recently, by immunohistochemical localization (47).

It has been suggested that patients with familial adenomatous polyposis have an increased incidence of nasopharyngeal angiofibroma (44). In one study of patients with adenomatous polyposis, nasopharyngeal angiofibromas were 25 times more frequent than in an age-matched population (44). If further studies bear out this association, the role of somatic mutations of the adenomatous polyposis gene in the development of nasopharyngeal angiofibromas should be sought.

Clinical Features. There is a sharp predilection for adolescent males with a mean age of 15 years. A small number occur in young children and older adults. Convincingly documented nasopharyngeal angiofibromas in females are vanishingly rare (62). Four large series of 216 cases from the Mayo Clinic, Memorial-Sloan Kettering, Barnes Hospital, and the University of Michigan included no female patients (36,50, 55,57), and the AFIP material, as of 1986, contained no female patients (51).

Patients with nasopharyngeal angiofibromas most often present with signs and symptoms of nasal obstruction (92 percent) (57). Epistaxis is also common (70 percent). Other frequent presenting features include nasal discharge (21 percent), facial deformity (19 percent), deafness or otitis (13 percent), bulging palate (10 percent), and proptosis (8 percent) (57). Facial deformity, in the form of bulging of the cheek, is usually due to growth through the sphenopalatine foramen into the pterygomaxillary fossa and the infratemporal fossa. Proptosis results from tumor extension into the inferior orbital fissure, often with destruction of the sphenoid wing and widening of the superior orbital fissure. Destruction of the pterygoid process may place the tumor against the dura covering the middle cranial fossa. Extension into the pterygomaxillary fossa, cheek, or maxillary antrum often makes complete excision difficult or impossible. Larger masses may fill the nasopharynx and extend downward to be visible in the upper portion of the oropharynx.

Radiographic Findings. Routine or sinus-view radiographs often show "bowing" of the posterior wall of the maxillary antrum. This is considered a highly characteristic, if not diagnostic, radiographic feature (58). Angiographic procedures are commonly performed; the arterial phase of nasopharyngeal angiofibroma has a characteristic appearance with large numbers of irregular, tortuous vessels in a pattern similar to that seen in meningiomas. In the proper clinical setting, this appearance is virtually diagnostic (fig. 9-13). Angiograms are also of considerable value to delineate vascular supply, which often derives from the internal maxillary artery. The blood supply may be quite diverse, however, with origins from the dural, sphenoidal, and ophthalmic branches of the internal carotid artery, as well as the vertebral and thyrocervical arteries (57). Selective, angiographically directed embolization of angiofibromas is associated with a considerable reduction in intraoperative blood loss (59).

Gross Findings. Grossly, nasopharyngeal angiofibromas may have a deceptively avascular, fibrous appearance. The innumerable blood vessels seen microscopically in large part escape gross detection (fig. 9-14). Somewhat larger vessels may be more obvious at the base of the lesion (fig. 9-15). Resected specimens typically consist of lobulated, firm, sessile or polypoid masses, which although unencapsulated may have a deceptively well-demarcated margin. Local invasion

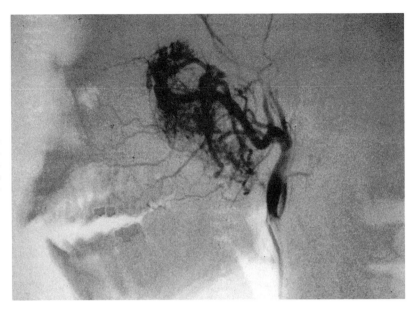

Figure 9-13
NASOPHARYNGEAL
ANGIOFIBROMA

The intense vascularity of this nasopharyngeal angiofibroma is clearly evident in a subtraction angiogram. In addition to being virtually diagnostic, the
angiographic studies also allow planning for surgery and embolization.

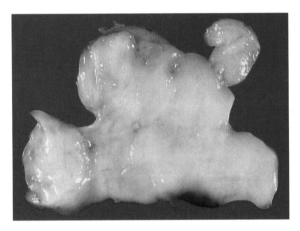

Figure 9-14
ANGIOFIBROMA

Grossly, angiofibromas are usually "fleshy," lobulated
masses with sharp borders. The vascular spaces are usually
too small to be appreciated grossly.

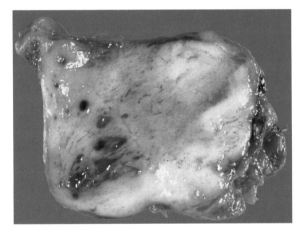

Figure 9-15
ANGIOFIBROMA

This cut section of an angiofibroma extends through the base
of the lesion where larger feeder vessels are grossly visible.

may be considerable, but is usually with a pushing rather than infiltrating border.

Microscopic Findings. The histologic hallmark of nasopharyngeal angiofibroma is a fibrocollagenous stroma containing numerous irregular vascular spaces that vary in size from small
slits to dilated structures. Usually, these spaces
are seen as defects in a stroma apparently lined
by a single layer of endothelial cells (figs. 9-16,
9-17). Vessels with thicker walls and an obvious
media are also present (fig. 9-18). There is often
increased vascularity around the periphery of

the lesion. In these regions, vessels may be
smaller and more densely packed, somewhat
resembling granulation tissue (fig. 9-19). Conversely, the central portions of the lesion may be
hypovascular (fig. 9-20). In such areas, the characteristic features of the stroma and stromal
cells still allow diagnosis. With the more widespread use of preoperative selective embolization, iatrogenic emboli of collagen and other embolization material are increasingly encountered
in resected specimens (fig. 9-21), often in association with areas of infarction.

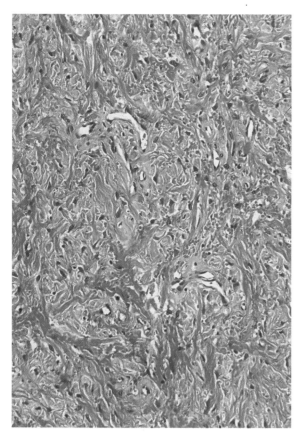

Figure 9-16
ANGIOFIBROMA

At low-power magnification, the haphazard stromal collagen and scattered small vascular spaces of angiofibroma can be seen. Many very small vascular spaces are present, some appearing as only tiny "defects" in the stroma.

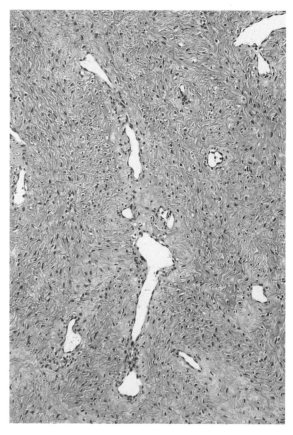

Figure 9-17
ANGIOFIBROMA

This angiofibroma is composed of both very small vascular spaces, just visible in this low-power image, as well as scattered larger vascular channels. The characteristic, haphazardly arranged stromal collagen is again seen.

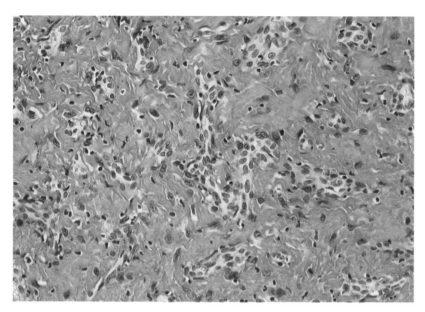

Figure 9-18
ANGIOFIBROMA

In most angiofibromas, pericytic cells cannot be clearly seen surrounding lumina, but in this example the vascular channels appear to be actively forming. Well-developed lumina are not present, but a prominent spindle cell pericytic component is clearly visible.

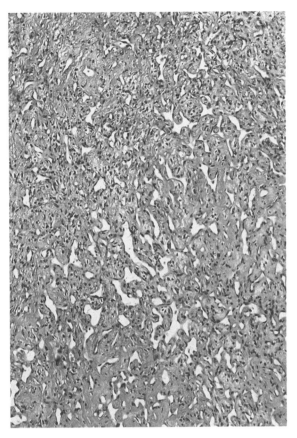

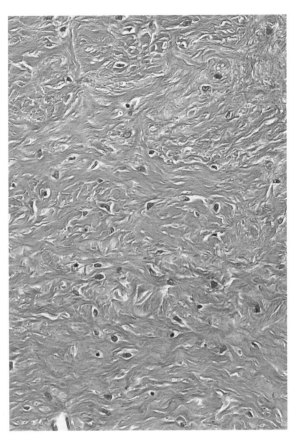

Figure 9-19
ANGIOFIBROMA

The more superficial portions of angiofibroma may be highly vascular and indistinguishable from a hemangioma or granulation tissue.

Figure 9-20
ANGIOFIBROMA

The deeper portions of angiofibroma, away from the central feeding vessels, may be hypovascular. Even in these regions, the distinct, haphazardly arranged stromal collagen is a key diagnostic feature.

Figure 9-21
ANGIOFIBROMA

The large vascular channel in the center of the illustration is filled with the microfibrillary collagen used in selective embolization prior to surgical resection.

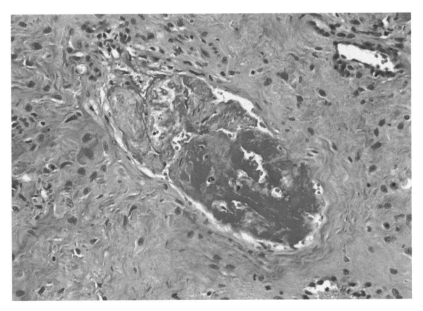

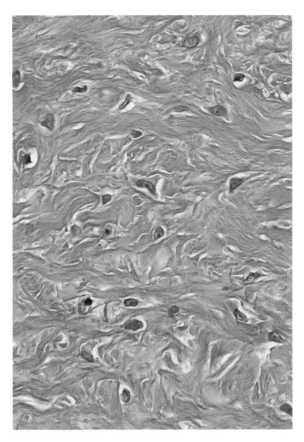

Figure 9-22
ANGIOFIBROMA

A high-power magnification of the stromal cells in angiofibroma shows the characteristic stellate configuration of the stromal nuclei.

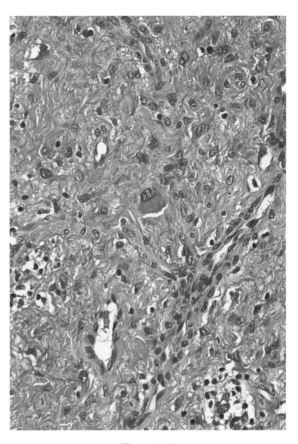

Figure 9-23
ANGIOFIBROMA

Occasional angiofibromas contain ganglion-like stromal cells with prominent, eosinophilic cytoplasm and enlarged, offset nuclei.

The stroma of nasopharyngeal angiofibroma consists of characteristic spindled and stellate mesenchymal cells, separated by wavy, haphazardly arranged collagen (fig. 9-22). The nuclei in the stromal cells vary from pyknotic and hyperchromatic to large and vesicular with prominent nucleoli. Mitotic figures are extremely rare. Occasional stromal cells possess abundant eosinophilic cytoplasm and resemble the "ganglion-like" cells of proliferative myositis (fig. 9-23). "Giant cell" multinucleated forms are also common. The stroma of nasopharyngeal angiofibroma often contains numerous mast cells. Except in foci of mucosal ulceration, other inflammatory cells are scarce.

Immunohistochemical Findings. Immunohistochemically, nasopharyngeal angiofibroma contains three prominent cell types. The vascular spaces are lined by endothelial cells that express appropriate vascular markers, including factor VIII–related antigen, *Ulex europeaus* I lectin, CD31, and CD34 (fig. 9-24). In our experience, even the small, slit-like, capillary-sized vascular spaces are surrounded, at least partially, by a layer of smooth muscle actin–positive pericytes (fig. 9-25) (38). The spindled to stellate, nonpericytic stromal cells express vimentin, but we and others have been unable to label them with smooth muscle markers (38). In our experience, the stromal cells of nasopharyngeal angiofibroma are strongly positive for testosterone receptors (fig. 9-26) (47).

Ultrastructural Findings. By electron microscopy, the stromal cells of nasopharyngeal angiofibroma contain large numbers of filaments, many of which appear to be actin filaments (fig. 9-27) (63). The stromal nuclei contain

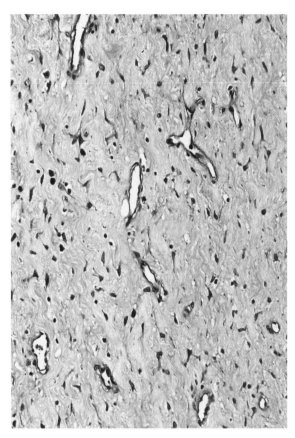

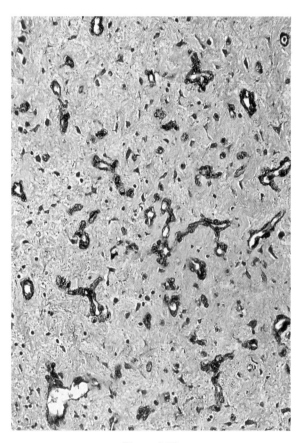

Figure 9-24
ANGIOFIBROMA
Immunohistochemical reactivity with endothelial cell markers highlights the numerous vascular channels in angiofibroma (anti-factor VIII–related antigen, hematoxylin).

Figure 9-25
ANGIOFIBROMA
Reactivity for actin highlights larger numbers of pericytic cells in angiofibroma that are often not recognized in H&E-stained sections (anti-smooth muscle actin, hematoxylin).

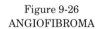

Figure 9-26
ANGIOFIBROMA
Reactivity for testosterone receptor is seen in the stromal cell nuclei of this angiofibroma (anti-testosterone receptor, hematoxylin). (Courtesy of Dr. A.M. Gown, Seattle, WA.)

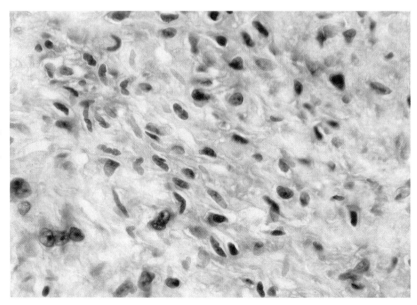

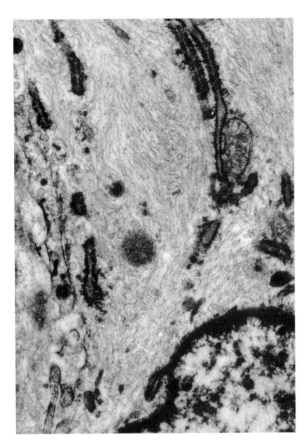

Figure 9-27
ANGIOFIBROMA
Ultrastructurally, the stromal cells of angiofibroma contain numerous actin-like filaments with occasional dense bodies and membrane attachment plaques. (Courtesy of Dr. J.B. Taxy, Chicago, IL.)

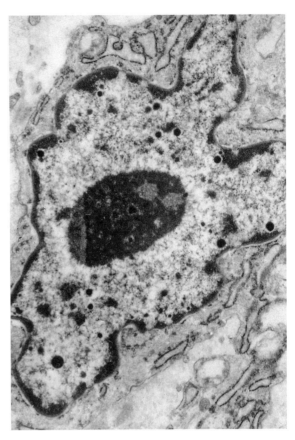

Figure 9-28
ANGIOFIBROMA
The stromal cell nuclei of angiofibroma contain characteristic dense granules. (Courtesy of Dr. J.B. Taxy, Chicago, IL.)

highly characteristic, electron-dense inclusions that vary from 20 to 300 nm in diameter (fig. 9-28) (62,64). Their exact nature is not known. They are not viral particles and probably represent aggregates of protein and nucleic acids.

Differential Diagnosis. *Lobular Capillary Hemangioma.* The advancing, highly vascular edge of an angiofibroma may contain plexiform capillaries in a loose, myxoid stroma. This nondiagnostic pattern may be seen at the edge of hemangiomas, including LCH. LCH involves the nasal cavity, but not the nasopharynx (56); in contrast, nasopharyngeal angiofibroma is a predominantly nasopharyngeal lesion. LCHs do not have the dense collagenized stroma with uniformly distributed, irregular, thin-walled vessels seen in nasopharyngeal angiofibroma. Angiofibromas lack the lobular arrangement of cap-

illaries that is characteristic of LCH. Because LCHs only superficially involve underlying tissue, only rarely recur, and are associated with minimal blood loss during resection, differentiation is clinically important.

Aggressive Fibromatosis. The central hypovascular portions of nasopharyngeal angiofibroma, taken out of context, could be confused with aggressive fibromatosis. However, nasopharyngeal angiofibroma does not form highly collagenized, compact bands of fibrous tissue that diffusely infiltrate and entrap surrounding tissues as seen in fibromatosis. The nuclei in fibromatosis tend to be spindled, and stellate forms are rare. We have not seen the multinucleated and ganglion-like stromal giant cells of angiofibroma in fibromatosis. Radiographically, fibromatosis lacks the prominent neovascularity that is the hallmark of nasopharyngeal angiofibroma.

Fibroma. Nasal fibromas are small, noninvasive polypoid lesions that typically occur on the nasal septum. They may represent the "end stage" of a prior lesion such as LCH. Their location, small size, and lack of stromal vascularity should allow easy distinction.

Solitary Fibrous Tumor. This lesion of the nasal cavity and paranasal sinuses microscopically resembles pleural benign fibrous mesothelioma (66). Unlike nasopharyngeal angiofibroma, it typically presents as a polypoid intranasal mass in a middle-aged patient of either sex. Microscopically, there is a patternless proliferation of spindled fibroblasts in a focally collagenized background. The degree of stromal cellularity is significantly greater than that seen in nasopharyngeal angiofibroma. Large blood vessels are prominent and areas resembling hemangiopericytoma are common. However, the smaller, slit-like spaces characteristic of nasopharyngeal angiofibroma are not present. Immunohistochemically, the spindle cells express vimentin, but are negative for muscle-specific actin or S-100 protein.

Frozen Section. Frozen section diagnosis of nasopharyngeal angiofibroma can be highly problematic. The small vascular spaces may be difficult to identify and their lumina may be constricted by frozen section artifact. Recognition of the distinctive, stellate stromal cells and haphazard, "wavy" stromal collagen may aid in diagnosis. This pattern differs, at least subtly, from the bipolar fibroblasts and the more organized collagen of scar tissue. The distinction is not always possible, however.

Treatment and Prognosis. The therapeutic cornerstone for nasopharyngeal angiofibroma is surgical excision, often requiring a transpalatal-transantral or lateral rhinotomy approach. Because of the inability to completely excise many of these lesions, multiple recurrences or, more accurately, persistence and regrowth are the rule. In one series, 42 percent of patients had one or more (mean, 3) recurrences (50). Recurrences seldom occur after a 2-year disease-free interval. Persistent tumor may regrow, remain asymptomatic, or even regress. In contrast, spontaneous regression of lesions that have not been partially excised, while stated to occur in past literature, has only rarely been adequately documented (40,65).

Angiofibromas may bleed extensively when excised (1000 to 3000 mL). Therefore, biopsies should be approached with caution, particularly when done as an office procedure without vascular access for fluid replacement. The clinical presentation, anatomic location, and radiographic findings are so classic that biopsy is seldom necessary. In several studies, administration of oral estrogens prior to surgery reduced the clinical vascularity of the tumor and operative blood loss. It has been postulated that estrogen exerts its "regressing" effect on these lesions by inhibiting the pituitary synthesis of luteinizing hormone, resulting in decreased testicular synthesis of testosterone (52). Estrogen also increases plasma sex steroid binding protein, which decreases the nonbound testosterone available for the tumor cells. Recently, preoperative regression in tumor size has been documented following treatment with the testosterone receptor blocker, flutamide (43): four of five patients treated experienced an average regression in size, measured radiographically, of 44 percent. No sequelae of the treatment could be detected 2 or more years following therapy and testosterone levels were normal, but this approach requires additional study. Microscopic changes following this therapy are not evident, however. Preoperative selective embolization is also commonly used to decrease operative bleeding (59).

Radiation therapy is of value in unresectable lesions (41,48,54), although there is the slight risk for subsequent sarcoma in the irradiated field. All purported examples of "malignant transformation" by nasopharyngeal angiofibroma are either misdiagnoses or postradiation sarcomas (37,39, 45,49,60). Chemotherapy has also been utilized for particularly aggressive, unresectable nasopharyngeal angiofibromas (46).

In spite of tumor persistence, patients with nasopharyngeal angiofibromas have a good prognosis. In the Mayo Clinic series that included a large number of advanced lesions, 9 percent of patients treated with a lateral rhinotomy surgical approach died from their disease (57). However, in the Barnes Hospital series of 30 cases, there were no deaths from tumor, and the estimated overall mortality was approximately 3 percent (55). Patients dying from nasopharyngeal angiofibroma usually do so as a result of intracranial extension or exsanguination.

MISCELLANEOUS VASCULAR NEOPLASMS

Glomus Tumor

Glomus tumors predilect the skin and subcutaneous tissues. Involvement of the noncutaneous head and neck structures, including the nasal cavity, buccal mucosa, tongue, hard palate, and trachea has been described but is rare (69–71). Although the term *glomangioma* is typically used for a variant of glomus tumor with larger, more ectatic vascular channels, in the head and neck this term and *glomus tumor* are often considered synonymous. Fewer than a dozen nasal and paranasal lesions have been described, and Fu and Perzin (69) noted only one example in a review of 256 nonepithelial neoplasms from this region.

Patients have ranged in age from young adults to the elderly. The nasal septum accounted for three of five intranasal tumors reviewed in one study (70). Two of the five lesions were painful, two were asymptomatic, and three presented with nasal obstruction.

The typical gross finding in the nasal cavity is that of a blue-red, polypoid mass usually less than a centimeter in diameter.

As in other locations, the typical microscopic pattern is one of prominent, variably sized vascular spaces surrounded by variably prominent pericytes. The latter typically assume an epithelioid appearance, with conspicuous eosinophilic cytoplasm (fig. 9-29). Immunohistochemical stains document actin positivity within the pericytic cells. Other immunohistochemical markers of myogenous differentiation (myoglobin, desmin) have been reported to be negative (67). Stains for S-100 protein highlight small nerve fibers between aggregates of glomus cells (67). Ultrastructural analysis on well-fixed material shows more evidence of myogenous differentiation than does immunohistochemistry. With this technique, the neoplastic cells exhibit thick and thin myofilaments (myosin and actin), well-formed basal lamina, membrane dense bodies (attachment plaques), and pinocytotic vesicles (68,72).

Laryngeal Hemangioma

Although hemangiomas can arise throughout the head and neck region, most do not differ significantly from hemangiomas occurring at

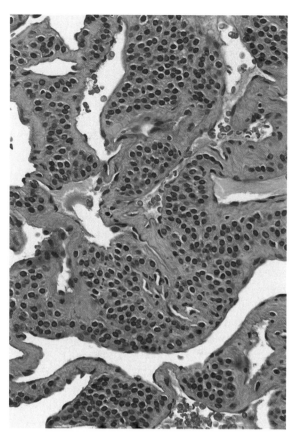

Figure 9-29
GLOMUS TUMOR
This glomus tumor contains large vascular channels separated by nests of epithelioid glomus cells.

any other anatomic site. Those arising in the larynx, however, have some distinct clinicopathologic features that warrant brief discussion. The larynx gives rise to two distinctive variants of hemangioma: the juvenile, infantile, or congenital variant and the adult variant.

Infantile Hemangioma. Infantile laryngeal hemangiomas invariably arise in the subglottic region (74–78). Symptoms are usually present at birth and 94 percent of patients are symptomatic by 6 months of age. There is a 2 to 1 female predominance. About half of affected children have associated cutaneous hemangiomas, and their presence should lead to a strong suspicion of laryngeal hemangioma in an infant with respiratory distress. The presenting symptom is usually inspiratory stridor, which is typically present at birth or shortly thereafter, and may be life threatening. Symptoms may wax and wane, perhaps in response to variations in the engorgement of the vascular channels. Endoscopic examination may be difficult or impossible, even under general anesthesia. If successful, endoscopy demonstrates a broad-based mass, fullness, or distortion of the subglottic larynx that may be localized or circumferential. The overlying intact mucosa may appear blue-violet. Endoscopic biopsy is generally avoided because of potential hemorrhage. Magnetic resonance imaging (MRI) and even frontal radiographs of the neck demarcate the lesion.

Microscopically, laryngeal lesions are identical in appearance to cutaneous *juvenile hemangiomas,* lesions known by a large number of variably appropriate synonyms including strawberry nevus, hypertrophic angioma of infancy, congenital hemangioma, and the particularly confusing term, benign hemangioendothelioma of infancy. The clinical involution of these lesions has a microscopic counterpart. "Early" lesions are highly cellular nodules composed of plump endothelial cells and pericytes with small, often inapparent vascular lumina. Mitotic rate is brisk and the overall image may be suggestive of malignancy. With time, the vascular channels enlarge, the endothelial cells become elongated, and mitotic rate greatly decreases, resulting in an image more typical of a conventional capillary hemangioma (fig. 9-30). Over further time, there is a progressive decrease in the number of vascular channels with increasing intralesional fibrous tissue.

Although once treated aggressively with low-dose radiation therapy, the natural history of these lesions is now known to be analogous to that of similar cutaneous lesions (74). They may enlarge during the first 6 months of life, but this is almost invariably followed by involution. Steroids may be of value for symptomatic treatment, and some patients require a low tracheostomy to maintain airway patency (78). The possible role of carbon dioxide laser excision for very large lesions is currently under study (78).

Adult Hemangioma. These are almost 10 times more common than the infantile form (73,76). Unlike the childhood lesion, the adult laryngeal hemangioma predilects the supraglottic and glottic larynx, and is more common in males. Symptoms are variable and include cough, hemoptysis, dysphagia, dyspnea, and hoarseness. Acute respiratory compromise is rare, and patients are often

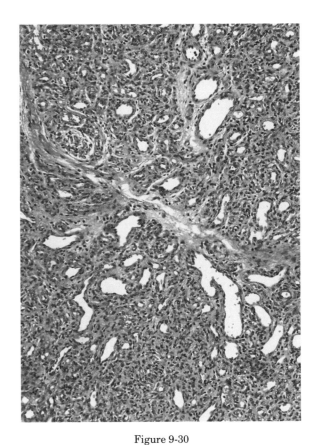

Figure 9-30
INFANTILE LARYNGEAL HEMANGIOMA
This infantile laryngeal hemangioma is composed of highly cellular aggregates of proliferating endothelial cells with developing vascular lumina.

symptomatic for many years. We are unaware of an association with cutaneous hemangiomas.

These lesions are typically more superficial in location that the infantile variant and may be polypoid or pedunculated. The color is commonly red to purple, and some have been said to resemble a raspberry. Small, pedunculated lesions have been successfully removed endoscopically, with little blood loss, but larger lesions may require more extensive surgery.

Microscopically, adult laryngeal hemangiomas are usually of the cavernous type (fig. 9-31). The stroma surrounding the dilated vascular spaces varies from edematous to fibrous. Endothelial cells are flattened and devoid of mitotic activity. When adult hemangiomas involve the glottis as a polypoid lesion, the distinction from vocal cord polyps with an angiomatous stroma is essentially arbitrary (fig. 9-32). Both laryngeal hemangiomas and angiomatous vocal cord polyps may exhibit changes of papillary endothelial hyperplasia within the dilated vascular spaces (figs. 9-33, 9-34). This reactive change has occasionally been misinterpreted as representing an angiosarcoma.

Polypoid Granulation Tissue

Granulation tissue is a common, reproducible reaction to trauma. Within the head and neck, the prototypical site for granulation tissue formation is along the margins of a tracheostomy stoma. The larynx is also a common site, and at that location the preceding trauma is usually a prior biopsy or prolonged intubation (80). Intubation-induced laryngeal granulation tissue may occur throughout the larynx, but usually involves the posterior portion of the true vocal cord, or overlies the vocal process of the arytenoid cartilage (79). In the larynx or a tracheostomy stoma, granulation tissue occasionally forms a distinctively polypoid mass (figs. 9-35, 9-36). The stroma underlying the polypoid granulation tissue of the vocal cords often shows distinct, sometimes diagnostically worrisome, reactive microscopic changes. These are discussed elsewhere in the section on laryngeal contact ulcers.

Microscopically, granulation tissue consists of radially oriented capillaries in a loosely edematous to more fibrotic, variably inflamed stroma (figs. 9-36, 9-37). The capillaries range from narrow

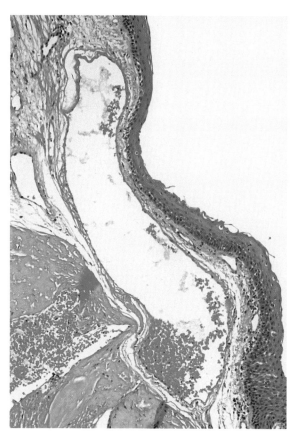

Figure 9-31
"ADULT TYPE" LARYNGEAL HEMANGIOMA
This "adult type" laryngeal hemangioma consists of large vascular channels just beneath intact surface mucosa.

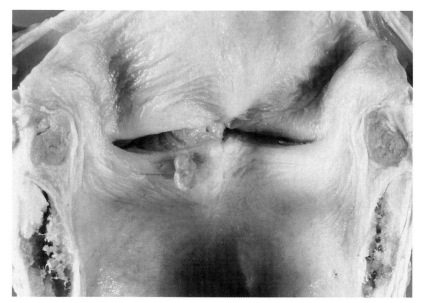

Figure 9-32
"ADULT TYPE"
LARYNGEAL HEMANGIOMA
This vascular vocal cord polyp involves the anterior portion of the right true vocal cord. The vascular nature of the lesion is not apparent in this fixed specimen.

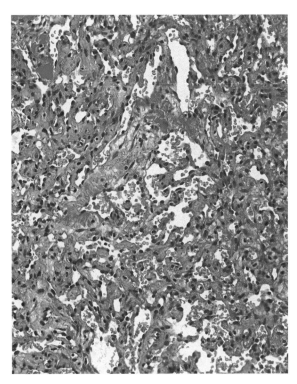

Figure 9-33
PAPILLARY ENDOTHELIAL HYPERPLASIA

Hemangiomas and angiomatous vocal cord polyps may contain papillary endothelial hyperplasia. The complex papillae and anastomosing vascular spaces must not be confused with angiosarcoma.

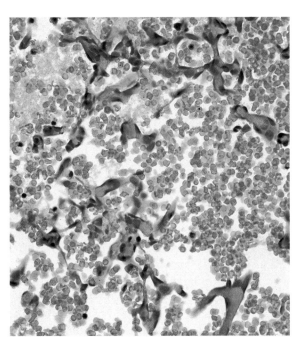

Figure 9-34
PAPILLARY ENDOTHELIAL HYPERPLASIA

This area of papillary endothelial hyperplasia from the specimen seen grossly in figure 9-32, shows delicate, anastomosing fibrous cores lined by proliferating endothelial cells.

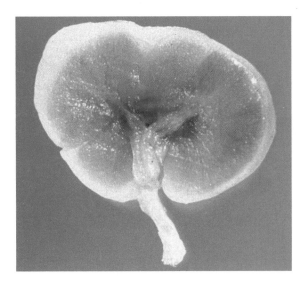

Figure 9-35
POLYPOID GRANULATION TISSUE

Granulation tissue from the region of a tracheostomy stoma forms a polypoid mass with an attenuated stalk. (Slide 75 from Mills SE, Fechner RE. Pathology of the larynx, Chicago: ASCP, 1985:55.)

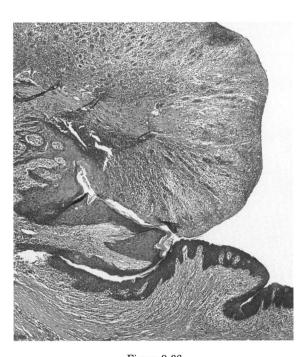

Figure 9-36
POLYPOID GRANULATION TISSUE

This low-power magnification of laryngeal granulation tissue shows a large polypoid mass of capillaries and edematous, inflamed stroma. There is no underlying vascular proliferation.

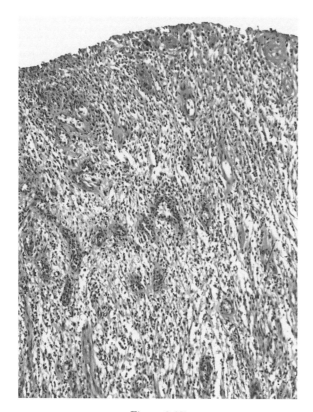

Figure 9-37
GRANULATION TISSUE
Radially oriented capillaries in an acutely inflamed, edematous stroma are typical of granulation tissue.

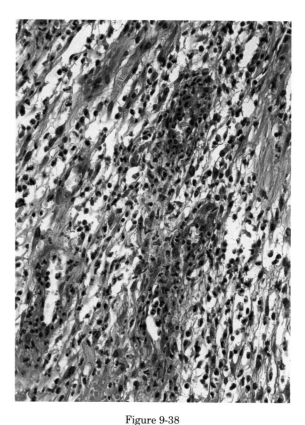

Figure 9-38
GRANULATION TISSUE
This higher power magnification shows the intense stromal inflammation present in granulation tissue.

vascular channels with prominent, reactive-appearing endothelial cells to more ectatic vascular spaces. The inflammatory reaction varies from acute to chronic (fig. 9-38). Often the process forms a pedunculated mass, with the base containing prominent, larger blood vessels and a hemosiderin-laden stroma. There is a natural progression from "early" granulation tissue with acute inflammation, large numbers of small capillaries, edematous stroma, and ulcerated surface mucosa to more mature granulation tissue with chronic inflammation, fibrotic stroma, fewer numbers of capillaries with larger lumina, and intact surface mucosa.

In spite of its reactive, non-neoplastic nature, granulation tissue may produce polypoid tumor-like masses, leading to biopsy of specimens to exclude the possibility of recurrent carcinoma. In addition, granulation tissue may recur, particularly if the source of trauma persists, leading to further concern regarding possible malignancy.

Lymphangioma (Cystic Hygroma)

Cystic lymphangiomas of the neck region (cystic hygromas) are relatively common childhood vascular tumors, accounting for 26 percent of all vascular lesions in this age range in one review (81). Considering lymphangioma arising in any anatomic location or age, the head and neck is the most common site, followed by the axilla. Most occur within the first year of life. Lymphangiomas of the head and neck are often centered in the posterior cervical triangle (fig. 9-39), or less often, in the anterior triangle just below the angle of the jaw. Tumors in this location, not surprisingly, have been associated with significant laryngo-tracheal and esophageal obstructive symptoms (82). About 10 percent of lymphangiomas of the head and neck extend into the mediastinum, emphasizing the need for thorough preoperative radiologic evaluation and planning of the surgical approach for the removal of these lesions.

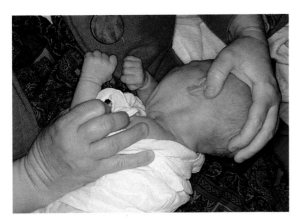

Figure 9-39
CAVERNOUS LYMPHANGIOMA
A slightly violaceous mass representing a cavernous lymphangioma (cystic hygroma) is seen in the left posterior cervical region of this young child.

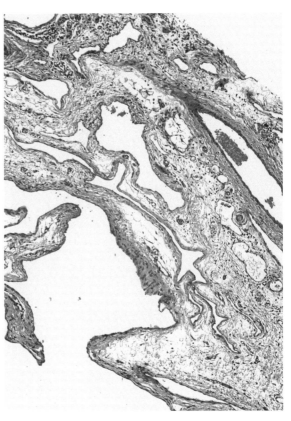

Figure 9-40
CAVERNOUS LYMPHANGIOMA
Cavernous lymphangioma (cystic hygroma) consists of dilated empty or blood-filled vascular channels. Diffuse infiltration of skeletal muscle and subcutaneous fat may be present (not seen).

Grossly, the tumors may be unicystic or multicystic, often quite large masses, measuring up to 15 cm (81). Some cystic lymphangiomas may be very sharply demarcated, but most have a rather poorly defined margin. The tumors arising in the neck are usually centered in the more superficial tissues, with growth outward, rather than invading deeper structures in the neck. About 20 percent of resected cavernous lymphangiomas of the neck recur. In our experience, evaluation of resection margins has been difficult or impossible, and has not correlated with subsequent recurrences.

Microscopically, cystic lymphangiomas consist of often irregularly shaped, thin-walled vascular channels lined by highly attenuated, often inapparent endothelial cells (fig. 9-40). Variably sized aggregates of lymphoid cells are often present within the walls between adjacent cystic spaces. The irregular vascular lumina, lymphoid aggregates, and inapparent widely spaced endothelial cells are features that help distinguish lymphangiomas with intraluminal hemorrhage from true hemangiomas. Lymphatic endothelial cells are much less reactive for vascular endothelial markers, such as factor VIII–related antigen, CD31, and *Ulex europeaus* lectin than their blood-vascular counterparts. Staining may occur with any of these markers, however, and this approach has very limited diagnostic value.

Kaposi's Sarcoma

Approximately 84 percent of patients with acquired immunodeficiency syndrome (AIDS) have one or more head and neck lesions, including Kaposi's sarcoma, lymphoma, reactive lymphadenopathy, oral hairy leukoplakia, and candidiasis (84). In many instances head and neck lesions may be the initial manifestation of illness. Once a rare lesion (83), Kaposi's sarcoma of the head and neck is now a common finding in patients with human immunodeficiency virus (HIV)-related disease. In this setting, Kaposi's sarcoma may be considerably more aggressive than in the "classic" form. Although HIV-related Kaposi's sarcoma of the head and neck is seldom fatal, it may contribute to significant patient morbidity (85). Common sites of disease include the oral mucosa (fig. 9-41), especially the palate and

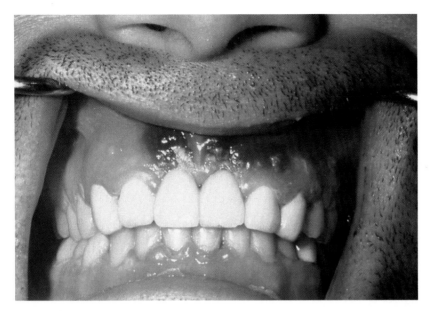

Figure 9-41
KAPOSI'S SARCOMA
Gingival involvement by Kaposi's sarcoma in this HIV-positive male produces multiple, deep blue nodules.

tonsils, as well as the skin of the face and neck (86). Depending on the site of involvement, treatment is directed toward relieving pain, bleeding, airway obstruction, difficulty swallowing, or disfigurement (85). Amelioration of the immunocompromise with alpha-interferon or chemotherapy is the usual treatment, but therapy is invariably individualized (85). Other immunodeficient conditions such as iatrogenic transplant-related immunosuppression, have also been associated with an increase in the frequency of Kaposi's sarcoma, although not nearly to the degree seen in HIV-positive patients.

Microscopically, HIV-related Kaposi's sarcoma is generally a well-developed, easily recognized lesion. An infiltrative proliferation of mildly pleomorphic, spindled cells separated by slit-like vascular spaces filled with erythrocytes is typical (fig. 9-42). Periodic acid–Schiff (PAS)-positive, diastase-resistant "globules" may be present within the spindled cells or in the extracellular stroma.

Immunohistochemical studies have demonstrated variable reactivity for endothelial-type markers including factor VIII–related antigen, *Ulex europeaus* lectin, and CD34. Many lesions are negative for endothelial markers, however, and this should not dissuade one from the diagnosis, given appropriate light microscopic and clinical findings. Kaposi's sarcoma must be distinguished from another HIV-related vascular lesion, bacillary angiomatosis (see below).

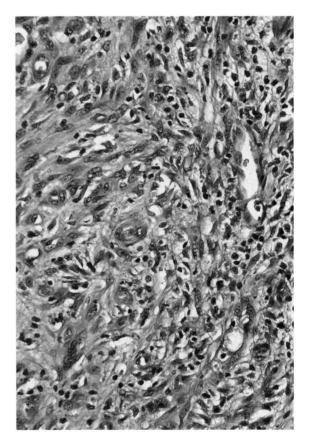

Figure 9-42
KAPOSI'S SARCOMA
Nodular Kaposi's sarcoma consists of proliferating spindle cells, with scattered, often slit-like vascular spaces and some associated inflammation.

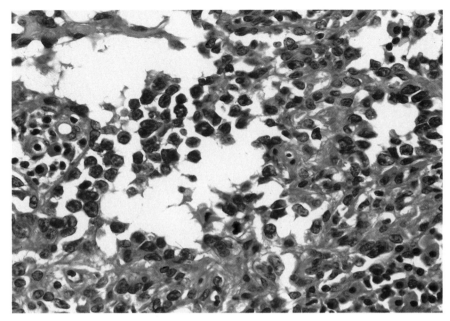

Figure 9-43
ANGIOSARCOMA
This low-grade angio-
sarcoma forms large vessel-
like spaces partially lined by
enlarged, hyperchromatic endothelial cells. Within the
larger lumen is an apparently
exfoliated aggregate of neoplastic endothelial cells.

Angiosarcoma

Angiosarcomas involving the skin and superficial soft tissues show a strong predilection for
the scalp, forehead, and upper facial region; involvement of the lower face is much less common.
Most patients are elderly and some studies show
a male predominance. Involvement is often multifocal, with microscopic disease frequently present
in clinically uninvolved areas. Treatment by radical surgical resection was typical up until the
1970s, but because of the associated high local
recurrence rate and overall abysmal prognosis
this aggressive approach has been replaced by a
combination of more limited surgical resection
and electron beam radiation (90–92).

Noncutaneous angiosarcomas of the head and
neck region are, in marked contrast, quite rare.
One review from 1968 could document only 15
reported angiosarcomas of the larynx (94), which
appears to be the most common site in the upper
aerodigestive tract (95). A separate study from
1979 documented only 14 examples from the sinonasal region (87); the maxillary antrum was the
most common site for the latter group of lesions.

Multiple systems for grading angiosarcomas
have been utilized. In our experience, tumors
interpreted as low-grade angiosarcoma in the
older literature are often better interpreted with
more recent terminology as epithelioid (histiocytoid) hemangiomas or epithelioid hemangio-
endotheliomas. True angiosarcomas of low or
intermediate grade are obviously vasoformative,
with complex, anastomosing and infiltrating
vascular spaces lined by enlarged, often hyperchromatic, obviously atypical endothelial cells.
Intraluminal papillae may be common (fig. 9-43).
With higher grade lesions, the vasoformative
features are more focal and the primary diagnostic problem is verifying their endothelial differentiation (fig. 9-44). In this regard, the currently
available endothelial markers, including CD31,
CD34, factor VIII–related antigen, and *Ulex europeaus* lectin are extremely helpful (89,93,98).
It should be noted that some endothelial neoplasms, particularly those with prominent cytoplasm, may express focal cytokeratin (99). Thus,
this marker, if taken out of context and applied
without an appropriate staining "panel," may
lead to an erroneous diagnosis of carcinoma.

In our experience with vascular lesions arising
from mucosal surfaces of the head and neck, lobular capillary hemangiomas and papillary endothelial hyperplasia (88,96,97) have been mistaken
for low-grade angiosarcoma. With regard to the
latter, we have encountered both laryngeal polyps
and inflammatory nasal polyps with prominent
papillary endothelial hyperplasia which had
been misinterpreted as low-grade angiosarcoma.

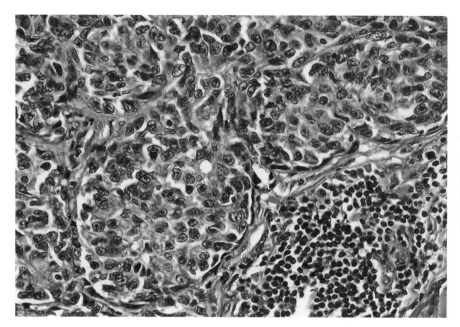

Figure 9-44
ANGIOSARCOMA
Some angiosarcomas may be less obviously vasoformative and consist of epithelioid nests of cells. Immunohistochemical studies may be needed to confirm the endothelial nature of the cells and scattered cytokeratin positivity should not be misinterpreted.

Bacillary Angiomatosis

This bacterial-induced vascular proliferation is strongly associated with immunosuppression, usually due to HIV infection. It was first described in 1982, and has subsequently been the subject of multiple reports (102). Patients typically present with numerous red to violet cutaneous and subcutaneous nodules, often associated with systemic symptoms such as fever, chills, headache, weight loss, and malaise (100). The face is a common site of involvement, but any portion of the skin may be affected. Confusion clinically with Kaposi's sarcoma is common and, indeed, the two lesions often occur together. Bacillary angiomatosis is now known to be due to infection with *Rochalimacea henselae,* an organism also associated with cat scratch disease in immunocompetent patients (100).

Microscopically, the more superficial lesions are often polypoid, with attenuated overlying epidermis and epithelial collarettes, features indicative of rapid growth. The low-power microscopic pattern is that of a well-circumscribed lobular capillary proliferation, most closely resembling a lobular capillary hemangioma. Within the lobules, small capillaries often surround ectatic ones. The capillary lumina are lined by variably protuberant endothelial cells (fig. 9-45). In some cases, the endothelial cells may be prominent and cuboidal, similar to those seen in epithelioid hemangioma. Cuboidal endothelial cells may appear singly or in small aggregates, without well-formed lumina. The nuclei display a range of nuclear atypia, including foci of "solid" endothelial cells with prominent pleomorphism and mitotic activity. A reticulin stain can define the vascular nature of the proliferation and the relationship of seemingly isolated endothelial cells.

Bands of variably edematous, mucinous, or fibrotic stroma separate the lobules of capillaries. The presence of neutrophils deep within the lesion is an important diagnostic clue. The neutrophils often aggregate in clusters, with or without neutrophilic debris, adjacent to the capillaries. Clumps of granular amphophilic material, corresponding to clusters of bacilli, are encountered in almost all cases (fig. 9-46). The granular bacillary clumps can easily be mistaken for fibrin. Unlike fibrin, in well-prepared sections the clumps are finely granular, rather than fibrillar. A Warthin-Starry stain or electron microscopic examination confirms the presence of characteristic bacilli (fig. 9-47) (101).

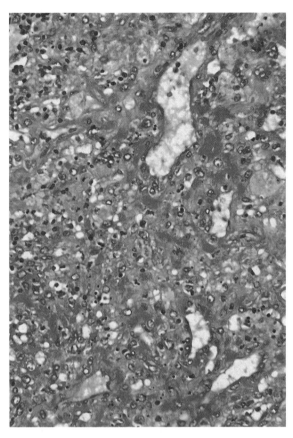

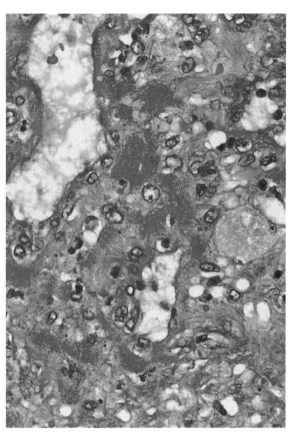

Figure 9-45
BACILLARY ANGIOMATOSIS
Complex vascular spaces, perivascular eosinophilic material, and prominent inflammation are typical features of bacillary angiomatosis. (Courtesy of Dr. M.H. Stoler, Charlottesville, VA.)

Figure 9-46
BACILLARY ANGIOMATOSIS
Higher magnification demonstrates prominent endothelial cells and perivascular eosinophilic material. The latter somewhat resembles fibrin, but actually represents clumps of organisms. (Courtesy of Dr. M.H. Stoler, Charlottesville, VA.)

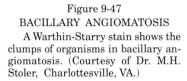

Figure 9-47
BACILLARY ANGIOMATOSIS
A Warthin-Starry stain shows the clumps of organisms in bacillary angiomatosis. (Courtesy of Dr. M.H. Stoler, Charlottesville, VA.)

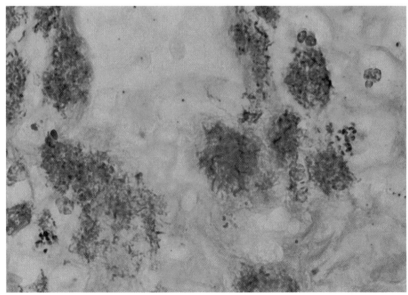

REFERENCES

Lobular Capillary Hemangioma

1. Compagno J, Hyams VJ. Hemangiopericytoma-like intranasal tumors. A clinicopathologic study of 23 cases. Am J Clin Pathol 1976;66:672–83.
2. Cooper PH, McAllister HA, Helwig EB. Intravenous pyogenic granuloma. A study of 18 cases. Am J Surg Pathol 1979;3:221–8.
3. Cooper PH, Mills SE. Subcutaneous granuloma pyogenicum. Lobular capillary hemangioma. Arch Dermatol 1982;118:30–3.
4. Fechner RE, Cooper PH, Mills SE. Pyogenic granuloma of the larynx and trachea. A causal and pathologic misnomer for granulation tissue. Arch Otolaryngol 1980;107:30–2.
5. Fu YS, Perzin KH. Non-epithelial tumors of the nasal cavity, paranasal sinuses and nasopharynx: a clinico-pathologic study. I. General features and vascular tumors. Cancer 1974;33:1275–88.
6. Hartzel MB. Granuloma pyogenicum (botryomycosis of French authors). J Cutan Dis 1904;22:520-3.
7. Mills SE, Cooper PH, Fechner RE. Lobular capillary hemangioma: the underlying lesion of pyogenic granuloma. A study of 73 cases from the oral and nasal mucous membranes. Am J Surg Pathol 1980;4:470–9.
8. Neel HB, Whicker JH, Devine KD, Weiland LH. Juvenile angiofibroma. Review of 120 cases. Am J Surg 1973;126:547–56.
9. Nichols GE, Gaffey MJ, Mills SE, Weiss LM. Lobular capillary hemangioma. An immunohistochemical study including steroid hormone receptor status. Am J Clin Pathol 1992;97:770–5.

Sinonasal Hemangiopericytoma

10. Battifora H. Hemangiopericytoma: ultrastructural study of five cases. Cancer 1973;31:1418–32.
11. Cantrell RW, Chew JY, Morioka WT. Hemangiopericytoma of the nasopharynx. Trans Am Acad Ophthalmol Otolaryngol 1976;82:551–9.
12. Compagno J. Hemangiopericytoma-like tumors of the nasal cavity: a comparison with hemangiopericytoma of soft tissues. Laryngoscope 1978;88:460–9.
13. Compagno J, Hyams VJ. Hemangiopericytoma-like intranasal tumors. A clinicopathologic study of 23 cases. Am J Clin Pathol 1976;66:672–83.
14. Dardick I, Hammar SP, Scheithauer BW. Ultrastructural spectrum of hemangiopericytoma: a comparative study of fetal, adult, and neoplastic pericytes. Ultrastruct Pathol 1989;13:111–54.
15. Enzinger FM, Smith BH. Hemangiopericytoma. An analysis of 106 cases. Hum Pathol 1976;7:61–82.
16. Fu YS, Perzin KH. Non-epithelial tumors of the nasal cavity, paranasal sinuses and nasopharynx: a clinico-pathologic study. I. General features and vascular tumors. Cancer 1974;33:1275–88.
17. Gorenstein A, Facer GW, Weiland LH. Hemangiopericytoma of the nasal cavity. Otolaryngology 1978;86:405–15.
18. Gudrun R. Haemangiopericytoma in otolarygology. J Laryngol Otol 1979;93:477–94.
19. Huvos AG, Rosen G, Dabska M, Marcove RC. Mesenchymal chondrosarcoma. A clinicopathologic analysis of 35 patients with emphasis on treatment. Cancer 1983;51:1230–7.
20. Kapadia SB, Meis JM, Wenig BM, Frisman DM, Heffner DK. Sinonasal hemangiopericytoma [Abstract]. Mod Pathol 1993;6:81A.
21. McMaster MJ, Soule EH, Ivins JC. Hemangiopericytoma. A clinicopathologic study and long-term followup of 60 patients. Cancer 1975;36:2232–44.
22. Nappi O, Ritter JH, Pettinato G, Wick MR. Hemangiopericytoma: histopathological pattern or clinicopathologic entity? Semin Diagn Pathol 1995;12:221–32.
23. O'Brien P, Brasfield RD. Hemangiopericytoma. Cancer 1965;18:249–52.
24. Perzin KH, Pushparaj N. Nonepithelial tumors of the nasal cavity, paranasal sinuses, and nasopharynx. A clinicopathologic study. XIII: Meningiomas. Cancer 1984;54:1860–9.
25. Porter PL, Bigler SA, McNutt M, Gown AM. The immunophenotype of hemangiopericytomas and glomus tumors, with special reference to muscle protein expression: an immunohistochemical study and review of the literature. Mod Pathol 1991;4:46–52.
26. Potter AJ Jr, Khatib G, Peppard SB. Intranasal glomus tumor. Arch Otolaryngol 1984;110:755–6.
27. Roth JA, Enzinger FM, Tannenbaum M. Synovial sarcoma of the neck: a follow-up study of 24 cases. Cancer 1975;35:1243–53.
28. Scheithauer BW, Rubinstein LJ. Meningeal mesenchymal chondrosarcoma. Report of 8 cases with review of the literature. Cancer 1978;42:2744–52.
29. Schurch W, Skalli O, Lagace R, Seemayer T, Gabbiani G. Intermediate filament proteins and actin isoforms as markers for soft tissue differentiation and origin: III. Hemangiopericytomas and glomus tumors. Am J Pathol 1990;136:771–86.
30. Stout AP. Hemangiopericytoma: a study of twenty-five new cases. Cancer 1949;2:1027–37.
31. Stout AP, Murray MR. Hemangiopericytoma: a vascular tumor featuring Zimmermann's pericytes. Ann Surg 1942;116:26–33.
32. Walike JW, Bailey BJ. Head and neck hemangiopericytoma. Arch Otolaryngol 1971;93:345–53.
33. Winek RR, Scheithauer BW, Wick MR. Meningioma, meningeal hemangiopericytoma and acoustic schwannoma: a comparative immunohistochemical study. Am J Surg Pathol 1989;13:251–61.
34. Witkin GB, Rosai J. Solitary fibrous tumor of the upper respiratory tract. A report of six cases. Am J Surg Pathol 1991;15:842–8.
35. Zukerberg LR, Rosenberg AE, Randolph G, Pilch BZ, Goodman ML. Solitary fibrous tumor of the nasal cavity and paranasal sinuses. Am J Surg Pathol 1991;15:126–30.

Nasopharyngeal Angiofibroma

36. Apostol JV, Frazell EL. Juvenile nasopharyngeal angiofibroma. A clinical study. Cancer 1965;18:869–78.

37. Batsakis JG, Klopp CT, Newman N. Fibrosarcoma arising in a "juvenile" nasopharyngeal angiofibroma following extensive radiation therapy. Am Surg 1955;21:786–93.

38. Beham A, Fletcher CD, Kainz J, Schmid C, Humer U. Nasopharyngeal angiofibroma: an immunohistochemical study of 32 cases. Virchows Arch [A] 1993;423:281–5.

39. Chen KT, Bauer FW. Sarcomatous transformation of nasopharyngeal angiofibroma. Cancer 1982;49:369–71.

40. Dohar JE, Duvall AJ. Spontaneous regression of juvenile nasopharyngeal angiofibroma. Ann Otol Rhinol Laryngol 1992;101:469–71.

41. Fields JN, Halverson KJ, Devineni VR, Simpson JR, Perez CA. Juvenile nasopharyngeal angiofibroma: efficacy of radiation therapy. Radiology 1990;176:263–5.

42. Fu YS, Perzin KH. Non-epithelial tumors of the nasal cavity, paranasal sinuses and nasopharynx: a clinicopathologic study. I. General features and vascular tumors. Cancer 1974;33:1275–88.

43. Gates GA, Rice DH, Koopmann CF Jr, Schuller DE. Flutamide-induced regression of angiofibroma. Laryngoscope 1992;102:641–4.

44. Giardiello FM, Hamilton SR, Krush AJ, Offerhaus JA, Booker SV, Petersen GM. Nasopharyngeal angiofibroma in patients with familial adenomatous polyposis. Gastroenterology 1993;105:1550–2.

45. Gisselsson L, Lindgren M, Stenram U. Sarcomatous transformation of a juvenile, nasopharyngeal angiofibroma. Acta Pathol Microbiol Scand 1958;42:305–12.

46. Goepfert H, Cangir A, Lee YY. Chemotherapy for aggressive juvenile nasopharyngeal angiofibroma. Arch Otolaryngol 1985;111:285–9.

47. Gown AM, Morihara J, Davie P, et al. Androgen receptor expression in angiofibromas of the nasopharynx [Abstract]. Mod Pathol 1993;6:81A.

48. Gudea F, Vega M, Canals E, Montserrat JM, Valdano J. Role of radiation therapy for "juvenile" angiofibroma. J Laryngol Otol 1990;104:725–6.

49. Hormia M, Koskinen O. Metastasizing nasopharyngeal angiofibroma. A case report. Arch Otolaryngol 1969;89:523–6.

50. Hubbard EM. Nasopharyngeal angiofibromas. Arch Otolaryngol 1958;65:192–204.

51. Hyams VJ, Batsakis JG, Michaels L. Lymphoreticular tissue neoplasia. In: Tumors of the upper respiratory tract and ear. Atlas of Tumor Pathology, 2nd Series, Fascicle 25. Washington DC: Armed Forces Institute of Pathology, 1988:207–25.

52. Johns ME, MacLeod RM, Cantrell RW. Estrogen receptors in nasopharyngeal angiofibromas. Laryngoscope 1980;90:628–34.

53. Johnsen S, Kloster JH, Schiff M. The action of hormones on juvenile nasopharyngeal angiofibroma. A case report. Acta Otolaryngol 1966;61:153–60.

54. Kasper ME, Parsons JT, Mancuso AA, et al. Radiation therapy for juvenile angiofibroma: evaluation by CT and MRI, analysis of tumor regression, and selection of patients. Int J Radiat Oncol Biol Phys 1993;25:689–94.

55. McGavran MH, Dorfman RF, Davis DO, Ogura JH. Nasopharyngeal angiofibroma. Arch Otolaryngol 1969;90:68–78.

56. Mills SE, Cooper PH, Fechner RE. Lobular capillary hemangioma: the underlying lesion of pyogenic granuloma. A study of 73 cases from the oral and nasal mucous membranes. Am J Surg Pathol 1980;4:470–9.

57. Neel HB, Whicker JH, Devine KD, Weiland LH. Juvenile angiofibroma. Review of 120 cases. Am J Surg 1973;126:547–56.

58. Sessions RB, Wills PI, Alford BR, Harrell JE, Evans RA. Juvenile nasopharyngeal angiofibroma: radiographic aspects. Laryngoscope 1976;86:2–18.

59. Siniluoto TM, Luotonen JP, Tikkakoski TA, Leinonen AS, Jokinen KE. Value of pre-operative embolization in surgery for nasopharyngeal angiofibroma. J Laryngol Otol 1993;107:514–21.

60. Spagnolo DV, Papadimitriou JM, Archer M. Postirradiation malignant fibrous histiocytoma arising in juvenile nasopharyngeal angiofibroma and producing alpha-1-antitrypsin. Histopathology 1984;8:339–52.

61. Sternberg SS. Pathology of juvenile nasopharyngeal angiofibroma–a lesion of adolescent males. Cancer 1954;7:15–28.

62. Svoboda DJ, Kirchner F. Ultrastructure of nasopharyngeal angiofibromas. Cancer 1966;19:1949–62.

63. Taxy JB. Juvenile nasopharyngeal angiofibroma. An ultrastructural study. Cancer 1977;39:1044–54.

64. Topilko A, Zakrzewski A, Pichard E, Viron A. Ultrastructural cytochemistry of intranuclear dense granules in nasopharyngeal angiofibroma. Ultrastruct Pathol 1985;6:221–8.

65. Weprin LS, Siemers PT. Spontaneous regression of juvenile nasopharyngeal angiofibroma. Arch Otolaryngol Head Neck Surg 1991;117:796–9.

66. Zukerberg LR, Rosenberg AE, Randolph G, Pilch BZ, Goodman ML. Solitary fibrous tumor of the nasal cavity and paranasal sinuses. Am J Surg Pathol 1991;15:126–30.

Glomus Tumor

67. Dervan PA, Tobbia IN, Casey M, O'Loughlin J, O'Brien M. Glomus tumors: an immunohistochemical profile of 11 cases. Histopathology 1989;14:483–91.

68. di Sant'Agnese PA, de Mesy Jensen KL. Thick (myosin) filaments in a glomus tumor. Am J Clin Pathol 1983;79:130–4.

69. Fu YS, Perzin KH. Non-epithelial tumors of the nasal cavity, paranasal sinuses and nasopharynx: a clinicopathologic study. I. General features and vascular tumors. Cancer 1974;33:1275–88.

70. Potter AJ Jr, Khatib G, Peppard SB. Intranasal glomus tumor. Arch Otolaryngol 1984;110:755–6.

71. Tajima Y, Weathers DR, Neville BW, Benoit PW, Pedley DM. Glomus tumor (glomangioma) of the tongue. A light and electron microscopic study. Oral Surg 1981;52:288–93.

72. Tsuneyoshi M, Enjoji M. Glomus tumor: a clinicopathologic and electron microscopic study. Cancer 1982;50:1601–7.

Laryngeal Hemangioma

73. Bridger GP, Nassar VH, Skinner HG. Hemangioma of the adult larynx. Arch Otolaryngol 1970;92:493–8.

74. Calcaterra TC. An evaluation of the treatment of subglottic hemangioma. Laryngoscope 1968;78:1956–64.

75. Cooper M, Slovis TL, Madgy DN, Levitsky D. Congenital subglottic hemangioma: frequency of symmetrical subglottic narrowing on frontal radiographs of the neck. AJR Am J Roentgenol 1992;159:1269–71.

76. Ferguson CF, Flake CG. Subglottic hemangioma as a cause of respiratory obstruction in infants. Ann Otol Rhinol Laryngol 1961;70:1095–112.

77. Ferguson GB. Hemangioma of the adult and of the infant larynx: a review of the literature and a report of two cases. Arch Otolaryngol 1944;40:189–95.

78. Seikaly H, Cuyler JP. Infantile subglottic hemangioma. J Otolaryngol 1994;23:135–7.

Polypoid Granulation Tissue

79. Barton RT. Observation on the pathogenesis of laryngeal granuloma due to endotracheal anesthesia. N Engl J Med 1953;248:1097–9.

80. Fechner RE, Cooper PH, Mills SE. Pyogenic granuloma of the larynx and trachea. A causal and pathologic misnomer for granulation tissue. Arch Otolaryngol 1980;107:30–2.

Lymphangioma (Cystic Hygroma)

81. Coffin CM, Dehner LP. Vascular tumors in children and adolescents: a clinicopathologic study of 228 tumors in 222 patients. Pathol Annu 1993;28:97–120.

82. Emery PJ, Bailey CM, Evans JN. Cystic hygroma of the head and neck: a review of 37 cases. J Laryngol Otol 1984;98:613–9

Kaposi's Sarcoma

83. Abramson AL, Simons RL. Kaposi's sarcoma of the head and neck. Arch Otolaryngol 1970;92:505–8.

84. Barzan L, Tavio M, Tirelli U, Comoretto R. Head and neck manifestations during HIV infection. J Laryngol Otol 1993;107:133–6.

85. Goldberg AN. Kaposi's sarcoma of the head and neck in acquired immunodeficiency syndrome. Am J Otolaryngol 1993;14:5–14.

86. Thomsen HK, Jacobsen M, Malchow-Moller A. Kaposi sarcoma among homosexual men in Europe [Letter]. Lancet 1981;2:688.

Angiosarcoma

87. Bankaci M, Myers EN, Barnes L, DuBois P. Angiosarcoma of the maxillary sinus: literature review and case report. Head Neck Surg 1979;1:274–80.

88. Corio RL, Brannon RB, Tarpley TM. Intravascular papillary endothelial hyperplasia of the head and neck. Ear Nose Throat J 1982;61:50–4.

89. De Young BR, Wick MR, Fitzgibbon JF, Sirgi KE, Swanson PE. CD31. An immunospecific marker for endothelial differentiation in human neoplasms. Appl Immunohistochem 1993;1:97–100.

90. Huerter CJ, Kunkel JR, Rouse JR. Angiosarcoma of the face and scalp. Cutis 1993;51:461–2.

91. Mark RJ, Tran LM, Sercarz J, Fu YS, Calcaterra TC, Juillard GF. Angiosarcoma of the head and neck. The UCLA experience 1955 through 1990. Arch Otolaryngol Head Neck Surg 1993;119:973–8.

92. Morrison WH, Byers RM, Garden AS, Evans HL, Ang KK, Peters LJ. Cutaneous angiosarcoma of the head and neck. A therapeutic dilemma. Cancer 1995;76:319–27.

93. Ordóñez NG, Batsakis JG. Comparison of Ulex europeaus I lectin and factor VIII-related antigen in vascular lesions. Arch Pathol Lab Med 1984;108:129–32.

94. Pratt LW, Goodof II. Hemangioendotheliosarcoma of the larynx. Arch Otolaryngol 1968;87:484–9.

95. Sciot R, Delaere P, Van Damme B, Desmet V. Angiosarcoma of the larynx. Histopathology 1995;26:177–80.

96. Stern Y, Braslavsky D, Segal K, Shpitzer T, Abraham A. Intravascular papillary endothelial hyperplasia in the maxillary sinus. A benign lesion that may be mistaken for angiosarcoma. Arch Otolaryngol Head Neck Surg 1991;117:1182–4.

97. Stern Y, Braslavsky D, Shpitzer T, Feinmesser R. Papillary endothelial hyperplasia in the tongue: a benign lesion that may be mistaken for angiosarcoma. J Otolaryngol 1994;23:81–3.

98. Traweek ST, Kandalaft PL, Mehta P, Battifora H. The human hematopoietic progenitor cell antigen (CD34) in vascular neoplasia. Am J Clin Pathol 1991;96:25–31.

99. Wenig BM, Abbondanzo SL, Heffess CS. Epithelioid angiosarcoma of the adrenal glands. A clinicopathologic study of nine cases with a discussion of the implications of finding "epithelial-specific" markers. Am J Surg Pathol 1994;18:62–73.

Bacillary Angiomatosis

100. Adal KA, Cockerell CJ, Petri WA Jr. Cat scratch disease, bacillary angiomatosis, and other infections due to Rochalimaea. N Engl J Med 1994;330:1509–15.

101. LeBoit PE, Berger TG, Egbert BM, Beckstead JH, Yen TS, Stoler MH. Bacillary angiomatosis. The histopathology and differential diagnosis of a pseudoneoplastic infection in patients with human immunodeficiency virus disease. Am J Surg Pathol 1989;13:909–20.

102. Stoler MH, Bonfiglio TA, Steigbigel RT, Pereira M. An atypical subcutaneous infection associated with acquired immune deficiency syndrome. Am J Clin Pathol 1983; 80:714–8.

10

FIBROUS TUMORS OF THE UPPER AERODIGESTIVE TRACT

NASAL FIBROMA

The diagnosis of "fibroma" should be approached with caution at most anatomic sites, and the head and neck area is no exception. Many lesions labeled as fibroma would be better interpreted as other reactive or neoplastic fibroblastic proliferations, including nodular fasciitis and aggressive fibromatosis. However, there are occasional lesions in the head and neck region, particularly in the nasal cavity, for which this term, or a variant such as *fibrous polyp,* seems warranted (1).

In their large review of nonepithelial tumors of the sinonasal region, Fu and Perzin (1) identified four fibromas. These were small, smooth surfaced, well-demarcated, polypoid nodules invariably measuring less than 1 cm in size (fig. 10-1). One was located on the posterior portion of the nasal vestibule, one was from the floor of the nasal cavity, and two were from the nasal septum. Each was an incidental finding. We have encountered several additional examples, also from the nasal cavity.

Microscopically, fibromas are composed of mature, heavily collagenized fibrous tissue, containing haphazardly oriented, mature spindle cells.

The spindle cells may show some nuclear enlargement and cytologic atypia, analogous to that seen in fibrous polypoid lesions from other anatomic sites, such as the skin (fig. 10-2). There is no evidence of infiltration at the periphery of the lesion, and local recurrences have not been documented (1). Fu and Perzin speculated that these fibromas may be the end stage of a prior polypoid lesion. We agree. It seems likely that preexistent inflammatory polyps or, perhaps, lobular capillary hemangiomas may involute over time, leaving a so-called fibroma or fibrous polyp.

SOLITARY FIBROUS TUMOR

Definition. This is a benign, variably cellular, fibroblastic proliferation affecting primarily the nose and paranasal sinuses. The light microscopic and immunohistochemical features are identical to those of solitary fibrous tumor of the pleura.

Clinical Features. Solitary fibrous tumors of the head and neck region occur in adults and, rarely, adolescents (6), with no predilection for men or women (8,9). The nasal cavity and paranasal sinuses are the most common anatomic sites. All patients with nasal lesions present with nasal obstruction or congestion. Symptoms have

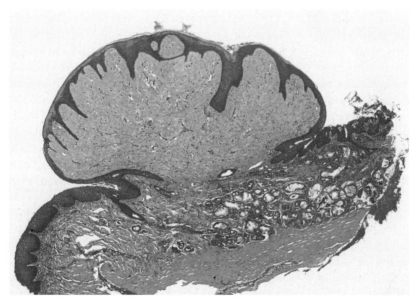

Figure 10-1
NASAL FIBROMA
Nasal "fibromas" or "fibrous polyps" typically consist of small, exophytic fibrous nodules covered by squamous epithelium, without invasion of the underlying nasal tissues.

273

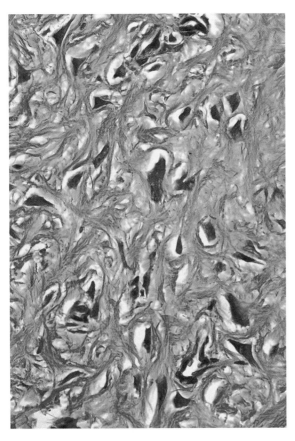

Figure 10-2
NASAL FIBROMA
The stroma of nasal "fibroma" is densely collagenized and may contain enlarged, slightly atypical stromal cells analogous to those seen in fibrous polyps or papules from other anatomic sites such as the skin.

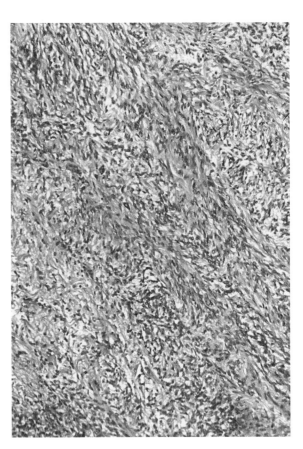

Figure 10-3
SOLITARY FIBROUS TUMOR
Solitary fibrous tumor is a cellular, partially collagenized spindle cell proliferation.

often been present for more than a year, and may have been noted for more than a decade. Physical examination demonstrates a polypoid mass which may cause perforation of the nasal septum or distortion of surrounding structures, without invasion of bone. Additional cases have been described in the parotid gland (5), sublingual gland (4), thyroid gland (2), orbit (3), parapharyngeal space (6), and epiglottis (6).

Gross Findings. Solitary fibrous tumors of the nasal cavity and sinuses are gray-white, polypoid fibrous masses measuring 3 to 7 cm in greatest dimension. Areas of hemorrhage and necrosis are not seen.

Microscopic Findings. The prototypical light microscopic feature is a haphazard proliferation of small spindled cells with scant or unapparent cytoplasm in a background of colla-

gen fibers (fig. 10-3) (8). Cellularity is often variable, with hypercellular sparsely collagenized areas in close approximation to densely collagenized, hypocellular regions. Nuclei are regular in size and shape. Mitotic figures are typically uncommon, and necrosis, mucosal ulceration, and invasion of surrounding structures are not seen (fig. 10-4) (9). Blood vessels may be focally prominent and often have thickened walls. In areas, the vascularity is reminiscent of an hemangiopericytoma, but the diffuse hypervascularity and "staghorn" vessels of the latter lesion are not uniformly present (8,9).

Immunohistochemical Findings. Solitary fibrous tumors are immunoreactive for vimentin and unreactive or weakly focally reactive for most other antigens, including S-100 protein, desmin, actin, factor VIII–related antigen, and neurofilament (4,8,9). Larger studies of solitary

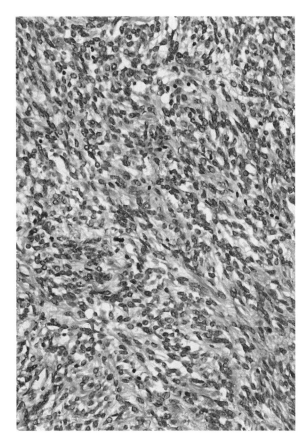

Figure 10-4
SOLITARY FIBROUS TUMOR
The high cellularity of solitary fibrous tumor may lead to initial concern regarding malignancy. Occasional mitotic figures may be present but the spindled cells show remarkable nuclear uniformity.

fibrous tumors from a wide variety of anatomic sites have shown uniform, strong positivity for CD34 (5,7). This may be helpful in differential diagnosis since neurofibromas, schwannomas, fibrosarcomas, and hemangiopericytomas have absent, focal, or weak staining for CD34 (7).

Differential Diagnosis. In our experience, hemangiopericytoma is most commonly confused with solitary fibrous tumor. Although solitary fibrous tumor may have a hemangiopericytoma-like appearance focally, it lacks this change as a diffuse feature. Conversely, hemangiopericytomas lack the prominent stromal collagenization of solitary fibrous tumor. Solitary fibrous tumors are also mistaken for neurofibromas, but they lack the S-100 protein positivity and other histologic features typical of the latter tumors (8). Distinction from angiofibroma is sel-

dom problematic; angiofibroma invariably involves the nasopharynx, always occurs in males, and usually occurs in adolescents. They are much less cellular than the more cellular regions of solitary fibrous tumor, and have distinctive small to medium-sized, thin-walled vascular spaces uniformly distributed in their haphazardly collagenized stroma.

Treatment and Prognosis. Polypoid solitary fibrous tumors involving the nasal cavity and paranasal sinuses are relatively easily resected. If they are completely removed, they do not appear to recur (8,9). Partially resected tumors at more problematic anatomic sites such as the nasopharynx or periorbital region have been noted to persist for years without associated mortality (8).

AGGRESSIVE FIBROMATOSIS

Definition. Aggressive fibromatosis is a locally infiltrative, frequently recurrent, nonmetastasizing and noninflammatory proliferation of mature fibrous tissue arising in the deep soft tissues. Histologically identical intraosseous lesions are referred to as desmoplastic fibromas. Single lesions are most common, but multifocal and diffuse disease has also been documented. Aggressive fibromatosis is one of the two major forms of so-called adult fibromatosis. It is more infiltrative, more locally destructive, and more deeply located than the other adult variant, Dupuytren's type fibromatosis (10,11). The terms *extra-abdominal desmoid tumor* and *extra-abdominal fibromatosis* are commonly used synonyms for aggressive fibromatosis not involving the abdominal wall. In the past, these lesions were also referred to as *well-differentiated fibrosarcoma, fibrosarcoma grade I,* or *nonmetastasizing fibromatosis.* These terms should be avoided, given the accepted nonmetastasizing nature of this proliferation.

General Features. A wide variety of fibroblastic proliferations occurs in the head and neck region. Many of these are apparently reactive fibroinflammatory processes that have been referred to by terms such as tumefactive fibroinflammatory lesion, inflammatory fibrous pseudotumor, and plasma cell granuloma. The presence of a prominent inflammatory component distinguishes such lesions from aggressive fibromatosis. Whether aggressive fibromatosis is a neoplasm or a reactive-type process seems to have been convincingly answered. The demonstration of multiple clonal genetic abnormalities, including an absence of the Y chromosome and a deletion from the "q" region of chromosome 5, argue convincingly that these are true neoplasms (13,21).

Clinical Features. From 12 to 22 percent of aggressive fibromatoses involve the head and neck region (16,24). In a review of 367 cases from the Armed Forces Institute of Pathology (AFIP) involving extra-abdominal sites, Enzinger and Weiss (16) noted that 35 examples involved the head and neck region, with 81 occurring in the shoulder. Of six cases from the sinonasal region reviewed by Fu and Perzin (18), the lesions tended to involve the nasal turbinates and maxillary antrum (fig. 10-5). Paraoral involvement favors the paramandibular soft tissues, tongue, and parotid region (12,17,29). Involvement of the oral soft tissues, including the lip, alveolar ridge, and floor of mouth, as well as the upper airway, is uncommon (12,17).

The primary clinical features of aggressive fibromatosis arising in the head and neck region are identical to those of analogous tumors arising at other extra-abdominal sites. The usual presenting complaints relate to a deeply seated mass with little or no associated pain. In the head and neck, specific complaints typically include nasal stuffiness, obstruction, or mass (18).

Aggressive fibromatosis is seen in about 10 percent of patients with Gardner's syndrome, and more recently it also has been associated with hereditary nonpolyposis colon cancer syndrome (20,23). In this setting the tumors almost invariably involve the mesentery, retroperitoneum, or abdominal wall. Unlike their counterparts involving the abdominal wall, which show a striking tendency to arise in women of child-bearing age, extra-abdominal aggressive fibromatoses show a less clear-cut sex predilection. Some studies have suggested a preponderance of female patients (12,24) and others have shown an equal sex distribution (14,26), or even a male predominance (17,30). The extra-abdominal tumors occur at any age, but they are less common in children or the elderly. Most patients are in their fourth or fifth decade of life.

Gross Findings. Tumor size is highly variable. On cut section these are uniform, firm, scar-like fibrous masses. Portions of the lesion

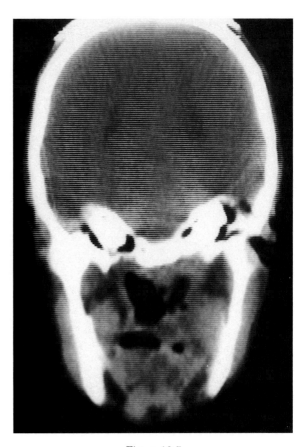

Figure 10-5
AGGRESSIVE FIBROMATOSIS
Aggressive fibromatosis involving the posterior lateral portion of the nasopharynx distorts the palate and extends into the masseter muscle.

may be sharply demarcated and some have a clearly invasive appearance. Areas of spontaneous hemorrhage or necrosis are not seen.

Microscopic Findings. There is a variably cellular proliferation of uniform spindle cells in a heavily collagenized stroma (fig. 10-6). The spindle cells are often oriented in broad, sweeping fascicles that intersect at varying angles. "Herring-bone" patterns typical of fibrosarcoma are not seen, but fascicles may occasionally intersect to form a storiform pattern. Any inflammatory component is always minor and consists, at most, of scattered collections of lymphocytes. The poorly circumscribed, infiltrative nature of the lesion is always discernable microscopically, even if not apparent grossly (fig. 10-7). Cell borders are difficult or impossible to delineate. Nuclei are small and uniform with occasional small

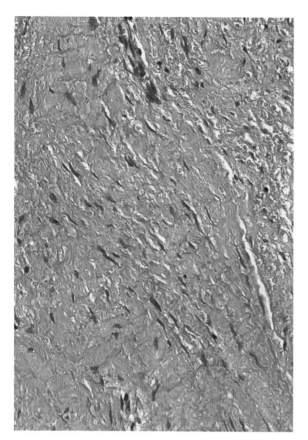

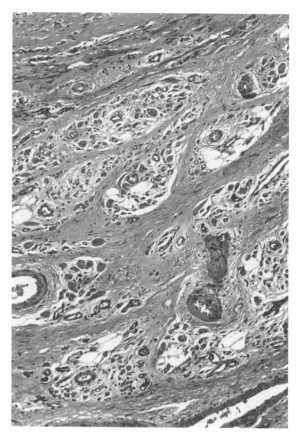

Figure 10-6
AGGRESSIVE FIBROMATOSIS

Aggressive fibromatosis is a hypocellular, densely collagenized lesion. Hyperchromatic, bipolar nuclei are widely separated by the collagenized stroma.

Figure 10-7
AGGRESSIVE FIBROMATOSIS

The infiltrative nature of aggressive fibromatosis is best seen at the periphery of the lesion. Here, strands of fibrous tissue surround bundles of partially atrophic skeletal (masseter) muscle.

nucleoli. Once other diagnostic entities have been excluded, grading aggressive fibromatosis with respect to cellularity, pleomorphism, or mitotic activity does not seem to correlate with clinical behavior (17).

Immunohistochemical Findings. As with most fibroblastic proliferations, the cells of aggressive fibromatosis often display focal myogenous differentiation in the form of localized reactivity for muscle-specific actin and smooth muscle actin. Immunoreactivity for desmin is less common, but may occur. As would be expected, there is typically strong reactivity for vimentin. Because of its infiltrative growth pattern, aggressive fibromatosis often entraps a variety of normal structures including smooth muscle, skeletal muscle, and peripheral nerve (fig. 10-7). Atrophic or regenerative changes may

alter the light microscopic appearance of these normal elements, although they retain their normal immunohistochemical reactivity. This can lead to potentially confusing "pockets" of immunoreactivity within aggressive fibromatosis.

Ultrastructural Findings. Aggressive fibromatosis is composed of uniform, spindled mesenchymal cells with abundant stromal collagen. The neoplastic cells often have convoluted nuclei with numerous infoldings. In addition to scattered mitochondria, Golgi complexes, and pinocytotic vesicles, the cytoplasm displays prominent rough endoplasmic reticulum with variably prominent aggregates of actin-type filaments. These filaments may be associated with membranous "dense bodies" (19,20). Thus, aggressive fibromatosis usually shows at least focal evidence of myofibroblastic differentiation, in

277

agreement with the immunohistochemical findings described above.

Differential Diagnosis. Aggressive fibromatosis lacks the cellularity, high mitotic rate, and focally distinctive "herring-bone" orientation of cell fascicles typical of fibrosarcoma. Distinction of aggressive fibromatosis from the heterogeneous group of "fibroinflammatory lesions" is based on the absence of prominent inflammation in the former tumors. Aggressive fibromatosis is histologically identical to desmoplastic fibroma of bone and this nomenclatural distinction is based solely on the epicenter of the lesion. As aggressive fibromatoses can erode and "saucerize" adjacent bones, this distinction may not always be straightforward. Aggressive fibromatosis lacks the distinctive clinical features, haphazard collagen deposition, stellate spindle cells, and characteristic vascularity of nasopharyngeal angiofibroma (see chapter 9). Central regions of angiofibroma may lack the prominent vascularity typical of the remainder of the lesion, and such areas, taken out of context, are histologically similar to aggressive fibromatosis. Unlike deep-seated aggressive fibromatosis, keloid is a proliferation of dermal collagen, with a characteristic gross appearance.

Treatment and Prognosis. Optimal treatment for aggressive fibromatosis is wide surgical resection. Unfortunately, this is often not an option in the head and neck region. Accordingly, the behavior in this location is more aggressive than in areas of easy resectability. The overall recurrence rate for all extra-abdominal locations is approximately 50 percent (29); in the head and neck, recurrence rates approach 60 to 70 percent (12), excluding oral and paraoral lesions which are more amenable to surgery and have a recurrence rate of approximately 25 percent (17). Because the mortality associated with these lesions is relatively low, radical, physically mutilating surgical procedures should be reserved for recurrent lesions that have failed lesser resections and radiation therapy (16). Incompletely excised and recurrent tumors benefit from radiation therapy, and radiation therapy as the primary treatment modality may yield acceptable responses, with local control rates of 75 to 83 percent (25,27). The role of antiestrogen and progesterone-like hormone chemotherapy remains to be fully understood. Partial or complete responses to proges-

terone have been documented in some studies (22), and not confirmed in others (15). Spontaneous regression is rare and tends to occur in children and individuals with multiple lesions (18). Adequately documented spontaneous conversion of aggressive fibromatosis not previously treated with radiation therapy to fibrosarcoma has not been reported (12).

FIBROSARCOMA

Definition. Fibrosarcoma is a malignant mesenchymal neoplasm composed of spindle cells, often growing in fascicles, and associated with variably prominent collagen deposition. By definition, other forms of differentiation are lacking, at least at the light microscopic level.

Clinical Features. In Fu and Perzin's (31) series of 13 sinonasal fibrosarcomas, there were 8 male and 5 female patients ranging in age from 10 to 77 years. Presenting complaints were typically related to a nasal mass: obstruction or epistaxis, nasal discharge, pain or swelling in the facial region, or sensory changes involving the regional nerves. Radiographic studies typically documented a nasal or paranasal sinus mass with some associated bone erosion. Several fibrosarcomas of the head and neck region have been reported to arise as long-term complications of radiation therapy (33,35).

Gross Findings. These may be sessile or polypoid, often grossly invasive masses. The cut surface is frequently tan, fibrous, and homogeneous, not unlike the appearance of aggressive fibromatosis. High-grade fibrosarcomas may be associated with areas of grossly obvious hemorrhage or necrosis.

Microscopic Findings. Unlike the fibromatoses, fibrosarcomas are highly cellular proliferations. The spindle cells are often oriented in well-formed fascicles that frequently intersect at approximately 90 degree angles, creating a "herringbone" pattern. Nuclear pleomorphism is usually not striking, but mitotic figures are often abundant, even in well-differentiated forms of the tumor. In the head and neck region, most fibrosarcomas are well-differentiated, low-grade neoplasms (see below). Regardless of the grade of the neoplasm, multinucleated giant cells or overtly bizarre cells are not a typical feature. Fibrosarcoma-like images may be encountered in a wide variety of neoplasms including synovial sarcoma, sarcomatoid carcinoma, mesenchymal chondrosarcoma, desmoplastic melanoma, malignant schwannoma, leiomyosarcoma, spindle cell rhabdomyosarcoma, and hemangiopericytoma. Therefore, the diagnosis is in large part exclusionary. Because of the closely adjacent bony structures in the sinonasal region, fibrosarcomas in this area often abut or erode adjacent bone, and biopsy or resection specimens may contain fragments of reactive bone (31). This should not lead to an erroneous diagnosis of fibroblastic osteosarcoma. In other instances the tumor may form a polypoid, exophytic mass entrapping seromucinous glands (fig. 10-8).

Microscopic Grading. Well-differentiated or low-grade fibrosarcomas are composed of very uniform spindle cells with fascicles oriented to produce obvious herringbone arrays. The amount of background collagen varies, but it may be focally prominent. Poorly differentiated or high-grade fibrosarcomas exhibit more striking nuclear pleomorphism, but overtly bizarre or giant neoplastic cells should suggest a malignant fibrous histiocytoma. The mitotic rate is quite brisk and abnormal forms may be identified. The well-oriented fascicles of spindle cells are less distinct in high-grade fibrosarcomas, and areas of hemorrhage and necrosis may be present.

Immunohistochemical Findings. The immunohistochemical reactivity of fibrosarcoma does not differ from that of aggressive fibromatosis. The neoplastic cells are often strongly reactive for vimentin and weakly reactive for actin. Negativity for epithelial markers (cytokeratin, epithelial membrane antigen) and S-100 protein is helpful in excluding differential diagnostic considerations.

Ultrastructural Findings. As with the immunohistochemical findings, the electron microscopic features of fibrosarcoma are similar to those noted for aggressive fibromatosis. In particular, the neoplastic cells may show evidence of myofibroblastic differentiation in the form of bundles of actin-type filaments and membranous "dense bodies."

Differential Diagnosis. The distinction of fibrosarcoma from aggressive fibromatosis is based on the markedly increased cellularity, mitotic activity, and well-formed fascicular or herringbone growth pattern of the former. In our

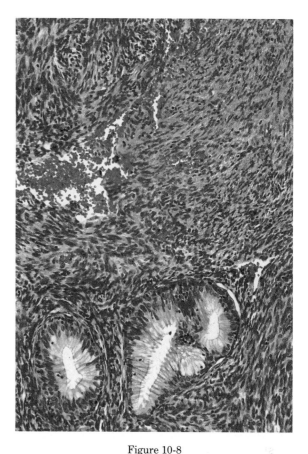

Figure 10-8
NASAL FIBROSARCOMA
Low-grade nasal fibrosarcoma consists of interlacing fascicles of spindle cells infiltrating around seromucinous glands.

experience, although aggressive fibromatoses may show a spectrum of cellularity, they invariably fall short, by a considerable margin, of the highly cellular appearance encountered in even well-differentiated fibrosarcoma. As noted above, the diagnosis of fibrosarcoma is in large part exclusionary. A large number of malignancies may have a spindle cell growth pattern. Fortunately, many of these neoplasms lack the cellular uniformity and well-formed fascicular growth pattern of fibrosarcoma. Distinction from a malignant peripheral nerve sheath tumor may be difficult on purely light microscopic grounds. A palisading growth pattern, myxoid stroma, and tendency to cuff blood vessels are features more typical of peripheral nerve sheath tumors. About half of the latter neoplasms are reactive for S-100 protein, whereas fibrosarcomas are uniformly negative with this marker. Lack of

S-100 protein or HMB-45 reactivity helps exclude desmoplastic malignant melanoma from diagnostic consideration. Monophasic synovial sarcomas often contain fibrosarcoma-like areas, but typically exhibit at least focal staining for cytokeratin or epithelial membrane antigen. Sarcomatoid carcinomas may also express epithelial markers, but usually exhibit considerably more pleomorphism than is typical of fibrosarcoma or synovial sarcoma.

Treatment and Prognosis. Surgical resection, with or without adjuvant therapy, is the treatment mainstay for these neoplasms. The most common indications for adjuvant radiation therapy are positive or suspicious surgical margins and high tumor grade. Failure to control disease locally is more problematic than distant metastases. In one series of sinonasal sarcomas, including 16 fibrosarcomas, the incidence of local and distant treatment failure was 76 percent and 12 percent, respectively (32). Regional lymph node metastases from fibrosarcomas are uncommon.

In a review of 29 patients with fibrosarcoma of the head and neck region the absolute 5-year survival after a 66-month follow-up was 62 percent (34); 80 percent of patients with low-grade lesions were ultimately rendered free of disease, whereas this was only true for 8 percent of patients with high-grade disease. The authors concluded that tumor grade was the most important prognostic feature for fibrosarcoma of the head and neck. Tumor size and the status of the surgical margins were additional prognostic factors.

INFLAMMATORY MYOFIBROBLASTIC (PSEUDO) TUMOR

Definition. This heterogeneous group of myofibroblastic proliferations has an associated prominent inflammatory component and may occur at virtually any anatomic site. Most lesions encompassed in this terminology are benign reactive proliferations, but occasional examples may represent benign or aggressive neoplasms. Terms generally considered synonymous with inflammatory myofibroblastic tumor include: *inflammatory pseudotumor, plasma cell granuloma,* and *pseudosarcomatous myofibroblastic lesion* (37). These lesions are generally considered distinct from so-called postoperative spindle cell nodules, inflammatory pseudotumor of lymph nodes, and

sclerotic fibroinflammatory lesions such as Reidel's thyroiditis, sclerosing mediastinitis, and retroperitoneal fibrosis. It seems likely that reported examples of inflammatory myofibroblastic tumor behaving in a malignant fashion are examples of inflammatory fibrosarcoma or malignant fibrous histiocytoma.

General Features. Although some apparently malignant forms of inflammatory myofibroblastic tumor have been reported, whether this lesion or group of lesions is a reactive process or a neoplasm remains to be fully clarified. Some tumors in this group appear to develop as a response to infection, particularly to *Mycobacterium avium intracellulare,* often in human immunodeficiency virus (HIV)-positive or other immunosuppressed patients (37). Others may be related to trauma or ongoing inflammation. Some examples of inflammatory myofibroblastic tumor, particularly those involving the liver and spleen, are clonal proliferations of the follicular dendritic cells associated with Epstein-Barr virus (36). It is likely that further study will subdivide these lesions into more distinct clinicopathologic entities.

Clinical Features. Patients have ranged in age from newborns to the elderly (38,41). There is no apparent sex predilection. In one review of 84 extrapulmonary lesions, 12 occurred in the head and neck region (38). Of these, 1 involved the skin of the face, 1 involved the meninges, and 1 arose in the orbit; the remaining 9 head and neck cases involved the larynx (3 patients), trachea (2 patients), nasopharynx (2 patients), and oropharynx (2 patients). Wenig et al. (41) reported a separate series of eight laryngeal cases: six arose from the vocal cords, one from the pyriform sinus, and one from the subglottic region. In addition to localized symptoms relating to a mass, patients may have more generalized complaints of fever, malaise, and weight loss; anemia and hypergammaglobulinemia also may be present (38). The laryngeal lesions, as would be expected, were associated with hoarseness and stridor. Of eight patients with laryngeal involvement, seven had no history of prior trauma, and one had been intubated 3 months previously. Additional cases have been described involving the oral cavity, cheek, maxilla, and mandible (39,40).

Gross Findings. The tumors are polypoid or pedunculated, fleshy to firm nodular masses (41).

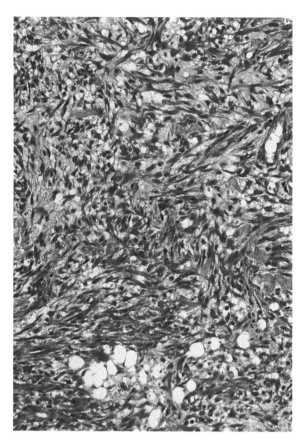

Figure 10-9
INFLAMMATORY MYOFIBROBLASTIC TUMOR
This inflammatory myofibroblastic tumor consists of haphazardly arranged spindled cells in a loose, inflamed stroma.

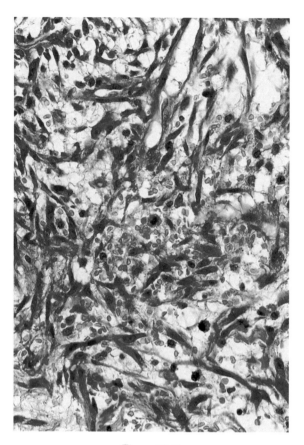

Figure 10-10
INFLAMMATORY MYOFIBROBLASTIC TUMOR
At higher magnification, extravasated erythrocytes are easily appreciated between the widely separated spindled cells.

Myxoid change, hemorrhage, necrosis, or focal calcification may also be present (38). Not surprisingly, the vocal cord lesions were usually 1.5 cm or less in size, although somewhat larger lesions have been described (41).

Microscopic Findings. Coffin et al. (38) described three microscopic patterns seen in inflammatory myofibroblastic tumor. The first pattern consists of loose, stellate to plump, spindle cells, haphazardly oriented in a myxoid background with numerous irregular small blood vessels and inflammatory cells (fig. 10-9). Extravasated erythrocytes may be present within the myxoid stroma (fig. 10-10). This pattern has been likened to granulation tissue and nodular fasciitis. The proliferating stromal cells in this pattern have enlarged vesicular nuclei, often with prominent nucleoli, and have prominent eosinophilic to amphophilic cytoplasm. Mitotic figures may be abundant, but in our experience and that of others, atypical forms are not present (38).

In the second pattern, there is a more compact proliferation of spindle cells with less intervening stroma (fig. 10-11). The proliferating cells may be oriented in well-formed, intersecting fascicles. Nuclear pleomorphism is minimal, but mitotic activity is highly variable. Atypical mitotic figures are not seen. A prominent inflammatory infiltrate insinuates between the fascicles of the spindle cells. Plasma cells typically predominate, but aggregates of lymphocytes may also be present. Without the inflammatory component, this pattern may easily be mistaken for a neoplasm.

The third pattern is characterized by large zones of hypocellular, scar-like collagen which entrap the proliferating spindle cells, as well as

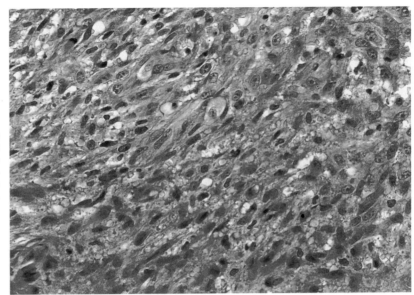

Figure 10-11
INFLAMMATORY
MYOFIBROBLASTIC TUMOR
Other microscopic foci from the lesion seen in figures 10-9 and 10-10 were more cellular with correspondingly less intervening stroma and inflammation. Extravasated erythrocytes are still plentiful in these areas.

an obvious inflammatory cell component. Zones of punctate or dystrophic calcification may be present within the sclerotic collagen. It has been suggested that these three stages, which may be present focally in a single specimen, represent stages in the chronologic progression of inflammatory myofibroblastic tumor.

Immunohistochemical Findings. The spindle cells of inflammatory myofibroblastic tumors show strong cytoplasmic reactivity for vimentin, with focal to diffuse immunoreactivity for smooth muscle actin and muscle-specific actin seen in about 90 percent of cases (38). About two thirds show focal immunoreactivity for desmin. Interestingly, in one study, 36 percent of the lesions were at least focally immunoreactive for cytokeratin (38).

Differential Diagnosis. The cellular form of inflammatory myofibroblastic tumor may be mistaken for fibrosarcoma or other spindle cell malignancies. Recognition of the prominent inflammatory component and the lack of significant cytologic atypia are helpful diagnostic features. The less cellular, more sclerotic form may be mistaken for aggressive fibromatosis. Again, the prominent inflammatory component is the critical distinguishing feature.

Treatment and Prognosis. Surgical excision is the usual therapy. Most laryngeal tumors have been treated by laryngoscopic excision or laser ablation (41). In the study by Wenig et al. (41), only one of eight patients with a laryngeal lesion treated by complete resection or ablation developed a recurrence.

REFERENCES

Nasal Fibroma

1. Fu YS, Perzin KH. Nonepithelial tumors of the nasal cavity, paranasal sinuses and nasopharynx: a clinicopathologic study. IV. Fibrous tissue tumors (fibroma, fibromatosis, fibrosarcoma). Cancer 1976;37:2912–28.

Solitary Fibrous Tumor

2. Cameselle-Teijeiro J, Varela-Duran J, Fonseca E, Villanueva JP, Sobrinho-Simoes M. Solitary fibrous tumor of the thyroid. Am J Clin Pathol 1994;101:535–8.
3. Dorfman DM, To K, Dickersin GR, Rosenberg AE, Pilch BZ. Solitary fibrous tumor of the orbit. Am J Surg Pathol 1994;18:281–7.
4. Gunhan O, Yildiz FR, Celasun B, Onder T, Finci R. Solitary fibrous tumour arising from sublingual gland: report of a case. J Laryngol Otol 1994;108:998–1000.
5. Hanau CA, Miettinen M. Solitary fibrous tumor: histological and immunohistochemical spectrum of benign and malignant variants presenting at different sites. Hum Pathol 1995;26:440–9.
6. Safneck JR, Alguacil-Garcia A, Dort JC, Phillips SM. Solitary fibrous tumour: report of two new locations in the upper respiratory tract. J Laryngol Otol 1993;107:252–6.
7. Westra WH, Gerald WL, Rosai J. Solitary fibrous tumor. Consistent CD34 immunoreactivity and occurrence in the orbit. Am J Surg Pathol 1994;18:992–8.
8. Witkin GB, Rosai J. Solitary fibrous tumor of the upper respiratory tract. A report of six cases. Am J Surg Pathol 1991;15:842–8.
9. Zukerberg LR, Rosenberg AE, Randolph G, Pilch BZ, Goodman ML. Solitary fibrous tumor of the nasal cavity and paranasal sinuses. Am J Surg Pathol 1991;15:126–30.

Aggressive Fibromatosis

10. Allen PW. The fibromatoses: a clinicopathologic classification based on 140 cases. Part 1. Am J Surg Pathol 1977;1:255–70.
11. Allen PW. The fibromatoses: a clinicopathologic classification based on 140 cases. Part 2. Am J Surg Pathol 1977;1:305–21.
12. Batsakis JG, Raslan W. Extra-abdominal desmoid fibromatosis. Ann Otol Rhinol Laryngol 1994;103:331–4.
13. Bridge JA, Sreekantaiah C, Mouron B, Neff JR, Sandberg AA, Wolman SR. Clonal chromosomal abnormalities in desmoid tumors. Implications for histogenesis. Cancer 1992;69:430–6.
14. Conley J, Healey WV, Stout AP. Fibromatosis of the head and neck. Am J Surg 1966;112:609–14.
15. Easter DW, Halasz NA. Recent trends in the management of desmoid tumors. Summary of 19 cases and review of the literature. Ann Surg 1989;210:765–9.
16. Enzinger FM, Weiss SW. Fibromatoses. In: Enzinger FM, Weiss SW, eds. Soft Tissue Tumors. St. Louis: Mosby, 1995:201–29.
17. Fowler CB, Hartman KS, Brannon RB. Fibromatosis of the oral and paraoral region. Oral Surg Oral Med Oral Pathol 1994;77:373–86.
18. Fu YS, Perzin KH. Nonepithelial tumors of the nasal cavity, paranasal sinuses and nasopharynx: a clinicopathologic study. IV. Fibrous tissue tumors (fibroma, fibromatosis, fibrosarcoma). Cancer 1976;37:2912–28.
19. Goellner JR, Soule EH. Desmoid tumors. An ultrastructural study of eight cases. Hum Pathol 1980;11:43–50.
20. Jones IT, Jagelman DG, Fazio VW, Lavery IC, Weakley FL, McGannon E. Desmoid tumors in familial polyposis. Ann Surg 1986;204:94–7.
21. Karlsson I, Mandahl N, Heim S, Rydholm A, Willen H, Mitelman F. Complex chromosome rearrangements in an extraabdominal desmoid tumor. Cancer Genet Cytogenet 1988;34:241–5.
22. Lanari A. Effect of progesterone on desmoid tumors (aggressive fibromatosis) [Letter]. N Engl J Med 1983;309:1523.
23. Maher ER, Morson B, Beach R, Hodgson SV. Phenotypic variation in hereditary nonpolyposis colon cancer syndrome. Association with infiltrative fibromatosis (desmoid tumor). Cancer 1992;69:2049–51.
24. Masson JK, Soule EH. Desmoid tumors of the head and neck. Am J Surg 1966;112:615–22.
25. McCollough WM, Parsons JT, van der Griend R, Enneking WF, Heare T. Radiation therapy for aggressive fibromatosis: the experience at the University of Florida. J Bone Joint Surg [Am] 1991;73:717–25.
26. Plaat BE, Balm AJ, Loftus BM, Gregor RT, Hilgers FJ, Keus RB. Fibromatosis of the head and neck. Clin Otolaryngol 1995;20:103–8.
27. Sherman NE, Romsdahl M, Evans H, Zagars G, Oswald MJ. Desmoid tumors: a 20-year radiotherapy experience. Int J Radiat Oncol Biol Phys 1990;19:37–40.
28. Stiller D, Katenkamp D. Cellular features of desmoid fibromatosis and well-differentiated fibrosarcomas. An electron microscopic study. Virchows Arch [A] 1975;369:155–64.
29. Vally IM, Altini M. Fibromatoses of the oral and paraoral soft tissues and jaws. Review of the literature and report of 12 new cases. Oral Surg Oral Med Oral Pathol 1990;69:191–8.
30. Wilkins SA Jr, Waldron CA, Mathews WH, Droulias CA. Aggressive fibromatosis of the head and neck. Am J Surg 1975;130:412–5.

Fibrosarcoma

31. Fu YS, Perzin KH. Nonepithelial tumors of the nasal cavity, paranasal sinuses and nasopharynx: a clinicopathologic study. IV. Fibrous tissue tumors (fibroma, fibromatosis, fibrosarcoma). Cancer 1976;37:2912–28.

32. Koka V, Vericel R, Lartigau E, Lusinchi A, Schwaab G. Sarcomas of nasal cavity and paranasal sinuses: chondrosarcoma, osteosarcoma and fibrosarcoma. J Laryngol Otol 1994;108:947–53.

33. Lalwani AK, Jackler RK, Gutin PH. Lethal fibrosarcoma complicating radiation therapy for benign glomus jugulare tumor. Am J Otol 1993;14:398–402.

34. Mark RJ, Sercarz JA, Tran L, Selch M, Calcaterra TC. Fibrosarcoma of the head and neck. The UCLA experience. Arch Otolaryngol Head Neck Surg 1991;117:396–401.

35. Nageris B, Elidan J, Sherman Y. Fibrosarcoma of the vocal fold: a late complication of radiotherapy. J Laryngol Otol 1994;108:993–4.

Inflammatory Myofibroblastic (Pseudo) Tumor

36. Arber DA, Kamel OW, van de Rijn M, et al. Frequent presence of the Epstein-Barr virus in inflammatory pseudotumor. Hum Pathol 1995;26:1093–8.

37. Chan JK. Inflammatory pseudotumor: a family of lesions of diverse nature and etiologies. Advances Anat Pathol 1996;3:156–69.

38. Coffin CM, Watterson J, Priest JR, Dehner LP. Extrapulmonary inflammatory myofibroblastic tumor (inflammatory pseudotumor). A clinicopathologic and immunohistochemical study of 84 cases. Am J Surg Pathol 1995;19:859–72.

39. Earl PD, Lowry JC, Sloan P. Intraoral inflammatory pseudotumor. Oral Surg Oral Med Oral Pathol 1993; 76:279–83.

40. Shek AW, Wu PC, Samman N. Inflammatory pseudotumor of the mouth and maxilla. J Clin Pathol 1996;49:164–7.

41. Wenig BM, Devaney K, Bisceglia M. Inflammatory myofibroblastic tumor of the larynx. A clinicopathologic study of eight cases simulating a malignant spindle cell neoplasm. Cancer 1995;76:2217–29.

11
OSSEOUS LESIONS PREDILECTING THE HEAD AND NECK REGION

Although some osseous neoplasms exclusively involve the long bones of the appendicular skeleton, most at least rarely occur in the flat bones of the craniofacial region. Osseous tumors are covered in far greater detail in a separate Fascicle devoted entirely to this topic, and the reader is referred to this publication for more detailed descriptions of these entities (5). The current chapter serves as a selected review of osseous lesions that have a strong predilection for the head and neck region or show distinctive biologic behavior when they involve this area.

Regardless of anatomic site, the associated radiograph provides critical information regarding the diagnosis of an osseous lesion. In some instances, as in the evaluation of low-grade cartilaginous lesions, the radiograph is considerably more valuable than the microscopic section. Only rarely, for example with acute osteomyelitis, will the radiograph be a potentially deceptive factor. The value of radiographs in osseous pathology is a well-established concept. In 1922, James Ewing (4) commented that, "the gross

anatomy (as revealed in radiographs) is often a safer guide to correct clinical conception of disease than the variable and uncertain nature of a small piece of tissue." Although the definitive evaluation of radiographic studies should be done by an experienced skeletal radiologist, pathologists with an interest in osseous neoplasia should examine the radiographs associated with their biopsy or resection specimens. Over time such individuals can become quite good at the differential diagnoses suggested by given radiographic images. Under virtually no circumstances should a pathologist render a diagnosis on an intraosseous lesion without knowledge of the radiographic interpretation. To do so is to court disaster. The eighth Fascicle in this series includes an introductory approach to the evaluation of radiographs that is suitable for pathologists with interest in this field (5).

OSTEOMA

General Features. In the head and neck, osteomas may arise from bone or soft tissue. Solitary osteomas of the facial bones are not rare, but when multiple, the diagnosis of Gardner's syndrome should be considered (2). Although there is predilection for mandibular bone, osteomas may also arise from the bones surrounding the sinonasal cavities. Osteomas of sinonasal bones most often grow into the frontal, ethmoid, or maxillary sinuses (figs. 11-1, 11-2) (1,6,7).

In a review of 39 oral osteomas from the literature (3), 85 percent occurred in the posterior dorsum of the tongue near the circumvallate papilla or the foramen cecum, 8 percent arose in the middle third of the dorsum of the tongue, 3 percent developed on the lingual aspect of the alveolar process of the anterior mandible, and 3 percent arose in the mandibular buccal vestibule.

Clinical Features. Osteomas of the sinonasal bones occur more often in men (ratio of 1.5-2.0 to 1) (1,7). They may be seen at any age, and are found as asymptomatic lesions detected by radiography. Occasionally there is blockage of the sinus ostium that results in symptoms of sinusitis. Over 70 percent of oral osteomas occur

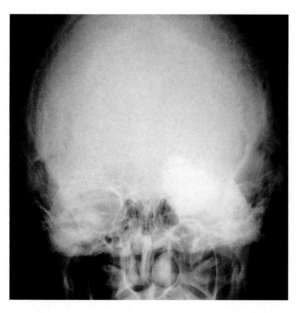

Figure 11-1
OSTEOMA

The left frontal sinus is filled with a sclerotic, radiodense osteoma.

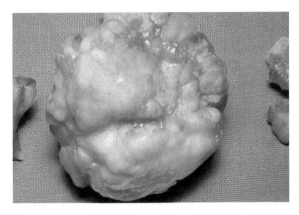

Figure 11-2
OSTEOMA

In this resection specimen from the tumor in figure 11-1, the osteoma is characterized by multilobulated "rock hard" fragments of densely sclerotic bone.

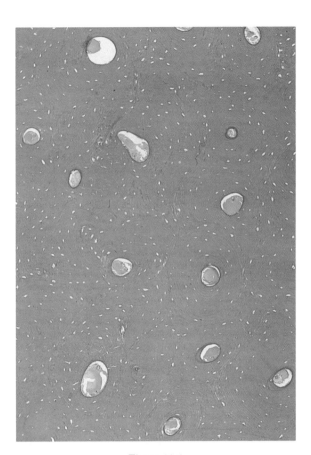

Figure 11-4
OSTEOMA

Some osteomas are composed entirely of "ivory-like" dense cortical bone.

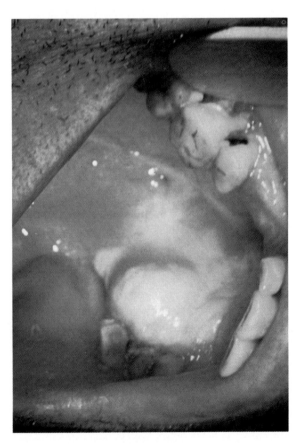

Figure 11-3
OSTEOMA

This osteoma of the palate is associated with considerable reactive keratosis of the overlying and adjacent epithelium, producing a large patch of "leukoplakia."

in women (3,8). Two thirds develop in patients in the third or fourth decade of life, with a mean age of 30 years; however, the age range is wide. Oral osteomas are usually asymptomatic, but occasionally patients may experience choking, gagging, nausea, or dysphagia. They are firm to hard, mobile, and well circumscribed (fig. 11-3).

Gross Findings. Osteomas typically range from 0.5 to 2.0 cm in greatest dimension. They are hard and spherical and require extensive decalcification prior to sectioning.

Microscopic Findings. A well-circumscribed nodule of mature dense bone is the characteristic feature (figs. 11-4, 11-5). Bony trabeculae sometimes are rimmed by osteoblasts. Between bony trabeculae there may be fibrous tissue (fig. 11-6) or fatty stroma with varying amounts of hematopoietic elements. Occasionally, there are foci of mature cartilage.

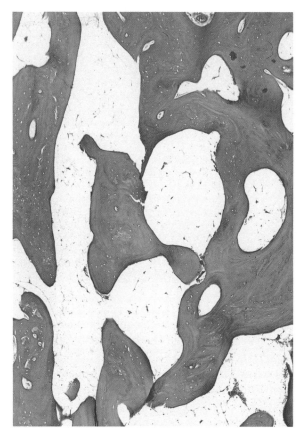

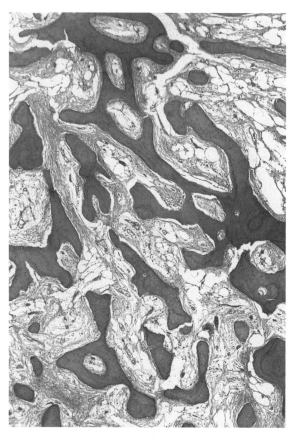

Figure 11-5
OSTEOMA
This soft tissue osteoma from the base of the tongue contains well-formed trabeculae of lamellar bone separated by fatty marrow-like stroma.

Figure 11-6
OSTEOMA
This osteoma from the frontal sinus contains trabeculae of lamellar bone with an intervening bland fibrous stroma.

Treatment and Prognosis. For oral lesions, simple excision is curative. For sinonasal osteomas, treatment is not indicated unless the patient is symptomatic or desires cosmesis. Recurrences typically do not develop.

OSTEOSARCOMA

Osteosarcoma is a malignant neoplasm of bone or occasionally soft tissue that demonstrates at least focal osteoid production by neoplastic cells. Patterns of fibrosarcoma, chondrosarcoma, or malignant fibrous histiocytoma may also be present. By definition and based on clinicopathologic features, production of osteoid by neoplastic cells warrants a designation of osteosarcoma, even if other matrix elements or microscopic patterns predominate.

Although most osteosarcomas involve the appendicular skeleton of adolescents, the head and neck region is occasionally affected, often in older individuals. In patients over 60 years of age 13 percent of osteosarcomas involve the craniofacial bones (15). One of several clinical scenarios occurs. Osteosarcoma of the jaw as a de novo lesion is not uncommon, accounting for about 7 percent of all osteosarcomas (11). As discussed below, these tumors have distinctive clinicopathologic features that warrant their separation from tumors involving the extragnathic bones. Because Paget's disease often affects the craniofacial bones, secondary sarcomas including osteosarcomas arising in this setting may occur in this location (13,14,16,23). Sarcomas of the craniofacial bones also occur as a late sequela of radiation therapy to this region (9,22).

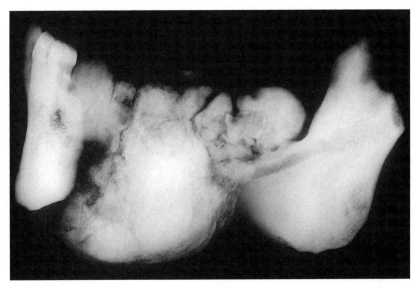

Figure 11-7
OSTEOSARCOMA
In this specimen radiograph from a hemi-mandibulectomy, an osteosarcoma involving the anterior portion of the mandible produces a densely sclerotic, destructive mass.

Osteosarcoma of the Jaws

Clinical Features. Patients with osteosarcoma of the jaws range in age from 4 to 79 years, with a mean of 33 years (11,12). This is more than a decade greater than the mean age of patients with osteosarcomas of the long bones. Men outnumber women by a ratio of 1.5 to 1. Of 122 total cases, 72 involved the mandible and 50 arose in the maxilla (11,12). Of the mandibular lesions, 41 involved the body, 10 occurred at the angle, 9 involved the symphysis, and 7 arose in the ramus. Of the maxillary lesions, 25 were located along the alveolar ridge, 20 involved the maxillary antrum, and 5 were in the anterior midline region or the hard palate.

Presenting complaints are typical of a space-occupying lesion in this region and include swelling, loosening of teeth, separation of teeth, paresthesia, and bleeding. Lesions in the maxilla may be associated with sinonasal symptoms including nasal obstruction and proptosis. Unlike conventional osteosarcomas of the long bones, patients may be symptomatic for more than a year.

Radiographic Findings. The earliest radiographic feature of osteosarcomas arising near the teeth is a widened periodontal membrane space (12), but it is unusual to encounter these lesions at this early stage. Usually, radiographs show an obviously malignant, expansile and permeative mass, with extraosseous extension noted in more than half of cases (11), and "ominous" periosteal reactions also frequently encountered (11). The mass may have a lytic, blastic, or mixed appearance (fig. 11-7).

Gross Findings. Grossly, the appearance is identical to that of conventional osteosarcoma of long bones. Because the gnathic tumors are often chondroblastic or osteoblastic, corresponding gross features of neoplastic cartilage or bone may be present (fig. 11-8).

Microscopic Findings. The spectrum of microscopic appearances manifest by long-bone osteosarcoma may also be seen in osteosarcoma of the jaws. In some studies, there has been a tendency towards better differentiation in the gnathic tumors (11), although others have not noted this trend (10). Chondroblastic (fig. 11-9) and osteoblastic (fig. 11-10) differentiation occur with approximately equal frequency (10,11). A fibrosarcoma-like pattern is also common. Chondroblastic variants may consist almost entirely of lobules of malignant cartilage, with only focal osteoid production. In our experience, areas of dense osteoblastic activity may contain deceptively bland, "normalized" osteoblasts that lack clear-cut features of malignancy (fig. 11-11). In such cases, areas of less prominent osteoid production often show more overtly malignant cells (fig. 11-12). In problematic cases, the infiltrative radiographic appearance of the lesion confirms the diagnosis of osteosarcoma.

Spread and Metastasis. Local recurrence is the most frequent form of treatment failure, occurring in about 85 percent of patients (10). Only 4 of

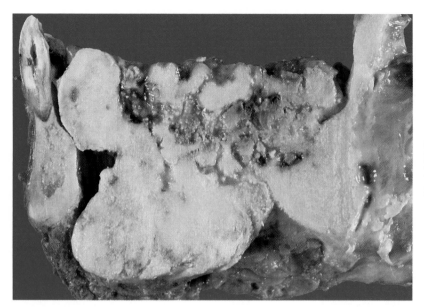

Figure 11-8
OSTEOSARCOMA
A gross photograph of the radiographic specimen in figure 11-7 shows a densely sclerotic, focally hemorrhagic mass which infiltrates the mandible and extends into the periodontal tissues.

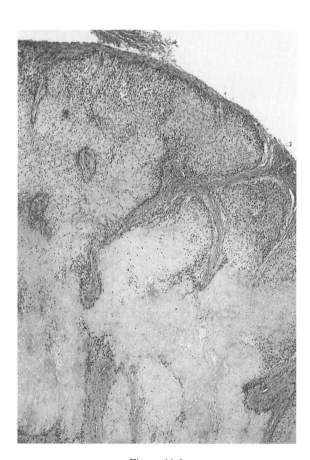

Figure 11-9
CHONDROBLASTIC OSTEOSARCOMA
This low-grade chondroblastic osteosarcoma of the jaw has a low-power lobular pattern typical of cartilage-containing neoplasms.

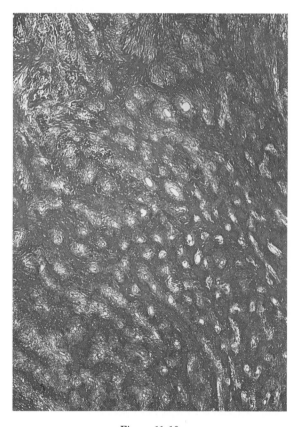

Figure 11-10
OSTEOBLASTIC OSTEOSARCOMA
This densely sclerotic osteoblastic osteosarcoma has a low-magnification appearance somewhat similar to that of an osteoma. Although features of malignancy may not be clearly present in such foci, the complex pattern of the osteoid (in comparison to figures 11-5 and 11-6) is a clue that this is an osteosarcoma.

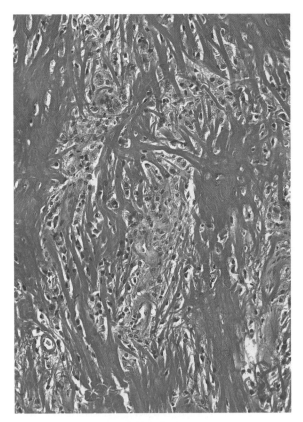

Figure 11-11
OSTEOSARCOMA
Dense, irregular islands of osteoid in this osteosarcoma are separated by a cellular but not overtly malignant stroma.

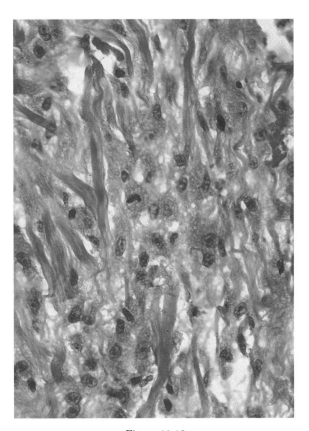

Figure 11-12
OSTEOSARCOMA
Other, less osteoblastic foci in the case seen in figure 11-11 consist of more variable, mitotically active spindled cells.

66 patients (6 percent) in the Mayo Clinic series (11) developed metastases, usually involving the lung (18). In another study, lung metastases were documented in 5 of 28 patients (18 percent) (10).

Treatment and Prognosis. Radical resection is the treatment of choice. In the series from the Mayo Clinic, 12 of 15 patient treated in this fashion were disease free from 2 to 12 years later (11,12). Radiation therapy was noted to have little affect on prognosis, and the overall 5-year survival was approximately 40 percent. In the series of 28 patients, however, the 5-year survival rate was 23 percent (10).

Osteosarcoma of the Extragnathic Bones

Osteosarcomas of the extragnathic craniofacial bones, including the skull bones, differ in several respects from osteosarcomas of the jaws and should be distinguished from them (19,20). These are typically extensive, high-grade lesions, often arising in association with a premalignant condition such as Paget's disease (13,14, 16,23), chronic osteomyelitis (19), multiple osteochondromas (19), fibrous dysplasia (fig. 11-13) (17), or prior radiation therapy (21,22). As with the gnathic tumors, most patients are older than those with conventional osteosarcomas.

Survival for patients with extragnathic tumors appears to be worse than for those with lesions of the jaws. In the Mayo Clinic series, only 2 of 21 patients survived for 5 years (19). This appears to be due in large part to the very poor prognosis associated with sarcomas arising in Paget's disease (17,23). In one study of Paget-related osteosarcomas of the skull, the median survival was only 4 months whereas patients with de novo sarcomas fared much better (17).

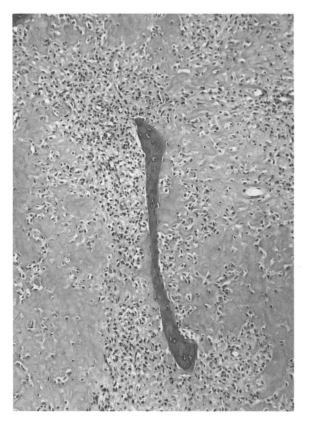

Figure 11-13
OSTEOSARCOMA

Rarely, osteosarcomas of the jaws and facial bones may arise from preexistent lesions such as fibrous dysplasia. In this example from the mandible, a trabecula of woven bone from fibrous dysplasia is used as a "scaffold" for the deposition of osteoid by a secondary osteosarcoma.

Sarcomas Arising in Paget's Disease

Sarcoma arising in preexistent Paget's disease is a well-recognized phenomenon (24–26, 29). In all studies, the predominant form of sarcoma in this setting has been osteosarcoma, accounting for about 85 percent of cases (24–26,29), but fibrosarcoma and chondrosarcoma have also been described. The overall risk of malignant transformation in Paget's disease of bone is low (1 percent) and is probably related to the severity of the disease (29); it may occur in up to 10 percent of patients with severe polyostotic Paget's disease. Because Paget's disease of bone is a relatively common lesion, associated sarcomas account for about 3 to 5 percent of all osteosarcomas (26,29). The skeletal involvement generally parallels that of the precursor lesion. In one series, 14 percent of the associated sarcomas involved the craniofacial bones (26).

Pain of increasing severity and less than 1 year's duration, often with a palpable mass is the most common complaint (29). Serum alkaline phosphatase is elevated in about 85 percent of patients (26) and distant metastases are present at the time of diagnosis in over 25 percent (29). The skull is the most common site of involvement in the head and neck region (25,27,28).

Microscopically, most tumors are conventional osteosarcomas, although telangiectatic and small cell variants have been described (29). Areas of chondroblastic, fibroblastic, fibrohistiocytic, or giant cell differentiation are common.

The overall 5-year survival for patients with sarcoma related to Paget's disease is only about 5 to 8 percent (26,28), which is considerably lower than that for de novo neoplasms. In part, this disparity in prognosis may relate to the tendency to involve flat bone sites of the axial skeleton that are difficult or impossible to resect. Other theories to account for the poorer prognosis include delay in diagnosis due to masking of the lesion by the pain of Paget's disease, more frequent metastases because of the highly vascular nature of the preexistent Paget's disease, and the generally older age of the affected individuals.

Postradiation Sarcomas

The flat bones of the head and neck are virtually always contained within the radiation fields used to treat carcinomas or lymphomas involving this region. Because of this, they are a common site for the development of postradiation sarcomas. Criteria for a radiation-related sarcoma were proposed by Cahen et al. in 1948 (31) and later modified by Arlen et al. (30). In several studies, the mean interval between radiation therapy and the detection of a secondary sarcoma has been 13 to 15 years (32,34,35).

The amount of absorbed radiation appears to directly correlate with the frequency of subsequent sarcoma (33). Approximately 0.2 percent of patients receiving radiation at the usual therapeutic dosage in the range of 7000 rads develop postradiation sarcomas. For highly unusual patients absorbing 20,000 rads, the frequency rises to over 20 percent (33). Below 1000 rads, the incidence of sarcoma within the radiated field is the same as that for de novo sarcomas in the same region (33).

Radiographs of postradiation intraosseous sarcoma usually show obvious features of malignancy, but the changes can be obscured by the non-neoplastic effects of the radiation, or the malignant features may be mistaken for a metastasis from the original malignancy.

Weatherby et al. (34) reviewed the Mayo Clinic experience with 78 postradiation sarcomas. Osteosarcomas were the most common and accounted for almost half the cases, followed by fibrosarcomas (41 percent); the remainder were chondrosarcomas. There were no morphologic features distinguishing postradiation and de novo sarcomas. In a study of postradiation osteosarcomas from Memorial Sloan-Kettering Cancer Center (32), radiation-related tumors accounted for 5.5 percent of cases, and 16 percent of the postradiation osteosarcomas arose in the head and neck.

The prognosis of patients with postradiation sarcomas is not clearly distinct from those with de novo sarcomas arising at the same anatomic site. Lesions of the vertebrae and shoulder girdle have an abysmal prognosis with virtually all patients dead of disease within 4 years, most within the first year postdiagnosis (34). Patients with tumors of the skull and jaw bones appear to fare considerably better, with an approximately 30 percent 5-year survival rate. Many of the survivors have had completely resected mandibular tumors (34).

CHORDOMA

Definition. This is an indolent but malignant neoplasm that arises along the axial skeleton in the region of the embryonic notochord, particularly near it's cranial and caudal ends. In addition to *classic* or *conventional chordomas,* two subtypes have been recognized, the *chondroid chordoma* and *"dedifferentiated" chordoma.* Although the existence of chondroid chordoma has been the subject of considerable debate, the overwhelming evidence supports that this is a microscopically distinct variant of chordoma and not a chondrosarcoma.

General Features. Chordomas account for approximately 1 to 4 percent of malignant osseous neoplasms. They arise along or near the spinal axis, the site of the embryologic notochord and its remnants. About 36 percent of chordomas arise in the spheno-occipital region, and a few additional tumors affect the cervical vertebrae. Conventional or classic chordomas light microscopically resemble fetal notochord and are probably derived from notochord remnants, or perhaps a common progenitor cell. At least some histochemical differences have been noted between notochord and chordoma (38). Lesions of the appendicular skeleton purported to be chordomas or having chordoma-like features are virtually always myxoid chondrosarcomas (58,59).

Clinical Features. Chordomas arising from the spheno-occipital region tend to occur 10 to 20 years earlier in life than sacrococcygeal lesions. Most patients with head and neck chordomas are in their third to fifth decades. Tumors may occur at any age, including in young children. Some reports of spheno-occipital chordomas have shown a male predominance of approximately 2 to 1 (44,52,54), and others have shown no predilection (53).

Signs and symptoms have typically been present for more than a year, due to the slow growth of the tumor. Diplopia is common secondary to involvement or compression of the sixth cranial nerve (44). Other common complaints include headache, palsies of other cranial nerves, visual field disturbances, and signs of endocrine imbalance due to compression of the pituitary gland. About 25 percent of patients with a spheno-occipital chordoma have a symptomatic intranasal mass (44).

Radiographic Appearance. Chordomas are expansile, destructive lesions that frequently extend extraosseously. Erosion of the clivus, sella turcica, and portions of the petrous or sphenoid bones is common. Intralesional calcifications are present in about 42 percent of chondroid chordomas and 14 percent of conventional chordomas (44). These may be due to dystrophic calcium deposits or entrapped fragments of non-neoplastic bone.

Gross Findings. Chordomas are multilobated, soft, myxoid gelatinous masses (fig. 11-14). This appearance may resemble a mucinous adenocarcinoma or myxoid chondrosarcoma. Soft tissue extensions of tumor may be surrounded, at least partially, by a rim of reactive periosteal bone, which has remained intact due to the slow growth of the tumor. Soft tissue

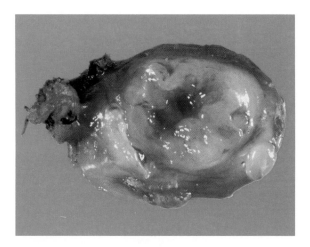

Figure 11-14
CHORDOMA
This chordoma within the upper posterior portion of the nasal cavity presented as a polypoid mass. On cut section its myxoid character is obvious.

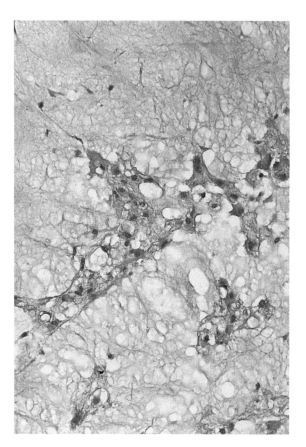

Figure 11-16
CHORDOMA
At higher magnification, the cells have vacuolated or "bubbly" cytoplasm and uniform nuclei.

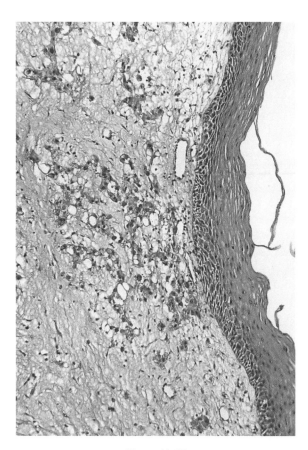

Figure 11-15
CHORDOMA
At low magnification, this chordoma consists of small cords of epithelioid cells in a myxoid matrix underlying intact squamous nasal mucosa.

margins may appear grossly discrete, belying an infiltrative microscopic appearance.

Microscopic Findings. The prototypical appearance of chordoma consists of lobules and cords of cells with vacuolated (physaliphorous) cytoplasm suspended in a prominent myxoid matrix (figs. 11-15–11-17). However, the spectrum of microscopic appearances is wide and many chordomas do not contain classic physaliphorous cells (57). Some cells have a distinctly epithelioid appearance with prominent, nonvacuolated eosinophilic cytoplasm (fig. 11-18); others have a single cytoplasmic vacuole, resembling a signet-ring cell adenocarcinoma. Nuclear pleomorphism is often minimal, but may occasionally be more striking (fig. 11-19) (57). Mitotic figures are rare unless the tumor has undergone "dedifferentiation" (see below). These cytologic variations, excluding dedifferentiation, do not appear to be associated with

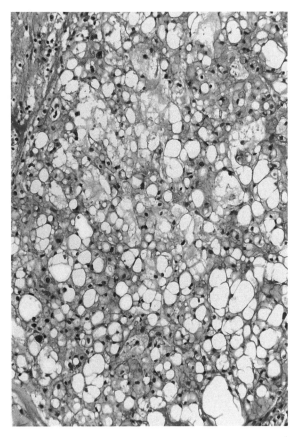

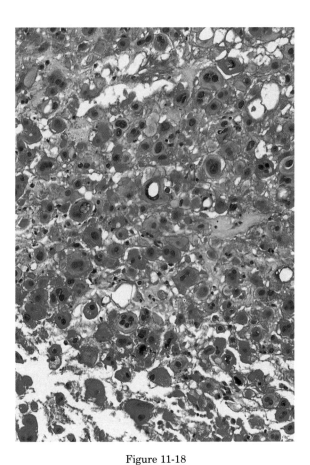

Figure 11-17
CHORDOMA
This more typical chordoma consists of sheets of highly vacuolated or "physaliphorous" cells.

Figure 11-18
CHORDOMA
Some chordomas are composed of nonvacuolated or minimally vacuolated cells with dense eosinophilic cytoplasm.

Figure 11-19
CHORDOMA
Occasional highly pleomorphic or overtly bizarre cells may be present in otherwise typical chordomas without altering the tumor-associated prognosis.

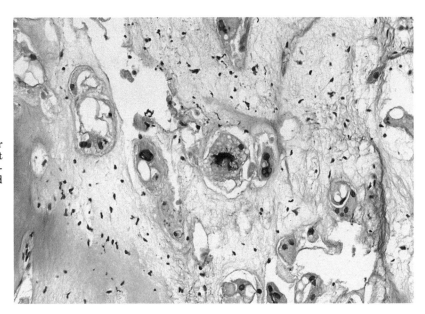

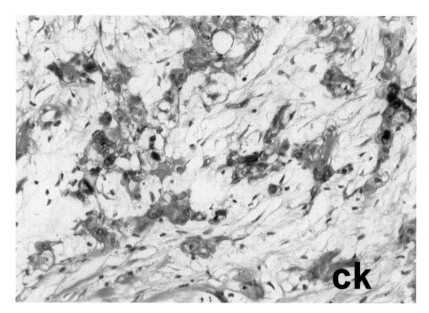

Figure 11-20
CHORDOMA
Immunoreactivity for cytokeratin can be a helpful diagnostic feature for distinguishing chordomas from other, cytokeratin-negative myxoid lesions (anticytokeratin, hematoxylin).

clinically significant differences in survival rates. The neoplastic cells of chordoma are typically "floating" in a prominent extracellular myxoid matrix, which consists of hyaluronidase-resistant sulfated mucopolysaccharides.

Immunohistochemical Findings. Conventional chordomas have been the subject of multiple immunohistochemical studies (37,46,49,52,55,56). Virtually all are immunoreactive for cytokeratin (fig. 11-20) (49,52), and 90 percent or more are reactive for epithelial membrane antigen (49,52). These stains are thus of considerable value for excluding chondrosarcomas or other myxoid mesenchymal neoplasms. Approximately 50 to 75 percent of conventional chordomas react for S-100 protein (36,49,52) and 10 to 38 percent label for carcinoembryonic antigen (49,52).

Treatment and Prognosis. (See below under Chondroid Chordoma.)

Chondroid Chordoma

Definition. This variant of chordoma includes foci of apparent cartilaginous differentiation, in association with areas of conventional chordoma.

General Features. Chondroid chordoma has been the subject of considerable controversy which appears to have resulted in a better understanding of this tumor. Chondroid chordomas were first described in 1968 (42), and documented in more detail in a subsequent series from the Mayo Clinic (44). Most arise in the spheno-occipital region (42,44,47,49,56,60) where they are at least one third as common as conventional chordomas (44). Two fundamental issues have surrounded this tumor. First, is it a distinctive variant of chordoma or a chondrosarcoma? Second, is its biologic behavior different from that of conventional chordoma or low-grade chondrosarcoma occurring in this region? The first of these questions has been convincingly answered, and there has been a recent revision in our understanding of the second.

Although some authors have doubted whether chondroid chordoma is microscopically distinct from chondrosarcoma (38,39), more recent studies have convincingly demonstrated that these tumors have clear-cut immunohistochemical differences (47,49,52,60).

Microscopic Findings. The distinctive microscopic feature of chondroid chordoma is the presence of areas of cartilaginous or cartilage-like differentiation (fig. 11-21). In these regions, the neoplastic cells occupy lacunar spaces within a hyalinized stromal matrix. The chondrocyte-like cells show minimal atypia and the overall appearance is similar to that of an enchondroma or low-grade chondrosarcoma (fig. 11-22). The amount of cartilaginous tissue may vary from scant to dominant. By definition, any such foci, in association with areas of conventional chordoma or appropriate immunohistochemical features, are sufficient to place the lesion in the category of

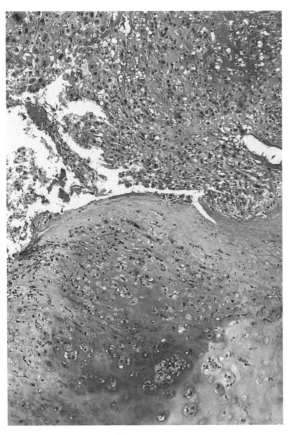

Figure 11-21
CHONDROID CHORDOMA
This chondroid chordoma contains areas of more typical chordoma (top), as well as sharply demarcated cartilaginous areas.

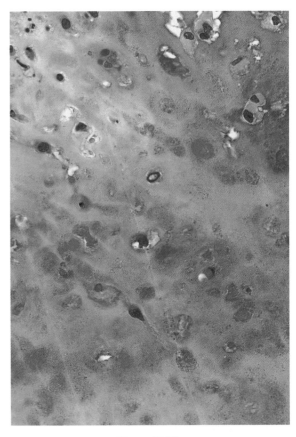

Figure 11-22
CHONDROID CHORDOMA
A higher magnification from the chondroid region seen in figure 11-21 shows chondrocytes in lacunar spaces within the chondroid matrix.

chondroid chordoma. The significance, or lack thereof, of this designation is discussed below.

Immunohistochemical Findings. Chondroid chordomas with areas of conventional chordoma express epithelial antigens (epithelial membrane antigen, cytokeratin), in most instances, in the areas of cartilaginous differentiation (49,52,55). In addition, as with conventional chordomas and chondrosarcomas, they express S-100 protein in a high percentage of cases (52). It has been suggested that cartilaginous lesions in this region that are positive for epithelial markers are chondroid chordomas, regardless of whether areas of conventional chordoma are identified. Conversely, epithelial marker–negative cartilaginous tumors, lacking areas of conventional chordoma, are chondrosarcomas.

Treatment and Prognosis. Early studies suggested that recognition of chondroid chordoma was important, because these tumors appeared to pursue a more indolent clinical course when compared to conventional chordomas (44). However, more recent studies from the same institution (Mayo Clinic) have shown that there is no statistically significant difference in survival for patients with spheno-occipital tumors with chondroid differentiation that are epithelial marker positive (chondroid chordoma), epithelial marker negative (chondrosarcoma), or lack cartilaginous features (classic chordoma) (52). The single factor that did show significant prognostic correlation was the age of the patient at the time of diagnosis: patients younger than 40 years of age had a significantly better outcome.

The treatment of chordoma, chondroid chordoma, or low-grade chondrosarcoma in the spheno-occipital region is surgical. Complete excision is rarely possible and, because of this, local recurrences are common. In the initial Mayo Clinic series, the mean survival was 4.1 years, with only 1 patient of 36 surviving 10 years (44). The more recent studies from that institution, based on a somewhat larger series of cases, demonstrated 5-year survival of 100 percent for patients under 40 years of age (52), while for those over 40 years of age, it was 22 percent with conventional condroma and 38 percent with chondroid chordoma (43,52). This difference is not statistically significant. DNA ploidy studies have not been of great value in prognostication. Approximately 75 percent of chordomas are diploid neoplasms (46). Chemotherapeutic agents have not been effective in the treatment of chordoma. Debulking and radiation therapy have been applied to recurrent or unresectable neoplasms. Newer modalities of radiation therapy, such as the "gamma knife" and proton beam therapy, are showing considerable promise.

Dedifferentiated Chordoma

Definition. This is a distinct, high-grade sarcoma that usually resembles a malignant fibrous histiocytoma and arises in association with a conventional chordoma, or less commonly, a chondroid chordoma.

General Features. Conventional chordomas may display moderate nuclear pleomorphism that is of no apparent clinical significance. However, the emergence of a distinct "dedifferentiated," high-grade sarcoma is associated with a considerably worsened prognosis. The presence of a high-grade sarcoma within or at the site of a prior chordoma was first described over 80 years ago (41), and has been well documented in subsequent studies (37, 44,46,48,50,51,57). Most of these have occurred in sacrococcygeal chordomas, but spheno-occipital lesions have been described (44).

Clinical Features. It is unusual for the dedifferentiated component to be present initially, and the typical history is for one or more recurrences of a conventional chordoma, followed by the development of a dedifferentiated component. Some patients with dedifferentiated chordomas have had prior radiation therapy and

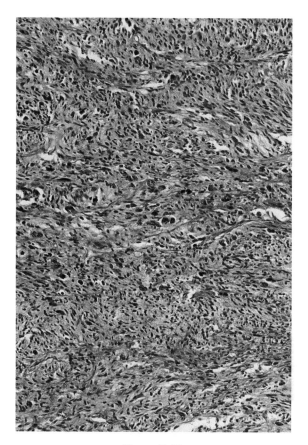

Figure 11-23
DEDIFFERENTIATED CHORDOMA
This high-grade spindle cell sarcoma resembling a malignant fibrous histiocytoma arose at the site of a previously excised conventional-type chordoma.

it can be argued strongly that the subsequent tumors are postradiation sarcomas. In other instances, however, the sarcomatous component has arisen following only surgery.

Microscopic Findings. Elements of conventional or chondroid chordoma may be present, but are typically a minor component. The sarcomatous elements usually resemble a malignant fibrous histiocytoma (fig. 11-23) (37,46,48,50,51), but areas resembling fibrosarcoma, high-grade chondrosarcoma, and osteosarcoma have also been documented (40,44,45,50). Immunohistochemical studies show that the areas of sarcomatous dedifferentiation show a marked decrease in the expression of epithelial markers, as compared to the areas of conventional or chondroid chordoma (46). There is an associated increase in vimentin expression in the sarcomatous components (46).

Treatment and Prognosis. The presence of foci of high-grade sarcoma is associated with a considerably worsened prognosis. Hematogenous metastases consisting entirely of the sarcomatous elements are common. Because of this considerable effect on prognosis, chordomas, especially longstanding or recurrent ones, should be carefully studied to exclude the presence of a dedifferentiated sarcomatous component.

EOSINOPHILIC GRANULOMA

Definition. This clonal proliferation of Langerhans cells is often associated with an inflammatory infiltrate composed of eosinophils, histiocytes, lymphocytes, plasma cells, and neutrophils. Other synonymous terms applied to this lesion have included *histiocytosis X, Langerhans cell histiocytosis,* and *Langerhans granulomatosis.*

General Features. Although eosinophilic granuloma has been viewed as a reactive process or immune system disorder by many, recent studies have indicated that the proliferating cells are, in fact, clonal (72,73). This suggests that eosinophilic granuloma is a neoplastic proliferation with a variable clinical course.

Virtually all organ systems may be affected by eosinophilic granuloma and purely extraosseous lesions occur. Most often, however, the disease involves bones or bones and extraosseous sites. The bones of the head and neck, particularly the skull and mandible, are common sites of involvement. For a more detailed general discussion of eosinophilic granuloma at all osseous sites please refer to the third series Fascicle dealing with osseous neoplasms (64).

Clinical Features. Although eosinophilic granuloma occurs in a broad age range from newborns to the elderly, about 85 percent of cases are detected in the first three decades of life, and 60 percent are diagnosed in the first decade of life. Males are affected about twice as frequently as females. Pain and a soft tissue swelling overlying the affected bone are the most common presenting complaints. Involvement of the temporal bone may result in a clinical presentation indistinguishable from that of otitis media or mastoiditis. In reported series, patients with solitary lesions outnumber those with multisite disease by between 2 to 1 and 5 to 1. This probably represents over-reporting from referral cen-

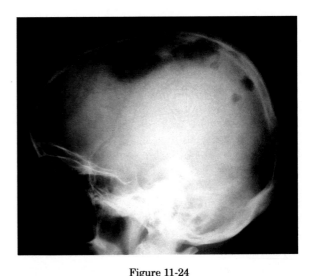

Figure 11-24
EOSINOPHILIC GRANULOMA
Eosinophilic granuloma produces multiple lytic skull lesions.

ters of patients with clinically problematic multifocal disease. The true ratio of solitary to polyostotic disease is greater than 5 to 1.

Radiographic Findings. Eosinophilic granuloma of bone typically results in a lytic medullary defect, usually with sharply defined margins, resulting in a "punched out" appearance. Lesions of the skull, in particular, often show "beveled" margins due to angulated destruction of the cortical bone margins. If multiple lesions are present, as is common in the skull, there may be considerable variation in appearance, with some of the lesions being lytic and sharply demarcated, and others having ill-defined sclerotic margins (fig. 11-24). Lesions of the latter type may undergo spontaneous resolution with reactive bone "infiltrating" the lesional defect.

Gross Findings. Specimens usually consist of curettings or small biopsies and have a nonspecific gross appearance. Older lesions associated with lipid accumulation may be yellow; other lesions may be gray, brown, or hemorrhagic in appearance.

Microscopic Findings. The diagnosis of eosinophilic granuloma requires recognition of the Langerhans cell. The latter are often dispersed in a background of characteristic, but nondiagnostic inflammatory cells, including prominent eosinophils (fig. 11-25). Langerhans cells have highly variable amounts of cytoplasm which may be eosinophilic, vacuolated due to

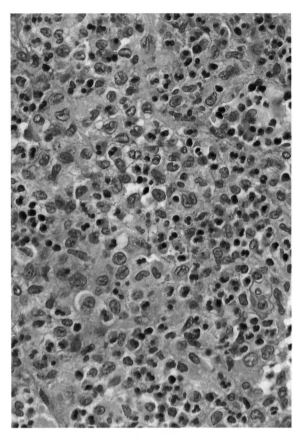

Figure 11-25
EOSINOPHILIC GRANULOMA
Eosinophilic granuloma consists of a mixture of Langerhans histiocytes and large numbers of eosinophils.

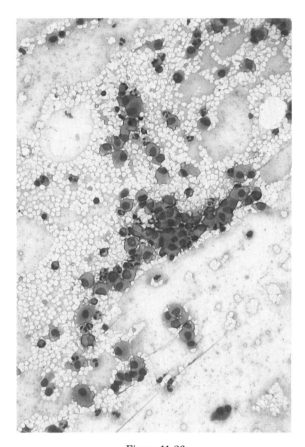

Figure 11-26
EOSINOPHILIC GRANULOMA
Fine needle aspiration cytologic specimen shows clusters of Langerhans histiocytes.

lipid accumulation, or contain other phagocytosed material such as hemosiderin (fig. 11-26). The nuclei are typically "bean shaped" or convoluted with nuclear grooves and indentations easily seen by focusing up and down through well-made hematoxylin and eosin (H&E)-stained sections. Nuclear chromatin is delicate and often condensed around the nuclear rim. Mitotic figures in Langerhans cells are variable in number, but fewer than 5 per high-power field are typical.

Ordinary histiocytes, as well as eosinophils, plasma cells, and neutrophils are common components of eosinophilic granuloma. The histiocytes may demonstrate prominent phagocytosis with some cells containing intracytoplasmic debris, lipid vacuoles, hemosiderin, or Charcot-Leyden crystals from degenerating eosinophils. In some microscopic fields, there may be large aggregates of eosinophils, some of which have central necrosis (eosinophilic microabscesses); other examples contain few if any eosinophils (71).

Osteoid and bone are typically lacking from the central regions of eosinophilic granuloma and, at the periphery of the lesion, there is usually intense osteoclastic activity. Langerhans cells have been shown to produce prostaglandins that are strong stimulators of bone resorption (65). During the resorbing or "healing" phase of eosinophilic granuloma, the stroma becomes increasingly fibrotic and Langerhans cells decrease in number. The presence of retained histiocytes with foamy cytoplasm may result in an appearance suggestive of nonossifying fibroma.

Immunohistochemical Findings. The characteristic Langerhans cells of eosinophilic granuloma have been the subject of multiple immunohistochemical studies (61–63,66–68). Strong labeling for S-100 protein has been well recognized

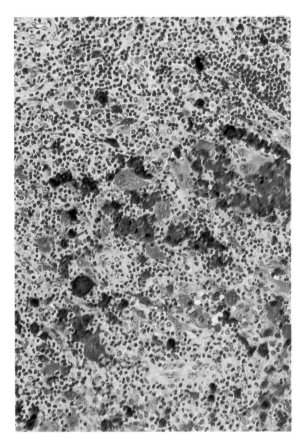

Figure 11-27
EOSINOPHILIC GRANULOMA
Langerhans histiocytes are strongly reactive for S-100 protein. Typical histiocytes are not immunoreactive (anti-S-100 protein, hematoxylin).

as a feature of Langerhans cells (fig. 11-27) (61–63,67). These cells also react with peanut agglutinin (70). More recent studies have shown staining with monoclonal antibody (Mab) O10, an antibody known to recognize the CD1 antigenic site (63). Malignant melanomas, nevi, neurofibromas, as well as non-Langerhans cell histiocytoses including juvenile xanthogranulomas and Rosai-Dorfman disease all react negatively with Mab O10 (63). Thus, this antibody appears to be a valuable diagnostic adjunct in association with S-100 protein. Langerhans cells also react with anti-T6 and anti-Ia antibodies, and are negative for anti-T3, anti-T8, anti-M1, and anti-lysozyme antibodies (66).

Differential Diagnosis. The differential diagnosis of eosinophilic granuloma includes granulomatous inflammation, xanthogranulomatous osteomyelitis, Hodgkin's disease, and Rosai-

Dorfman disease. These entities are discussed in detail in Fascicle 8, Tumors of the Bones and Joints (64). In essence, a high index of suspicion for eosinophilic granuloma is warranted when dealing with cranial or craniofacial osseous lesions, particularly multiple lesions with a lytic, punched-out appearance. If necessary, immunohistochemical reactions for S-100 protein or with Mab O10 aid in the diagnostic evaluation. It should be remembered that many of the histiocyte-like cells in eosinophilic granuloma are not Langerhans cells and do not label with these markers, but a sizeable population of immunoreactive cells should be present.

Treatment and Prognosis. Some radiographically typical examples of eosinophilic granuloma have been noted to spontaneous regress and disappear over time. Other lesions may develop irregular sclerotic margins, suggestive of partial regression or "healing." Isolated osseous lesions of eosinophilic granuloma are usually cured by simple curettage or by injection of steroids into the lesion (69). Radiation therapy is generally avoided, but may be utilized at low levels to treat isolated lesions at immediate risk of causing fracture and not amenable to resection. Systemic chemotherapy has been used in patients with multifocal osseous and extraosseous disease.

GIANT CELL GRANULOMA

Definition. This benign, apparently reactive, intraosseous and extraosseous proliferation is characterized by granuloma-like aggregates of giant cells in a fibrovascular stroma. In the head and neck region, the mandible and maxilla are most commonly involved. This lesion is also referred as *giant cell reaction of bone* and *giant cell reparative granuloma*.

General Features. Jaffe (82a) first described giant cell granulomas of the jaws in 1953, and there have been numerous subsequent publications further describing involvement of the jaws, as well as other craniofacial sites (74,83,90, 91,94,95). This lesion also shows a predilection for the small tubular bones of the hands and feet. The uncommon inherited childhood condition of cherubism (figs. 11-28, 11-29) is due to bilateral, symmetrical involvement of the jaws by giant cell granulomas (80,94). True giant cell tumors involving the craniofacial bones are quite rare, but

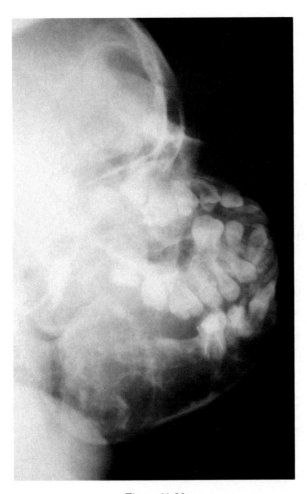

Figure 11-28
GIANT CELL GRANULOMA
Bilateral giant cell granulomas involve the gnathic bones (cherubism). Note the distortion of the mandible by an expansile, vacuolated mass.

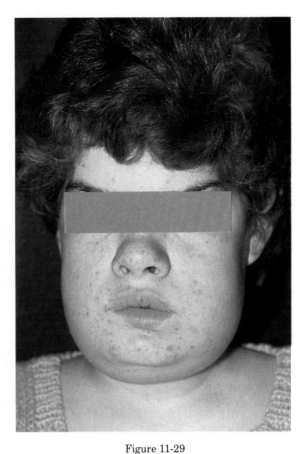

Figure 11-29
GIANT CELL GRANULOMA
Bilateral giant cell granulomas of the jaws creates facial features of cherubism.

have been described (77,89). It has been suggested that many of the giant cell lesions arising in Paget's disease of bone are giant cell granulomas and not true giant cell tumors, but this point remains controversial (93).

Several other uncertainties surround these lesions. The microscopic appearance of giant cell granuloma is indistinguishable from that of the so-called solid variant of aneurysmal bone cyst (76,87,96). In addition, giant cell granulomas may have areas of associated aneurysmal bone cyst. Thus, these are at minimum closely related, occasionally indistinguishable lesions. To add to the controversy surrounding this lesion, Mirra (86) has noted that giant cell granulomas of the jaws

are indistinguishable from nonossifying fibromas and suggests that jaw lesions with these microscopic features be labeled as nonossifying fibromas. We consider giant cell granulomas as a distinct entity, acknowledging their close relationship to, or virtual identity with, the solid variant of aneurysmal bone cyst.

Clinical Features. Pain and swelling are the most common complaints. Lesions involving the sphenoid bone may be associated with optic nerve symptoms (diplopia) or frontal headaches. Temporal bone lesions may produce conductive or sensory hearing loss, or inner ear–related symptoms such as vertigo and tinnitus. Most patients with giant cell granuloma of the head and neck bones are under 20 years of age, and many of the remainder are under 30 years. Female patients are more commonly affected than males, with a female to male ratio of about 2 to 1 in some series

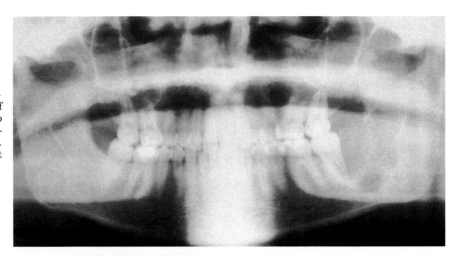

Figure 11-30
GIANT CELL GRANULOMA
This panorex radiograph of the jaws shows a lytic "soap bubble" lesion in the left anterior portion of the mandible. Curettings documented a giant cell granuloma.

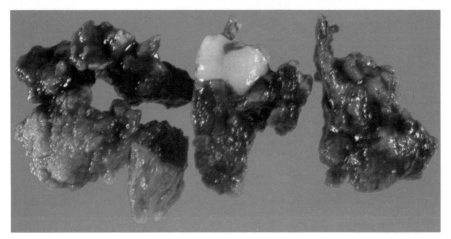

Figure 11-31
GIANT CELL GRANULOMA
Tissue fragments and tooth from a resected giant cell granuloma. These lesions are often grossly hemorrhagic.

(94). It has been suggested that giant cell granulomas are hormonally influenced and tend to enlarge during pregnancy (84,85).

In the head and neck region, these lesions most commonly occur in the anterior portion of the maxilla or, slightly less commonly, in the same portion of the mandible (94). Excluding the jaws, osseous involvement is common in the skull, particularly the sphenoid and temporal bones (82). The term *peripheral giant cell reparative granuloma* is applied to soft tissue tumors arising around the gums and in the nasal cavity that are histologically identical to the intraosseous lesions.

Radiographic Findings. Radiographically, these are expansile, lytic lesions, often with a "soap bubble" or trabeculated internal structure. The edges of the lesion tend to be well-demarcated, without prominent perilesional sclerosis

(fig. 11-30). Cortical breakthrough with soft tissue extension is rare.

Gross Findings. The specimens are usually curetted, both for diagnostic and therapeutic purposes. The resultant tissue fragments have a nondescript, pink-tan to hemorrhagic appearance (fig. 11-31). Cystic components noted radiographically or at the time of surgery are destroyed by the curettage procedure.

Microscopic Findings. The microscopic hallmark of giant cell granuloma is a cellular, fibroblastic stroma containing granuloma-like aggregates of giant cells (figs. 11-32, 11-33). The latter are often associated with foci of hemorrhage. Giant cells may also be diffusely dispersed in the stroma. The multinucleated cells tend to be considerably smaller than those of true giant cell tumor, with correspondingly fewer nuclei. Typical-appearing

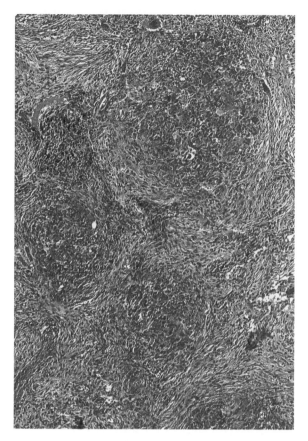

Figure 11-32
GIANT CELL GRANULOMA
At low magnification, giant cell granuloma consists of granuloma-like aggregates of histiocytes with associated clumps of hemosiderin.

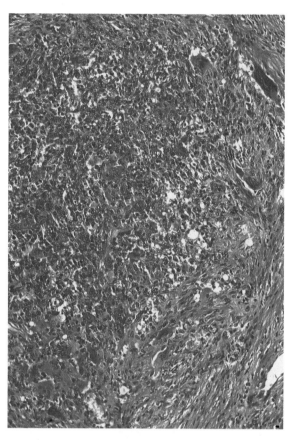

Figure 11-33
GIANT CELL GRANULOMA
At higher magnification, a histiocytic aggregate typical of giant cell granuloma contains scattered multinucleated cells and is surrounded by a fibrous tissue stroma.

mitotic figures are easily identified in the stromal fibroblasts, but are not seen in the multinucleated giant cells. Trabeculae of reactive bone and unmineralized osteoid are commonly seen in giant cell granulomas, but unless there has been an associated fracture, areas of cartilaginous differentiation are lacking.

Immunohistochemical Findings. The multinucleated cells of giant cell granuloma express macrophage-associated markers, and label immunohistochemically for alpha-1-antitrypsin, alpha-1-antichymotrypsin, and lysozyme (88).

Differential Diagnosis. Giant cell granuloma is microscopically indistinguishable from the so-called brown tumor of hyperparathyroidism. Accordingly, the diagnosis should not be made without confirmation of normal serum calcium, phosphate, and alkaline phosphatase lev-

els. Parathyroid hormone levels should also be determined if the serum calcium is marginally elevated. There is general, but not unanimous agreement that giant cell granuloma is microscopically distinct from giant cell tumor (75,80,82). This distinction is important because of the more aggressive local behavior and occasional limited metastatic potential associated with giant cell tumor and not seen with giant cell granuloma. True giant cell tumor of the craniofacial bones is rare in comparison to giant cell granuloma, but well-documented cases have been described (92). Most lesions from the head and neck region reported in the older literature as "giant cell tumor" (78) are, in reality, giant cell granulomas. Giant cell tumors are characterized by a more diffuse component of larger giant cells, some with literally dozens of nuclei, and a distinct polygonal-shaped mononuclear cell that differs from the fibroblastic background of giant cell granuloma. These distinguishing features are discussed in more detail in the in third series Fascicle, Tumors of the Bones and Joints (79).

Treatment and Prognosis. The usual treatment approach to giant cell granuloma is curettage, with or without packing the lesional cavity with bone chips. Approximately 15 percent of the intraosseous jaw lesions recur following initial curettage (94), and these are cured by a second procedure. "Benign" metastases of the type occasionally encountered in the lungs of patients with true giant cell tumors have not been described. Soft tissue or "peripheral" giant cell lesions of the oral or nasal cavity have an even lower recurrence rate.

FIBROUS DYSPLASIA

Definition. Fibrous dysplasia is a benign, monostotic or polyostotic proliferation of fibrous tissue and predominantly woven bone showing little or no osteoblastic rimming. About 10 percent of cases contain a cartilaginous component, which can be prominent (*fibrocartilaginous dysplasia*).

General Features. The exact nature of fibrous dysplasia has been the subject of considerable discussion. At various times and by various authors it has been considered to represent a true neoplasm, a hamartomatous malformation, and a localized failure of woven bone to mature into lamellar bone. Most examples of fibrous dysplasia are monostotic, but about 20 percent affect multiple osseous sites. It must be emphasized that benign fibro-osseous lesions of the craniofacial bones often display a histologic spectrum of appearances, and may well represent a continuum rather than distinct clinicopathologic entities (97). At opposite ends of the spectrum are lesions conventionally labeled fibrous dysplasia and ossifying fibroma.

Clinical Features. About one third of cases of monostotic fibrous dysplasia involve the craniofacial bones. Patients may be virtually any age at the time of diagnosis, but about 75 percent are diagnosed before 30 years of age, and usually within the first two decades of life. In one well-studied series (101), nearly all patients were symptomatic before 20 years of age. There is no sex predilection. Gnathic lesions usually result in ob-

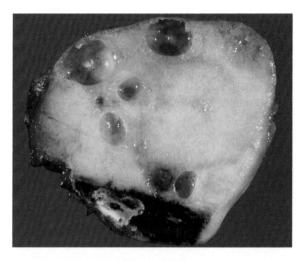

Figure 11-34
FIBROUS DYSPLASIA
This example of fibrous dysplasia from the maxilla has a dense fibrous appearance and multiple small cysts. The latter are common in this lesion.

vious facial deformity, but may be painless and otherwise asymptomatic. The maxilla is involved slightly more often than the mandible (101). Untreated, fibrous dysplasia may continue to enlarge or stabilize over time. It has been suggested that most monostotic lesions stabilize and become inactive following puberty (98).

Radiographic Findings. Fibrous dysplasia can usually be diagnosed, or at least strongly suspected, on the basis of its radiographic appearance. Involvement of the craniofacial bones typically produces a somewhat ill-defined, "ground glass" or "orange peel" density that expands and deforms the involved bone. The lesion may be more or less radiodense, overall, than the surrounding bone. The lack of perilesional sclerosis and blurring of the margins is particularly common in craniofacial lesions, whereas long bone lesions may be more sharply demarcated.

Gross Findings. Fibrous dysplasia is typically a firm, tan to hemorrhagic mass, with a gritty consistency due to variable amounts of interposed mineralized woven bone (fig. 11-34). Cartilage nodules may be grossly visible, and secondary cyst formation is common.

Microscopic Findings. The prototypical appearance of fibrous dysplasia consists of irregularly shaped trabeculae of osteoid and woven bone diffusely embedded in a variably cellular

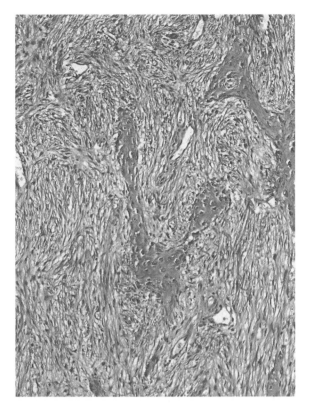

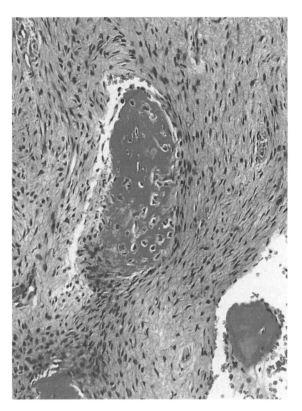

Figure 11-35
FIBROUS DYSPLASIA
Irregular islands of woven bone in a cellular fibrous stroma are characteristic of fibrous dysplasia.

Figure 11-36
FIBROUS DYSPLASIA
The islands of woven bone in fibrous dysplasia typically contain numerous entrapped osteoblasts. Osteoblastic rimming is not prominent.

fibrous tissue stroma (fig. 11-35). The osteoid appears to "emerge" from the associated fibrous tissue and often contains entrapped osteoblast-like cells (fig. 11-36). Alignment of osteoblasts around the margins of the osteoid trabeculae (osteoblastic rimming), as is typical of reactive lesions and so-called ossifying fibroma, is absent or focal. Although much of the bone in fibrous dysplasia is of the woven type, areas of lamellar bone, easily identified under polarized light, are often present. These may represent areas of reactive host bone surrounding the fibrous dysplasia or an intrinsic portion of the lesion. Sharply defined microscopic nodules of benign cartilage may be embedded in the fibro-osseous lesion. These are more likely to be encountered in younger children. The ill-defined margin seen radiographically has a microscopic counterpart in the form of infiltration of surrounding normal bone by the lesional tissue.

Differential Diagnosis. The occasionally impossible distinction from the opposite end of the fibro-osseous spectrum, the ossifying fibroma, is discussed below. Fibrous dysplasia is occasionally confused with a quite different lesion, osteofibrous dysplasia, primarily because of the similarities in nomenclature. However, osteofibrous dysplasia almost exclusively involves the tibia and fibula, and has none of the radiographic or microscopic features of fibrous dysplasia.

The fibrous stroma of fibrous dysplasia may have areas devoid of osteoid, leading to confusion with desmoplastic fibroma. However, these regions lack the heavily collagenized stroma typical of true desmoplastic fibroma. Conversely, the infiltrating margin of desmoplastic fibroma places fibrous tissue and reactive trabeculae of bone in close approximation, leading to potential confusion with fibrous dysplasia. The latter areas, however, have the intense osteoblastic rimming characteristic of reactive bone and lack the "metaplastic bone" appearance of fibrous dysplasia.

Occasionally, fibrous dysplasia may be confused with intraosseous well-differentiated osteosarcoma because the latter lesion also contains short trabeculae of well-formed bone. However, the stroma of fibrous dysplasia lacks the cellularity and nuclear enlargement typical of well-differentiated osteosarcoma. As always, radiographs are very helpful, as the latter lesions, unlike fibrous dysplasia, are typically heavily mineralized with a more permeative margin.

Treatment and Prognosis. The treatment options for fibrous dysplasia are multiple and depend on a wide variety of factors including the site and extent of the lesion, and the age of the patient. Recurrences following curettage or limited resection are not uncommon, or unexpected, given the tendency for infiltration at the lesional periphery. Some lesions apparently stabilize with the onset of puberty. Radiation is considered a last resort, but may be used in otherwise intractable cases.

Sarcomas have been reported to arise in approximately 0.5 percent of patients with fibrous dysplasia (100,102). Slightly more than half these patients had monostotic fibrous dysplasia, and the remainder had polyostotic disease (99). There is considerable reason to believe that this reported frequency is much higher than reality. Most important in this regard, many examples of monostotic fibrous dysplasia are minimally symptomatic and go undiagnosed and unreported. Second, some purported examples of malignant transformation of fibrous dysplasia are better interpreted as "dedifferentiation" in well-differentiated intraosseous osteosarcoma.

The gnathic bones are most commonly involved in true malignant transformations in preexistent fibrous dysplasia (see fig. 11-13). About one third of patients have had prior radiation therapy, making it likely that these are postradiation sarcomas (99,100).

OSSIFYING FIBROMA

Definition. This is a benign, fibro-osseous proliferation with an often characteristic radiographic appearance that is composed, microscopically, of fibrous tissue and mineralized bone, and, in many instances, contains scattered cementum-like or "psammomatoid" spherules. Also included under this category are histologic variants of ossifying fibroma with a more prominent cementum-like

matrix. Terms applied to these latter lesions include: *cemento-ossifying fibroma, juvenile active ossifying fibroma, cementifying fibroma,* and *psammomatoid ossifying fibroma.* Lesions described in the older literature as ossifying fibroma of long bones, are examples of an unrelated entity now termed osteofibrous dysplasia.

General Features. As discussed elsewhere in this chapter, ossifying fibroma can be viewed as one extreme of a spectrum of fibro-osseous proliferations. Although usually occurring close to the teeth and predilecting the mandible over the maxilla, ossifying fibroma is a nonodontogenic lesion. Histologically similar or identical lesions occur in the skull and other extragnathic craniofacial bones. Variants with prominent psammomatoid calcification have been described in the paranasal sinuses, nasopharynx, orbit, palate, and anterior cranial fossa (104,105,107).

Clinical Features. Patients with ossifying fibroma are typically older than those with fibrous dysplasia. In one series, those affected ranged in age from 15 to 70 years, with more than half in their third or fourth decade of life (106). Unlike fibrous dysplasia, ossifying fibroma shows a strong female predilection; in the series by Waldron and Giansanti (106), 84 percent of patients were women. Many patients with ossifying fibroma are asymptomatic. Ossifying fibroma has been said to predilect black women, and, indeed, in one series of over 400 cases studied radiographically, 8 percent of black women had asymptomatic gnathic defects interpreted as ossifying fibromas (103).

Radiographic Findings. Ossifying fibromas tend to be sharply demarcated, usually lytic lesions, most commonly involving the mandible or maxilla and often closely associated with the roots of normal teeth (fig. 11-37). The sharp, smooth contour of the lesion contrasts with the blurred, permeative margin of "classic" fibrous dysplasia. Over time, ossifying fibromas may become mineralized and less lytic. Some lesions, particularly those with prominent psammomatoid calcifications, may be focally or diffusely radiodense (107). Lesions involving the sinuses may show large, polypoid extensions into the sinus cavities with remodeling and distortion of the surrounding walls.

Gross Findings. Specimens from gross curettings have a nondescript, fibrous, tan appearance

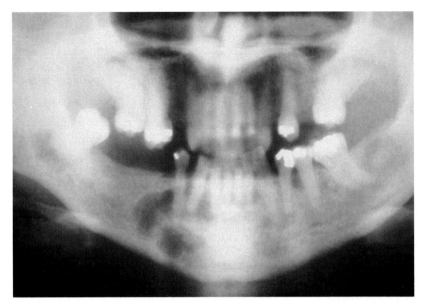

Figure 11-37
OSSIFYING FIBROMA
An ossifying fibroma involving the
right anterior portion of the mandible
produces a sharply defined lytic lesion.

with a gritty consistency due to the presence of numerous calcified trabeculae and spicules.

Microscopic Findings. In its relatively pure or "classic" form, ossifying fibroma consists of evenly spaced, interconnected trabeculae of bone within a fibrous stroma. Osteoblastic rimming is focally obvious, but diffusely prominent rimming of trabeculae is rare (fig. 11-38). Osteoclasts are also present in variable numbers. Most of the bone is woven, but scattered trabeculae of lamellar bone are usually demonstrable. Mitotic figures are rare or absent (105). On detailed study, most examples of classic ossifying fibroma contain scattered, calcified, cementum-like or psammomatoid spherules. When the latter predominate, terms such as cemento-ossifying fibroma or aggressive psammomatoid ossifying fibroma have been used. We consider the psammomatoid lesions a part of the spectrum of ossifying fibroma, which, in turn, is part of the larger spectrum of benign fibro-osseous lesions.

Treatment and Prognosis. Most ossifying fibromas are amenable to curettage or complete surgical excision, usually with a favorable result. Recurrences and locally aggressive behavior have been described, and may or may not be more common with the "psammomatoid" variant (105, 107). In one series of 56 fibro-osseous lesions of all types including mixed lesions, pure fibrous

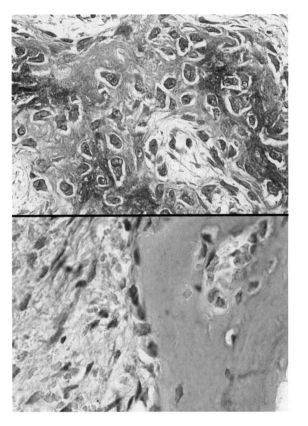

Figure 11-38
FIBROUS DYSPLASIA VERSUS OSSIFYING FIBROMA
Woven bone of fibrous dysplasia with entrapped osteo-blasts (top) contrasts with lamellar bone showing osteoblastic rimming (bottom) typical of ossifying fibroma. Many fibro-osseous lesions, however, exhibit a spectrum of microscopic features including both of the extremes seen here.

dysplasia, and pure ossifying fibroma, the histologic features of the lesion did not influence the rate of recurrence or overall prognosis (105).

BENIGN FIBRO-OSSEOUS LESION

Having described the prototypical features of fibrous dysplasia and ossifying fibroma, it must be acknowledged that in many instances in the craniofacial region, the microscopic features of the two entities will be blurred in any given lesion. For example, it is quite common to find foci of lamellar bone and osteoblastic rimming in lesions that otherwise resemble fibrous dysplasia. In many, but by no means all such cases, the radiographic features may be of considerable value (110,111). Boysen et al. (108) emphasized the importance of radiologic criteria in attempting to distinguish these lesions. Fechner, Waldron, and Dehner (109,110,112) have each noted the potentially conflicting, overlapping nature of the histologic features, and suggested that pathologists must sometimes make a diagnosis of "benign fibro-osseous" lesion in the absence of clear-cut radiographic features.

Waldron and Giansanti (113,114), in a two-part study, applied a somewhat different approach. A series of 65 lesions was first classified as fibrous dysplasia or ossifying fibroma based on radiographic features. As noted above, the radiographs showing ill-defined, "ground glass" or "orange peel" defects were considered as fibrous dysplasia. Lesions classified radiographically as ossifying fibroma had a sharply demarcated, "punched out" lytic appearance. Microscopically, about one third of the lesions interpreted as fibrous dysplasia consisted of purely woven bone and the remainder showed varying amounts of lamellar bone deposition. The bony trabeculae tended to be irregular but small, and did not interconnect. The lesions classified radiographically as ossifying fibromas typically consisted of interconnecting trabeculae of bone with osteoblastic rimming. Importantly, Waldron and Giansanti noted that even though two thirds of the ossifying fibromas contained lamellar bone, it was never prominent, and most of the lesions were composed of woven bone. Most of the ossifying fibromas contained foci of spherical mineralization interpreted as cementum-like material.

REFERENCES

Osteoma

1. Atallah N, Jay MM. Osteomas of the paranasal sinuses. J Laryngol Otol 1981;95:291–304.
2. Bulow S, Sondergaard JO, Witt I, Larsen E, Teters G. Mandibular osteomas in familial polyposis coli. Dis Col Rectum 1984;27:105–8.
3. Chou L, Hansen LS, Daniels TE. Choristomas of the oral cavity: a review. Oral Surg Oral Med Oral Pathol 1991;72:584–93.
4. Ewing J. A review and classification of bone sarcomas. Arch Surg 1922;4:485–533.
5. Fechner RE, Mills SE. Tumors of the bones and joints. Atlas of tumor pathology, 3rd series, Fascicle 8. Armed Forces Institute of Pathology: Washington, D.C., 1993.
6. Fu YS, Perzin KH. Non-epithelial tumors of the nasal cavity, paranasal sinuses, and nasopharynx: a clinicopathologic study. II. Osseous and fibro-osseous lesions, including osteoma, fibrous dysplasia, ossifying fibroma, osteoblastoma, giant cell tumor, and osteosarcoma. Cancer 1974;33:1289–305.
7. Samy LL, Mostafa H. Osteomata of the nose and paranasal sinuses with a report of twenty one cases. J Laryngol Otol 1971;85:449–69.
8. Wasserstain MH, SunderRaj M, Jain R, Yamane G, Chaudry AP. Lingual osseous choristoma. J Oral Med 1983;38:87–9.

Osteosarcoma

9. Arlen M, Higinbotham NL, Huvos AG, Marcove RC, Miller T, Shah IC. Radiation-induced sarcoma of bone. Cancer 1971;28:1087–99.
10. Bertoni F, Dallera P, Bacchini P, Marchetti C, Campobassi A. The Istituto Rizzoli-Beretta experience with osteosarcoma of the jaw. Cancer 1991;68:1555–63.
11. Clark JL, Unni KK, Dahlin DC, Devine KD. Osteosarcoma of the jaw. Cancer 1983;51:2311–6.
12. Garrington GE, Scofield HH, Cornyn J, Hooker SP. Osteosarcoma of the jaws. Analysis of 56 cases. Cancer 1996;20:377–91.
13. Hadjipavlou A, Lander P, Srolovitz H, Enker IP. Malignant transformation of Paget disease of bone. Cancer 1992;70:2802–8.
14. Haibach H, Farrell C, Dittrich FJ. Neoplasms arising in Paget's disease of bone: a study of 82 cases. Am J Clin Pathol 1985;83:594–600.
15. Huvos AG. Osteogenic sarcoma of bones and soft tissues in older persons. A clinicopathologic analysis of 117 patients older than 60 years. Cancer 1986;57:1442–9.
16. Huvos AG, Butler A, Bretsky SS. Osteogenic sarcoma associated with Paget's disease of bone. A clinicopathologic study of 65 patients. Cancer 1983;52:1489–95.
17. Huvos AG, Sundaresan N, Bretsky SS, Butler A. Osteogenic sarcoma of the skull. A clinicopathologic study of 19 patients. Cancer 1985;56:1214–21.
18. Kyriakos M, Berlin BP, DeSchryver-Kecskemeti K. Oat-cell carcinoma of the larynx. Arch Otolaryngol 1978;104:168–76.
19. Nora FE, Unni KK, Pritchard DJ, Dahlin DC. Osteosarcoma of extragnathic craniofacial bones. Mayo Clin Proc 1983;58:268–72.
20. Salvati M, Ciappetta P, Raco A. Osteosarcomas of the skull. Clinical remarks on 19 cases. Cancer 1993;71:2210–6.
21. Tountas AA, Fornasier VL, Harwood AR, Leung PM. Postirradiation sarcoma of bone: a perspective. Cancer 1979;43:182–7.
22. Weatherby RP, Dahlin DC, Ivins JC. Postradiation sarcoma of bone: review of 78 Mayo Clinic cases. Mayo Clin Proc 1981;56:294–306.
23. Wick MR, Siegal GP, Unni KK, McLeod RA, Greditzer HG III. Sarcomas of bone complicating osteitis deformans (Paget's disease): fifty years' experience. Am J Surg Pathol 1981;5:47–59.

Sarcomas Arising in Paget's Disease

24. Hadjipavlou A, Lander P, Srolovitz H, Enker IP. Malignant transformation of Paget disease of bone. Cancer 1992;70:2802–8.
25. Haibach H, Farrell C, Dittrich FJ. Neoplasms arising in Paget's disease of bone: a study of 82 cases. Am J Clin Pathol 1985;83:594–600.
26. Huvos AG, Butler A, Bretsky SS. Osteogenic sarcoma associated with Paget's disease of bone. A clinicopathologic study of 65 patients. Cancer 1983;52:1489–95.
27. Huvos AG, Sundaresan N, Bretsky SS, Butler A. Osteogenic sarcoma of the skull. A clinicopathologic study of 19 patients. Cancer 1985;56:1214–21.
28. Salvati M, Ciappetta P, Raco A. Osteosarcomas of the skull. Clinical remarks on 19 cases. Cancer 1993; 71:2210–6.
29. Wick MR, Siegal GP, Unni KK, McLeod RA, Greditzer HG III. Sarcomas of bone complicating osteitis deformans (Paget's disease): fifty years' experience. Am J Surg Pathol 1981;5:47–59.

Postradiation Sarcomas

30. Arlen M, Higinbotham NL, Huvos AG, Marcove RC, Miller T, Shah IC. Radiation-induced sarcoma of bone. Cancer 1971;28:1087–99.
31. Cahan WG, Woodard HQ, Higinbotham NL, Stewart FW, Coley BL. Sarcoma arising in irradiated bone: report of eleven cases. Cancer 1948;1:3–29.
32. Huvos AG, Woodard HQ, Cahan WG, et al. Postradiation osteogenic sarcoma of bone and soft tissues. A clinicopathologic study of 66 patients. Cancer 1985;55:1244–55.
33. Tountas AA, Fornasier VL, Harwood AR, Leung PM. Postirradiation sarcoma of bone: a perspective. Cancer 1979;43:182–7.
34. Weatherby RP, Dahlin DC, Ivins JC. Postradiation sarcoma of bone: review of 78 Mayo Clinic cases. Mayo Clin Proc 1981;56:294–306.
35. Wiklund TA, Blomqvist CP, Raty J, Elomaa I, Rissanen P, Miettinen M. Postirradiation sarcoma. Analysis of a nationwide cancer registry material. Cancer 1991;68:524–31.

Chordoma

36. Abenoza P, Sibley RK. Chordoma: an immunohistochemical study. Hum Pathol 1987;17:744–7.
37. Belza MG, Urich H. Chordoma and malignant fibrous histiocytoma. Evidence for transformation. Cancer 1986;58:1082–7.
38. Bottles K, Beckstead JH. Enzyme histochemical characterization of chordomas. Am J Surg Pathol 1984;8:443–7.
39. Brooks JJ, LiVolsi VA, Trojanowski JQ. Does chondroid chordoma exist? Acta Neuropathol (Berl) 1987;72:229–35.
40. Chambers PW, Schwinn CP. Chordoma. A clinicopathologic study of metastasis. Am J Clin Pathol 1979;72:765–76.
41. Debernardi L. Cordoma sarcomatose del sacro contributo alla conoscenza istologica e clinica dei tumori di origine cordale. Arch Sci Med (Torino) 1913; 37:404–42.
42. Falconer MA, Bailey IC, Duchen LW. Surgical treatment of chordoma and chondroma of the skull base. J Neurosurg 1968;29:261–75.

43. Forsyth PA, Cascino TL, Shaw EG, et al. Intracranial chordomas: a clinicopathological and prognostic study of 51 cases. J Neurosurg 1993;78:741–7.

44. Heffelfinger MJ, Dahlin DC, MacCarty CS, Beabout JW. Chordomas and cartilaginous tumors of the skull base. Cancer 1973;32:410–20.

45. Hruban RH, May M, Marcove RC, Huvos AG. Lumbosacral chordoma with high-grade malignant cartilaginous and spindle cell components. Am J Surg Pathol 1990;14:384–9.

46. Hruban RH, Traganos F, Reuter VE, Huvos AG. Chordomas with malignant spindle cell components. A DNA flow cytometric and immunohistochemical study with histogenetic implications. Am J Pathol 1990;137:435–47.

47. Jeffrey PB, Biava CG, Davis RL. Chondroid chordoma. A hyalinized chordoma without cartilaginous differentiation. Am J Clin Pathol 1995;103:271–9.

48. Makek M, Leu HJ. Malignant fibrous histiocytoma arising in recurrent chordoma. Case report and electron microscopic findings. Virchows Arch [A] 1982;397:241–50.

49. Meis JM, Giraldo AA. Chordoma. An immunohistochemical study of 20 cases. Arch Pathol Lab Med 1988;112:553–6.

50. Meis JM, Raymond AK, Evans HL, Charles RE, Giraldo AA. "Dedifferentiated" chordoma. A clinicopathologic and immunohistochemical study of three cases. Am J Surg Pathol 1987;11:516–25.

51. Miettinen M, Lehto VP, Virtanen I. Malignant fibrous histiocytoma within a recurrent chordoma. A light microscopic, electron microscopic, and immunohistochemical study. Am J Clin Pathol 1984;82:738–43.

52. Mitchell A, Scheithauer BW, Unni KK, Forsyth PJ, Wold LE, McGivney DJ. Chordoma and chondroid neoplasms of the spheno-occiput. An immunohistochemical study of 41 cases with prognostic and nosologic implications. Cancer 1993;72:2943–9.

53. O'Connell JX, Renard LG, Liebsch NJ, Efird JT, Munzenrider JE, Rosenberg AE. Base of skull chordoma. A correlative study of histologic and clinical features of 62 cases. Cancer 1994;74:2261–7.

54. Perzin KH, Pushparaj N. Nonepithelial tumors of the nasal cavity, paranasal sinuses, and nasopharynx. A clinicopathologic study. XIV: Chordomas. Cancer 1986;57:784–96.

55. Rutherfoord GS, Davies AG. Chordomas—ultrastructure and immunohistochemistry: a report based on the examination of six cases. Histopathology 1987;11:775–87.

56. Salisbury JR, Isaacson PG. Demonstration of cytokeratins and an epithelial membrane antigen in chordomas and human fetal notochord. Am J Surg Pathol 1985;9:791–7.

57. Volpe R, Mazabraud A. A clinicopathologic study of 25 cases of chordoma (a pleomorphic and metastasizing neoplasm). Am J Surg Pathol 1983;7:161–70.

58. Weiss SW. Ultrastructure of the so-called "chordoid sarcoma." Evidence supporting cartilaginous differentiation. Cancer 1976;37:300–6.

59. Wick MR, Burgess JH, Manivel JC. A reassessment of "chordoid sarcoma." Ultrastructural and immunohistochemical comparison with chordoma and skeletal myxoid chondrosarcoma. Mod Pathol 1988;1:433–43.

60. Wojno KJ, Hruban RH, Garin-Chesa P, Huvos AG. Chondroid chordomas and low-grade chondrosarcomas of the craniospinal axis. An immunohistochemical analysis of 17 cases. Am J Surg Pathol 1992;16:1144–52.

Eosinophilic Granuloma

61. Azumi N, Sheibani K, Swartz WG, Stroup RM, Rappaport H. Antigenic phenotype of Langerhans cell histiocytosis: an immunohistochemical study demonstrating the value of LN-2, LN-3, and vimentin. Hum Pathol 1988;19:1376–82.

62. Beckstead JH, Wood GS, Turner RR. Histiocytosis X cells and Langerhans cells: enzyme histochemical and immunologic similarities. Hum Pathol 1984;15:826–33.

63. Emile JF, Wechsler J, Brousse N, et al. Langerhans' cell histiocytosis. Definitive diagnosis with the use of monoclonal antibody O10 on routinely paraffin-embedded samples. Cancer 1995;76:2471–84.

64. Fechner RE, Mills SE. Tumors of the bones and joints. Atlas of tumor pathology, 3rd series, Fascicle 8. Armed Forces Institute of Pathology: Washington, D.C., 1993.

65. Gonzalez-Crussi F, Hsueh W, Wiederhold MD. Prostaglandins in histiocytosis-X. PG synthesis by histiocytosis-X cells. Am J Clin Pathol 1981;75:243–53.

66. Harrist TJ, Bhan AK, Murphy GF, et al. Histiocytosis-X: in situ characterization of cutaneous infiltrates with monoclonal antibodies. Am J Clin Pathol 1983;79:294–300.

67. Ide F, Iwase T, Saito I, Umemura S, Nakajima T. Immunohistochemical and ultrastructural analysis of the proliferating cells in histiocytosis X. Cancer 1984;53:917–21.

68. Lieberman PH, Jones CR, Steinman RM, et al. Langerhans cell (eosinophilic) granulomatosis. A clinicopathologic study encompassing 50 years. Am J Surg Pathol 1996;20:519–52.

69. Nauert C, Zornoza J, Ayala A, Harle TS. Eosinophilic granuloma of bone: diagnosis and management. Skeletal Radiol 1983;10:227–35.

70. Ree HJ, Kadin ME. Peanut agglutinin. A useful marker for histiocytosis X and interdigitating reticulum cells. Cancer 1986;57:282–7.

71. Risdall RJ, Dehner LP, Duray P, Kobrinsky N, Robinson L, Nesbit ME Jr. Histiocytosis X (Langerhans' cell histiocytosis). Prognostic role of histopathology. Arch Pathol Lab Med 1983;107:59–63.

72. Willman CL. Detection of clonal histiocytes in Langerhans cell histiocytosis: biology and clinical significance. Br J Cancer Suppl 1994;23:S29–33.

73. Willman CL, Busque L, Griffith BB, et al. Langerhans'-cell histiocytosis (histiocytosis X)—a clonal proliferative disease. N Engl J Med 1994;331:154–60.

Giant Cell Granuloma

74. Alappat JP, Pillai AM, Prasanna D, Sambasivan M. Giant cell reparative granuloma of the craniofacial complex: case report and review of the literature. Br J Neurosurg 1992;6:71–4.
75. Auclair PL, Cuenin P, Kratochvil JJ, Slater LJ, Ellis GL. A clinical and histomorphologic comparison of the central giant cell granuloma and the giant cell tumor. Oral Surg Oral Med Oral Pathol 1988;66:197–208.
76. Bertoni F, Bacchini P, Capanna R, et al. Solid variant of aneurysmal bone cyst. Cancer 1993;71:729–34.
77. Bertoni F, Unni KK, Beabout JW, Ebersold MJ. Giant cell tumor of the skull. Cancer 1992;70:1124–32.
78. Emley WE. Giant cell tumor of the sphenoid bone. A case report and review of the literature. Arch Otolaryngol 1971;94:369–74.
79. Fechner RE, Mills SE. Tumors of the bones and joints. Atlas of tumor pathology, 3rd series, Fascicle 8. Armed Forces Institute of Pathology: Washington, D.C., 1993.
80. Franklin CD, Craig GT, Smith CJ. Quantitative analysis of histologic parameters in giant cell lesions of the jaws and long bones. Histopathology 1979;3:511–22.
81. Hamner JE III, Ketcham AS. Cherubism: an analysis of treatment. Cancer 1969;23:1133–43.
82. Hirschl S, Katz A. Giant cell reparative granuloma outside the jaw bone. Diagnostic criteria and review of the literature with the first case described in the temporal bone. Hum Pathol 1974;5:171–81.
82a. Jaffe HL. Giant-cell reparative granuloma, traumatic bone cyst, and fibrous (fibro-osseous) dysplasia of the jawbones. Oral Surg Oral Med Oral Pathol 1953;6:159–75.
83. Koay CB, Whittet HB, Ryan RM, Lewis CE. Giant cell reparative granuloma of the concha bullosa. J Laryngol Otol 1995;109:555–8.
84. Littler BO. Central giant-cell granuloma of the jaw—a hormonal influence. Br J Oral Surg 1979;17:43–6.
85. McGowan DA. Central giant cell tumours of the mandible occurring in pregnancy. Br J Oral Surg 1969;7:131–5.
86. Mirra JM. Bone tumors: clinical, radiologic, and pathologic correlations. Philadelphia: Lea & Febiger, 1989:733–5.
87. Oda Y, Tsuneyoshi M, Shinohara N. "Solid" variant of aneurysmal bone cyst (extragnathic giant cell reparative granuloma) in the axial skeleton and long bones. A study of its morphologic spectrum and distinction from allied giant cell lesions. Cancer 1992;70:2642–9.
88. Regezi JA, Zarbo RJ, Lloyd RV. Muramidase, alpha-1 antitrypsin, alpha-1 antichymotrypsin, and S-100 protein immunoreactivity in giant cell lesions. Cancer 1987;59:64–8.
89. Saleh EA, Taibah AK, Naguib M, et al. Giant cell tumor of the lateral skull base: a case report. Otolaryngol Head Neck Surg 1994;111:314–8.
90. Sidhu MS, Parkash H, Sidhu SS. Central giant cell granuloma of jaws–review of 19 cases. Br J Oral Maxillofac Surg 1995;33:43–6.
91. Sidoni A, Monico S, D'Errico P, Simoncelli C. Giant cell reparative granuloma of the maxillary bone: case report and review of diagnostic criteria. Pathologica 1994;86:552–6.
92. Smith GA, Ward PH. Giant-cell lesions of the facial skeleton. Arch Otolaryngol 1978;104:186–90.
93. Upchurch KS, Simon LS, Schiller AL, Rosenthal DI, Campion EW, Krane SM. Giant cell reparative granuloma of Paget's disease of bone: a unique clinical entity. Ann Intern Med 1983;98:35–40.
94. Waldron CA, Shafer WG. The central giant cell reparative granuloma of the jaws. An analysis of 38 cases. Am J Clin Pathol 1966;45:437–47.
95. Wise AJ, Bridbord JW. Giant cell granuloma of the facial bones. Ann Plast Surg 1993;30:564–8.
96. Wold LE, Dobyns JH, Swee RG, Dahlin DC. Giant cell reaction (giant cell reparative granuloma) of the small bones of the hands and feet. Am J Surg Pathol 1986;10:491–6.

Fibrous Dysplasia

97. Fechner RE. Problematic lesions of the craniofacial bones. Am J Surg Pathol 1989;13(Suppl 1):17–30.
98. Henry A. Monostotic fibrous dysplasia. J Bone Joint Surg (Br) 1969;51:300–6.
99. Huvos AG, Higinbotham NL, Miller TR. Bone sarcomas arising in fibrous dysplasia. J Bone Joint Surg (Am) 1972;54:1047–56.
100. Taconis WK. Osteosarcoma in fibrous dysplasia. Skeletal Radiol 1988;17:163–70.
101. Waldron CA, Giansanti JS. Benign fibro-osseous lesions of the jaws: a clinical-radiologic-histologic review of sixty-five cases. I. Fibrous dysplasia of the jaws. Oral Surg 1973;35:190–201.
102. Yabut SM Jr, Kenan S, Sissons HA, Lewis MM. Malignant transformation of fibrous dysplasia. A case report and review of the literature. Clin Orthop 1988;228:281–9.

Ossifying Fibroma

103. Neville BW, Albenesius RJ. The prevalence of benign fibro-osseous lesions of periodontal ligament origin in black women: a radiographic survey. Oral Surg 1986;62:340–4.
104. Slootweg PJ, Panders AK, Nikkels PG. Psammomatoid ossifying fibroma of the paranasal sinuses. An extragnathic variant of cemento-ossifying fibroma. Report of three cases. J Craniomaxillofac Surg 1993;21:294–7.
105. Voytek TM, Ro JY, Edeiken J, Ayala AG. Fibrous dysplasia and cemento-ossifying fibroma. A histologic spectrum. Am J Surg Pathol 1995;19:775–81.
106. Waldron CA, Giansanti JS. Benign fibro-osseous lesions of the jaws: a clinical-radiologic-histologic review of sixty-five cases. II. Benign fibro-osseous lesions of periodontal ligament origin. Oral Surg 1973;35:340–50.
107. Wenig BM, Vinh TN, Smirniotopoulos JG, Fowler CB, Houston GD, Heffner DK. Aggressive psammomatoid ossifying fibromas of the sinonasal region. A clinicopathologic study of a distinct group of fibro-osseous lesions. Cancer 1995;76:1155–65.

311

Benign Fibro-Osseous Lesion

108. Boysen ME, Olving JH, Vatne K, Koppang HS. Fibro-osseous lesions of the cranio-facial bones. J Laryngol Otol 1979;93:793–807.

109. Dehner LP. Pediatric surgical pathology. Baltimore: Williams & Wilkins, 1996:142.

110. Fechner RE. Problematic lesions of the craniofacial bones. Am J Surg Pathol 1989;13(Suppl 1):17–30.

111. Voytek TM, Ro JY, Edeiken J, Ayala AG. Fibrous dysplasia and cemento-ossifying fibroma. A histologic spectrum. Am J Surg Pathol 1995;19:775–81.

112. Waldron CA. Fibro-osseous lesions of the jaws. J Oral Maxillofac Surg 1985;43:249–62.

113. Waldron CA, Giansanti JS. Benign fibro-osseous lesions of the jaws: a clinical-radiologic-histologic review of sixty-five cases. I. Fibrous dysplasia of the jaws. Oral Surg 1973;35:190–201.

114. Waldron CA, Giansanti JS. Benign fibro-osseous lesions of the jaws: a clinical-radiologic-histologic review of sixty-five cases. II. Benign fibro-osseous lesions of periodontal ligament origin. Oral Surg 1973;35:340–50.

12

GERM CELL NEOPLASMS

TERATOMA

General Features. Of all germ cell neoplasms occurring in children, approximately 6 percent arise in the soft tissues of the head and neck, 5 percent occur within the cranial cavity (2), and 2 percent arise in the face, orbit, upper aerodigestive tract, and basocranial area (1). With few exceptions, germ cell tumors of the upper aerodigestive tract are teratomas. When arising in the upper aerodigestive tract, these neoplasms most often involve the nasopharynx, but have been described in the oropharynx, palate, tongue, tonsil, sinonasal tract, mandible, maxilla, and external and middle ear including the temporal bone. In a review of reported series of pediatric teratomas, only 3 of 850 tumors involved the nasopharynx (9). Teratomas of the upper aerodigestive tract may be extensive, involving adjacent anatomic sites. Massive intracranial extension may be seen in stillborn infants (3). Historically, *epignathus* has been used to describe a large, often grotesque teratomatous neoplasm arising in the upper aerodigestive tract, although technically, it should be applied only to a teratoma arising in the alveolus of the mandible. Its incorrect usage and the early if not fanciful speculations regarding its pathogenesis are reasons that the term should probably be abandoned. One author recommended that the term be dropped due to its etymological imprecision (4). The related terms, epicranium, episphenoid, and epipalatus, serve only to note the anatomic location of the teratoma (7).

Clinical Features. Teratomas of the upper aerodigestive tract occur almost exclusively in children. In stillborn infants the teratomas are extensive with striking skull and facial bone deformities. Minor developmental defects of facial structures may be found in other patients. Sometimes, massive teratomas arising in the soft tissues of the neck extend to adjacent structures of the upper aerodigestive system. In a report of one patient and review of 27 other patients with nasopharyngeal teratomas, Tharrington and Bossen (9) noted 9 of 20 had been premature and 8 of 13 had had maternal hydramnios. Twenty-three of the teratomas were noted at birth, 2 were found in children less than 1 year of age, and 2 occurred in children more than 1 year old. There was no sex predilection. The main symptom was airway obstruction caused by a protruding mass. In a report of one case and review of six other teratomas arising in the tongue, all neoplasms presented at birth as masses up to 12 cm in greatest diameter (5). Of 10 teratomas occurring in the tonsil, 8 were noted in infants (8). There was an equal sex distribution for patients with lingual and tonsillar teratomas.

Gross Findings. Tumor size ranges from a few centimeters to a large, polypoid, and grotesque mass. Neoplasms can involve multiple adjacent sites in the head and neck area. They may appear circumscribed, and on cut section are cystic, solid, or both. The gross appearance resembles that of teratomas located in gonadal sites and elsewhere.

Microscopic Findings. Endodermal, ectodermal, and mesodermal components are present (fig. 12-1). Epithelial differentiation includes squamous (with or without keratinization), columnar, and ciliated respiratory cells. There may be cutaneous adnexal structures and minor salivary glands. Mesodermal tissues include fat, bone, cartilage, and smooth muscle. Neural tissue including immature elements is commonly present (fig. 12-2). Foci of calcification are also frequent and were described in 18 of 23 nasopharyngeal neoplasms (9).

Differential Diagnosis. Teratomas must be distinguished from dermoid cyst, hairy polyp, encephalocele, and glial heterotopia. Unlike dermoid cyst and hairy polyp, teratomas consist of ectodermal, endodermal, and mesodermal tissues. Malignant germ cell tumor elements were found in only one teratoma and this was an endodermal sinus tumor (4).

Foci of endodermal sinus tumor differentiation have been described in two adult patients with nonkeratinizing squamous (transitional cell) carcinomas of the nasopharynx and paranasal sinus (6). Immunohistochemical support for endodermal sinus differentiation included staining for alpha-1-antitrypsin and alpha-fetoprotein. Both neoplasms were biologically aggressive.

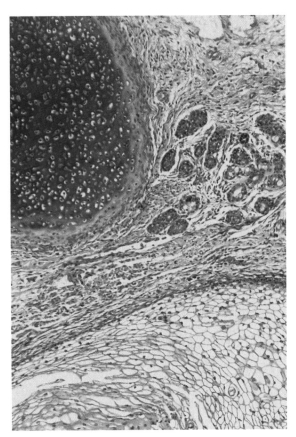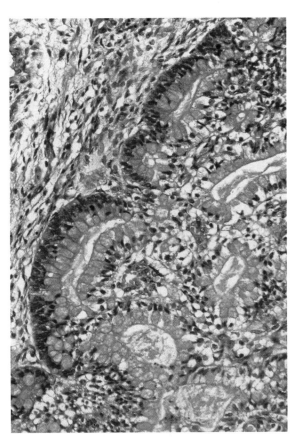

Figure 12-1
TERATOMA
Nodules of cartilage, squamous epithelium (left), and columnar epithelium (right) are commonly present.

Treatment and Prognosis. Complete surgical excision of teratoma may be difficult when the tumor is large and involves multiple facial structures. More than one surgical procedure for tumor eradication may be necessary. Adjuvant therapy for teratomas with immature elements is unnecessary.

If a neoplasm is completely removed, recurrences usually' are absent. The presence of immature areas has no prognostic meaning. Tumor related deaths, including stillbirths, result from large unresectable neoplasms. For nasopharyngeal teratomas, only one liveborn infant died as a direct result of the tumor, and this occurred prior to operative intervention (9). Only two nasopharyngeal teratomas from the literature recurred, but both may actually have been incompletely resected (9). Teratomas of the tongue or tonsil have not recurred after surgical resection (5,8).

TERATOCARCINOSARCOMA

General Features. This malignant sinonasal neoplasm has features of both teratoma and carcinosarcoma. Previous terms for sinonasal neoplasms consisting of mixed components include *malignant teratoma, teratocarcinoma, blastoma, mixed mesodermal tumor,* and *malignant mixed tumor.* Prior to the initial detailed description in 1984 (10), there were seven probable cases reported in the English literature. Another series of cases of teratocarcinosarcoma was described recently (11).

Clinical Features. Of the 29 patients reported in two series (10,11), 25 were male. The age range was 18 to 79 years, with a median in the sixth decade of life. Patients usually had a short history of nasal obstruction or epistaxis, or both. Less common symptoms included pain,

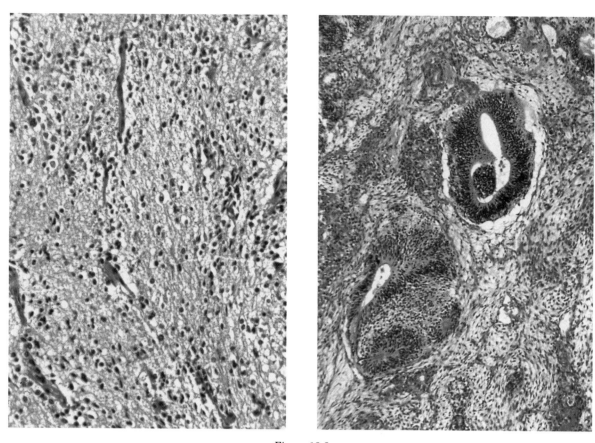

Figure 12-2
TERATOMA
Foci of mature (left) or immature (right) neural tissue have no adverse prognostic significance.

headache, and proptosis. The nasal cavity was involved by tumor in all but 2 patients. Involvement of the ethmoid sinus occurred in 14 patients and the maxillary antrum was involved in 14 as well. Neoplasm extended into the sphenoid sinus in 1 case. One neoplasm not involving the nasal cavity arose in the roof of the nasopharynx, while another developed in the maxillary antrum. One teratocarcinosarcoma was mentioned as arising on the dorsum of the tongue (10). Sinonasal radiographs sometimes show bone destruction, a nasal mass, or opaque sinuses.

Gross Findings. The neoplasms tend to be large, friable to firm, and red or red-purple.

Microscopic Findings. Teratocarcinosarcoma typically shows a combination of features of teratoma and carcinosarcoma. Irregular glandular and ductal structures are set in a stromal background. Most cases contain stroma consist-

ing, in part, of benign smooth and striated muscle, while other foci show atypical or overtly malignant myogenous elements. Glandular and ductal structures surrounded by bland-appearing smooth muscle sometimes resemble primitive bronchial or gastrointestinal tract structures. The glandular or ductal structures are often lined by benign-appearing epithelium (fig. 12-3). Often, the squamous epithelium that is commonly present has a fetal, clear cell appearance and contains abundant glycogen (fig. 12-4). Foci of overt squamous cell carcinoma, adenocarcinoma, or poorly differentiated carcinoma are typically present. Additional fibroblastic, myofibroblastic, and cartilaginous components range from benign to overtly malignant. Osteoid may also be observed. Neural tissue consisting of poorly differentiated neuroepithelial elements, sometimes with neural rosettes and a neurofibrillary matrix,

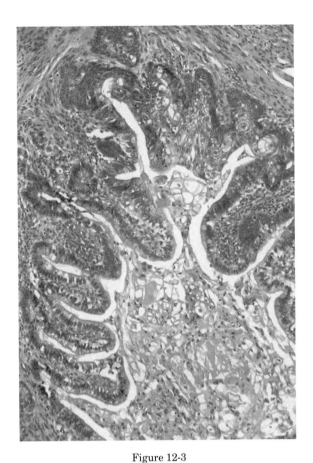

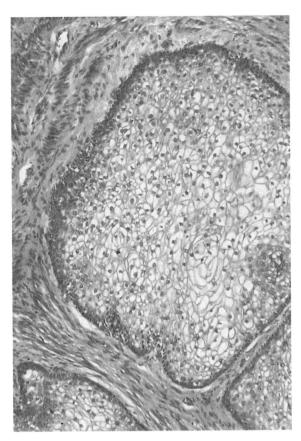

Figure 12-3
TERATOCARCINOSARCOMA
Benign glandular structures in this case have features of intestinal epithelium.

Figure 12-4
TERATOCARCINOSARCOMA
Large nests of benign squamous epithelium are commonly present.

are frequently present (figs. 12-5, 12-6). Teratocarcinosarcomas characteristically lack areas of seminoma, choriocarcinoma, yolk sac tumor, and embryonal carcinoma.

Immunohistochemical Findings. Immunohistochemical results depend upon the specific components present, but usually there is immunopositivity for cytokeratin, epithelial membrane antigen, S-100 protein, chromogranin, Ber-EP4, Leu-7, neuron-specific enolase, desmin, vimentin, and glial fibrillary acidic protein. The neoplasm lacks immunoreactivity for human chorionic gonadotropin and alphafetoprotein.

Ultrastructural Findings. The features in one case included fibroblastic and myofibroblastic differentiation of the stromal components (12). Squamous and glandular differentiation were also observed.

Differential Diagnosis. Small biopsy specimens that fail to show the heterogeneity of teratocarcinosarcoma may suggest a number of other entities. These include squamous cell carcinoma, adenocarcinoma, olfactory neuroblastoma, mixed tumor, teratoma, rhabdomyosarcoma, and craniopharyngioma, among others. While there is a predominance of neuroepithelial tissues, teratocarcinosarcoma may closely resemble olfactory neuroblastoma. The recognition of the presence of multiple components that are benign, atypical, and malignant is important for the diagnosis of teratocarcinosarcoma.

Treatment and Prognosis. Aggressive radical surgery and radiotherapy are indicated. There is no information regarding the effect of chemotherapy. In the largest study, 6 of 17 patients with follow-up developed metastatic disease to cervical lymph nodes (10). Sixty percent

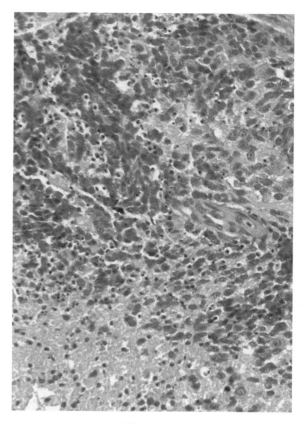

Figure 12-5
TERATOCARCINOSARCOMA
Poorly differentiated cells with neuroepithelial features are surrounded by a neurofibrillary matrix.

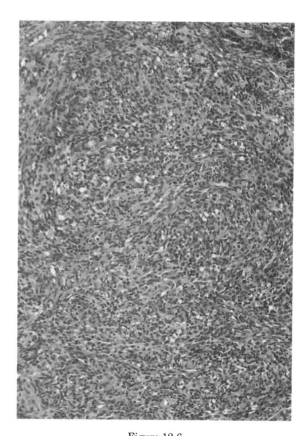

Figure 12-6
TERATOCARCINOSARCOMA
Sheets of poorly differentiated malignant cells have some areas without overt neuroepithelial features.

of patients in this study died within 3 years of diagnosis. Recurrences were common and local invasion was extensive. Three of nine patients in a smaller series died of disease within 3 years, while four with at least 2 years of follow-up were alive without evidence of tumor (11).

ENDODERMAL SINUS TUMOR

General Features. Endodermal sinus tumors arising in the upper aerodigestive tract are very rare. Lack (2) reported three examples in children; one arose in the nasopharynx, one in the oropharynx, and one in the oral cavity near the midline. Two cases of endodermal sinus tumor of the ear in young children have been described (13,15).

Clinical Features. Of the five patients described above, one was a newborn, while each of the four others was less than 1 year of age. All were females.

Microscopic Findings. The appearance of the neoplasms was similar to that for gonadal endodermal sinus tumors (14). This includes a loose papillary arrangement of neoplastic cells with surrounding connective tissue containing delicate capillary channels. One of the three cases reported by Lack (14) apparently began as a teratoma, while the other four were pure endodermal sinus tumors.

Treatment and Prognosis. Of the three cases described by Lack (14), there was incomplete resection or biopsy only in each case. Two patients received chemotherapy and all three had radiotherapy. All three patients died, however, at 7, 9, and 15 months after diagnosis. One patient died of a massive recurrence, two had lung metastases, one had lymph node metastasis, and one had brain metastasis. The two children with endodermal sinus tumor of the ear were alive without evidence of disease slightly over 1 year after surgery and chemotherapy (13,15).

REFERENCES

Teratoma

1. Dehner LP. Gonadal and extragonadal germ cell neoplasia of childhood. Hum Pathol 1983;14:493–511.
2. Dehner LP, Mills A, Talerman A, Billman GF, Krous HF, Platz CE. Germ cell neoplasms of head and neck soft tissues: a pathologic spectrum of teratomatous and endodermal sinus tumors. Hum Pathol 1990;21:309–18.
3. Ehrich WE. Teratoid parasites of the mouth (episphenoids, epipalati [epurani], epignathi). Am J Orthodont Oral Surg 1945;31:650–9.
4. Lack EE. Extragonadal germ cell tumors of the head and neck region: review of 16 cases. Hum Pathol 1985;16:56–64.
5. Lalwani AK, Engel TL. Teratoma of the tongue: a case report and review of the literature. Int J Pediatr Otorhinolaryngol 1992;24:261–8.
6. Manivel C, Wick MR, Dehner LP. Transitional (cylindric) cell carcinoma with endodermal sinus tumor-like features of the nasopharynx and paranasal sinuses. Clinicopathologic and immunohistochemical study of two cases. Arch Pathol Lab Med 1986;110:198–202.
7. Sciubba JJ, Younai F. Epipalatus: a rare intraoral teratoma. Oral Surg Oral Med Oral Pathol 1991;71:476–81.
8. Shah BL, Vasan U, Raye Jr. Teratoma of the tonsil in a premature infant. Case report and review of the literature. Am J Dis Child 1979;133:79–80.
9. Tharrington CL, Bossen EH. Nasopharyngeal teratomas. Arch Pathol Lab Med 1992;116:165–7.

Teratocarcinosarcoma

10. Heffner DK, Hyams VJ. Teratocarcinosarcoma (malignant teratoma?) of the nasal cavity and paranasal sinuses. A clinicopathologic study of 20 cases. Cancer 1984;53:2140–54.
11. Malpica A, Luna MA, Lyos AT, Silva EG. Sinonasal teratocarcinosarcoma: a clinicopathologic study of 9 cases [Abstract]. Mod Pathol 1995;8:103A.
12. Patterson SD, Ballard RW. Nasal blastoma: a light and electron microscopic study. Ultrastruct Pathol 1980;1:487–94.

Endodermal Sinus Tumor

13. Fukunaga M, Miyazawa Y, Harada T, Ushigome S, Ishikawa E. Yolk sac tumour of the ear. Histopathology 1995;27:563–7.
14. Lack EE. Extragonadal germ cell tumors of the head and neck region: review of 16 cases. Hum Pathol 1985;16:56–64.
15. Stanley RJ, Scheithauer BW, Thompson EI, et al. Endodermal sinus tumor (yolk sac tumor) of the ear. Arch Otolaryngol Head Neck Surg 1987;113:200–3.

13

METASTATIC NEOPLASMS

General Features. In a study of metastatic deposits in the sinonasal tract, approximately half occurred in the maxillary sinus, while a near equal number were found in the nasal cavity, frontal sinus, and ethmoid sinus (3); the sphenoid sinus was the least common site of metastatic disease to the paranasal sinuses. Approximately 60 percent of the primary neoplasms arose in the kidney, while most of the remainder developed in the lung, breast, or elsewhere in the urogenital tract (3). Additional anatomic sites of origin included the gastrointestinal tract, thyroid, pancreas, and adrenal gland (3,8,9). Malignant melanoma rarely metastasizes to the nasal cavity and paranasal sinuses, and, when present in the sinonasal tract, typically represents a primary neoplasm.

Metastatic neoplasms to the larynx involve the soft tissue and mucosa or the laryngeal skeleton (1,5,12). They may be present in the supraglottic, glottic, or subglottic larynx. Metastases to the laryngeal skeleton are not rare, but may not produce symptoms. Such metastases involve ossified cartilage, and are usually a manifestation of generalized bony metastatic disease. In a study of patients with bone metastases, Ehrlich (5) found that 22 percent had involvement of the thyroid and cricoid cartilages. The most common neoplasm metastatic to the larynx is melanoma, followed by carcinomas of the kidney, breast, lung, prostate, and gastrointestinal tract. In one series of metastatic neoplasms to the larynx, melanoma constituted 40 percent of the cases (12).

Neoplasms metastasize to the bones of the jaw more frequently than to the soft tissues of the oral cavity. Metastases to the latter most often involve the gingiva or tongue, followed by the lips, buccal mucosa, and palate (6,7). The most common primary sites are kidney and lung (6,7,14). In addition, melanoma and carcinomas of the breast, liver, and gastrointestinal tract also sometimes metastasize to the oral cavity (6,7,13). Metastasis to the tonsil is unusual. Bilateral tonsillar involvement by melanoma is more common than that by renal cell carcinoma (4).

Most metastases to the upper aerodigestive tract from renal cell carcinoma are found in the nasal cavity or paranasal sinuses. The first presentation of a renal cell carcinoma may occur in the upper aerodigestive tract (2,14); conversely, renal cell carcinoma may metastasize to head and neck sites many years after nephrectomy (10,11).

Clinical Features. Metastases to the nasal cavity result in nasal obstruction, pain, swelling, or bleeding (2). Metastatic renal cell carcinoma to the sinonasal tract typically presents as epistaxis (2). In 50 to 65 percent of these cases, nasal and sinus symptoms precede the discovery of the primary renal neoplasm (2). The mean age of patients with renal cell carcinoma metastatic to the sinonasal tract is over 65 years (2). This mean age is similar to that for patients with sinonasal metastatic breast cancer, but is approximately 10 years more than for patients with metastases from the lung or gastrointestinal tract.

Metastatic neoplasms to the oral cavity present as rapidly growing masses that ulcerate and hemorrhage (6). In a literature review of 12 cases of renal cell carcinoma metastatic to the tongue, the age range was 41 to 84 years (14). Ten patients were male; they often complained of a lump, oral discomfort, or hemorrhage.

Hoarseness is the most common complaint of patients with metastasis to the larynx, although stridor or airway obstruction may also occur (1,12). Sometimes laryngeal symptoms are absent, particularly when there is supraglottic involvement.

Gross Findings. Metastasis to the upper aerodigestive tract appears as a mass that is often tan-white and has areas of hemorrhage and necrosis. Ulceration is frequent.

Microscopic Findings. The metastatic deposits recapitulate the appearance of the neoplasm at its anatomic site of origin. The correct diagnosis is readily apparent when the primary site of origin is known. When presenting in the upper aerodigestive tract, however, the diagnosis may be difficult or even erroneous. Primary neoplasms of the upper aerodigestive tract may be mimicked by metastatic deposits from the breast (fig. 13-1), gastrointestinal tract, lung, and kidney (fig. 13-2). Renal cell carcinoma may simulate paraganglioma, acinic cell carcinoma,

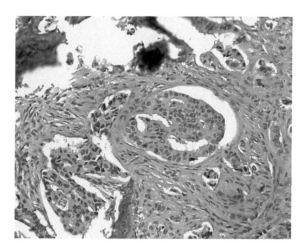

Figure 13-1
METASTATIC MAMMARY CARCINOMA
A cellular fibrotic stroma surrounds the glands and nests of metastatic ductal carcinoma to the sinonasal tract.

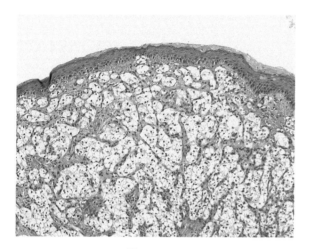

Figure 13-2
METASTATIC RENAL CELL CARCINOMA
Packets of tumor cells with abundant clear cytoplasm are characteristic of renal cell carcinoma metastatic to the upper aerodigestive tract.

and mucoepidermoid carcinoma. The knowledge that renal cell carcinoma is notorious for its presentation at distant sites, including the oral cavity and sinonasal tract, assists in the interpretation of an unusual clear cell neoplasm appearing in the head and neck.

Treatment and Prognosis. For metastatic neoplasms to the upper aerodigestive tract, palliative therapy is indicated. In an exceptional case of renal cell carcinoma, removal of the metastasis and nephrectomy may result in a favorable out-

come. For the most part, however, metastatic neoplasms to the oral cavity and sinonasal tract represent generalized disease (2). Hence, the interval between symptoms referable to the head and neck and death is usually short, regardless of the tumor type. For instance, 7 of 10 patients with renal cell carcinoma metastatic to the tongue died of disease less than 8 months after diagnosis (14). One patient, however, was alive without evidence of disease 18 months following local excision, nephrectomy, and chemotherapy (14).

REFERENCES

1. Abemayor E, Cochran AJ, Calcaterra TC. Metastatic cancer to the larynx. Diagnosis and management. Cancer 1983;52:1944–8.
2. Batsakis JG, McBurney TA. Metastatic neoplasms to the head and neck. Surg Gynecol Obstet 1971;133:673–7.
3. Bernstein JM, Montgomery WW, Balogh K Jr. Metastatic tumors to the maxilla, nose, and paranasal sinuses. Laryngoscope 1966;76:621–50.
4. Brownson RJ, LaMonte SE, Jaques WE, Zollinger WK. Hypernephroma metastatic to the palatine tonsils. Ann Otol 1979;88:235–40.
5. Ehrlich A. Tumor involving the laryngeal cartilages. Arch Otolaryngol 1954;59:178–85.
6. Hatziotis JC, Constantinidou H, Papanayotou PH. Metastatic tumors of the oral soft tissues. Review of the literature and report of a case. Oral Surg 1973;36:544–50.
7. Hirshberg A, Buchner A. Metastatic tumours to the oral region. An overview. Oral Oncol Eur J Cancer 1995;31B:355–60.
8. Kent SE, Majumdar B. Metastatic tumours in the maxillary sinus. A report of two cases and a review of the literature. J Laryngol Otol 1985;99:459–62.
9. McClatchey KD, Lloyd RV, Schaldenbrand JD. Metastatic carcinoma to the sphenoid sinus. Case report and review of the literature. Arch Otorhinolaryngol 1985;241:219–24.
10. Miyamoto R, Helmus C. Hypernephroma metastatic to the head and neck. Laryngoscope 1973;83:898–905.
11. Schantz JC, Miller SH, Graham WP III. Metastatic hypernephroma to the head and neck. J Surg Oncol 1976;8:183–90.
12. Whicker JH, Carder GA, Devine KD. Metastasis to the larynx. Report of a case and review of the literature. Arch Otolaryngol 1972;96:182–4.
13. Zegarelli DJ, Tsukada Y, Pickren JW, Greene GW Jr. Metastatic tumor to the tongue. Report of twelve cases. Oral Surg 1973;35:202–11.
14. Ziyada WF, Brookes JD, Penman HG. Expectorated tissue leading to diagnosis of renal adenocarcinoma. J Laryngol Otol 1994;108:1108–10.

14

MISCELLANEOUS SOFT TISSUE NEOPLASMS

LIPOMA

General Features. Lipomas in the head and neck region are usually solitary lesions: in a review of 24 hypopharyngeal lipomas, only 6 were multiple (4). Of the 18 solitary lipomas, 39 percent arose in the aryepiglottic fold, 28 percent were postcricoid, 11 percent were in the pyriform fossa, 11 percent were in the lateral wall, and 11 percent occurred in the arytenoid. In other reviews, approximately three fourths of laryngeal lipomas have involved the extrinsic larynx (8,11). Laryngeal involvement by adipose tissue has also been described in benign symmetrical lipomatosis (5). In the oral cavity, between one third and half of reported lipomas have arisen in the buccal mucosa of the cheek (3,8); the remainder occurred in the tongue, floor of mouth, palate, lips, or gingiva. Lingual lipomas usually arise on the lateral edge of the anterior two thirds of the tongue (7,8). Retropharyngeal lipomas are unusual, but can grow to a large size (8). In their series of 256 nonepithelial tumors of the nasal cavity, paranasal sinus, and nasopharynx, Fu and Perzin (2) saw only one lipoma.

Clinical Features. Hypopharyngeal lipomas usually occur in patients over 40 years of age (4),

more often in men. Most are asymptomatic, although some cause dysphagia, change in voice, or dyspnea. Hypopharyngeal lipomas may be pedunculated, and two patients have died of suffocation from pedunculated lesions (4). Oral lipomas are usually painless masses that are soft, mobile, and asymptomatic. Although an oral lipoma may occur at almost any age, as with hypopharyngeal lesions, most patients are over 40 years of age (3). There is a slight male predominance. Congenital oral lipomas have been described, and they chiefly involve the buccal mucosa (10).

Gross Findings. Hypopharyngeal lesions are often polypoid and measure from 2 to 23 cm in greatest dimension (4). The size of oral lesions is variable.

Microscopic Findings. Lipomas of the upper aerodigestive tract are identical to those occurring in other anatomic sites (fig. 14-1). A lesion purported to be a lipoma with a prominent myxoid component (myxolipoma) has been described in the aryepiglottic fold (1). One case of spindle cell lipoma has been described (6).

Differential Diagnosis. Unlike well-differentiated (lipoma-like) liposarcoma, lipomas do not infiltrate, and lack pleomorphic nuclei and lipoblasts (9). Purported examples of laryngeal

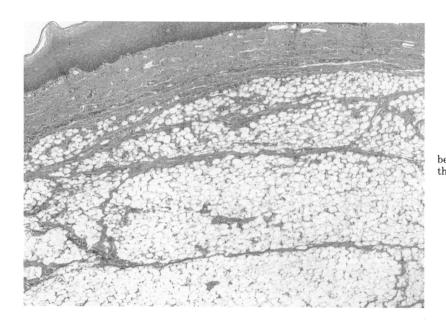

Figure 14-1
LIPOMA
Lobules of mature fat are located beneath the squamous epithelium of the buccal mucosa.

lipomas with myxoid foci need to be distinguished from vocal fold polyps with myxoid features, myxoma, and myxoid liposarcoma (9).

Treatment and Prognosis. Surgical excision is curative. A "recurrent lesion" is likely to represent a new primary lipoma or, perhaps, an incompletely excised lesion (9). A true recurrence of an excised hypopharyngeal or laryngeal fatty neoplasm would indicate that the original lesion was a well-differentiated (lipoma-like) liposarcoma, whose features may be subtle and difficult to distinguish from lipoma (9).

LEIOMYOMA

General Features. In a literature review of 257 head and neck leiomyomas, 92 arose in the cervical esophagus, 22 in the larynx, 14 in the lips, 13 in the tongue, 11 in the palate, 8 in the buccal mucosa, and 6 in the nasal cavity (12). Other head and neck sites including the trachea were also represented. Of 256 nonepithelial neoplasms of the sinonasal tract or nasopharynx, there were 2 leiomyomas and 6 leiomyosarcomas (14). Oral *vascular leiomyoma (angiomyoma)* most often occurs in the palate, cheek, or lip (15). In addition to the oral cavity, vascular leiomyomas may arise elsewhere in the upper aerodigestive tract.

Clinical Features. The age range is wide, but leiomyoma most often develops in adults from 40 to 70 years of age (12). Oral lesions are usually asymptomatic and found as a painless, nonulcerated nodule (13,15). Sinonasal leiomyomas are sometimes small incidental lesions in nasal polypectomy specimens (14).

Gross Findings. Oral vascular leiomyomas range from 0.3 to 3.0 cm in greatest dimension (15). Sinonasal lesions are usually less than 2.0 cm in greatest diameter (14). Laryngeal leiomyoma appears as a round or oval nodule covered by a smooth surfaced epithelial lining. They most often develop in the vestibular folds and may be pedunculated (16).

Microscopic Findings. The well-circumscribed nodule consists of well-differentiated smooth muscle cells (fig. 14-2). Pleomorphism is typically absent, and mitotic figures are also usually not observed. Vascular leiomyoma (angiomyoma) contains conspicuous thick-walled vessels. The outer layers of these vessels merge

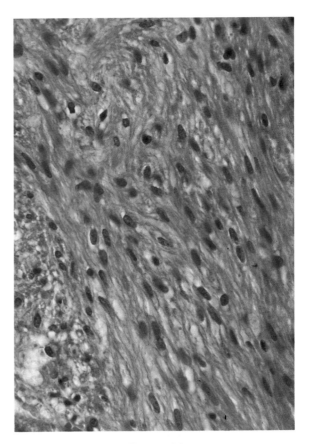

Figure 14-2
LEIOMYOMA
Smooth muscle cells with uniform, elongated nuclei characterize this neoplasm from the sinonasal tract.

with the proliferating bundles of smooth muscle cells. Although vessels with thickened walls resemble arteries, they characteristically lack both internal and external elastic laminae.

Treatment and Prognosis. Simple excision is curative.

RHABDOMYOMA

General Features. Benign skeletal muscle proliferations occurring in the head and neck include the *adult and fetal types of rhabdomyoma* and *rhabdomyomatous mesenchymal hamartoma.* Unlike cardiac rhabdomyomas, the adult type of rhabdomyoma arising the upper aerodigestive tract has no association with tuberous sclerosis (30). The most common sites of involvement of this type of rhabdomyoma include the pharynx, floor of mouth, base of tongue, and larynx (20,27,30,31,

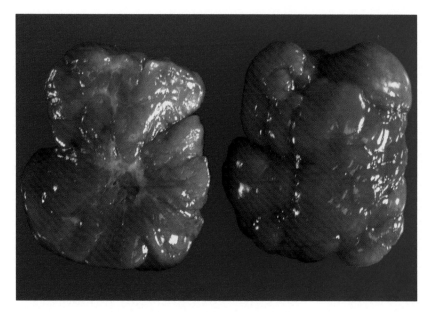

Figure 14-3
RHABDOMYOMA
The adult type typically is lobulated, firm, and red-brown.

38,39); less frequent sites include soft palate, uvula, nasopharynx, lower lip, and buccal mucosa (19,23,25,30,37). The fetal type of rhabdomyoma may be subclassified into myxoid and intermediate variants (26,28). The myxoid variant usually arises in the lamina propria or subcutaneous tissue of the head and neck, especially in the preauricular and postauricular areas and the nasopharynx. The intermediate variant occurs most often around the orbit or in the tongue, nasopharynx, and soft palate.

Rhabdomyomas of the head and neck must be distinguished from rhabdomyomatous mesenchymal hamartoma (17,33,34). This lesion occurs as solitary or multiple small papules in the skin of the face or neck of newborns or infants. It most often arises around the eye or ear and is composed of well-differentiated skeletal muscle with interposed foci of fat, fibrous tissue, and, occasionally, nerves. Rhabdomyoma must also be distinguished from benign masseter muscle hypertrophy, a unilateral or bilateral muscle enlargement that is usually accompanied by a bony overgrowth at the angle of the mandible (18). This rare condition is seen most often in adolescents or young adults and is familial or acquired.

Clinical Features. The adult type of rhabdomyoma occurs as a solitary, spherical and well-demarcated mass without accompanying tenderness or pain. There may be displacement or compression of oropharyngeal structures. Symptoms sometimes include hoarseness or difficulty in breathing or swallowing. Most patients are over 40 years of age (median, 60 years) (24); males predominate 3 to 1. Approximately 20 percent of lesions are multifocal (24). Only rare cases of the adult type of rhabdomyoma have been described in children (36).

In one study of 24 fetal rhabdomyomas, 6 were congenital, while 11 developed in patients who were at least 15 years of age (29). The age range was 3 days to 58 years (median, 4.5 years). The myxoid variant tends to occur in males in the first year of life, while the intermediate variant occurs more often in adults. Fetal rhabdomyomas are nontender, firm, movable solitary masses that, depending upon the location, may cause obstructive symptoms.

Gross Findings. Adult rhabdomyomas are circumscribed, round or lobulated masses that are usually less than 10 cm in greatest dimension. They are often red-brown and resemble the cortical surface of the kidney (fig. 14-3).

Fetal rhabdomyomas are well-circumscribed. Most are 2 to 3 cm in greatest diameter but some pedunculated masses can measure up to 12.5 cm (29). They are gray-white to pink and often have a glistening surface. They are typically solitary and located superficially.

Microscopic Findings. The adult type consists of large polyhedral cells that are demarcated by thin bands of fibrous stroma. The finely

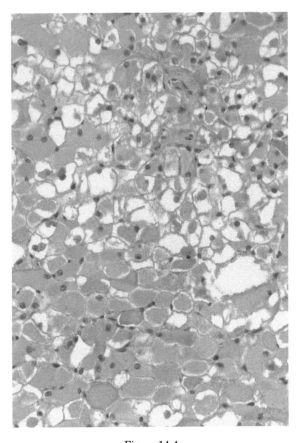

Figure 14-4
RHABDOMYOMA
Cells with abundant granular, eosinophilic cytoplasm as well as cells with vacuolated cytoplasm characterize the adult type.

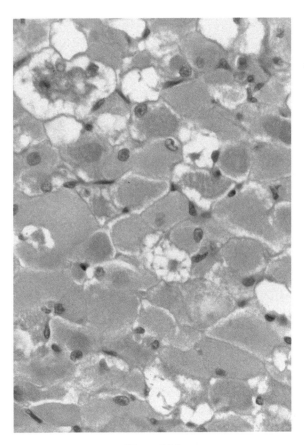

Figure 14-5
RHABDOMYOMA
So-called spider cells have a condensed core of eosinophilic cytoplasm with thin strands of cytoplasm radiating from the center.

granular cytoplasm is eosinophilic and abundant. Nuclei are vesicular and contain one or more small nucleoli. The cytoplasm of many cells, at least in part, contains vacuolated spaces which represent the intracellular glycogen that was removed during processing (fig. 14-4). The so-called spider cells are vacuolated and contain a central portion of cytoplasm with thin strands radiating to the cell membrane (fig. 14-5). Cross striations are seen in the majority of cases, but may be present in only a few cells (fig. 14-6). Intracytoplasmic rod-like or "jackstraw"-like crystalline structures are also characteristically present. Cross striations are highlighted by phosphotungstic acid hematoxylin (PTAH) and Masson trichrome stains. PTAH also highlights the intracytoplasmic crystalline structures (24). Mitotic figures are generally absent.

The myxoid variant of the fetal subtype of rhabdomyoma contains undifferentiated round or oval cells with interspersed muscle fibers set in a conspicuously myxoid matrix (fig. 14-7) (29). The muscle fibers contain small oval nuclei with evenly dispersed chromatin and inconspicuous nucleoli. The fibers may occasionally form slender fascicles (fig. 14-8). Cross striations are seen in most cases, but typically occur in only a few cells. The intermediate variant of fetal rhabdomyoma contains numerous well-formed muscle fibers (fig. 14-9). There are also spindle-shaped mesenchymal cells, but little or no myxoid intercellular material. The muscle cells are usually spindle shaped, but sometimes they simulate ganglion cells. They have abundant eosinophilic cytoplasm with central uniform vesicular nuclei. Cross striations are found in numerous cells (fig. 14-10).

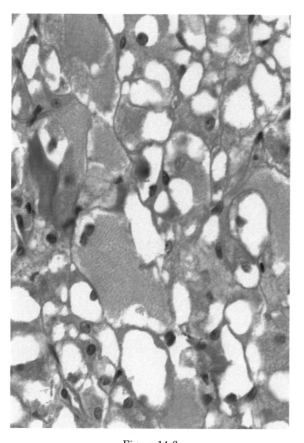

Figure 14-6
RHABDOMYOMA
Cells whose cytoplasm contains cross striations are present in most cases.

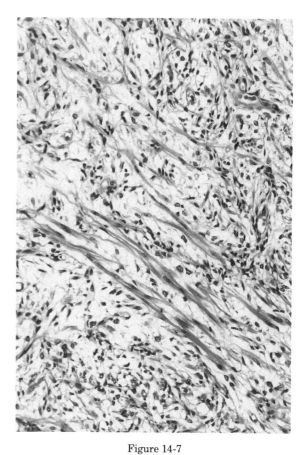

Figure 14-7
RHABDOMYOMA
The myxoid (classic) variant of fetal rhabdomyoma consists of a mixture of undifferentiated small cells and elongated muscle cells. (Courtesy of Dr. S.B. Kapadia, Pittsburgh, PA.)

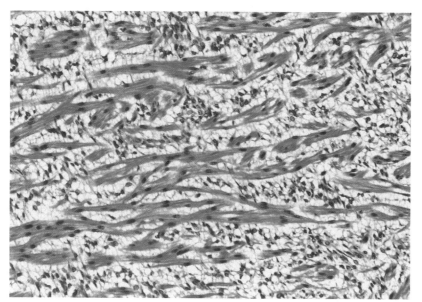

Figure 14-8
RHABDOMYOMA
Slender fascicles of muscle cells are present in this myxoid (classic) variant of fetal rhabdomyoma. (Courtesy of Dr. S.B. Kapadia, Pittsburgh, PA.)

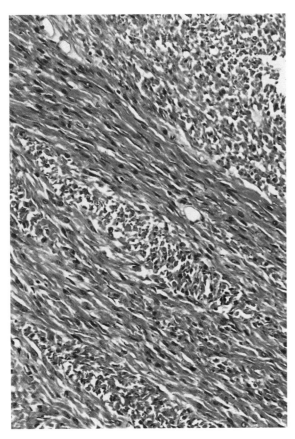

Figure 14-9
RHABDOMYOMA
Well-formed fascicles of skeletal muscle cells character-ize the intermediate variant of fetal rhabdomyoma. (Cour-tesy of Dr. S.B. Kapadia, Pittsburgh, PA.)

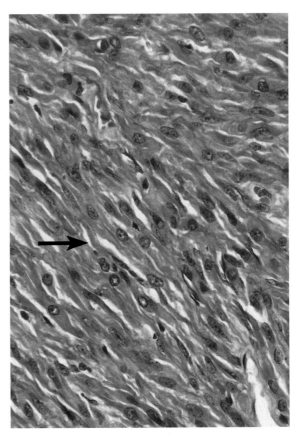

Figure 14-10
RHABDOMYOMA
Cross striations are conspicuous in cells of the interme-diate variant of fetal rhabdomyoma. (Courtesy of Dr. S.B. Kapadia, Pittsburgh, PA.)

Cytoplasmic vacuoles (glycogen) may also be pres-ent, and occasional spider-like cells are seen (28). There may be transitional forms between the myxoid and intermediate variants of rhabdo-myoma, which may represent differentiation of the myxoid to the intermediate variant (24). Fetal rhabdomyomas are sometimes associated with peripheral nerves and focal fibroblastic prolifer-ation, raising the possibility that they may be related to benign Triton tumor (neuromuscular hamartoma) (24). In a series of 24 cases, 19 fetal rhabdomyomas lacked mitotic figures, while 5 had 1 to 40 mitotic figures per 50 high-power fields (28). Fetal rhabdomyomas lack a cambium layer, conspicuous necrosis, and pleomorphism.

Immunohistochemical Findings. Adult rhabdomyomas are usually reactive for muscle-specific actin, desmin, alpha-smooth muscle actin, and myoglobin (30). In one study, 6 of 17 were immunoreactive for vimentin, 14 of 21 for S-100 protein, and 10 of 20 for Leu-7 (30). They typi-cally lack staining for cytokeratin, epithelial membrane antigen, CD68, and glial fibrillary acidic protein (GFAP). Fetal rhabdomyomas are immunoreactive for myoglobin, desmin, and muscle-specific actin (29). Sometimes they show immunopositivity for vimentin, smooth muscle actin, S-100 protein, GFAP, and Leu-7. They lack staining for cytokeratin, epithelial membrane antigen, and CD68.

Ultrastructural Findings. The cells of the adult type of rhabdomyoma are surrounded by a thin basal lamina and their cytoplasm is filled with mitochondria, thick and thin myofilaments, and distinct Z lines within I bands (19,21,31,35). Sometimes A, H, M, and N bands are also noted.

Crystalline structures are formed by hypertrophic Z bands. Fetal rhabdomyomas contain organized thick and thin myofilaments with characteristic banding (22,29). Rod-like inclusions and hypertrophied Z bands are less common than in the adult variant. As in the adult variant, glycogen may be present. The spindle-shaped cells in fetal rhabdomyoma show little differentiation.

Other Special Techniques. Clonal cytogenetic changes have been described in a case of adult rhabdomyoma (27). This consisted of a reciprocal translocation of chromosomes 15 and 17 and an abnormality of chromosome 10.

Differential Diagnosis. The microscopic features of adult rhabdomyoma are characteristic. Although it typically does not lead to other differential diagnostic considerations, neoplasms that might potentially be considered include granular cell tumor, hibernoma, rhabdomyosarcoma, oncocytoma, paraganglioma, and alveolar soft part sarcoma. Rhabdomyoma may be mimicked by crystal-storing histiocytosis associated with lymphoplasmacytic neoplasms (28). This rare condition has involved the upper aerodigestive tract in a few cases, and manifests as a neoplastic lymphoplasmacytic infiltrate that is masked by sheets of benign histiocytes filled with sheaves of crystals. Unlike rhabdomyoma, crystal-storing histiocytosis contains atypical monoclonal lymphoplasmacytic cells, and the histiocytes are immunoreactive for CD68, but lack staining for muscle-specific actin, desmin, and myoglobin (28).

Fetal rhabdomyomas must be distinguished from rhabdomyosarcoma, in particular the embryonal and spindle cell types. Unlike rhabdomyosarcoma, rhabdomyoma is superficially located, is well circumscribed, and often lacks mitotic figures. Significant pleomorphism, necrosis, invasion, and a cambium layer are absent. There are rare cases of possible transformation from fetal rhabdomyoma to sarcoma (24,32).

Treatment and Prognosis. Local excision for fetal rhabdomyoma is curative; recurrences are exceptional (29). For adult rhabdomyoma, excision is usually curative, although recurrence may develop if it is incomplete. In one series, 8 of 19 adult rhabdomyomas recurred from 2 to 11 years after diagnosis (30). Some "recurrences" may actually represent a second primary rhabdomyoma; an additional rhabdomyoma may be found many years after removal of the initial neoplasm.

CHONDROMA

General Features. Benign cartilaginous lesions of the upper aerodigestive tract include *extraskeletal chondroma, chondroid choristoma,* and *chondromatous metaplasia.* In one study of 128 cartilaginous lesions of the sinonasal tract or oropharynx, 50 percent arose in the nasal cavity and ethmoids; 17 percent in the nasal septum; 18 percent in the maxilla and antrum; 6 percent in the hard palate; 6 percent in the oropharynx, sphenoid sinus, and eustachian tube; and 3 percent in the alar cartilages (48). Some nasal or nasopharyngeal lesions might actually represent hypertrophy of nasal septal cartilage or heterotopic islands of cartilage in the nasopharyngeal mucosa (choristoma) (43). Hence, some small and incidental cartilaginous lesions may be metaplastic or hamartomatous. When present in the oral cavity, extraskeletal chondroma has a propensity for developing in the tongue (41,51). When benign cartilaginous foci are found in the tonsils or tissues underneath ill-fitting dentures, it is likely that they represent metaplastic changes secondary to chronic inflammation and fibrosis (40,42). Chondromatous metaplasia beneath dentures more often occurs in the maxilla than in the mandible. It is present more frequently anteriorly than posteriorly and is found more commonly in women (42).

The majority of cartilaginous neoplasms of the larynx are malignant, but are of low grade. True chondromas of the larynx are rare, and arise from preexisting cartilage (45,47,49,50). Cartilaginous metaplasia may be seen in the soft tissues of the true cords (44). The solitary, small focus may be secondary to laryngeal trauma. It should be remembered that bilateral cartilaginous nodules are present normally in the anterior portion of the thyroarytenoid ligament (fig. 14-11) (46).

Clinical Features. Sinonasal and pharyngeal chondromas are usually asymptomatic and are found incidentally (43). The smooth surfaced nodules occur in patients with a wide age range. Benign chondromatous foci in the tonsil are typically incidental findings that are unilateral (40). Cartilaginous metaplasia beneath dentures appears as a raised and erythematous ulcer or a firm, movable, and pale polyp (42). It is usually solitary, and is found more often in women. Of 11 lingual chondromas reviewed in one study, patients

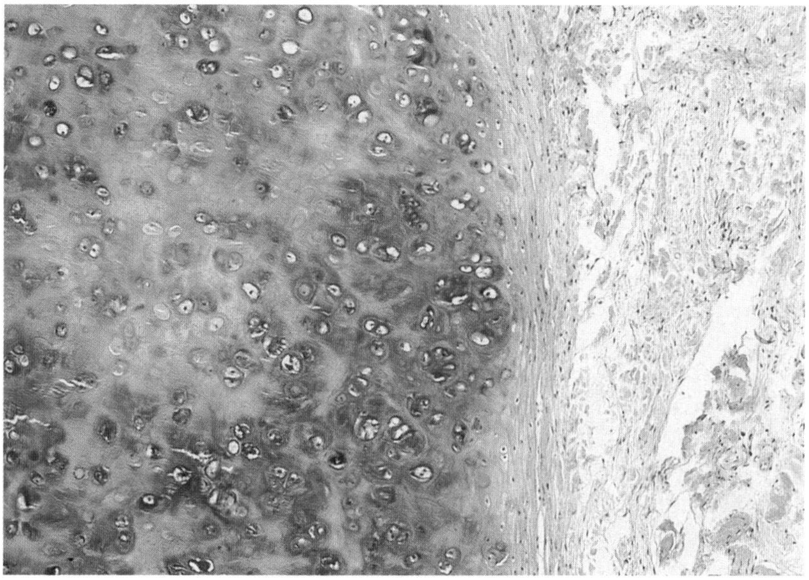

Figure 14-11
THYROARYTENOID LIGAMENT
Bilateral cartilaginous nodules in this location should not be misinterpreted as a benign or a low-grade malignant cartilaginous neoplasm.

ranged in age from 2 to 52 years and there was no sex predilection (51). Nine of the 11 were present on the lateral portion of the tongue. They appeared as mobile, hard, painless nodules. Patients with laryngeal chondromas usually present with hoarseness, but occasionally there is dyspnea.

Gross Findings. Sinonasal or nasopharyngeal chondromas are usually 0.5 to 2.0 cm in greatest dimension (43). They are firm and well circumscribed. Laryngeal lesions also tend to be small, while lingual tumors can be up to 5 cm in greatest dimension (51). Chondromatous metaplasia of the vocal cord is typically less than 1 cm and is single (44). All chondromas are typically covered by smooth surfaced epithelium.

Microscopic Findings. Chondromas are composed of circumscribed mature hyaline cartilage that may be surrounded by perichondrium-like connective tissue (fig. 14-12). Cellular atypia is absent and mitotic figures are absent or rare. Foci of calcification or bone may be present. Cartilaginous foci in the tonsil are present in the connective tissue and not in the lymphoid component (fig. 14-13) (40). Cartilaginous metaplasia of the larynx appears as central chondrocytes surrounded by peripheral fibroblasts (44); there is initial accumulation of acid mucopolysaccharides between strands of collagen and subsequent metaplasia into chondrocytes. Cartilaginous metaplastic foci beneath dentures may show foci of calcification and bone (42). Mitotic figures are

typically absent. Occasionally there is mild hyperchromatism and nuclear enlargement.

Differential Diagnosis. Benign laryngeal proliferations must be distinguished from well-differentiated chondrosarcoma. Cartilaginous lesions greater than 2 cm in diameter that possess nuclear atypicality and show local extension are malignant.

Treatment and Prognosis. Simple excision of benign cartilaginous lesions at any site is curative.

OSSIFYING FIBROMYXOID TUMOR

General Features. This mesenchymal lesion has features suggestive of Schwann cell differentiation and most often arises in the deep subcutaneous tissue or skeletal muscle of the extremities. Two of the nine head and neck neoplasms that have been reported arose in the upper aerodigestive tract; one tumor occurred beneath the gingival mucosa while the other developed below the palatal mucosa (52).

Clinical Features. One of the two upper aerodigestive tract tumors occurred in a 67-year-old female and the other developed in a 37-year-old man.

Gross Findings. A white-tan, firm mass was observed below the oral mucosa. The larger lesion measured 4.5 cm.

Microscopic Findings. Small, uniform, round cells in nests or cords are present in tumor lobules. Neoplastic lobules are moderately cellular

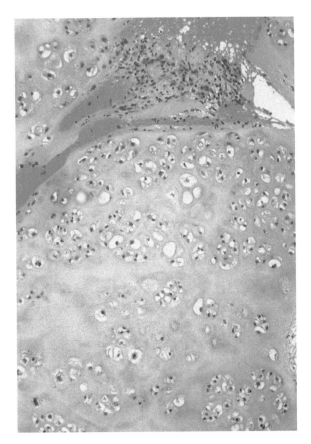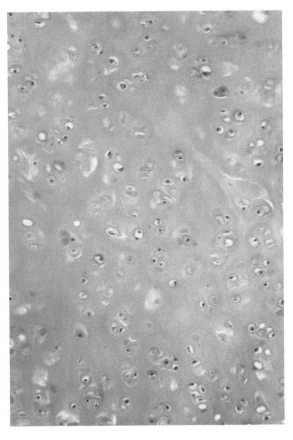

Figure 14-12
CHONDROMA
Mature chondrocytes set in an abundant cartilaginous matrix are seen in these examples from the sinonasal tract (left) and tongue (right).

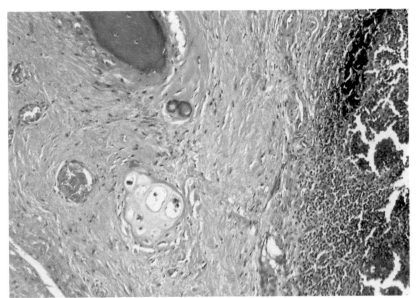

Figure 14-13
CARTILAGINOUS AND
OSSEOUS METAPLASIA
Metaplastic foci of cartilage and bone are present in the connective tissue component of the tonsil.

and consist of cells having nuclei with inconspicuous nucleoli. The stroma within the lesion is myxoid or hyalinized, and is surrounded in part by dense fibrous connective tissue. The amount of chondro-osseous matrix is variable. The lobules are sometimes delimited by a thin, incomplete shell of lamellar bone. Mitotic figures are infrequent.

Immunohistochemical Findings. Ossifying fibromyxoid tumors of the head and neck are sometimes positive for S-100 protein, neuron-specific enolase, and Leu-7 (52). Occasionally they stain for GFAP, smooth muscle actin (1A8), and muscle-specific actin (HHF 35). They are typically immunoreactive for vimentin, but do not stain for cytokeratin, epithelial membrane antigen, and neurofilament.

Treatment and Prognosis. After the lesion was excised, each patient was without evidence of disease 1.5 and 3 years, respectively, after treatment.

ECTOMESENCHYMAL CHONDROMYXOID TUMOR

General Features. Nineteen cases of this new clinicopathologic entity were reported in 1995 (53). Each lesion arose in the anterior dorsum of the tongue.

Clinical Features. The patients ranged in age from 9 to 78 years (median, 32 years). There was no race or sex predilection. The lesions appeared as slowly growing nodules, typically without inducing pain or discomfort. Their duration ranged from a few months up to 8 to 10 years. They ranged in size from 0.3 to 2.0 cm.

Gross Findings. The neoplasms were submucosal and pale gray, tan, or yellow. They were small and rubbery. On cut surface, they often had a gelatinous appearance and sometimes showed foci of hemorrhage.

Microscopic Findings. The well-circumscribed lobules of tumor were set in the superficial lingual musculature (fig. 14-14). Sometimes normal muscle fibers and nerve branches were entrapped within the neoplastic lobules. The myxoid background consisted of cells distributed as cords, strands, or net-like sheets (fig. 14-15). Neoplastic cells were round, fusiform, or polygonal, and had regular small nuclei and small amounts of slightly basophilic cytoplasm (fig. 14-16). The background often had chondroid or

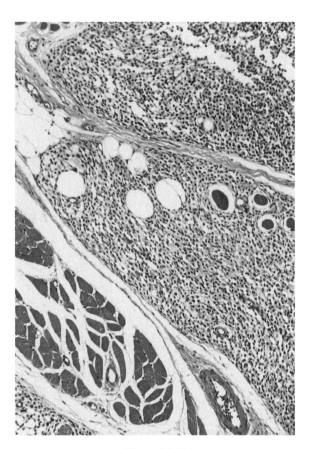

Figure 14-14
ECTOMESENCHYMAL CHONDROMYXOID TUMOR
Lobules of neoplasm separate and sometimes entrap lingual skeletal muscle.

hyalinized foci. A few tumors had focal cytologic atypia manifested by nuclear pleomorphism, hyperchromatism, and multinucleation. Mitotic figures were scarce. When present, nucleoli were single and inconspicuous. Some cup-shaped nuclei had eosinophilic fibrillary material along concave surfaces. Pseudocystic spaces or clefts were sometimes found in the mucinous stroma. The neoplasms also contained small capillaries, some of which were dilated. Hemosiderin granules were sometimes present.

The overlying squamous epithelial rete ridges were often flattened, but were usually separated from the neoplasm by a band of connective tissue. A few tumors abutted the basal layer of the squamous epithelium. Focal ulceration was uncommon.

Aldehyde fuchsin stains were positive, indicating the presence of highly acidic sulfated mucosubstances. Positivity with the alcian blue stain

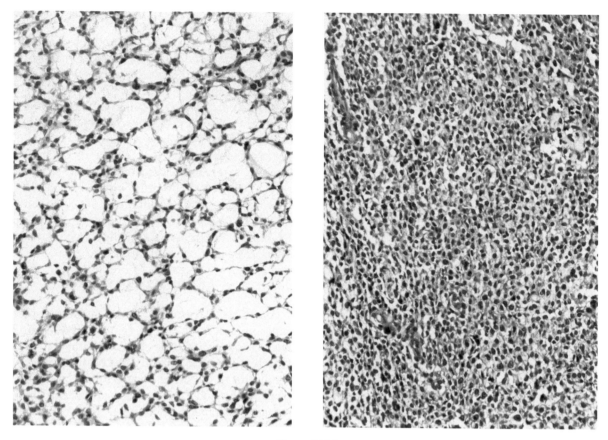

Figure 14-15
ECTOMESENCHYMAL CHONDROMYXOID TUMOR
Small cells with scant cytoplasm are typically present in a myxoid matrix (left) or, less often, are packed together with less intercellular connective tissue (right).

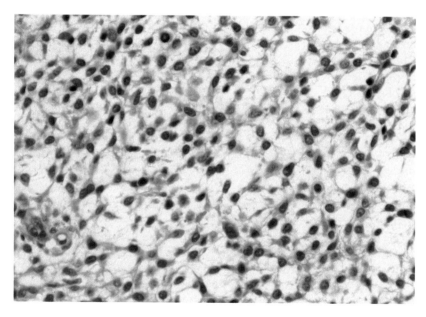

Figure 14-16
ECTOMESENCHYMAL
CHONDROMYXOID TUMOR
Most often, the small cells are uniform, lack prominent nuclei, and have scant cytoplasm. Mitotic figures are rare.

was also indicative of the presence of acidic mucosubstances, which were resistant to bovine testicular hyaluronidase. Tumor cells lacked staining with periodic acid–Schiff (PAS).

Immunohistochemical Findings. Immunopositivity with polyclonal anti-GFAP was seen in each of 13 examined tumors, while monoclonal anti-GFAP was positive in 8 of 11 neoplasms. An anticytokeratin antibody cocktail showed immunoreactivity in 12 of 13 cases. At least focal positivity for S-100 protein was observed in 9 of 15 tumors. Variable immunoreactivity for CD57 occurred in 8 of 9. Scattered tumor cells in 7 of 13 cases were positive for smooth muscle actin, but none of the tumors studied was immunoreactive for desmin and none of 5 tumors examined was immunoreactive for epithelial membrane antigen.

Ultrastructural Findings. Neoplastic cells had bilobated and concave nuclei with evenly distributed chromatin. Nucleoli were small and single or double. Some cells were surrounded by partial basal lamina. Desmosomes and condensations of thin filaments, features of myoepithelial cells, were absent.

Differential Diagnosis. Unlike ectomesenchymal chondromyxoid tumor, mucocele results from spillage of salivary mucin into connective tissue, and occurs in the ventral part of the tongue. Oral focal mucinosis, very rarely occurring in the tongue, lacks a lobular architecture and the histochemical and immunohistochemical findings of ectomesenchymal chrondromyxoid tumor. Intraoral soft tissue myxomas are rare, if they occur, while ossifying fibromyxoid tumor of soft parts has not been reported to arise in the tongue. Extraskeletal myxoid chondrosarcoma, very rarely arising in the tongue, generally lacks immunoreactivity for cytokeratin and GFAP. Additional lesions in the differential diagnosis include heterotopic glial tissue, chondroid chordoma, and nerve sheath myxoma. Ectomesenchymal chrondromyxoid tumor must also be distinguished from pleomorphic adenoma and myoepithelioma. Immunoreactivity for GFAP and cytokeratin plus the variable immunopositivity for S-100 protein and smooth muscle actin are similar for neoplastic myoepithelial cells and the cells of ectomesenchymal chondromyxoid tumor. However, salivary neoplasms arising in the tongue are expected to be ventral rather than dorsal lingual nodules. Also, the appearance of ecto-

mesenchymal chondromyxoid tumor does not simulate that of any salivary gland tumor seen elsewhere. The unique aspects of the neoplasm include the lingual location, histologic features, and immunohistochemical profile.

Treatment and Prognosis. The follow-up interval for the 11 patients with available information ranged from 2 months to 19 years (mean, 15 months). One patient had a recurrence 3 months after initial excision, while another tumor recurred at the site of an excision done 20 years previously. The remainder of the patients have been free of disease. Although the follow-up is somewhat limited, the clinical behavior appears to be that of a benign tumor.

LIPOSARCOMA

General Features. This neoplasm represents approximately 1 percent of all head and neck sarcomas (56). It is rare in the upper aerodigestive tract. In a study of 256 nonepithelial neoplasms of the nasal cavity, sinuses, and nasopharynx, Fu and Perzin (55) reported only 1 liposarcoma (sinonasal). Additional cases have been described in the pharynx, parapharyngeal area, cheek, soft palate, floor of the mouth, tongue, larynx, lip, mastoid, and nasopharynx (54,57,58). Ten liposarcomas of the oral cavity were collected from the literature by Saddik et al. (57). Of 76 head and neck liposarcomas collected by Golledge et al. (56), 28 percent arose in the neck, 20 percent in the larynx, and 18 percent in the pharynx.

Clinical Features. Wenig and colleagues (58) described the clinicopathologic features of 10 laryngeal and hypopharyngeal liposarcomas; they also reviewed the literature and found 10 additional cases. For the 10 cases described by Wenig and colleagues, the age range was 37 to 77 years. Nine of the 10 neoplasms occurred in men. The tumors arose in the supraglottic larynx or pyriform sinus. Some of the patients complained of airway obstruction. Overall for head and neck liposarcoma, the median age for patients is in the seventh decade with a male predominance (56).

Gross Findings. The findings are similar to those for liposarcomas appearing in soft tissue. Well-differentiated tumors tend to be lobulated. Most arising in the oral cavity are less than 3 cm in greatest dimension (57).

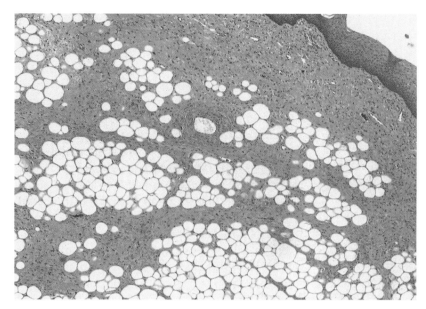

Figure 14-17
LIPOSARCOMA
This well-differentiated laryngeal neoplasm consists of lobules of adipocytes separated by fibrous connective tissue.

Microscopic Findings. The neoplasms may be myxoid, round cell, or pleomorphic, but most are well differentiated. All of the laryngeal and hypopharyngeal lesions in the series of Wenig and colleagues were well differentiated and sclerosing (58). They consisted of mature adipocytes separated by fibrous bands (fig. 14-17). Some of the adipocytes contained atypical nuclei, and lipoblasts were also present (fig. 14-18). The neoplasms were uncircumscribed. Similarly, oral cavity liposarcomas are typically well differentiated (57), and have little or no mitotic activity.

Differential Diagnosis. Laryngeal and hypopharyngeal liposarcomas may be difficult to distinguish from lipoma. The presence of cells with atypical nuclei and infiltrating tumor margins are important for the diagnosis for liposarcoma. "Atypical lipoma" was felt to be a less desirable term than liposarcoma for the group of lesions of the larynx and hypopharynx described by Wenig and colleagues (58). As oral cavity liposarcomas are also typically well differentiated, they may be confused with atypical lipomas and spindle cell lipomas (57). Hence, well-differentiated "atypical" lipomatous tumors of the upper aerodigestive tract should generally be regarded as low-grade liposarcomas.

Treatment and Prognosis. In the study of 10 laryngeal and hypopharyngeal lesions, no cases metastasized after surgery, but some resulted in multiple recurrences (58). A sinonasal liposarcoma extended to the cranial cavity and resulted

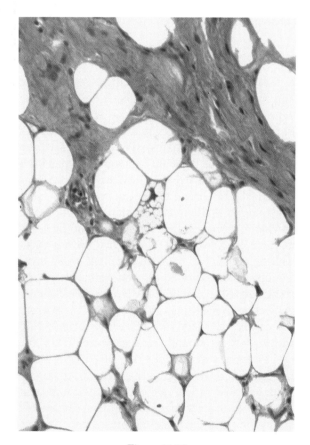

Figure 14-18
LIPOSARCOMA
Occasional lipoblasts are interspersed between mature-appearing adipocytes.

in the death of the patient (55). Oral cavity neoplasms have a high recurrence rate, but almost no tendency for metastasis (57). There may be a long interval between the primary diagnosis and recurrence. Wide local excision is appropriate therapy for primary well-differentiated liposarcomas as well as their local recurrences.

In the review of head and neck liposarcomas by Golledge et al. (56), the overall 5-year survival rate was 67 percent. The survival rate for patients with well-differentiated tumors was 100 percent; for those with myxoid neoplasms, 73 percent; for patients with pleomorphic tumors, 42 percent; and 0 percent for patients with round cell liposarcoma. The 5-year survival rate for patients with oral cavity liposarcoma was 50 percent (despite the low-grade appearance of each of the neoplasms), while it was 89 percent for patients with laryngeal neoplasms (56). Surgery is the most important treatment modality; radiotherapy and chemotherapy are reserved for those neoplasms that are not well differentiated.

CHONDROSARCOMA

General Features. When involving the head and neck, this sarcoma may arise from craniofacial bones or soft tissue of the upper aerodigestive tract. In the nasal cavity the neoplasm has developed in the septum and turbinates, paranasal sinuses, and nasopharynx (62,63,66,69). Sometimes when it involves the sinonasal area it is difficult to determine the exact site of origin because of its extent. Chondrosarcoma is the most common sarcoma of the larynx; in addition, it comprises most of the cartilaginous neoplasms of the larynx. In the past, well-differentiated chondrosarcomas were occasionally misinterpreted as chondroma, only to be recognized as sarcoma at recurrence. Most laryngeal chondrosarcomas (75 percent) arise from the cricoid cartilage and project anteriorly into the airway as smooth masses (60,61,64,65,67, 68), 17 percent arise in the thyroid cartilage, and the remainder develop in the corniculate, arytenoid, or epiglottic cartilage. Computed tomography (CT) scan of laryngeal chondrosarcoma often shows calcified foci within a mass that involves one or more of the cartilages (68).

Clinical Features. In a series of 56 chondrosarcomas of the jaw and facial bones from the Mayo Clinic (69), 45 percent involved the alveolar portion of the maxilla and maxillary sinus; 41 percent involved the nasal septum, ethmoid sinus, and sphenoid sinus; 11 percent involved the mandible; and 3 percent involved the nasal tip. The age range of patients in two other series of sinonasal or nasopharyngeal chondrosarcomas that included 23 cases was 20 months to 74 years (62,63). There was no sex predilection. Patients present with nasal obstruction, swelling, epistaxis, or a mass. Those with laryngeal chondrosarcoma complain of dyspnea, dysphagia, stridor, or hoarseness. The duration of symptoms ranges from a few weeks to several years. Most patients are over 50 years of age. The majority of patients with laryngeal chondrosarcoma are men, in a ratio of 3-4 to 1 (60,61,64,65,67,68). Chondrosarcomas may develop in the nasal cavity and paranasal sinuses of children, however. In fact, 81 percent of craniofacial chondrosarcomas reported in children involved the sinonasal tract (69).

Gross Findings. The neoplasm has a cartilaginous appearance, as it is firm, lobulated, gray, and glistening. The overlying surface mucosa is usually smooth. Most lesions measure over 2 cm in greatest dimension; chondrosarcomas of the jaw or facial bones range from 1 to 12 cm (median, 4 cm) (69).

Microscopic Findings. Most laryngeal chondrosarcomas are low grade (fig. 14-19). They are composed of lobules of well-differentiated hyaline cartilage that may have foci of calcification and ossification. The neoplasm may invade adjacent cartilage, but the borders typically are pushing. Nuclei are moderately hyperchromatic and may be enlarged. A lack of necrosis is usual, and mitotic figures appear absent or are sparse. Rarely, there are areas of dedifferentiation (59). In one study of 10 sinonasal chondrosarcomas, 6 were well differentiated, 3 were moderately differentiated, and 1 was poorly differentiated (fig. 14-20) (63).

Most chondrosarcomas of the jaw or facial bones have a lobulated growth pattern consisting of hyaline cartilage (69). Of the 56 tumors in the series from the Mayo Clinic, 43 were grade 1, 13 were grade 2, and none were grade 3 (69).

Immunohistochemical Findings. In general, immunoreactivity for S-100 protein and vimentin is usual. Chondrosarcoma lacks immunoreactivity for cytokeratin, epithelial membrane antigen, and carcinoembryonic antigen.

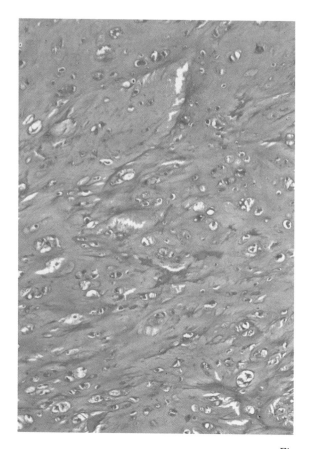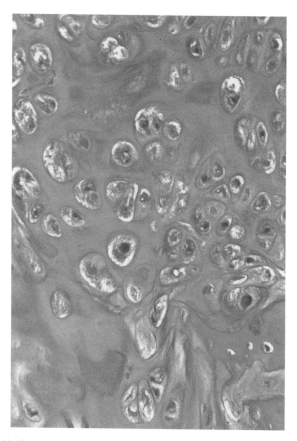

Figure 14-19
CHONDROSARCOMA

Most cartilaginous neoplasms of the larynx are low grade, and consist of an abundant matrix that surrounds chondrocytes showing only mild nuclear irregularities.

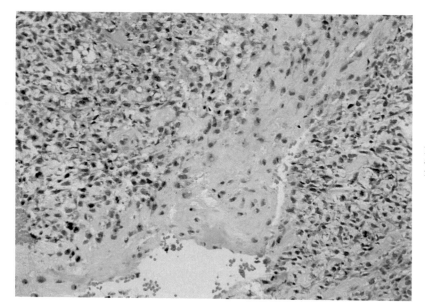

Figure 14-20
CHONDROSARCOMA

Sinonasal cartilaginous neoplasms sometimes are hypercellular and contain cells with more marked nuclear irregularities.

Differential Diagnosis. The most important neoplasms to distinguish from chondrosarcoma are chondroblastic osteosarcoma, pleomorphic adenoma (mixed tumor), and chondroma. In chondroblastic osteosarcoma of the jaw, sheets of spindle cells, spindling of tumor cells toward the periphery of lobules, and osteoid are typically present (69). The finding of epithelial areas within a sinonasal or laryngeal neoplasm containing well-differentiated cartilage is characteristic of pleomorphic adenoma (mixed tumor). Although well-differentiated laryngeal chondrosarcomas may be difficult to distinguish microscopically from chondromas, it should be kept in mind that most cartilaginous neoplasms of the larynx are malignant. The finding of cells with some nuclear atypia in a neoplasm involving several sites in the larynx is diagnostic of chondrosarcoma. The diagnosis of chondroma should be reserved for small, well-circumscribed cartilaginous nodules. Enchondroma is extremely rare or even nonexistent in the jaw and facial bones (69).

Treatment and Prognosis. Radical resection, even for recurrent tumors, is appropriate for sinonasal neoplasms. Recurrences relate to positive resection margins, tumor location, and tumor grade (63). Patients with lesions arising in the nasopharynx, posterior nasal cavity, and sphenoid sinus typically have a poor prognosis. For laryngeal chondrosarcoma, the success of complete excision may vary according to tumor location and size. As most neoplasms are well-differentiated, conservative surgery, if possible, is recommended (61). Total laryngectomy is suggested when the primary neoplasm is high grade or when conservative surgery is not feasible. Many laryngeal chondrosarcomas can be managed without laryngectomy. Laryngectomy may be indicated for recurrent lesions.

Sinonasal chondrosarcoma typically has a slow progressive course. Recurrences may be multiple, and death results from uncontrollable local growth. Metastases occur typically in less than 10 percent of cases. Approximately 60 percent of patients with sinonasal or nasopharyngeal tumors died of disease or were alive with tumor (63). Death may occur more than 10 years after treatment. Laryngeal chondrosarcoma behaves similarly, as the neoplasm tends to recur locally (60,61,64,65,67,68). Local recurrence may prove fatal. Less than 10 percent of reported cases have

metastasized, usually to the lungs or cervical lymph nodes. As expected, metastases are more apt to develop from high-grade neoplasms.

In the Mayo Clinic series of chondrosarcomas of the jaw and facial bones (69), one third of the patients had local recurrence. There were no cases of distant metastasis. The overall actuarial 10-year survival rate was 65 percent. No differences in survival were noted according to tumor location, size, or histologic grade.

MESENCHYMAL CHONDROSARCOMA

General and Clinical Features. This rare variant of chondrosarcoma arises from bone or soft tissue. It predilects sites in the head and neck, especially the orbit, skull, and jaws. Approximately 25 percent of skeletal mesenchymal chondrosarcomas arise in craniofacial bones (72, 74). Rare examples have been reported in the upper aerodigestive tract and involved the ethmoid sinus, palate, nasopharynx, nasal cavity, and paramandibular soft tissue (70,74). Although the age range is wide, the neoplasm tends to occur in adolescents or young adults of 10 to 30 years of age. One has been described in a neonate as a congenital nasal polyp (73). There seems to be no sex predilection.

Gross Findings. The multinodular neoplasm appears fleshy and gray-white. Gritty foci may be noted upon sectioning, while specimen X rays sometimes show stippled or flocculent calcifications. Hemorrhage and necrosis may be observed.

Microscopic Findings. Sheets of closely packed, small blue cells are present with occasional interspersed islands of well-differentiated cartilaginous tissue (fig. 14-21). The small blue cells have round or oval hyperchromatic nuclei with scant cytoplasm. Sometimes they are arranged in a hemangiopericytoma-like pattern (fig. 14-22) (71) or as spindle-shaped cells forming a herringbone pattern. The number of cartilaginous nodules is variable and sometimes only a few are present (fig. 14-23). The cartilaginous component may be calcified or ossified. Osteoid is absent. Mitotic figures range from sparse to numerous.

Immunohistochemical Findings. For typical cases, an antibody to S-100 protein labels the cells of the cartilaginous component only, while vimentin is present in cells of the cartilaginous component and those of the small cell component

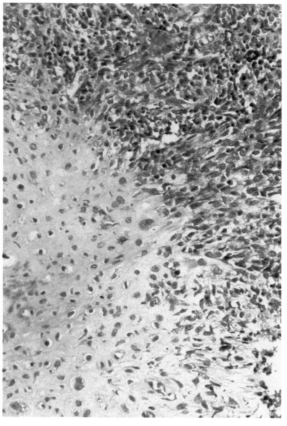

Figure 14-21
MESENCHYMAL CHONDROSARCOMA
Densely packed small cells with scant cytoplasm abut a nodule of cells in a cartilaginous matrix.

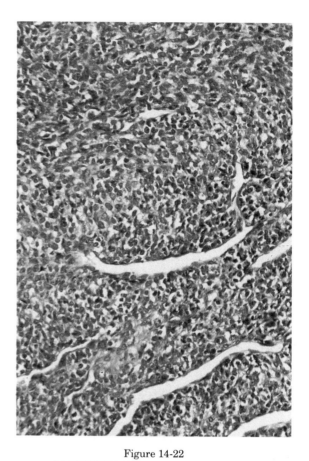

Figure 14-22
MESENCHYMAL CHONDROSARCOMA
Small cells with hyperchromatic nuclei are interspersed between vessels imparting a hemangiopericytoma-like pattern.

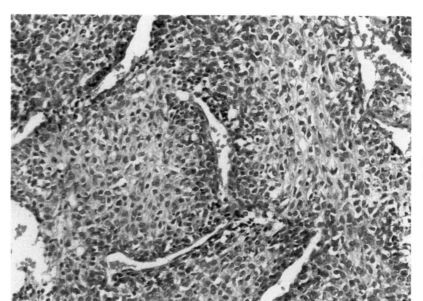

Figure 14-23
MESENCHYMAL
CHONDROSARCOMA
Small nodules of cells that are loosely packed suggest an attempt at cartilaginous differentiation.

(75). The small cells are also immunoreactive for neuron-specific enolase and Leu-7. Cytokeratin, epithelial membrane antigen, and desmin are typically absent.

Differential Diagnosis. Numerous small blue cell neoplasms may enter into the differential diagnosis when the cartilaginous component is absent in small biopsy specimens. They include hemangiopericytoma, synovial sarcoma, Ewing's sarcoma, peripheral neuroectodermal tumor, olfactory neuroblastoma, rhabdomyosarcoma, small cell osteosarcoma, undifferentiated carcinoma, granulocytic sarcoma, and malignant lymphoma. Selected immunohistochemical stains are useful in establishing the proper diagnosis.

Treatment and Prognosis. Radical surgery is the usual therapeutic modality. There is a general tendency for metastasis to regional lymph nodes and bones (72). Overall, the behavior of the neoplasm is variable, but often it is fatal (74). Recurrences may be late.

EXTRASKELETAL MYXOID CHONDROSARCOMA

General and Clinical Features. This neoplasm usually develops in the deep soft tissues of the extremities or in bone. Although it is typically classified as a low-grade sarcoma, it sometimes results in recurrence or metastasis. In the upper aerodigestive tract, reported cases have arisen in the maxillary sinus, epiglottis, arytenoid cartilage, and tongue (76,78–80). An epiglottic neoplasm occurred in a 15-year-old male (80), while a neoplasm of the arytenoid cartilage developed in a 61-year-old female (78).

Gross Findings. The epiglottic neoplasm was gelatinous and tan-gray, and measured 4.8 cm in diameter.

Microscopic Findings. The neoplasm, consisting of circumscribed lobules, contains oval or stellate cells within a variably mucoid matrix. Nuclei are small and hyperchromatic, and are surrounded by deeply eosinophilic cytoplasm. The cells are arranged in anastomosing cords and strands. Mitotic figures are typically few. The cytoplasm may contain glycogen. Foci consisting of differentiated cartilaginous cells are rare. The myxoid stroma stains with colloidal iron and alcian blue, and is not inhibited by hyaluronidase.

Immunohistochemical Findings. In an examination of 26 cases arising in the trunk or extremities, immunostaining for S-100 protein was present in 27 percent, epithelial membrane antigen in 26 percent, and cytokeratin in 9 percent (77); vimentin was positive in 91 percent.

Differential Diagnosis. Neoplasms containing a myxoid stroma such as pleomorphic adenoma (mixed tumor), myxoma, myxoid liposarcoma, and ectomesenchymal chondromyxoid tumor may be considered in small biopsy specimens. Larger biopsy specimens may be required for the proper diagnosis.

Treatment and Prognosis. After supraglottic laryngectomy for the epiglottic neoplasm, the patient was alive without evidence of disease at 30 months (80). The neoplasm of the arytenoid cartilage was rapidly fatal, as there were pulmonary and cerebral metastases (78).

RHABDOMYOSARCOMA

General Features. This sarcoma, characterized by rapid and infiltrative growth, is probably the most common sarcoma arising in the head and neck. Of 999 rhabdomyosarcomas in patients younger than 21 years of age entered in the Intergroup Rhabdomyosarcoma Study II (97), 8 percent arose in the orbit, 18 percent were parameningeal (nasopharynx, nasal cavity, middle ear, mastoid, paranasal sinuses, pterygopalatine-infratemporal fossa), and 8 percent developed in other head and neck sites. Of 558 rhabdomyosarcomas collected at the Armed Forces Institute of Pathology (AFIP) (91), 44 percent arose in the head and neck, of which 13 percent were located in the nasal cavity, nasopharynx, palate, oral cavity, or pharynx; 4 percent developed in the paranasal sinuses, cheek, or neck; and 3 percent arose in the ear or mastoid. In a literature review of 777 head and neck rhabdomyosarcomas (83), 36 percent occurred in the orbit, 15 percent in the nasopharynx, 14 percent in the middle ear or mastoid, 8 percent were sinonasal, 4 percent arose in the larynx, 3 percent in the soft palate, and 1 to 2 percent each for tongue, hypopharynx, and pharynx. Less than 1 percent each arose in the tonsil, buccal mucosa, gingiva, floor of mouth, and lip.

Clinical Features. The age of patients developing rhabdomyosarcoma relates to the particular microscopic type *(embryonal, alveolar, botryoid,* *pleomorphic).* Embryonal and botryoid neoplasms typically arise in young children, alveolar rhabdomyosarcoma develops in preadolescents to young adults, and pleomorphic neoplasms usually arise in adults. Thirty-five percent of patients in the Intergroup Rhabdomyosarcoma Study II were less than 5 years of age, while 12 percent were between 15 and 20 years old (97). Of the 999 patients in this study, 58 percent were male. The spindle cell type of embryonal rhabdomyosarcoma most often occurs in children; in one series, 18 of 21 such tumors developed in males (86); 6 of the 21 neoplasms arose in the head and neck area.

Botryoid rhabdomyosarcoma appears as a polypoid, grape-like mass arising in a cavity of the upper aerodigestive tract. It may simulate a nasal, oral, or aural polyp. Symptoms of rhabdomyosarcoma depend upon tumor site, and are reflective of the fact that the neoplasm tends to be destructive, often invading adjacent bones of the palate, paranasal sinuses, and floor of the orbit. Patients may experience pain, facial swelling, bleeding, proptosis, hoarseness, or difficulty breathing (91). Those with neoplasms arising in or near the ear may present with symptoms of otitis media (91). Rhabdomyosarcoma of the larynx has a tendency to arise in the glottis, often as a bulky mass.

Gross Findings. Rhabdomyosarcoma has the usual appearance of a sarcoma: soft, white or tan, and sometimes gelatinous. There may be foci of hemorrhage and necrosis. The size is variable.

Microscopic Findings. Approximately 80 to 85 percent of head and neck rhabdomyosarcomas are embryonal or botryoid, 10 to 15 percent are alveolar, and 5 percent or less are pleomorphic (83). The embryonal subtype is composed of round, oval, or spindle-shaped cells with scant to sometimes prominent cytoplasm (fig. 14-24). Many have the appearance of a small blue cell tumor, but sometimes there is striking skeletal muscle differentiation. They are quite cellular when composed of sheets of packed small cells, but are much less cellular when there is a conspicuous edematous or myxoid stroma. The nuclei of the small blue cells are hyperchromatic and nucleoli may not be prominent (fig. 14-25). Mitotic figures are readily identified. Scattered rhabdomyoblasts are also observed. Well-differentiated skeletal muscle cells are spindle shaped, have

conspicuous eosinophilic cytoplasm, and, at times, cross striations. They are sometimes quite prominent after chemotherapy. The spindle cell subtype of embryonal rhabdomyosarcoma simulates a fibrosarcoma or leiomyosarcoma (86).

The botryoid subtype consists of small blue cells set in an abundant myxoid stroma. It typically has a cambium layer, a linear band of more compact cells just beneath the epithelial surface. Rhabdomyoblasts are often scattered within the loose matrix.

Alveolar rhabdomyosarcoma contains small, round or oval dark cells set on bands of fibroconnective tissue (fig. 14-26). Characteristically, there is a central loss of cell cohesion with a layer of cells resting on the connective tissue stroma. Cells with loss of cohesion may show degenerative features or overt necrosis. The solid form of alveolar rhabdomyosarcoma consists of sheets of packed cells with an inconspicuous or near absent alveolar pattern. The nuclei are hyperchromatic, with small and often inapparent nucleoli; the cytoplasm is scant. Mitotic figures are numerous. Multinucleated bizarre tumor giant cells are often seen, and rhabdomyoblasts are sometimes scattered.

Pleomorphic rhabdomyosarcoma, by far the least common variant, cannot be diagnosed in the absence of strong immunohistochemical evidence of skeletal muscle differentiation or the presence of overt cytoplasmic cross striations. The cells are characteristically large and pleomorphic, with bizarre nuclei and abundant amounts of cytoplasm. They are polygonal shaped or spindled. Anaplastic (pleomorphic) cells are sometimes scattered in or a striking component of embryonal rhabdomyosarcoma (95). When anaplastic cells are present in aggregates or diffuse sheets in embryonal rhabdomyosarcoma, a poorer survival results.

The classification of rhabdomyosarcomas in children has been recently refined (100). The proposed classification includes: I. superior prognosis, botryoid and spindle cell types; II. intermediate prognosis, embryonal; III. poor prognosis, alveolar and undifferentiated types; and IV. subtypes whose prognosis is not presently evaluable, rhabdomyosarcoma with rhabdoid features.

Immunohistochemical Findings. Although vimentin is characteristically present, it is typically not helpful for the diagnosis. Important stains, however, include antibodies to desmin (81,

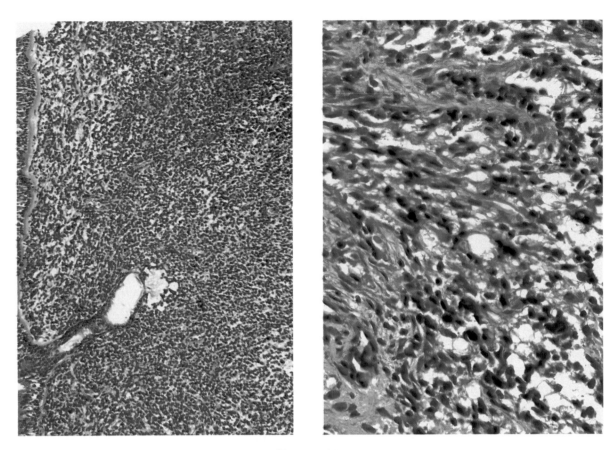

Figure 14-24
RHABDOMYOSARCOMA
Embryonal rhabdomyosarcoma growing beneath the respiratory epithelium of the nasal cavity (left) sometimes is composed of spindle-shaped cells (right).

Figure 14-25
RHABDOMYOSARCOMA
The embryonal subtype some-times contains a few large cells, some of which have abundant eosinophilic cytoplasm.

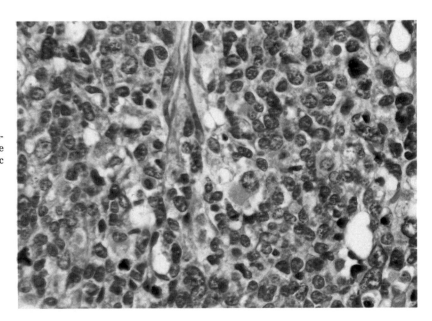

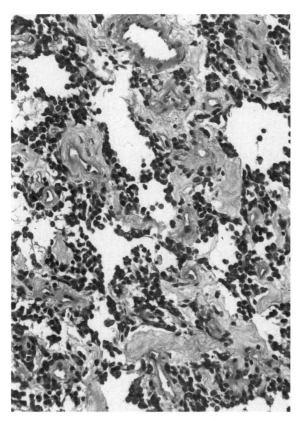

Figure 14-26
RHABDOMYOSARCOMA
The alveolar subtype consists of small cells with
hyperchromatic nuclei set on a scaffold of connective tissue.

82,98,101), muscle-specific actin (82,101,103), and myoglobin (88,94). An antibody to myosin is less sensitive (89,92). Immunostaining for myoD1, a regulatory protein in skeletal muscle differentiation, can be helpful but is not specific (90). Rhabdomyosarcomas at times are also immunoreactive for neuron-specific enolase (103), cytokeratin (87,99), and S-100 protein (87).

Ultrastructural Findings. The electron microscopic appearance reflects the state of differentiation of the neoplasm and, hence, a spectrum from undifferentiated to well-differentiated skeletal muscle cells may be observed. In some cells, there may be thin (6 to 8 nm) and thick (12 to 15 nm) alternating parallel filaments (91). Z bands may also be present. It is important that entrapped non-neoplastic skeletal muscle not be interpreted as neoplastic cells.

Other Special Techniques. A characteristic cytogenetic abnormality is seen in the alveolar

variant consisting of t(2;13)(q35-37;q14) (84, 102,105). A less common recurrent abnormality is t(1;13)(p36.1;q14) (105). The t(2;13) translocation disrupts the PAX3 paired box gene on chromosome 2 and places it beside the forkhead domain gene on chromosome 13, resulting in a fusion transcript that encodes a putative chimeric transcription factor (85,93,104).

Differential Diagnosis. When a small blue cell neoplasm is seen in a biopsy specimen from the head and neck of a child, rhabdomyosarcoma should be very high on the list of differential diagnostic possibilities. It should be included in the differential diagnosis for adults also, but occasionally it is not considered. Small blue cell neoplasms included in the differential diagnosis are malignant lymphoma, olfactory neuroblastoma, undifferentiated carcinoma, peripheral neuroectodermal tumor, melanoma, synovial sarcoma, and extramedullary myeloid cell tumor. Immunohistochemical stains are often crucial in separating rhabdomyosarcoma from other small blue cell neoplasms. A useful initial battery includes antibodies to desmin, muscle-specific actin, myoglobin, leukocyte common antigen, synaptophysin, cytokeratin, S-100 protein, and epithelial membrane antigen. The spindle cell variant of embryonal rhabdomyosarcoma may simulate fibrosarcoma or leiomyosarcoma. In addition, this subtype should be distinguished from fetal rhabdomyoma. The pleomorphic variant, undiagnosable without immunohistochemical stains in most cases, should be distinguished from malignant fibrous histiocytoma, melanoma, and leiomyosarcoma. Finally, it is important to distinguish rhabdomyosarcoma, particularly the botryoid variant, from nasal polyps having scattered stromal cells with large, atypical nuclei (see chapter 15).

Staging. The clinical staging for patients with rhabdomyosarcoma has been developed by the Intergroup Rhabdomyosarcoma Study (96). Patients in group I have completely resectable localized disease. Regional nodal involvement is absent. The neoplasm is confined to muscle or its site of origin, but there may be contiguous involvement with tumor infiltration outside the muscle or organ of origin through fascial planes. Patients in group II have grossly resectable neoplasms with microscopic evidence of residual disease, with or without regional lymph node involvement, or have completely resectable regional disease and resectable positive nodes without residual microscopic disease. Group III patients have incompletely resectable tumor or biopsy with grossly visible neoplasm. Group IV patients have distant metastatic tumor present at diagnosis.

Treatment and Prognosis. Tremendous progress in treatment has been accomplished by the Intergroup Rhabdomyosarcoma Group Studies which have collected and analyzed these neoplasms for over 20 years. Therapy is typically multimodal, with surgery, chemotherapy, and radiation. The most common chemotherapeutic agents employed are vincristine, dactinomycin, cyclophosphamide, and doxorubicin. The prognosis depends on stage, site, patient age, tumor size, and histologic type. In the 1993 Intergroup Rhabdomyosarcoma Study II (97) in which patients had complete surgical removal and varying regimens of chemotherapy and radiotherapy, patients with orbital tumors had the best prognosis, a 92 percent survival rate at 5 years; those with nonorbital head and neck tumors followed with an 80 percent 5-year survival rate; and those with parameningeal rhabdomyosarcomas had an approximately 70 percent survival rate at 5 years. For all sites, the prognosis was best for patients with the botryoid type without metastatic disease who had a 5-year survival rate of 89 percent. For patients with embryonal or alveolar rhabdomyosarcoma and no metastasis, the 5-year survival rates were 74 percent and 66 percent, respectively.

LEIOMYOSARCOMA

General Features. Of 94 head and neck leiomyosarcomas collected from the literature, 18 involved the sinonasal tract, 7 arose in the larynx, 6 developed in the buccal mucosa, and 5 arose in the gingiva (106). Additional primary sites included hypopharynx, tongue, trachea, palate, and floor of the mouth. Of 602 soft tissue tumors involving the sinonasal tract seen at the AFIP, 9 were leiomyosarcomas (108).

Clinical Features. When arising in the oral cavity, leiomyosarcoma usually presents as a painless mass that sometimes is ulcerated. The age range is 11 months to 88 years (107). Of 30 sinonasal neoplasms described in the literature, 10 were confined to the nasal cavity (108). The age range in that series was 18 to 87 years, with the mean

in the sixth decade. There was no sex predilection. Sinonasal symptoms were not specific.

Gross Findings. When occurring in the upper aerodigestive tract, this sarcoma is a firm, polypoid or bulky, gray-white mass. Hemorrhage, necrosis, or both are sometimes present. Sinonasal neoplasms range from 0.3 to 7.0 cm in greatest dimension (108). There may be invasion of adjacent bony structures.

Microscopic Findings. The neoplasm consists of infiltrating fascicles of spindle-shaped cells having smooth muscle features (fig. 14-27). Elongated, blunt-ended nuclei are surrounded by moderate amounts of eosinophilic cytoplasm (fig. 14-28). Nucleoli vary from inconspicuous to prominent. Pleomorphism is sometimes marked and the mitotic rate is variable. Sometimes there appears to be an association between the neoplastic cells and the endothelium of blood vessels within the tumor. Leiomyosarcoma having an epithelioid appearance is rare in the upper aerodigestive tract.

Immunohistochemical Findings. The neoplasm is usually immunoreactive for muscle-specific actin and smooth muscle actin (fig. 14-29). Desmin immunopositivity is also observed, but less often. Immunoreactivity for keratin or S-100 protein is unusual.

Differential Diagnosis. Spindle-shaped malignant neoplasms to be considered in the differential diagnosis include fibrosarcoma, malignant fibrous histiocytoma, malignant peripheral sheath tumor, melanoma, and sarcomatoid carcinoma. In some instances, immunohistochemical staining is required for the proper diagnosis.

Treatment and Prognosis. Complete resection is the mainstay of therapy. Of 17 patients with oral cavity leiomyosarcoma, 2 were alive with disease, while 7 died of disease from 8 to 39 months after treatment (106). Of 10 patients with leiomyosarcoma confined to the nasal cavity, none experienced recurrent disease (108). On the other hand, 70 percent of 20 neoplasms involving one or more paranasal sinuses exhibited aggressive behavior; only 5 of these metastasized, however (108).

MALIGNANT FIBROUS HISTIOCYTOMA

General Features. This is chiefly a sarcoma of older adults and usually develops in the extremities or retroperitoneum, but 3 to 10 percent of all cases arise in the head and neck area

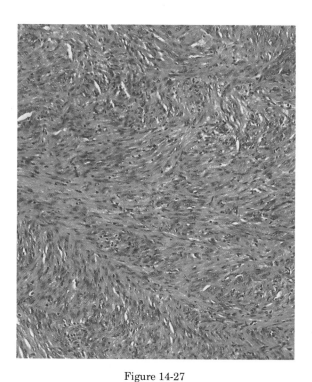

Figure 14-27
LEIOMYOSARCOMA
This neoplasm from the nasal cavity consists of fascicles of
spindle-shaped cells with conspicuous eosinophilic cytoplasm.

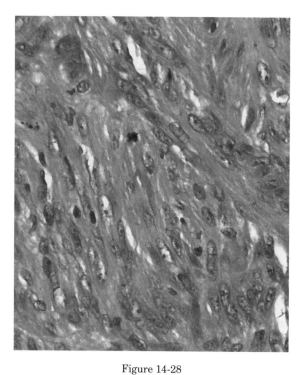

Figure 14-28
LEIOMYOSARCOMA
This nasal cavity neoplasm has cells with mildly pleomorphic
nuclei. Mitotic figures were present but were not numerous.

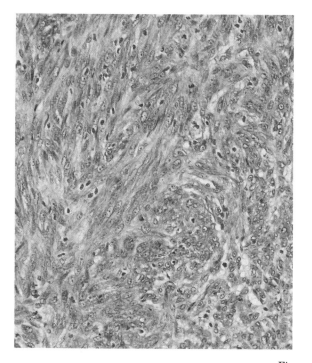

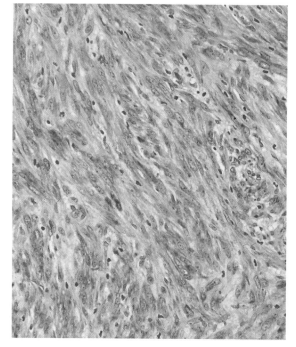

Figure 14-29
LEIOMYOSARCOMA
This neoplasm is immunoreactive for both muscle-specific actin (left) and desmin (right).

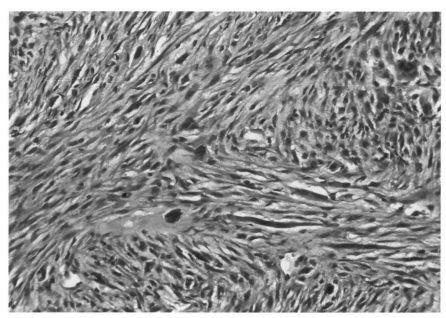

Figure 14-30
MALIGNANT FIBROUS
HISTIOCYTOMA
This sinonasal neoplasm consists of a predominance of spindle-shaped cells and a few that are polygonal.

(110,114,116,118,119). The most common upper aerodigestive tract site for malignant fibrous histiocytoma is the sinonasal tract, accounting for approximately 30 percent of head and neck cases; 10 to 15 percent occur in the larynx; and 5 to 15 percent arise in the oral cavity (109–111,113). In one well-documented series of 12 cases of head and neck malignant fibrous histiocytoma, 4 arose in the sinonasal tract, 2 in the oral cavity, and 1 in the larynx (110). Seven of the 12 neoplasms developed in soft tissue, while the remaining 5 either arose in bone or invaded it secondarily.

Clinical Features. Malignant fibrous histiocytoma of the upper aerodigestive tract sometimes occurs in young adults, but is rare in children (110). Symptoms are related to tumor site and size. Sinonasal tract symptoms include nasal obstruction, epistaxis, facial swelling, pain, and headache (117). Laryngeal involvement results in hoarseness, airway obstruction, or both (115). Of nine sinonasal or nasopharyngeal tumors reported in one study, seven arose in women (117); the age range was 28 to 67 years; and the most frequently involved sinus was the maxillary antrum. In a review of 16 laryngeal malignant fibrous histiocytomas from the literature, the age range was 8 to 68 years (115); 12 of the neoplasms arose in men. Of 16 oral malignant fibrous histiocytomas, the age range was 20 to 93 years (mean, 61 years); male to female ratio was 2.2 to 1 (112). In the oral cavity, the neoplasm is a painless mass, but extension to adjacent bone is sometimes observed.

Gross Findings. The majority of tumors measure 4 to 5 cm in greatest dimension, but some are over 10 cm (110,112). Their appearance is similar to that of malignant fibrous histiocytoma at other sites.

Microscopic Findings. The majority of malignant fibrous histiocytomas of the upper aerodigestive tract are of the storiform-pleomorphic type, composed of spindle-shaped fibroblastic-type cells as well large polygonal cells that superficially resemble bizarre histiocytes (fig. 14-30) (110,112). The cells are present in bundles imparting the typical storiform appearance. Nuclei are pleomorphic and hyperchromatic, and often contain one or more prominent nucleoli. Mitotic figures, including atypical forms, are commonly observed. Foci of necrosis are also common. Varying proportions of collagen, benign inflammatory cells, and xanthoma cells are intermixed with the malignant population. Myxoid, giant cell, and inflammatory subtypes of malignant fibrous histiocytoma are rarely observed in the upper aerodigestive tract.

Immunohistochemical Findings. Staining for vimentin is typical, while the neoplasms also may be immunoreactive for alpha-1-

antichymotrypsin (110). Keratin and S-100 protein are negative.

Differential Diagnosis. Sarcomas consisting largely of spindle-shaped cells, such as fibrosarcoma and leiomyosarcoma, are included in the differential diagnosis. The most important considerations, however, are melanoma and sarcomatoid carcinoma. Primary malignant melanoma of the upper aerodigestive tract may be composed almost entirely of spindle-shaped cells, and, at times, may also contain intermixed bizarre polygonal cells. Spindle-shaped cells may be distributed in a storiform pattern similar to that seen in malignant fibrous histiocytoma. The diagnosis of melanoma is secure when there is overt junctional change, melanin pigment, or immunoreactivity for HMB-45. Strong immunostaining for S-100 protein even in the absence of HMB-45 immunoreactivity is strongly suggestive of melanoma. Sarcomatoid carcinoma may also resemble malignant fibrous histiocytoma, but the diagnosis of the former can be made when there is overt squamous differentiation, surface squamous dysplasia, or immunoreactivity for cytokeratin. Unfortunately, some putative spindle cell carcinomas lack evidence of dysplasia or squamous cell carcinoma and are negative or only focally positive for cytokeratin. Although they may seem to lack evidence of epithelioid differentiation, most if not all of these tumors behave as spindle cell carcinomas. Hence, malignant fibrous histiocytoma can only be diagnosed when there is no evidence whatsoever to support a diagnosis of spindle cell carcinoma.

Treatment and Prognosis. Radical resection, with or without postoperative radiation therapy, has been most commonly employed. Chemotherapy has been used for extensive local recurrences or metastatic neoplasms. Of 21 sinonasal or nasopharyngeal neoplasms in the literature, 14 percent recurred locally, 14 percent resulted in cervical lymph node metastases, 10 percent metastasized systemically, and 10 percent of the patients died (117). Of 16 tumors arising in the oral cavity, 60 percent recurred, 38 percent metastasized to cervical lymph nodes, 44 percent metastasized systemically, and 63 percent of the patients died (112). Of 16 laryngeal malignant fibrous histiocytomas from the literature, 38 percent locally recurred, 6 percent metastasized to cervical lymph nodes, 19 percent metastasized to distant sites, and 25 percent of the patients died (115).

SYNOVIAL SARCOMA

General Features. This sarcoma, most often arising in the para-articular area of the extremities (particularly the lower thigh and knee) in adolescents and young adults, may arise in a wide variety of head and neck sites. The most common location in the latter area is the cervical prevertebral connective tissue (133). Of 345 synovial sarcomas studied by Enzinger and Weiss (126), 7 arose in the pharynx and an additional 7 arose in the larynx. Other reported sites of synovial sarcoma in the upper aerodigestive tract include the maxillofacial area (131,136), tonsil (136), soft palate (129), tongue (136), cheek (136), and mastoid (133).

Clinical Features. Sarcomas in the cervical prevertebral space typically manifest as solitary retropharyngeal or cervical triangle mass lesions. Of the 24 patients with cervical prevertebral space tumors in one study, hoarseness and difficulties in swallowing and breathing were noted (133). The age range for these patients was 10 to 51 years (median, 19 years). There were 10 females and 14 males.

Gross Findings. The tumor is often well circumscribed and solid, but there may be cystic foci. It is firm, soft, or mucoid; tan, white, or yellow; and may have areas of hemorrhage and necrosis. Head and neck synovial sarcomas range from 1 to 12 cm in greatest dimension (121,129,136).

Microscopic Findings. The neoplasm may be biphasic (having both spindle and epithelial components) (fig. 14-31), monophasic fibrous, monophasic epithelial, or poorly differentiated. Epithelial cells are cuboid or columnar and are arranged in cords, whorls, or nests. They may also form pseudoglandular spaces (fig. 14-32) that sometimes contain eosinophilic secretions. The cells have large, round to oval, vesicular nuclei and ample cytoplasm. Spindle-shaped cells are uniform and have hyperchromatic nuclei and scant cytoplasm. Although some foci resemble fibrosarcoma, the cells of monophasic synovial sarcoma more often are arranged in a nodular pattern (126). Usually, there are one or two mitotic figures per high-power field, but they may be more numerous in poorly differentiated neoplasms. Biphasic foci may be seen in poorly differentiated neoplasms, which consist predominantly of sheets of oval or

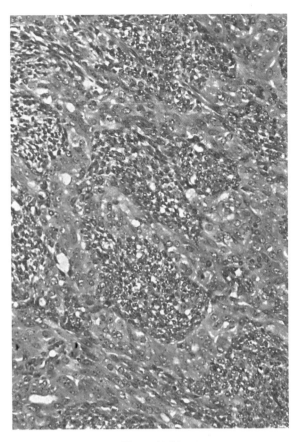

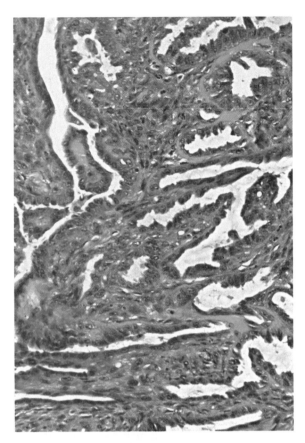

Figure 14-31
SYNOVIAL SARCOMA
This biphasic sarcoma consists of cords of epithelial cells
with interspersed bundles of spindle-shaped cells.

Figure 14-32
SYNOVIAL SARCOMA
Epithelial cells lining spaces impart a papillary appearance.

spindle-shaped cells with little cytoplasm and hyperchromatic nuclei.

Synovial sarcoma contains varying amounts of collagen and connective tissue mucin. Foci of calcification may also be present (126). The collagen is dispersed evenly or consists of thick bands or dense, hyalinized plaques (fig. 14-33). Calcified foci sometimes become ossified. Mast cells are characteristically numerous.

The secretions within pseudoglandular spaces stain with PAS, colloidal iron, alcian blue, and mucicarmine (126). The secretory material is resistant to both diastase and hyaluronidase. The stromal mucin surrounding spindle cells is negative for PAS, but stains with colloidal iron and alcian blue, and is sensitive to hyaluronidase digestion. The reticulin stain assists in delineating the biphasic pattern, which may be inconspicuous on H&E-stained sections. Reticu-

lin surrounds the spindle-shaped cells, while it is less apparent around epithelial foci.

Immunohistochemical Findings. Cytokeratin and epithelial membrane antigen are present in both components of synovial sarcoma, although more intense staining is seen in epithelial foci (124,127,130,132,134,137). Only focal immunoreactivity for cytokeratin may be seen in the monophasic spindle cell variant. Immunostaining for vimentin is characteristically present in the spindle-shaped cells, while it is usually absent in the epithelial foci. Immunostaining for S-100 protein (128,135) and Leu-7 (120) may also be observed. In a study of 50 synovial sarcomas from diverse anatomic sites, 62 percent were immunoreactive for the MIC-2 gene product (CD99) using either antibody 013 or 12E7 (125).

Special Techniques. Although multiple karyotypic abnormalities have been reported in

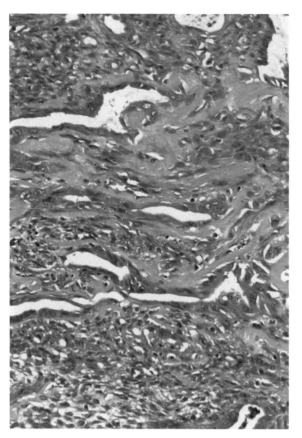

Figure 14-33
SYNOVIAL SARCOMA
The finding of collagenous foci sometimes is an important diagnostic clue in synovial sarcoma.

consist chiefly of spindle-shaped cells may simulate spindle cell carcinoma, fibrosarcoma, or leiomyosarcoma. Those that are poorly differentiated may raise the diagnostic possibilities of undifferentiated carcinoma, angiosarcoma, hemangiopericytoma, or peripheral neuroectodermal tumor. Key microscopic findings assisting in the proper diagnosis of synovial sarcoma include the biphasic pattern, hyalinized collagen, foci of calcification, and mast cells. Although the immunohistochemical findings may overlap those of other neoplasms, the characteristic staining pattern for cytokeratin and epithelial membrane antigen should provide confirmatory evidence.

Treatment and Prognosis. Wide or radical excision is the standard treatment. This may be supplemented by preoperative or postoperative radiotherapy. Occasionally, multidrug chemotherapy is used in the adjuvant setting. Of 50 patients with head and neck synovial sarcomas from the literature, almost one third had local recurrence and approximately one fourth had metastatic disease (122). Metastases developed an average of 3 1/2 years after diagnosis. One patient had cervical lymph node metastasis. Twenty-eight percent of the patients died of disease, 80 percent of these within 4 years. Hence, patients need to be followed long term, as late metastases can occur (121). The most common metastatic site is the lung. Tumor size and location are important prognostic factors since they affect the surgical approach.

ALVEOLAR SOFT PART SARCOMA

General Features. This rare sarcoma, whose cells possibly differentiate toward skeletal muscle or the muscle spindle, most often occurs in adolescents or young adults, and most commonly develops in the lower extremity (139,142). Of 143 cases seen at the AFIP, 44 percent were located in the lower extremity while 27 percent occurred in the head and neck area (139). In a 1989 review of the literature (149), there were 24 orbital and 20 nonorbital head and neck alveolar soft part sarcomas; 14 of the 20 nonorbital tumors arose in the tongue, while the remainder were located in the posterior triangle of the neck, jugulodigastric area, temporal region, masseter muscle, infratemporal fossa, and nasoethmoid area.

synovial sarcoma, there is a characteristic balanced translocation between X and 18 (t) (X;18) (p11.2;q.11.2). This translocation is seen in synovial sarcomas regardless of site and has been reported in a lingual example (123).

Differential Diagnosis. The differential diagnosis for head and neck synovial sarcoma is wide. Its appearance may be particularly troublesome in biopsy specimens; hence, the clinical findings and histochemical and immunohistochemical stains may be essential. When synovial sarcoma presents as a biphasic neoplasm, the proper diagnosis is made more readily. However, the sarcoma may raise diagnostic possibilities that include metastatic neoplasms, melanoma, epithelioid sarcoma, malignant peripheral nerve sheath tumor, and salivary gland neoplasms such as benign and malignant mixed tumor and spindle cell myoepithelioma. Synovial sarcomas that

Miscellaneous Soft Tissue Neoplasms

347

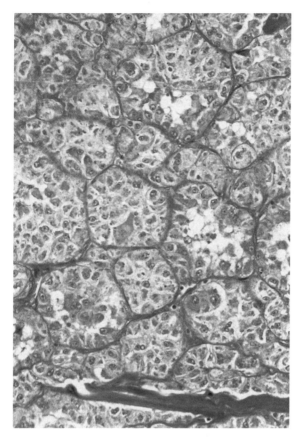

Figure 14-34
ALVEOLAR SOFT PART SARCOMA
Nests of cells are delimited by delicate fibrovascular tissue in this neoplasm from the tongue.

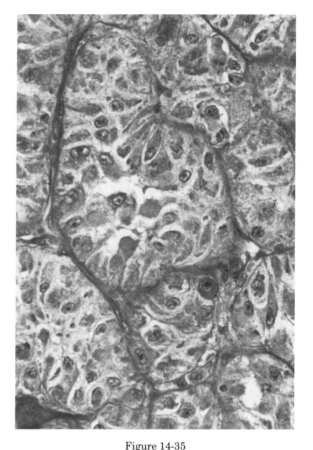

Figure 14-35
ALVEOLAR SOFT PART SARCOMA
The neoplastic cells have abundant eosinophilic cytoplasm, fairly uniform vesicular nuclei, and conspicuous nucleoli.

Clinical Features. Of 43 orbital and nonorbital head and neck neoplasms, 31 arose in females (149). The mean age for the 24 patients with orbital tumors was 23 years (range, 1 to 69 years), while for patients with neoplasms at other head and neck sites, the mean age was 14 years (range, 1 to 28 years). The tumor usually presents as a soft to firm, painless, slowly growing mass (139).

Gross Findings. The sarcoma is firm or soft, and gray or yellow. It may show areas of hemorrhage and necrosis (139,142). Most nonorbital head and neck neoplasms range from 2 to 5 cm in greatest dimension.

Microscopic Findings. The neoplasm has a distinctive appearance, consisting of packets of cells separated by fibrous bands. The packets are subdivided into cell nests which are delimited by thin-walled vascular channels (fig. 14-34). There may be cellular degeneration, necrosis, and loss of cohesion within the centers of the cell nests, imparting a pseudoalveolar pattern (139,142). The nesting pattern may not be conspicuous if the neoplasm consists chiefly of solid sheets of large granular cells. The cells are characteristically large and polygonal (fig. 14-35). Usually there is little pleomorphism. The cells contain one or more vesicular nuclei with small to prominent nucleoli. Multinucleated cells are sometimes seen. The cytoplasm is abundant, eosinophilic, and granular, and occasionally contains vacuoles. Mitotic figures are rare. Vascular invasion may be observed.

The PAS stain shows that the cells contain varying amounts of glycogen. This stain highlights the presence of diastase-resistant rhomboid or rod-shaped crystals, which sometimes are present in a stacked pattern (139,142). The identification of these crystals may be diagnostically quite important.

Immunohistochemical Findings. The neoplasm lacks immunoreactivity for epithelial membrane antigen, neurofilament, GFAP, chromogranin, synaptophysin, and myoglobin (138, 142,144,145,147). There is variable immunoreactivity for S-100 protein, neuron-specific enolase, vimentin, cytokeratin, muscle-specific actin, and desmin (138,140–142,144–147,151). Immunostaining for more specific muscle markers such as the beta-subunit of enolase (144), the MM isoenzyme of creatine kinase (144), and myoD1 (148) has been reported. In a recent study of 12 alveolar soft part sarcomas (151), 6 were positive for desmin, but immunostaining for muscle actin, myoglobin, myoD1 (nuclear), and myogenin (nuclear) was absent. Eleven of the neoplasms showed granular cytoplasmic immunoreactivity with anti-myoD1 monoclonal antibody; however, there was evidence to suggest that this represented a nonspecific crossreactivity with an unknown cytoplasmic antigen.

Ultrastructural Findings. The large nuclei have dispersed chromatin and one or two nucleoli. The cytoplasm contains well-developed Golgi complex, vesicles, numerous mitochondria, and rough endoplasmic reticulum. Glycogen and lipid droplets may also be present. Cell junctions are rudimentary, and occasionally there is a focal, thin basement membrane at the cell base (142). The cytoplasm also contains 200- to 400- nm secretory granules, which usually contain finely granular substance, but may also show crystallization of their contents (142). With crystallization, the granules assume a rectangular or rhomboid shape, and contain parallel rigid "fibers" (142). The number of crystals is variable, and they are not be present in all neoplasms. The tumor typically lacks evidence of true lumen formation with microvilli and desmosomes.

Differential Diagnosis. The distinctive microscopic features and its location in the tongue of a child are characteristic of alveolar soft part sarcoma. Neoplasms that show some histologic similarities include paraganglioma, granular cell tumor, renal cell carcinoma, melanoma, rhabdomyoma, and rhabdomyosarcoma. If necessary, immunohistochemical stains readily discriminate between most of these neoplasms.

Treatment and Prognosis. Surgery is the mainstay of therapy, as the role for adjuvant chemotherapy and radiotherapy is limited. The prognosis for patients with head and neck tumors is more favorable than that for patients with alveolar soft part sarcoma of the extremity. The 5-year survival rate for patients with nonorbital head and neck neoplasms is approximately 50 percent, while for orbital tumors it is greater than 90 percent (149). Alveolar soft part sarcoma rarely metastasizes from the tongue, but this has been reported (143,150).

REFERENCES

Lipoma

1. Dinsdale RC, Manning SC, Brooks DJ, Vuitch F. Myxoid laryngeal lipoma in a juvenile. Otolaryngol Head Neck Surg 1990;103:653–7.
2. Fu YS, Perzin KH. Non-epithelial tumors of the nasal cavity, paranasal sinuses and nasopharynx: a clinicopathologic study. VIII. Adipose tissue tumors (lipoma and liposarcoma). Cancer 1977;40:1314–7.
3. Hatziotis JC. Lipoma of the oral cavity. Oral Surg 1971;31:511–24.
4. Mansson I, Wilske J, Kindblom LG. Lipoma of the hypopharynx. A case report and a review of the literature. J Laryngol Otol 1978;92:1037–43.
5. Moretti JA. Laryngeal involvement in benign symmetric lipomatosis. Arch Otolaryngol 1973;97:495–6.
6. Nonako S, Enomoto K, Kawabovi S, Unno T, Muraoko S. Spindle cell lipoma within the larynx: a case report with correlated light and electron microscopy. ORL 1993;55:147–9.
7. Orlian AI. Lipomas of the tongue. NY State Dent J 1961;27:337.
8. Som PM, Scherl MP, Rao VM, Biller HF. Rare presentations of ordinary lipomas of the head and neck: a review. AJNR Am J Neuroradiol 1986;7:657–64.
9. Wenig BM. Lipomas of the larynx and hypopharynx: a review of the literature with the addition of three new cases. J Laryngol Otol 1995;109:353–7.
10. Yoshimura Y, Miyagi K, Shoju M, Matsumura T, Kawakatsu K, Yoshioka W. Lipoma in the infant and child: report of cases. J Oral Surg 1972;30;690–3.
11. Zakrzewski A. Subglottic lipoma of the larynx. Case report and literature review. J Laryngol Otol 1965;79:1039–48.

Leiomyoma

12. Barnes L. Tumors and tumor-like lesions of the soft tissues. In: Barnes L, ed. Surgical pathology of the head and neck. New York: Marcel Dekker, 1985:725–880.

13. Cherrick HM, Dunlap CL, King OH Jr. Leiomyomas of the oral cavity. Review of the literature and clinicopathologic study of seven new cases. Oral Surg 1973;35:54–66.

14. Fu YS, Perzin KH. Nonepithelial tumors of the nasal cavity, paranasal sinuses, and nasopharynx: a clinico-pathologic study. IV. Smooth-muscle tumors (leiomyoma, leiomyosarcoma). Cancer 1975;35:1300–8.

15. Gutmann J, Cifuentes C, Balzarini MA, Sobarzo V, Vicuna R. Angiomyoma of the oral cavity. Oral Surg 1974;38:269–73.

16. Kleinsasser O, Glanz H. Myogenic tumours of the larynx. Arch Otorhinolaryngeal 1979;225:107–19.

Rhabdomyoma

17. Ashfaq R, Timmons CF. Rhabdomyomatous mesenchymal hamartoma of skin. Pediatr Pathol 1992;12:731–5.

18. Batsakis JG. Tumors of the head and neck. 2nd ed. Baltimore: Williams & Wilkins, 1979:289.

19. Bock D, Bock P. Rhabdomyoma of the soft palate. Fine structural details of a highly differentiated muscle tumor. Histol Histopathol 1987;2:285–9.

20. Corio RL, Lewis DM. Intraoral rhabdomyomas. Oral Surg 1970;48:525–31.

21. Cornog JL Jr, Gonatas NK. Ultrastructure of rhabdomyoma. J Ultrastruct Res 1967;20:433–50.

22. Crotty PL, Nakleh RE, Dehner LP. Juvenile rhabdomyoma: an intermediate form of skeletal muscle tumor in children. Arch Pathol Lab Med 1993;117:43–7.

23. Czernobilsky B, Cornog JL Jr, Enterline HT. Rhabdomyoma. Report of a case with ultrastructural and histochemical studies. Am J Clin Pathol 1968;49:782–9.

24. Enzinger FM, Weiss SW. Soft tissue tumors. 3rd ed. St. Louis: Mosby, 1995:523–37.

25. Fu YS, Perzin KH. Nonepithelial tumors of the nasal cavity, paranasal sinuses, and nasopharynx: a clinicopathologic study. V. Skeletal muscle tumors (rhabdomyoma and rhabdomyosarcoma). Cancer 1976;37:364–76.

26. Gardner DG, Corio RL. Fetal rhabdomyoma of the tongue, with a discussion of the two histologic variants of this tumor. Oral Surg Oral Med Oral Pathol 1983;56:293–300.

27. Gibas Z, Miettinen M. Recurrent parapharyngeal rhabdomyoma: evidence of neoplastic nature of the tumor from cytogenetic study. Am J Surg Pathol 1992;16:721–8.

28. Kapadia SB, Enzinger FM, Heffner DK, Hyams VJ. Crystal-staining histiocytosis associated with lymphoplasmacytic neoplasms. Report of three cases mimicking adult rhabdomyoma. Am J Surg Pathol 1993;17:461–7.

29. Kapadia SB, Meis JM, Frisman DM, Ellis GL, Heffner DK. Fetal rhabdomyoma of the head and neck: a clinicopathologic and immunophenotypic study of 24 cases. Hum Pathol 1993;24:754–65.

30. Kapadia SB, Meis JM, Frisman DM, Ellis GL, Heffner DK, Hyams VJ. Adult rhabdomyoma of the head and neck: a clinicopathologic and immunophenotypic study. Hum Pathol 1993;24:608–17.

31. Kay S, Gerszten E, Dennison SM. Light and electron microscopic study of a rhabdomyoma arising in the floor of the mouth. Cancer 1969;23:708–15.

32. Kodet R, Fajstavr J, Kabelka Z, et al. Is fetal cellular rhabdomyoma an entity or a differentiated rhabdomyosarcoma? A study of patients with rhabdomyoma of the tongue and sarcoma of the tongue enrolled in the Intergroup Rhabdomyosarcoma Studies I, II, and III. Cancer 1991;67:2907–13.

33. Mills AE. Rhabdomyomatous mesenchymal hamartoma of skin. Am J Dermatopathol 1989;11:58–63.

34. Sahn EE, Garen PD, Pai GS, Levkoff AH, Hagerty RC, Maize JC. Multiple rhabdomyomatous mesenchymal hamartomas of skin. Am J Dermatopathol 1990;12:485–91.

35. Silverman JF, Kay S, Chang CH. Ultrastructural comparison between skeletal muscle and cardiac rhabdomyomas. Cancer 1978;42:189–93.

36. Solomon MP, Tolete-Velcek F. Lingual rhabdomyoma (adult variant) in a child. J Pediatr Surg 1979;14:91–4.

37. Tandler B, Rossi EP, Stein M, Mutt MM. Rhabdomyoma of the lip. Light and electron microscopical observations. Arch Pathol Lab Med 1970;89:118–27.

38. Tanner NS, Carter RL, Clifford P. Pharyngeal rhabdomyoma: an unusual presentation. J Laryngol Otol 1978;92:1029–36.

39. Winther LK. Rhabdomyoma of the hypopharynx and larynx. Report of two cases and a review of the literature. J Laryngol Otol 1976;90:1041–51.

Chondroma

40. Barnes L. Tumors and tumor-like lesions of the soft tissues. In: Barnes L, ed. Surgical pathology of the head and neck. New York: Marcel Dekker, 1985:725–880.

41. Chou LS, Hansen LS, Daniels TE. Choristomas of the oral cavity: a review. Oral Surg Oral Med Oral Pathol 1991;72:584–93.

42. Cutright DE. Osseous and chondromatous metaplasia caused by dentures. Oral Surg Oral Med Oral Pathol 1972;34:625–33.

43. Fu YS, Perzin KH. Non-epithelial tumors of the nasal cavity, paranasal sinuses, and nasopharynx: a clinicopathologic study. III. Cartilaginous tumors (chondroma, chondrosarcoma). Cancer 1974;34:453–63.

44. Hill MJ, Taylor CL, Scott GB. Chondromatous metaplasia in the human larynx. Histopathology 1980;4:205–14.

45. Huizenga C, Balogh K. Cartilaginous tumors of the larynx. A clinicopathologic study of 10 new cases and a review of the literature. Cancer 1970;26:201–10.

46. Hyams VJ, Batsakis JG, Michaels L. Tumors of the upper respiratory tract and ear. Atlas of Tumor Pathology. Fascicle 25, 2nd Series. Washington, DC: AFIP, 1988:169.

47. Hyams VJ, Rabuzzi DD. Cartilaginous tumors of the larynx. Laryngoscope 1969:80:755–67.

48. Kilby D, Ambegoakar AG. The nasal chondroma. Two case reports and a survey of the literature. J Laryngol Otol 1977;91:415–26.

49. Neel HB III, Unni KK. Cartilaginous tumors of the larynx: a series of 33 patients. Otolaryngol Head Neck Surg 1982;90:201–7.

50. Swerdlow RS, Som ML, Biller HF. Cartilaginous tumors of the larynx. Arch Otolaryngol 1974;100:269–72.

51. Zegarelli DJ. Chondroma of the tongue. Oral Surg Oral Med Oral Pathol 1977;43:738–45.

Ossifying Fibromyxoid Tumor

52. Williams SB, Ellis GL, Meis JM, Heffner DK. Ossifying fibromyxoid tumor (of soft parts) of the head and neck: a clinicopathological and immunohistochemical study of nine cases. J Laryngol Otol 1993;107:75–80.

Ectomesenchymal Chondromyxoid Tumor

53. Smith BC, Ellis GL, Meis-Kindblom JM, Williams SB. Ectomesenchymal chondromyxoid tumor of the anterior tongue. Nineteen cases of a new clinicopathologic entity. Am J Surg Pathol 1995;19:519–30.

Liposarcoma

54. Baden E, Newman R. Liposarcoma of the oropharyngeal region. Review of the literature and report of two cases. Oral Surg 1977;44:889–902.

55. Fu YS, Perzin KH. Non-epithelial tumors of the nasal cavity, paranasal sinuses and nasopharynx: a clinicopathologic study. VIII. Adipose tissue tumors (lipoma and liposarcoma). Cancer 1977;40:1314–7.

56. Golledge J, Fisher C, Rhys-Evans PH. Head and neck liposarcoma. Cancer 1995;76:1051–8.

57. Saddik M, Oldring DJ, Mourad WA. Liposarcoma of the base of tongue and tonsillar fossa: a possibly underdiagnosed neoplasm. Arch Pathol Lab Med 1996;120:292–5.

58. Wenig BM, Weiss SW, Gnepp DR. Laryngeal and hypopharyngeal liposarcoma. A clinicopathologic study of 10 cases with a comparison to soft-tissue counterparts. Am J Surg Pathol 1990;14:134–41.

Chondrosarcoma

59. Bleiweiss IJ, Kaneko M. Chondrosarcoma of the larynx with additional malignant mesenchymal component (dedifferentiated chondrosarcoma). Am J Surg Pathol 1988;12:314–20.

60. Burkey BB, Hoffman HT, Baker SR, Thornton AF, McClatchey KD. Chondrosarcoma of the head and neck. Laryngoscope 1990;100:1301–5.

61. Cantrell RW, Jahrsdoerfer RA, Reibel JF, Johns ME. Conservative surgical treatment of chondrosarcoma of the larynx. Ann Otol Rhinol Laryngol 1980;89:567–71.

62. Coates HL, Pearson BW, Devine KD, Unni KK. Chondrosarcoma of the nasal cavity, paranasal sinuses, and nasopharynx. Tr Am Acad Ophth Otol 1977;84:919–26.

63. Fu YS, Perzin KH. Non-epithelial tumors of the nasal cavity, paranasal sinuses, and nasopharynx: a clinicopathologic study. III. Cartilaginous tumors (chondroma, chondrosarcoma). Cancer 1974;34:453–63.

64. Goethals PL, Dahlin DC, Devine KD. Cartilaginous tumors of the larynx. Surg Gynecol Obstet 1963;117:77–82.

65. Hyams VJ, Rabuzzi DD. Cartilaginous tumors of the larynx. Laryngoscope 1970;80:755–67.

66. Kragh LV, Dahlin DC, Erich JB. Cartilaginous tumors of the jaws and facial regions. Am J Surg 1960;99:852–6.

67. Neel HB III, Unni KK. Cartilaginous tumors of the larynx: a series of 33 patients. Otolaryngol Head Neck Surg 1982;90:201–7.

68. Nicolai P, Sasaki CT, Ferlito A, Kirchner JA. Laryngeal chondrosarcoma: incidence, pathology, biological behavior, and treatment. Ann Otol Rhinol Laryngol 1990;99:515–23.

69. Saito K, Unni KK, Wollan PC, Lund BA. Chondrosarcoma of the jaw and facial bones. Cancer 1995;76:1550–8.

Mesenchymal Chondrosarcoma

70. Bloch DM, Bragoli AJ, Collins DN, Batsakis JG. Mesenchymal chondrosarcomas of the head and neck. J Laryngol Otol 1979;93:405–12.

71. Enzinger FM, Weiss SW. Soft tissue tumors. 3rd ed. St. Louis: Mosby, 1995:991–1011.

72. Huvos AG, Rosen G, Dabska M, Marcove RC. Mesenchymal chondrosarcoma. A clinicopathologic analysis of 35 patients with emphasis on treatment. Cancer 1983;51:1230–7.

73. Roland NJ, Kline MM, Clarke R, Van Velzen D. A rare congenital nasal polyp: mesenchymal chondrosarcoma of the nasal region. J Laryngol Otol 1992;106:1081–3.

74. Salvador AH, Beabout JW, Dahlin DC. Mesenchymal chondrosarcoma: observations on 30 new cases. Cancer 1971;28:605–15.

75. Swanson PE, Lillemoe TJ, Manivel JC, Wick MR. Mesenchymal chondrosarcoma. An immunohistochemical study. Arch Pathol Lab Med 1990;114:943–8.

Extraskeletal Myxoid Chondrosarcoma

76. Jawad J, Lang J, Leader M, et al. Extraskeletal myxoid chondrosarcoma of the maxillary sinus. J Laryngol Otol 1991;105:676–7.

77. Meis JM, Martz KL. Extraskeletal myxoid chondrosarcoma (EMC): a clinicopathologic study of 120 cases [Abstract]. Mod Pathol 1992;5:9A.

78. Moran CA, Suster S, Carter D. Laryngeal chondrosarcomas. Arch Pathol Lab Med 1993;117:914–7.

79. Smith BC, Ellis GL, Meis-Kindblom JM, Williams SB. Ectomesenchymal chondromyxoid tumor of the anterior tongue. Nineteen cases of a new clinicopathologic entity. Am J Surg Pathol 1995;19:519–30.

80. Wilkinson AH, Beckford NS, Babin RW, Parham DM. Extraskeletal myxoid chondrosarcoma of the epiglottis: case report and review of the literature. Otolaryngol Head Neck Surg 1991;104:257–60.

Rhabdomyosarcoma

81. Altmannsberger M, Weber K, Droste R, Osborn M. Desmin is a specific marker for rhabdomyosarcomas of human and rat origin. Am J Pathol 1985;118:85–95.

82. Azumi, N, Ben-Ezra J, Battifora H. Immunophenotypic diagnosis of leiomyosarcomas and rhabdomyosarcomas with monoclonal antibodies to muscle-specific actin and desmin in formalin fixed tissue. Mod Pathol 1988;1:469–74.

83. Barnes L. Tumors and tumor-like lesions of the soft tissues. In: Barnes L, ed. Surgical pathology of the head and neck. New York: Marcel Dekker, 1985:725–880.

84. Barr FG, Biegel JA, Sellinger B, Womer RB, Emanuel BS. Molecular and cytogenetic analysis of chromosomal arms 2q and 13q in alveolar rhabdomyosarcoma. Genes Chromosomes Cancer 1991;3:153–61.

85. Barr FG, Galili N, Holick J, Biegel JA, Ravera G, Emanuel BS. Rearrangement of the PAX3 paired box gene in the pediatric solid tumor alveolar rhabdomyosarcoma. Nature Genet 1993;3:113–17.

86. Cavazzana AO, Schmidt D, Ninfov, et al. Spindle cell rhabdomyosarcoma. A prognostically favorable variant of rhabdomyosarcoma. Am J Surg Pathol 1992;16:229–35.

87. Coindre JM, de Muscarel A, Trojani M, de Muscarel I, Pages A. Immunohistochemical study of rhabdomyosarcoma. Unexpected staining with S-100 protein and cytokeratin. J Pathol 1988;155:127–32.

88. Corson JM, Pinkus GS. Intracellular myoglobin—a specific marker for skeletal muscle differentiation in soft tissue sarcomas. An immunoperoxidase study. Am J Pathol 1981;103;384–9.

89. deJong AS, vanVark M, Albus-Lutter CE, van Raamsdonk W, Voute PA. Myosin and myoglobin as tumor markers in the diagnosis of rhabdomyosarcoma. A comparative study. Am J Surg Pathol 1984;8:521–28.

90. Dias P, Parham DM, Shapiro DN, Webber BL, Houghton PJ. Myogenic regulatory protein (MyoD1) expression in childhood solid tumors: diagnostic utility in rhabdomyosarcoma. Am J Pathol 1990;137:1283–91.

91. Enzinger FM, Weiss SW. Soft tissue tumors. 3rd ed. St. Louis: Mosby, 1995:539–77.

92. Eusebi V, Rilke F, Ceccarelli C, Fedeli F, Schiaffino S, Bussolati G. Fetal heavy chain skeletal myosin. An oncofetal antigen expressed by rhabdomyosarcoma. Am J Surg Pathol 1986;10:680–86.

93. Galili N, Davis RJ, Fredericks WJ, et al. Fusion of a forkhead gene to PAX3 in the solid tumour alveolar rhabdomyosarcoma. Nature Genet 1993;5:230-5.

94. Kindblom LG, Seidal T, Karlsson K. Immuno-histochemical localization of myoglobin in human muscle tissue and embryonal and alveolar rhabdomyosarcoma. Acta Pathol Microbiol Immunol Scand A 1982;90:167–74.

95. Kodet R, Newton WA Jr, Hamoudi AB, Asmar L, Jacobs, DL, Mauer HM. Childhood rhabdomyosarcoma with anaplastic (pleomorphic) features. A report of the Intergroup Rhabdomyosarcoma Study. Am J Surg Pathol 1993;17;443–53.

96. Maurer HM, Beltangady M, Gehan EA, et al. The Intergroup Rhabdomyosarcoma Study-I: a final report. Cancer 1988;61:209–20.

97. Maurer HM, Gehan EA, Beltangady M, et al. The Intergroup Rhabdomyosarcoma Study-II. Cancer 1993;71:1904–22.

98. Miettinen M, Lehto VP, Badley RA, Virtanen I. Alveolar rhabdomyosarcoma. Demonstration of the muscle type of intermediate filament protein, desmin, as a diagnostic aid. Am J Pathol 1982:108:246–51.

99. Miettinen M, Rapola J. Immunohistochemical spectrum of rhabdomyosarcoma and rhabdomyosarcoma-like tumors. Expression of cytokeratin and the 68-kD neurofilament protein. Am J Surg Pathol 1989;13:120–32.

100. Newton WA Jr, Gehan EA, Webber BL, et al. Classification of rhabdomyosarcomas and related sarcomas. Pathologic aspects and proposal for a new classification: an Intergroup Rhabdomyosarcoma Study. Cancer 1995;76:1073–85.

101. Rangdaeng S, Truong LD. Comparative immunohistochemical staining for desmin and muscle specific actin: a study of 576 cases. Am J Clin Pathol 1991;96:32–45.

102. Roberts P, Browne CF, Lewis IJ, et al. 12q13 abnormality in rhabdomyosarcoma. A nonrandom occurrence? Cancer Genet Cytogenet 1992;60:135–40.

103. Schmidt RA, Cone R, Haas JE, Gown AM. Diagnosis of rhabdomyosarcomas using HHF-35, a monoclonal antibody directed against muscle actins. Am J Pathol 1988;131:15–28.

104. Shapiro DN, Sublett JE, Li B, Downing JR, Naeve CW. Fusion of PAX3 to a member of the forkhead family of transcription factors in human alveolar rhabdomyosarcoma. Cancer Res 1993;53:5108–12.

105. Whang-Peng J, Knutsen T, Theil K, Harowitz ME, Triche T. Cytogenetic studies in subgroups of rhabdomyosarcoma. Genes Chromosomes Cancer 1992;5:299–310.

Leiomyosarcoma

106. Barnes L. Tumors and tumor-like lesions of the soft tissues. In: Barnes L, ed. Surgical pathology of the head and neck. New York: Marcel Dekker, 1985:725–880.

107. Farman AG, Kay S. Oral leiomyosarcoma. Report of a case and review of the literature pertaining to smooth-muscle tumors of the oral cavity. Oral Surg 1977;43:402–9.

108. Kuravilla A, Wenig BM, Humphrey DM, Heffner DK. Leiomyosarcoma of the sinonasal tract. A clinicopathologic study of nine cases. Arch Otolaryngeal Head Neck Surg 1990;166:1278–86.

Malignant Fibrous Histiocytoma

109. Barnes L. Tumors and tumor-like lesions of the soft tissue. In: Barnes L, ed. Surgical pathology of the head and neck. New York: Marcel Dekker, 1985:728–880.

110. Barnes L, Kanbour A. Malignant fibrous histiocytoma of the head and neck. A report of 12 cases. Arch Otolaryngeal Head Neck Surg 1988;114:1149–56.

111. Blitzer A, Lawson W, Zak FG, Biller HF, Som ML. Clinical-pathological determinants in prognosis of fibrous histiocytomas of head and neck. Laryngoscope 1981:91:2053–70.

112. Bras J, Batsakis JG, Luna MA. Malignant fibrous histiocytoma of the oral soft tissues. Oral Surg Oral Med Oral Pathol 1987;64:57–67.

113. Daou RA, Attia EL, Viloria JB. Malignant fibrous histiocytomas of the head and neck. J Otolaryngol 1983:12:783–8.

114. Enjoji M, Hashimoto H, Tsuneyoshi M, Iwasaki H. Malignant fibrous histiocytoma. A clinicopathologic study of 130 cases. Acta Pathol Jpn 1980:30:727–41.

115. Ferlito A, Nicolai P, Recher G, Narnes. Primary laryngeal malignant fibrous histiocytoma: review of the literature and report of seven cases. Largyngoscope 1983;93:1351–8.

116. Huvos AG, Heilweil M, Bretsky SS. The pathology of malignant fibrous histiocytoma of bone: a study of 130 patients. Am J Surg Pathol 1985;9:853–71.

117. Perzin KH, Fu YS. Non-epithelial tumors of the nasal cavity, paranasal sinuses and nasopharynx: a clinicopathologic study. XI. Fibrous histiocytomas. Cancer 1980;45:2616–26.

118. Russell WO, Cohen J, Enzinger FM, et al. A clinical and pathological staging system for soft tissue sarcomas. Cancer 1977;40:1562–70.

119. Weiss SW, Enzinger FM. Malignant fibrous histiocytoma: an analysis of 200 cases. Cancer 1978;41:2250–66.

Synovial Sarcoma

120. Abenoza P, Manivel JC, Swanson PE, Wick MR. Synovial sarcoma: ultrastructural study and immunohistochemical analysis by a combined peroxidase-antiperoxidase/avidin-biotin-peroxidase complex procedure. Hum Pathol 1986;17:1107–15.

121. Amble FR, Olsen KD, Nascimento AG, Foote RL. Head and neck synovial cell sarcoma. Otolaryngol Head Neck Surg 1992;107:631–7.

122. Barnes L. Tumors and tumor-like lesions of the soft tissues. In: Barnes L, ed. Surgical pathology of the head and neck. New York: Marcel Dekker, 1985:725–880.

123. Bridge JA, Bridge RS, Borek DA, Shaffer B, Norris CW. Translocation t(X;18) in orofacial synovial sarcoma. Cancer 1988;62:935–7.

124. Corson JM, Weiss LM, Banks-Schlegel SP, Pinkus GS. Keratin proteins and carcinoembryonic antigen in synovial sarcomas: an immunohistochemical study of 24 cases. Hum Pathol 1984;15:615–21.

125. Dei Tos AP, Wadden C, Calonje E, et al. Immunohistochemical demonstration of glycoprotein p30/32MIC2 (CD99) in synovial sarcoma. A potential cause of diagnostic confusion. Appl Immunohistochem 1995;3:168–73.

126. Enzinger FM, Weiss SW. Soft tissue tumors. 3rd ed. St. Louis: Mosby, 1995:757–86.

127. Fisher C. Synovial sarcoma: ultrastructural and immunohistochemical features of epithelial differentiation in monophasic and biphasic tumors. Hum Pathol 1986;17:996–1008.

128. Fisher C, Schofield JB. S-100 protein positive synovial sarcoma. Histopathology 1991;19:375–7.

129. Massarelli G, Tanda F, Salis B. Synovial sarcoma of the soft palate: report of a case. Hum Pathol 1978;9:341–5.

130. Miettinen M, Lehto VP, Virtanen I. Monophasic synovial sarcoma of spindle-cell type. Epithelial differentiation as revealed by ultrastructural features, content of prekeratin and binding of peanut agglutinin. Virchows Arch [Cell Pathol] 1983;44:187–99.

131. Nunez-Alonso C, Gashti EN, Christ ML. Maxillofacial synovial sarcoma. Light and electron microscopic study of two cases. Am J Surg Pathol 1979;3:23–30.

132. Ordonez NG, Mahfouz SM, Mackay B. Synovial sarcoma: an immunohistochemical and ultrastructural study. Hum Pathol 1990;21:733–49.

133. Roth JA, Enzinger FM, Tannenbaum M. Synovial sarcoma of the neck: a follow-up study of 24 cases. Cancer 1975;35:1243–53.

134. Salisbury JR, Isaacson PG. Synovial sarcoma: an immunohistochemical study. J Pathol 1985;147:49–57.

135. Schmidt D, Thum P, Harms D, Treuner J. Synovial sarcoma in children and adolescents. A report from the Kiel Pediatric Tumor Registry. Cancer 1991;67:1667–72.

136. Shmookler BM, Enzinger FM, Brannon RB. Orofacial synovial sarcoma: a clinicopathologic study of 11 new cases and review of the literature. Cancer 1982;50:269–76.

137. Sumitono M, Hirose T, Kudo E, Sano T, Shinomiya S, Hizawa K. Epithelial differentiation in synovial sarcoma. Correlation with histology and immunophenotypic expression. Acta Pathol Jpn 1989;39:381–7.

Alveolar Soft Part Sarcoma

138. Auerbach HE, Brooks JJ. Alveolar soft part sarcoma. A clinicopathologic and immunohistochemical study. Cancer 1987;60:66–73.

139. Enzinger FM, Weiss SW. Soft tissue tumors. 3rd ed. St. Louis: Mosby, 1995:1067–93.

140. Foschini MP, Ceccarelli C, Eusebi V, Skalli O, Gabbiani G. Alveolar soft part sarcoma: immunological evidence of rhabdomyoblastic differentiation. Histopathology 1988;13:101–8.

141. Hirose T, Kudo E, Hasegawa T, Abe JI, Hizawa K. Cytoskeletal properties of alveolar soft part sarcoma. Hum Pathol 1990;21:204–11.

142. Lieberman PH, Brennan MF, Kimmel M, Erlandson RA, Garin-Chesa P, Flehinger BY. Alveolar soft part sarcoma. A clinicopathologic study of half a century. Cancer 1989;63:1–13.

143. Master K, Berkmen YM. Pulmonary metastases 15 years after removal of alveolar soft part sarcoma of the tongue. Rev Interam Radiol 1979;4:43–5.

144. Matsuno Y, Mukai K, Itabashi M, et al. Alveolar soft part sarcoma. A clinicopathologic and immunohistochemical study of 12 cases. Acta Pathol Jpn 1990;40:199–205.

145. Miettinen M, Ekfors T. Alveolar soft part sarcoma: immunohistochemical evidence of muscle cell differentiation. Am J Clin Pathol 1990;93:32–8.

146. Mukai M, Torikata C, Iri H, et al. Histogenesis of alveolar soft part sarcoma. An immunohistochemical and biochemical study. Am J Surg Pathol 1986;10:212–8.

147. Ordonez NG, Ro JY, Mackay B. Alveolar soft part sarcoma. An ultrastructural and immunocytochemical investigation of its histogenesis. Cancer 1989;63:1721–36.

148. Rosai J, Dias P, Parham DM, Shapiro DN, Houghton P. MyoD1 protein expression in alveolar soft part sarcoma as confirmatory evidence of its skeletal muscle nature. Am J Surg Pathol 1991;15:974–81.

149. Simmons WB, Haggerty HS, Ngan B, Anonsen CK. Alveolar soft part sarcoma of the head and neck. A disease of children and young adults. Int J Pediatr Otorhinolaryngol 1989;17:139–53.

150. Spector R, Travis L, Smith J. Alveolar soft part sarcoma of the head and neck. Laryngoscope 1979;89:1301–6.

151. Wang NP, Bacchi CE, Jiang JJ, McNutt MA, Gown AM. Does alveolar soft-part sarcoma exhibit skeletal muscle differentiation? An immunocytochemical and biochemical study of myogenic regulatory protein expression. Mod Pathol 1996;9:496–506.

❖❖❖

15

MISCELLANEOUS TUMOR-LIKE LESIONS

NASAL POLYPS

Definition. A nasal polyp is a non-neoplastic, inflammatory, polypoid mass comprised of edematous to fibrotic, inflamed stroma and entrapped epithelium.

General Features. Typical nasal polyps are invariably multiple and usually bilateral, involving both the nasal cavity and the paranasal sinuses. Nasal polyps are frequently associated with asthma and, less commonly, with chronic rhinitis; in some cases, a predisposing condition cannot be identified. About 7 percent of longstanding asthmatics develop nasal polyps, as do about 2 percent of patients with chronic rhinitis (9). The clinical triad of inflammatory nasal polyps, asthma, and bronchospastic aspirin intolerance is well recognized (7); about 14 percent of asthmatics with nasal polyps develop a bronchospastic reaction to aspirin (9,11).

The pathogenesis of nasal polyps is not well understood. The role of allergic reactions is unclear, although immunoglobulins have been shown to be present within the stroma of the polyps in concentrations higher than would be expected due to passive diffusion (2). Other studies have suggested that an alteration in carbohydrate metabolism, with deposition of short-chain polysaccharides, might lead to increased osmotic pressure and fluid accumulation (10). In a similar fashion, evaporation of fluid from the mucosal surface of the polyp might lead to passive accumulation of normal proteins in the stroma with a similar osmotic gradient developing.

Clinical Features. Typical inflammatory nasal polyps are uncommon in patients under 20 years of age (3,5). The exception is the 7 to 20 percent of patients with cystic fibrosis (mucoviscidosis) who develop nasal polyps in childhood or early adolescence (9,11). The polyps may precede the clinical diagnosis of cystic fibrosis by several years, and the presence of multiple nasal polyps in a child or adolescent should lead to tests for cystic fibrosis (1). It has been suggested that the nasal polyps in cystic fibrosis have some microscopic distinctions from typical inflammatory nasal polyps (see Microscopic Findings below).

Although most nasal polyps are indolent lesions, rare examples have eroded bone and even extended into the cranial cavity (8,12).

Gross Findings. Grossly, inflammatory nasal polyps are soft, fleshy, and translucent gray to pink. They are typically sessile lesions lacking a long stalk. Often the cut surface "weeps" clear liquid or mucoid fluid. Most examples are one to several centimeters in size. Any areas of opaque tissue should be carefully sectioned for microscopic examination to exclude a schneiderian papilloma or malignancy.

Microscopic Findings. The surface of a nasal polyp may be covered with respiratory, mucinous, or squamous epithelium, or, most commonly, by a mixture of these cell types. The underlying basement membrane may be normal, but often appears as a thick eosinophilic band beneath the surface epithelium (fig. 15-1). The stroma is primarily edematous with an often prominent inflammatory cell component. Eosinophils may be present in striking numbers and the term, *allergic polyp* has been applied to such lesions, although this designation has no clearcut clinical significance (fig. 15-2). Mast cells, lymphocytes, and plasma cells may also be present in large numbers. Blood vessels are often prominent in the edematous stroma (fig. 15-3), and there may be areas of stromal fibrosis. Amyloid-like material, or, rarely, islands of cartilage or osteoid may also be present within the stroma of longstanding polyps. Scattered enlarged, variably atypical stromal cells may be seen in nasal polyps. In some examples they are characterized by large, hyperchromatic or smudged, multilobated nuclei. Others have eccentric vesicular nuclei and prominent cytoplasm, resembling ganglion cells (fig. 15-4). This phenomenon, discussed in more detail below under antrochoanal polyps, is of no clinical consequence, but must not be misdiagnosed as a stromal malignancy. Frequently, glandular structures are embedded within the stroma of nasal polyps. The mixture of respiratory, mucinous, and squamous epithelium is identical to that seen covering the polyp surface, and these glands presumably arise due to invagination of the

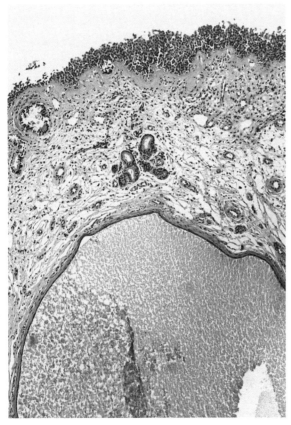

Figure 15-1
INFLAMMATORY NASAL POLYP
This inflammatory nasal polyp is lined by respiratory epithelium, with an underlying thickened basement membrane. The stroma is edematous and contains a large intralesional cyst.

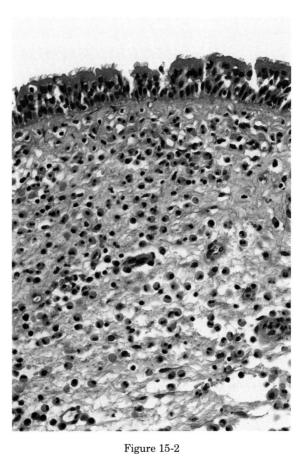

Figure 15-2
INFLAMMATORY NASAL POLYP
Beneath the slightly thickened basement membrane, the underlying stroma contains numerous eosinophils.

Figure 15-3
INFLAMMATORY NASAL POLYP
Inflammatory nasal polyps may contain prominent capillaries or larger blood vessels.

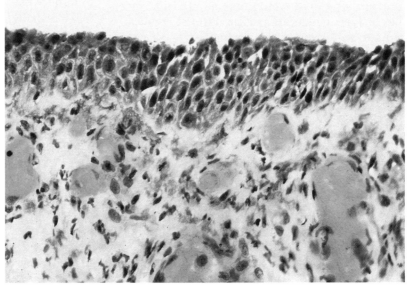

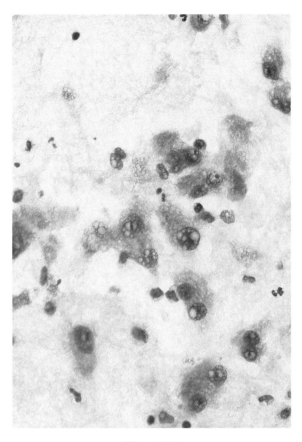

Figure 15-4
INFLAMMATORY NASAL POLYP
Inflammatory nasal polyps may contain enlarged, atypical stromal cells. In this instance, the enlarged cells resemble ganglion cells.

surface mucosa. Occasionally, the glandular component may be striking, leading to confusion with a glandular neoplasm.

Nasal polyps in patients with cystic fibrosis lack the basement membrane thickening and prominent stromal eosinophils typical of inflammatory polyps (6). In addition, the polyps in cystic fibrosis have acidic mucin in the cysts, mucous glands, and mucous blanket of the polyps (9) Differential staining with alcian blue and periodic acid–Schiff stains has been used to distinguish these features.

Differential Diagnosis. The distinction between typical nasal polyps and antrochoanal polyps is discussed below, under the latter topic. Also discussed in that section is the distinction between polyps with stromal atypia and a polypoid sarcoma such as the botryoid variant of

embryonal rhabdomyosarcoma. Nasal polyps may contain gaping vascular channels in a variably fibrous stroma, leading to some potential for confusion with angiofibroma. This is an easy misdiagnosis to avoid. Angiofibromas virtually always arise in the nasopharynx and have a uniformly fibrous stroma. More importantly, on higher magnification, they are comprised of innumerable small, irregular vascular spaces within the fibrous stroma. Nasal polyps may have prominent larger vessels, but they lack these delicate small vessels. In addition, the intralesional mucous glands seen in nasal polyps are not encountered in angiofibromas. Nasal polyps may undergo secondary ulceration with a prominent granulation tissue response, but areas of stromal edema and residual glandular inclusions usually allow for correct interpretation.

Treatment and Prognosis. Initial therapy for nasal polyps is usually aimed at treating an underlying allergic condition with topical or systemic steroids, and possible elimination of allergens (4). The most common form of surgical treatment is simple avulsion of the polyp(s) with a wire snare (3,4). Surgery is often planned for the time of year when offending allergens are less prevalent (4).

Recurrent disease is a common problem with nasal polyps and up to 50 percent of patients develop new lesions following initial polypectomy (3). Patients with aspirin intolerance and asthma have the highest rates of recurrence (3).

RESPIRATORY EPITHELIAL ADENOMATOID AND GLANDULAR (SEROMUCINOUS) HAMARTOMAS

General and Clinical Features. Although a few earlier examples of so-called hamartomatous nasopharyngeal lesions were documented, a case arising in the nasopharynx in 1974 was termed glandular (seromucinous) hamartoma (13). The 26-year-old retarded black male complained of epistaxis and difficulty in nasal breathing. On clinical examination there was subtotal obstruction of the right nasal cavity by a smooth, round, circumscribed mass that measured 4 cm. Additional hamartomatous lesions in the nasopharynx and sinonasal tract have been described (14,16), including 31 cases of respiratory epithelial adenomatoid hamartoma by Wenig and Heffner (15).

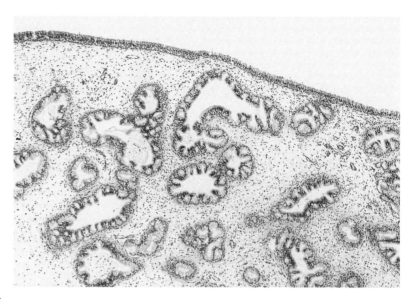

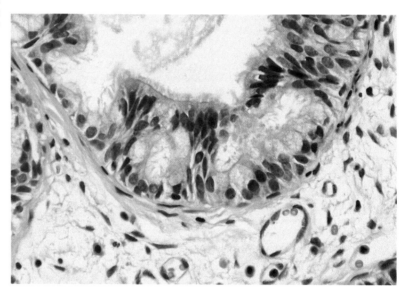

Figure 15-5
RESPIRATORY EPITHELIAL
ADENOMATOID HAMARTOMA
Well-formed, branching glands set
within an edematous stroma (top) are
lined chiefly by ciliated respiratory epithelial cells (bottom).

Over 80 percent of the patients with hamartomas are men (13–16). The age range is from
the third to ninth decade of life. Symptoms, of
months' or years' duration, are nasal obstruction,
stuffiness, epistaxis, postnasal drainage, and
chronic rhinosinusitis (15). Sites of occurrence
include nasal septum, ethmoid sinus, frontal
sinus, and nasopharynx. Approximately 70 percent of respiratory epithelial adenomatoid hamartomas occur in the nasal cavity, often along the
posterior nasal septum (15). These lesions may
result from stimulation by an inflammatory process (15). It is possible that some of them actually
represent an exuberant hyperplasia of epithelium in an inflammatory polyp.

Gross Findings. The lesions are circumscribed and polypoid, and measure up to 5 cm. A
stalk may be present. On cut surface, there are
firm, tan-white solid areas and, on occasion,
cystic foci that measure a few millimeters in size.

Microscopic Findings. Well-developed,
branching glands are composed chiefly of ciliated
respiratory epithelial cells (fig. 15-5) (15). Sometimes the epithelium is cuboid or flat. Mucous
gland metaplasia may also be present. Numerous glands with mucinous luminal contents may

be observed. The surface of the lesion is lined by ciliated respiratory epithelium which is in direct continuity with some of the glands (15). There may be stromal hyalinization. Other changes that are present as well in sinonasal inflammatory polyps include stromal edema, seromucous gland proliferation, increased vascularity, and a mixed acute and chronic inflammatory infiltrate. Inverted papilloma and solitary fibrous tumor have been found coincidentally (15). Lymphangiomatous proliferation and osseous metaplasia have rarely been seen within the respiratory epithelial adenomatoid hamartoma.

In a few instances the glandular component consists of seromucous glands (13–16). These *glandular hamartomas* also arise in the sinonasal tract and nasopharynx. The glands may be surrounded by basement membrane-like material. Cystic glands often contain eosinophilic material. Foci of squamous metaplasia may be present (16). The fibrovascular stroma sometimes has foci of metaplastic bone or lymphoid follicles.

One *mesenchymal hamartoma* composed of skeletal muscle has been described (14). It arose from the nasal surface of the soft palate. It also was lined by respiratory-type epithelium with focal squamous metaplasia. The polyp base had dense collagen with numerous blood vessels and some seromucinous glands.

The differential diagnosis for epithelial hamartoma includes inverted papilloma, teratoma, and adenocarcinoma.

Treatment and Prognosis. Complete excision is curative.

ANTROCHOANAL POLYP

Definition. This is a clinically and to a lesser extent microscopically distinctive variant of nasal polyp that originates from the maxillary antrum, extends into the nasal cavity through a maxillary ostium, and often protrudes through the nasal choana into the nasopharynx or oropharynx.

General Features. Antrochoanal polyps were first described in 1753, but it was not until 1906 that Killian (21) documented their origin within the maxillary antrum. These polyps originate from a wall of the maxillary antrum and enter the nasal cavity in the region of the middle meatus, usually through an accessory maxillary ostium, a structure that appears to be important

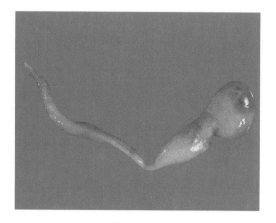

Figure 15-6
ANTROCHOANAL POLYP
This small antrochoanal polyp retained a long stalk from its point of origin in the maxillary sinus.

to the development of antrochoanal polyps and present in about 10 percent of the population (18,20). Once within the nasal cavity, the polyp enlarges, usually protruding through the nasal choana to become visible in the nasopharynx. The portion of the polyp within the maxillary antrum may continue to enlarge as well, producing an "hour glass" shaped structure with a constriction at the maxillary ostium.

Clinical Features. Antrochoanal polyps may occur at any age. Unlike typical nasal polyps, childhood cases are frequent. Thus, the presence of an antrochoanal polyp in a child should not raise undue concern regarding the possibility of cystic fibrosis. Whereas typical nasal polyps are often bilateral and multiple, 92 percent of antrochoanal polyps are solitary lesions (26). About 8 percent of patients with antrochoanal polyps also have typical nasal polyps. Antrochoanal polyps are less common than the typical nasal variants, and account for only about 4 to 6 percent of all nasal polyps (20,24). The majority of patients with typical nasal polyps have a documented allergic condition, but this is less common (16 to 40 percent) in patients with antrochoanal polyps (18,24).

Gross Findings. Antrochoanal polyps may grossly resemble typical nasal polyps, but often have a more fibrous, less edematous or translucent cut surface. Often, there is a long, attenuated stalk in the resected specimen as a result of the origin in the maxillary antrum (fig. 15-6). Some antrochoanal polyps are large multilobated

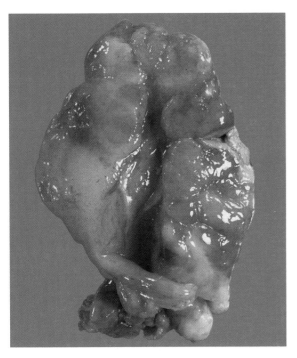

Figure 15-7
ANTROCHOANAL POLYP
Antrochoanal polyps may be large, multilobated, "fleshy" masses causing concern among both clinicians and pathologists that they may represent malignant neoplasms.

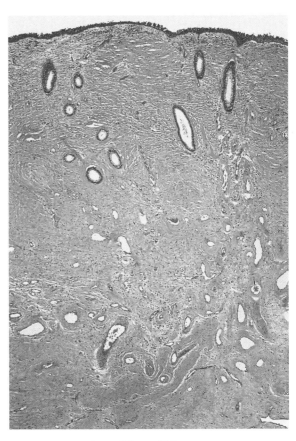

Figure 15-8
ANTROCHOANAL POLYP
Antrochoanal polyps typically have prominent fibrous stroma containing scattered blood vessels. Entrapped seromucinous glands are usually present superficially.

masses, leading to a clinical suspicion of malignancy (fig. 15-7).

Microscopic Findings. Antrochoanal polyps share some microscopic features with typical nasal polyps. There may be focal thickening of the subepithelial basement membrane and about 20 percent have prominent stromal eosinophils (19). Other examples may have prominent lymphocytes and plasma cells. Although the stroma of antrochoanal polyps may be quite edematous, often it has a more fibrotic appearance (fig. 15-8). Glandular epithelium may be present within the polyp, and is usually concentrated just below the surface epithelium. As with typical nasal polyps, the surface mucosa may consist of mixtures of squamous, mucinous, and respiratory epithelial cells.

Stromal Atypia. Scattered, atypical to overtly bizarre stromal cells, often with convoluted and "smudged" or hyperchromatic nuclei, may be encountered in both antrochoanal and typical nasal polyps (fig. 15-9) (17,22,23,25). These cells lack mitotic activity and resemble the atypical stro-

mal fibroblasts seen following radiation therapy. Other than their potential to confuse pathologists, these atypical cells are of no clinical significance. Similar or identical cells have also been described in polypoid lesions from other anatomic sites, including the vagina. In our experience, antrochoanal polyps are more prone to develop this change and, because they can occur in younger children, this benign change has occasionally been catastrophically misinterpreted as a botryoid rhabdomyosarcoma (25). Differential diagnostic features are briefly reviewed below.

Differential Diagnosis. Antrochoanal polyps should be distinguished from typical nasal polyps whenever possible, particularly if the lesion arises in a child or adolescent. Typical nasal polyps in this age range should lead to concern regarding cystic fibrosis. Differentiation is usually obvious

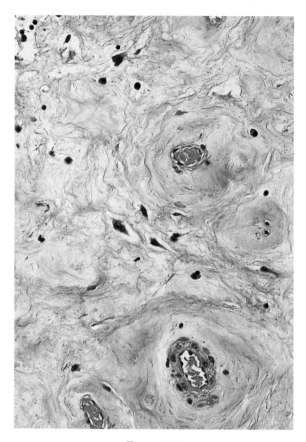

Figure 15-9
ANTROCHOANAL POLYP
Scattered, enlarged, hyperchromatic stromal cells are common in antrochoanal polyps and should not be confused with malignancy.

clinically, but the presence of a single polyp with a fibrous stroma and long stalk should alert the pathologist to this diagnostic possibility.

Polypoid, translucent nasal or nasopharyngeal masses in young children may be suspected, clinically, of representing the botryoid subtype of embryonal rhabdomyosarcoma, and this concern may be indicated on the pathology request card. Armed with this information, unwary pathologists may overdiagnose the scattered atypical stromal cells often encountered in antrochoanal (and typical) polyps as a sarcoma. The potential for error is enhanced by the fact that these stromal cells can express actin (23). Although the degree of individual cell atypia may be striking, the overall cellularity is sparse. Mitotic figures are extremely rare and the atypical cells are dispersed in a loose, edematous stroma without evidence of neovas-

cularity or a well-formed cambium layer as is encountered in embryonal rhabdomyosarcoma. Furthermore, the presence of scattered mature glands within the polypoid mass should alert the pathologist to the correct diagnosis. Although the atypical stromal cells may express muscle-specific actin and smooth muscle actin, they lack staining for desmin or myoglobin (23). Interestingly, they also have been shown to express cytokeratin (23). The latter may lead to confusion with a sarcomatoid carcinoma, but the features outlined above should aid in this distinction.

Treatment and Prognosis. Recurrences of antrochoanal polyps following snare excision develop in 20 to 33 percent of patients. Intervals between recurrences range from 1 to 10 years (24). Virtually all patients with recurrent antrochoanal polyps have a history of allergic disease (20). Patients treated with a medial maxillectomy (Caldwell-Luc procedure) with removal of the polyp base almost never develop recurrent disease.

VOCAL CORD NODULE/POLYP

Vocal cord nodules usually develop after prolonged misuse or overuse of the voice (27–30). They commonly occur in young children, singers, and others who chronically stress their vocal cords. *Vocal cord polyps* are larger masses that occupy most of the true vocal cord (fig. 15-10). They are commonly seen in smokers and also may be associated with voice abuse. Vocal cord nodules and polyps have virtually identical histologic features, differing only in extent of disease.

Microscopically, the initial change is an accumulation of edema fluid or blood in Reinke's space. Due to the underlying rigid elastic tissue barrier, this space can only expand outward. The outward bulge and fluid within the space alters the acoustic properties of the vocal cord, producing hoarseness or other variations in voice quality. Vocal cord nodules and polyps exhibit a large spectrum of microscopic appearances. There may be some relationship between the age of the lesion and its microscopic features.

Patients with shorter clinical histories tend to have nodules or polyps with prominent edematous or myxoid stroma, whereas longstanding examples tend to show more prominent stromal fibrosis. Variable degrees of vascular proliferation may be seen. In some instances there may be

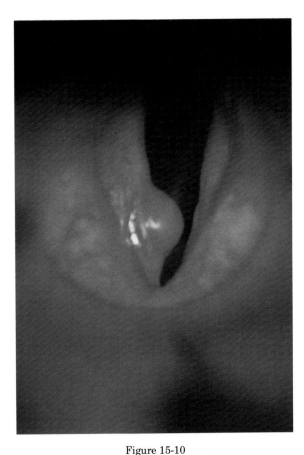

Figure 15-10
VOCAL CORD NODULE
A vocal cord nodule is located along the anterior portion of the vocal cord.

florid papillary endothelial hyperplasia, and we have seen this exuberant reaction misdiagnosed as angiosarcoma. The stroma of vocal cord nodules and polyps may contain aggregates of eosinophilic, proteinaceous material (fig. 15-11). In the past, this has been misinterpreted as amyloid, but it lacks appropriate staining with Congo red. Hemosiderin deposits are common in the stroma, particularly in longstanding polyps. Vocal cord nodules and polyps are usually covered by normal squamous mucosa. There may be some associated surface keratosis (fig. 15-11). Nodules and polyps removed from smokers may show the full spectrum of mucosal dysplastic changes including invasive carcinoma; this appears to be a coincidental process.

Smaller vocal cord nodules are treated non-surgically with voice rest. Larger nodules and vocal cord polyps may require surgical removal (30).

CONTACT/POSTINTUBATION ULCER OF THE LARYNX

Contact and postintubation ulcers differ only in their etiology (31,33). The latter term is applied to patients developing this lesion following endotracheal intubation, and the former is applied to identical lesions occurring without prior surgery, but often associated with vocal abuse or, possibly, acid regurgitation secondary to an esophageal hiatal hernia. Grossly, these are usually tan to hemorrhagic mucosal defects that measure from 1 mm to 3 cm and show a strong tendency to

Figure 15-11
VOCAL CORD NODULE
Left: This vocal cord nodule has reactive, hyperkeratotic overlying squamous mucosa. The stroma is vascular and edematous.
Right: Vocal cord nodules and polyps often contain eosinophilic proteinaceous material that should not be confused with amyloid.

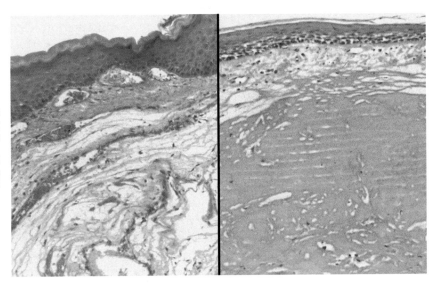

involve the posterior portion of one or both vocal cords (fig. 15-12) (33). Associated granulation tissue may produce a polypoid mass. The posterior area of the vocal cord appears to be predilected because of the thin mucosa covering the vocal process of the arytenoid, the fact that this portion of the cord moves the most during phonation, and the tendency for the vocal processes to strike each other during vocal abuse. Much less commonly the middle or, rarely, anterior portion of the vocal cord(s) may be affected.

Microscopically, most examples show overt mucosal ulceration with associated exuberant granulation tissue. The latter consists of closely spaced, radially oriented capillaries in an acutely inflamed stroma (32). Over time, if the causative factor is chronic, the surface will re-epithelialize, often with associated epithelial hyperplasia. More florid examples of such hyperplasia may lead to confusion with squamous cell carcinoma, although the posterior portion of the vocal cord is not a common site for such neoplasms. Chronic changes in the stroma may lead to the formation of larger blood vessels and a prominent fibroblastic proliferation. Mildly pleomorphic, multinucleated stromal giant cells may also be present (33). These may show a "floret-like" annular orientation of the nuclei.

DERMOID CYST

General Features. The term "teratoid" has been used for a solid or cystic growth in the upper aerodigestive tract that is not a true neoplasm but is composed of one or more germinal layers. The term has most often been applied to dermoid cysts or hairy polyps, both of which are not true neoplasms, but arise as congenital inclusions. McAvoy and Zuckerbraun (36) have classified four types of dermoid cyst that develop in the head and neck area. Fifty to 70 percent of these cysts occur as periorbital inclusions between the maxillary and mandibular processes in the naso-optic groove or pit (36,38,41); they appear retro-orbital, supraorbital, or canthal. Eight to 13 percent of head and neck dermoid cysts overlie the dorsum of the nose, and develop from displaced ectoderm at the time of ossification of the frontonasal plate (38). Approximately one fourth of dermoid cysts occur in the floor of the mouth and may appear as a submental mass (38,41);

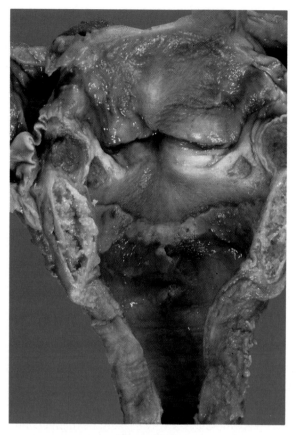

Figure 15-12
POSTINTUBATION ULCER
Bilaterally symmetrical subglottic ulcers secondary to prolonged intubation are noted just beneath the posterior portion of the vocal cords, near the lateral margins of the opened specimen. Another area of more diffuse mucosal hyperplasia and ulceration is located below this, near the laryngotracheal junction.

they result from enclavement of midline epithelium during closure of mandibular and hyoid branchial arches. The cyst occurs between the geniohyoid muscle and the oral mucosa, deeper between the geniohyoid and mylohyoid muscles, or below the mylohyoid muscle (39). The fourth type of dermoid cyst arises as a midventral and middorsal fusion in suprasternal, thyroidal, and suboccipital areas (36,38,41).

Clinical Features. Oral dermoid cysts may simulate a ranula, thyroglossal duct cyst, or lymphangioma (39). They are seldom present at birth, and are found chiefly in young adults (39). There is no sex predilection. A swelling in the anterior floor of the mouth is often present, sometimes with elevation of the tongue. Difficulties in eating and talking due to the painless mass may occur (39). Oral dermoid cysts occasionally become infected and a sinus tract may develop. Computed tomograms or ultrasonic images reveal an obviously cystic lesion.

Nasal dermoid cysts are seen most often at birth, but the mean age at surgery is 12 years (40). Such lesions have been reported in adults, especially those in the sixth decade of life (35). There is a slight male predilection. Sometimes nasal dermoid cysts are familial or are associated with other congenital abnormalities (35). They usually cause no discomfort, but may become infected. The cysts occur almost exclusively in the midline, most often in the dorsum of the nose; they may also be found on the septum, tip of the nose, glabella, or columella. Multiple sites of involvement may occur. A nasal dermoid cyst most often appears as a small midline pit or depression on the bridge of the nose from which hairs sometimes protrude. In fact, protruding hairs with or without sebaceous drainage at the nasal dorsum is pathognomonic (34). Two thirds of patients have bony or cartilaginous destruction, while about half have a sinus tract (37). Deep dermoid cysts may present as an obstructing nasal mass. Such cysts may have a dumbbell shape above and below the suture line of the nasal bones. The rates reported for intracranial extension have varied from 19 to 45 percent (34). It is important to distinguish a nasal dermoid cyst from an encephalocele. When a nasal dermoid cyst is suspected, radiographic studies of the facial bones and skull are essential.

Gross Findings. Cystic lesions range from a few millimeters to several centimeters in size. On cut section, the contents consist of hair and greasy, grumous material.

Microscopic Findings. The cyst is lined by keratinized squamous epithelium (fig. 15-13). The wall is often thickened and contains fibrovascular tissue. Sebaceous glands, hair follicles, and sweat glands are typically present. Endodermal tissue and the mesodermal components of bone and cartilage are absent.

Treatment and Prognosis. Surgical excision is indicated to obtain a pathologic diagnosis, prevent subsequent infection, and ensure cosmesis. Several surgical options are available, depending upon the cyst location. For nasal dermoid cysts, surgery includes complete excision,

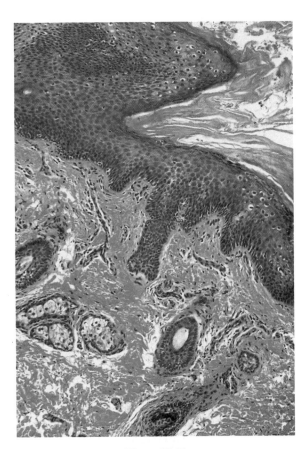

Figure 15-13
DERMOID CYST
Sebaceous glands and hair follicles lead to the cyst, which is lined by keratinized squamous epithelium.

repair of the cribriform plate defect (if present), and reconstruction of the nasal dorsum (34). Although recurrences are not typical for oral dermoid cysts (39), nasal lesions may return if they are incompletely resected (35,40), and more than one surgical attempt at eradication of a nasal dermoid cyst is not unusual.

HAIRY POLYP

General Features. This developmental lesion composed of ectoderm and mesoderm occurs chiefly in the nasopharynx (60 percent), but may also arise in the tonsil, eustachian tube, oropharynx, or middle ear (42,43). It may fill the nasal cavity or protrude into the oral cavity. Sometimes there is intracranial extension through a skull perforation. Hairy polyps likely represent developmental anomalies arising from the first

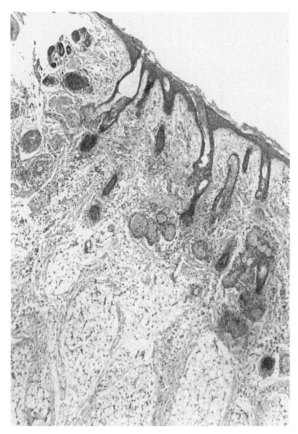

Figure 15-14
HAIRY POLYP
Sebaceous glands and sweat glands lie below the surface squamous epithelium.

branchial cleft area, and, hence, represent heterotopic accessory ears (auricles) (43).

Clinical Features. Hairy polyp is usually seen in newborns, but may be found in children or young adults (42). It occurs more often in females. It appears as a pedunculated mass, often causing nasal obstruction. Clinical symptoms depend on its size and location, but include dyspnea, cough, and difficulty in swallowing. Rarely it is associated with other congenital malformations such as cleft palate (42).

Gross Findings. The pedunculated mass may be up to 6 cm in greatest dimension. It is sausage, pear, or club shaped. It has a gray or white surface that is slightly corrugated and skin-like. The site of attachment of the polyp may appear as normal mucosa.

Microscopic Findings. The polyp is covered by keratinized squamous epithelium and con-

tains sebaceous glands, sweat glands, and hair follicles (fig. 15-14). Minor salivary glands may occasionally be present below the skin surface. Underlying the epithelium, the connective tissue consists of collagen, lobules of adipose tissue, and smooth and skeletal muscle. Cartilage and bone may also be present (42). The cartilage appears as a plate of uniform thickness, and is about as thick as normal auricular cartilage (43). Some polyps have well-developed elastic cartilage. In addition, a few nerve fibers may be found embedded in the polyp.

Treatment and Prognosis. Simple excision is adequate therapy. Recurrences generally are absent.

AMYLOID DEPOSITION

Amyloid deposition can occur throughout the head and neck, either as an apparently isolated phenomenon or as a part of systemic amyloidosis. The tongue is a very common site of involvement in systemic disease, while the larynx is a common location for isolated amyloid deposits (44–49,51,54,55). Any portion of the larynx may be involved, but the false cords and ventricles, followed by the true cords and subglottic region, are the usual sites. Adults are most often affected, although the age range is quite broad and occasional children with laryngeal amyloid nodules have been described (49). There is no male or female predilection. Localized amyloid deposition has also been described in the nose and paranasal sinuses (52).

Grossly, amyloid often forms distinct, tumor-like nodules of yellow, gray, or red, covered by intact mucosa (44). Occasionally, the infiltration is more diffuse. Microscopically, amyloid most often forms amorphous submucosal masses (fig. 15-15). It may also expand the walls of blood vessels or basement membranes of minor salivary glands. In standard hematoxylin and eosin (H&E)-stained sections, amyloid is a strongly eosinophilic, "glassy," fragmented material. As noted elsewhere in this chapter, the fibrinoid material deposited in a vocal cord polyp may superficially resemble amyloid. This material lacks the glassy, shattered, refractile appearance of true amyloid, however. Given the appropriate setting, a positive Congo red stain (fig. 15-15) with associated "apple-green" birefringence

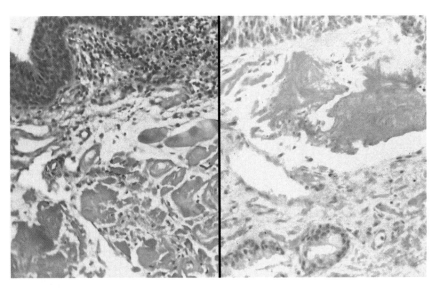

Figure 15-15
AMYLOID DEPOSITION
Left: Beneath a lining of respiratory mucosa and some associated inflammatory cells are aggregates of acellular eosinophilic material typical of amyloid.
Right: The aggregates of amyloid stain with Congo red.

under polarized light is diagnostic of amyloid. Metachromatic staining with crystal violet or fluorescent staining with the thioflavin-T technique may also be of value. The aggregates of amyloid are usually associated with a variable inflammatory reaction that often includes numerous plasma cells. Foreign body giant cells may be seen "engulfing" fragments of amyloid (amyloid granuloma). Ultrastructurally, this material has the same fibrillar pattern seen in systemic amyloidosis (55). Immunohistochemically, it contains lambda or, less commonly, kappa immunoglobulin light chains (49,50).

Limited surgical or laser resection is the treatment of choice for symptomatic localized laryngeal amyloid deposition (49,50,53). Local recurrences may develop, often after a protracted period of time, but conversion to systemic disease is extremely rare (45,50,53).

LARYNGEAL RHEUMATOID ARTHRITIS AND NODULES

Up to 25 percent of patients with rheumatoid arthritis develop symptomatic laryngeal involvement (57,58), and autopsy studies show that 50 to 80 percent of patients with rheumatoid arthritis have microscopic evidence of laryngeal disease. Either the cricoarytenoid or cricothyroid joints are involved, but damage to the former is more functionally significant. The small diarthrodial joints undergo pathologic changes identical to those en-

countered in larger joints elsewhere in the body. A vascular, inflamed, synovial proliferation covers and destroys articulating cartilaginous surfaces, forming a pannus that ultimately replaces the joint space. Fibrous tissue bridges the previous joint, producing a deformed, immobile structure. Such immobility of the arytenoids may lead to respiratory obstruction and require an emergency tracheostomy; in a nonemergency situation, the cord may be surgically lateralized to preserve the airway lumen.

Rheumatoid nodules of the larynx are less common than in the joints. Any portion of the larynx may be involved and there may or may not be associated joint disease. Patients with laryngeal rheumatoid nodules often have rheumatoid pulmonary disease. Microscopically, well-developed rheumatoid nodules consist of a central zone of fibrinoid necrosis, surrounded by palisading histiocytes (fig. 15-16). The overlying mucosa usually remains intact. Newly developing nodules are highly vascular, leading to possible confusion with granulation tissue (59). Laryngeal rheumatoid nodules or cricoarytenoid arthritis may also occur in patients with lupus erythematosus and ankylosing spondylitis (56,60).

RHINOSCLEROMA

Rhinoscleroma is a mass-forming lesion caused by bacterial infection with *Klebsiella rhinoscleromatis*. The disease often produces

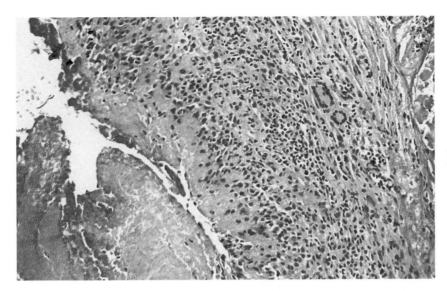

Figure 15-16
LARYNGEAL
RHEUMATOID NODULE
A laryngeal rheumatoid nodule
has an area of fibrinoid necrosis at
the lower left surrounded by a
zone of inflammatory cells including histiocytes and multinucleated giant cells.

large, deforming, tumorous masses that fill the
nasal cavity, paranasal sinuses, or involve the oral
cavity (61,64,65,67,68). The disease typically occurs in underdeveloped regions and is prevalent in
Egypt, portions of South America, portions of Af-
rica, and areas in the eastern regions of Europe. It
has traditionally been a rare disease in the United
States, but the increasing mobility of world populations has made this disease more commonly
encountered. There is no sex predilection and
patients are usually in their first four decades of
life. The nasal septum is the most common site
of disease, followed by the remainder of the nasal
cavity, nasopharynx, ethmoid sinuses, orbit, larynx, trachea, bronchi, and middle ear (63).

Grossly, there is typically a fungating or polypoid mass with a partially intact squamous mucosal covering. The gross appearance may be suggestive of a fungating malignancy. Microscopically, the
well-developed, "florid" phase of the lesion is characterized by prominent pseudoepitheliomatous
hyperplasia overlying an intense mixed inflammatory infiltrate containing lymphocytes, plasma
cells, polymorphonuclear leukocytes, and characteristic foamy histiocytes, often referred to as
Mikulicz cells (fig. 15-17). This appearance may
be quite similar to that of leprosy. A tissue Gram
stain, or, optimally, a Warthin-Starry or Steiner
silver stain reveals numerous Gram-negative
bacillary organisms within the cytoplasm of the
foamy histiocytes (fig. 15-18). The organisms
may also be identified by the immunoperoxidase
technique (66).

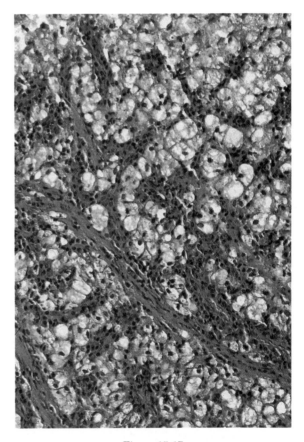

Figure 15-17
NASAL RHINOSCLEROMA
This example of nasal rhinoscleroma contains large num-
bers of vacuolated histiocytes (Mikulicz cells).

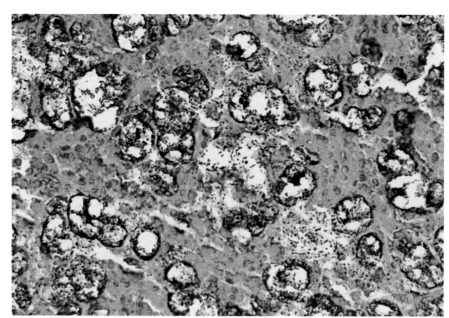

Figure 15-18
NASAL RHINOSCLEROMA
A Steiner silver stain shows large numbers of organisms within the vacuolated cells.

Without treatment, rhinoscleroma may progress to cause significant local destruction and death due to airway occlusion. The lesion usually responds to broad spectrum antibiotics such as tetracycline and may respond even more favorably to newer generation drugs (69). Lesions in danger of causing acute airway obstruction have been treated successfully with carbon dioxide laser ablation (67). There have been rare reports of squamous cell carcinomas arising in long-standing lesions (62).

RHINOSPORIDIOSIS

Rhinosporidiosis is a chronic infection predilecting the upper respiratory tract, conjunctiva, tracheobronchial tract and, less commonly, other anatomic sites (70–74). It is caused by the fungus, *Rhinosporidium seeberi*. Identical lesions occur in horses, mules, and cattle, presumably due to the same organism. Knowledge of the pathogenesis of this organism is limited by its only sporadic occurrence outside of India and Sri Lanka, its inability to grow in artificial media, and the failure of inoculated laboratory animals to produce infection.

The lateral wall of the nasal cavity is most commonly affected, with the formation of multiple polypoid masses that may clinically resemble inflammatory nasal polyps. The surface of the polyps contain small, grossly visible, yellow cysts which easily rupture, presumably providing a mechanism for disease dissemination.

Although pathologists often confuse rhinoscleroma and rhinosporidiosis because they are both seldom encountered, have similar sounding names, and share a tendency to produce nasal masses, they are quite distinct microscopically. The surface of the polypoid mass is typically covered by hyperplastic squamous epithelium. Occasionally, the surface mucosa may exhibit florid, pseudoepitheliomatous hyperplasia, leading to potential confusion with squamous cell carcinoma. Beneath this surface mucosa is a chronically inflamed stroma containing double-walled, cystic structures called sporangia, that vary in size from 20 to 300 µm (fig. 15-19). Each sporangium may contain up to several thousand endospores, the infectious particles of rhinosporidiosis. Scattered stromal giant cells may be present, but the foamy histiocytes characteristic of rhinoscleroma are absent.

Antibiotics and antifungal medications have not been effective in treating rhinosporidiosis and therapy is confined to surgical resection. Repeated procedures may be necessary because of the tendency for recurrent disease.

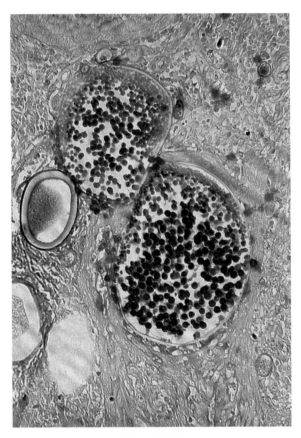

Figure 15-19
NASAL RHINOSPORIDIOSIS
Two sporangia of nasal rhinosporidiosis contain large numbers of endospores (periodic acid-Schiff stain).

LARYNGOCELE/LARYNGEAL CYST

Laryngocele

Laryngoceles are air-filled cysts that arise as outpouchings of the laryngeal saccule. As such, they retain a connection with the laryngeal ventricle. Laryngoceles have been divided into internal and external types. The *internal variant* is confined within the larynx and occurs beneath the false vocal cord, producing a bulging mass within the laryngeal lumen. *External laryngoceles* extend through the hyothyroid membrane to produce a mass in the neck, usually in the region of the hyoid bone. In a review of 131 laryngoceles, Canalis and colleagues (77) found that 44 percent of patients had a combined internal and external laryngocele, 30 percent had only the internal variant, and 26 percent had

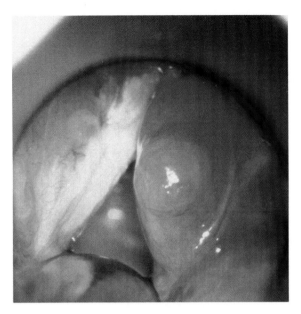

Figure 15-20
INTERNAL LARYNGOCELE
This internal laryngocele produces a cystic, air-filled mass in the region of the false vocal cord. The true cord below the lesion is obscured.

only an external laryngocele; bilateral laryngoceles were present in 23 percent.

Laryngoceles are believed by some to develop secondary to longstanding increases in intraglottic pressure, possibly in association with a predisposing abnormally enlarged or elongated sacculus (83). Macfie (83) noted that over half of musicians who play wind instruments had laryngoceles. The association between squamous cell carcinoma of the larynx and laryngocele has been the subject of multiple publications (78,79,84,86). Reviews of larynges removed for squamous cell carcinoma have noted an associated laryngocele in 4.9 to 28.8 percent of cases (78,84). The question of whether laryngoceles predispose to carcinoma or vice versa has been the subject of some discussion, but most authors currently feel that carcinomas of the larynx predispose to laryngocele formation, possibly by obstructing the sacculus (76,79).

In a laryngectomy specimen, an internal laryngocele may grossly be recognized as a mass or bulge of the mucosa in the lateral supraglottic region (fig. 15-20). Sectioning through this area shows that the mass is an air-filled cyst which is in direct communication with the laryngeal lumen via the ventricle. In external laryngoceles the air-filled cyst passes through the thyrohyoid

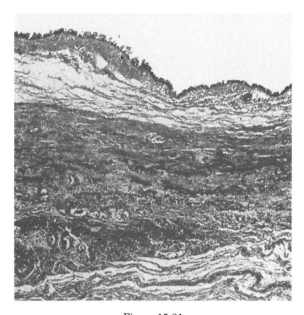

Figure 15-21
INTERNAL LARYNGOCELE
Microscopically, this internal laryngocele is lined by ciliated, respiratory-type epithelium.

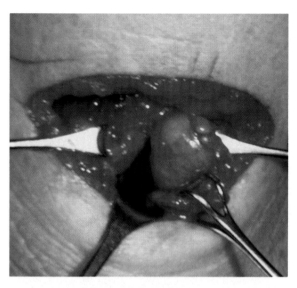

Figure 15-22
SACCULAR CYST OF THE LARYNX
This external, mucin-filed saccular cyst of the larynx is being resected via an anterior cutaneous incision. Grossly, an external laryngocele would have a similar or identical appearance, but would be filled with air.

membrane at the point of weakness where this membrane is penetrated by the superior laryngeal nerve and blood vessels. Microscopically, laryngoceles, like the sacculus from which they originate, are lined by respiratory-type epithelium (fig. 15-21).

Laryngeal Cysts

Laryngeal cysts have been divided into two major subtypes, saccular and ductal (81). Cysts of the sacculus (*saccular cysts*) are similar to laryngoceles in their origin, but differ in that the connection to the ventricle is absent or markedly stenotic, leading to accumulation of mucin rather than air within the cystic space (fig. 15-22). Saccular cysts may be congenital or acquired lesions (82). Acquired saccular cysts secondary to squamous cell carcinoma of the supraglottic larynx are analogous to the association between laryngoceles and carcinoma. Acute infections in saccular cysts are rare, but represent medical emergencies due to the potential for airway obstruction (80).

Ductal cysts of the larynx appear to be related to seromucinous gland ducts, which are particularly prominent in the false vocal cord region. These cysts are about three times more common

than saccular cysts. Often, ductal cysts are rather large and are lined by oncocytoid cells (fig. 15-23) (87). Terms such as *oncocytic cyst* and *oncocytic cystadenoma* have been applied to these lesions. Identical cysts have been described in the nasopharynx (75,85). Because these are not true neoplasms, we prefer to label them as oncocytic cysts. Microscopic sections through the false vocal cords of adults often reveal minimally dilated ducts with oncocytoid metaplasia of the lining epithelium. Further expansion of such structures in a few patients presumably leads to symptomatic disease. Ductal cysts in this region also may have a squamous epithelial lining.

MEDIAN RHOMBOID GLOSSITIS

Median rhomboid glossitis is a term applied to an ovoid or rhomboid-shaped, 1- to 2-cm area of induration located on the dorsal midline of the tongue, just anterior to the foramen cecum (90). The lesion is typically erythematous, but may be gray-white (90). It has been estimated that approximately 1 in 500 individuals have median rhomboid glossitis; men are said to be more often affected and the lesion may occur in childhood. The cause of median rhomboid glossitis has been

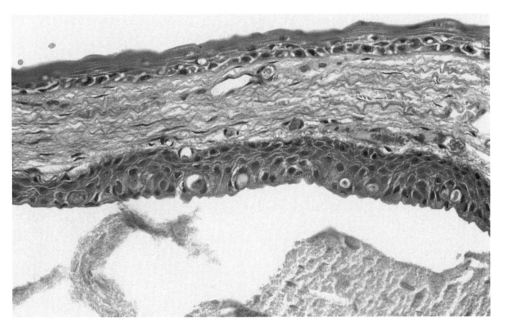

Figure 15-23
DUCTAL CYST OF LARYNX
This ductal cyst of the larynx arose in the region of the false vocal cords and has a prominent oncocytic lining. It could also be labelled as an oncocytic cyst of the false vocal cord.

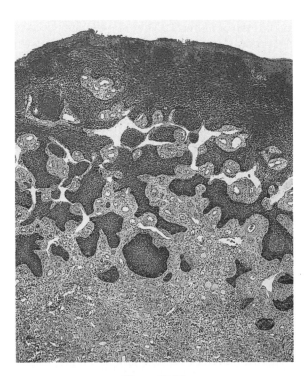

Figure 15-24
MEDIAN RHOMBOID GLOSSITIS
Median rhomboid glossitis is characterized microscopically by loss of surface papillations and underlying pseudoepitheliomatous hyperplasia.

the subject of considerable discussion, with both inflammatory and congenital theories suggested. More recently, it has been shown that the lesion appears to be associated with chronic infection with Candida species (89,91–93). There is a strong association with immunosuppression, particularly human immunodeficiency virus (HIV) infection (92), and there may be a localized immunologic defect in otherwise healthy individuals with the lesion (93).

The grossly indurated, erythematous appearance of median rhomboid glossitis may lead general physicians or inexperienced otolaryngologists to suspect carcinoma. Unfortunately, the features of the resultant biopsy specimen may add to the confusion. Microscopically, median rhomboid glossitis shows a loss of the normal surface papillations with an underlying, complex squamous hyperplasia (pseudoepitheliomatous hyperplasia) (figs. 15-24, 15-25). Adjacent seromucinous glands may show changes of squamous metaplasia (90). Awareness of the microscopic features of median rhomboid glossitis and the lack of convincing cytologic pleomorphism allows distinction. True squamous cell carcinomas arising in the dorsal midline of the tongue are quite

371

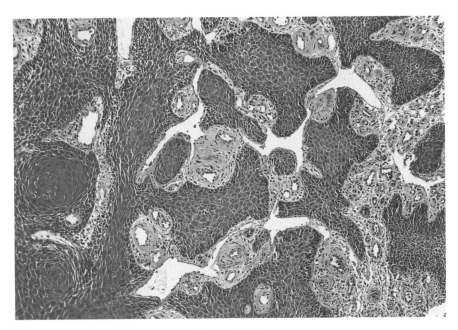

Figure 15-25
MEDIAN RHOMBOID GLOSSITIS
The interdigitating nests of hyperplastic squamous epithelium in median rhomboid glossitis may be confused with well-differentiated squamous cell carcinoma, particularly at the time of frozen section or in suboptimal tissue sections.

rare, although occasional cases have been described (88). It is unlikely that median rhomboid glossitis has any greater tendency to undergo malignant transformation than the surrounding normal mucosa.

JUXTAORAL ORGAN OF CHIEVITZ

Several decades ago, Lutman (96) found that small epithelial nests were often associated with nerves located in the buccal soft tissue near the angle of the mandible. He emphasized that these nests could be confused with squamous cell carcinoma, particularly at the time of frozen section. Shortly after the publication of his article, Krammer and Zenker (95) noted that these structures had been described almost 100 years earlier in the German literature by Chievitz (94). In fact, these epithelial nests were referred to as the "organ of Chievitz" by Ramsay in 1935 (98). There have been several additional studies dealing with these structures (97,99). Tschen and Fechner (99) examined tissue blocks obtained at autopsy transorally from the mucosa and soft tissue overlying the mandibular ramus of 25 adults of varying ages. Juxtaoral organs were found in 14 cases (11 unilateral, 3 bilateral). They were located deep to the internal pterygoid muscle and distinct from more superficial minor salivary glands. The organs consisted of 2 to 10 sharply demarcated nests of nonkeratinizing squamoid epithelial cells. Nuclei were moderately pleomorphic with irregular chromatin distribution. In one instance, the epithelial cell nests had a central lumen-like space. In all cases, small nerve twigs, representing branches of the buccal nerve, were closely associated with the epithelioid cell nests. Often, the nests were surrounded by a delicate, loose fibrous tissue distinct from the denser, more heavily collagenized fibrous tissue of the surrounding stroma.

Whether the juxtaoral organ of Chievitz is a functional structure or an embryologic remnant is unclear and less important than the very real potential for these epithelial nests to be mistaken for squamous cell carcinoma, particularly at the time of frozen section. The risk of this mistake may be enhanced by the presence of closely associated nerve twigs, mimicking perineural invasion. A high index of suspicion when dealing with deep soft tissue from the region of the angle of the mandible (retromolar trigone) is most important to avoid this pitfall. Other helpful features

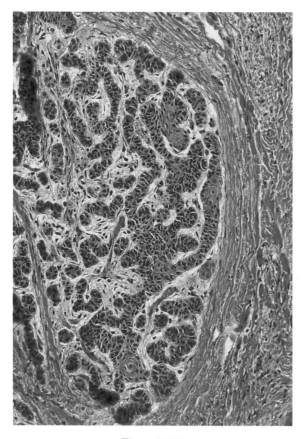

Figure 15-26
"ORGAN OF CHIEVITZ"
The "organ of Chievitz" typically consists of cords of nonkeratinized squamous cells in a loose stroma.

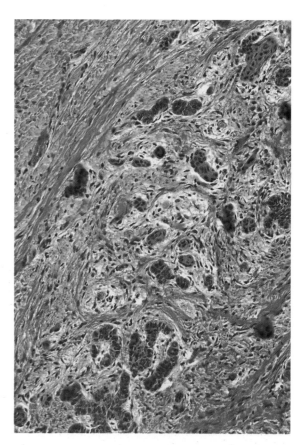

Figure 15-27
"ORGAN OF CHIEVITZ"
The cords of squamoid cells in the "organ of Chievitz" may be more widely separated. The characteristic loose stroma is present around each of the squamous nests.

include the sharp demarcation of the nests, lack of mitotic activity, lack of keratinization, absence of true perineural invasion, and looseness of the stroma surrounding the nests (figs. 15-26, 15-27).

NECROTIZING SIALOMETAPLASIA

This inflammatory, metaplastic process is discussed in more detail in the 3rd series Fascicle, Tumors of the Salivary Glands (102). It is briefly reviewed here as well because of its frequent occurrence in the minor salivary and seromucinous glands of the head and neck, and the ease with which it can be misdiagnosed as squamous cell carcinoma.

Necrotizing sialometaplasia was first described by Abrams et al. in 1973 (100). From the outset, its ability to simulate a malignancy was emphasized. The lesion can occur wherever there are salivary (seromucinous) glands. It may be apparently spontaneous, or develop in a setting of prior surgery, radiation therapy, or obvious trauma (101, 103,105,106,108). The spontaneous cases predilect the hard palate and have been presumed to be due to vascular compromise (101). There is a male predilection. On physical examination of the spontaneous cases, there is usually an obvious mucosal ulcer that may have been present for days or weeks (fig. 15-28). Healing occurs at a variable rate, depending on the size of the ulcer (fig. 15-29). Other sites of involvement include the soft palate, lip (104), oral mucosa, tongue, nasal cavity, paranasal sinuses, larynx, and rarely, the major salivary glands (107,108). Lesions secondary to surgery or radiation therapy may be smaller and without obvious mucosal ulcerations.

Microscopically, the edges of the ulcer, if present, and the surrounding tissues reveal features

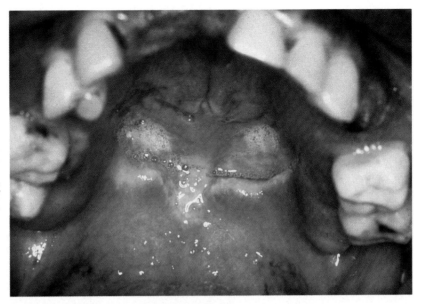

Figure 15-28
NECROTIZING
SIALOMETAPLASIA,
HARD PALATE
Spontaneously occurring necrotizing sialometaplasia often arises in the hard palate, where it presents as a symmetrical ulcer with heaped up margins. Biopsy specimens from the edge of the lesion show a mixture of glandular infarction and squamous metaplasia.

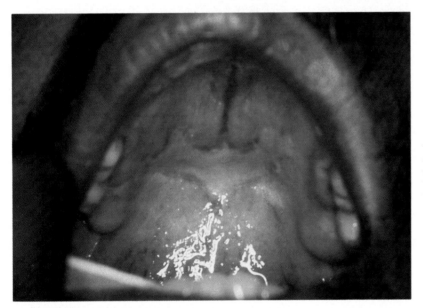

Figure 15-29
NECROTIZING
SIALOMETAPLASIA,
HARD PALATE
Without definitive therapy, the ulcer seen in figure 15-28 spontaneously re-epithelialized over a 2 week interval. There is a persistent defect in the area due to the loss of underlying seromucinous glands from the central portion of the ulcer.

which are both diagnostic and potentially misleading. Necrotizing sialometaplasia is an evolving process which begins with coagulative, infarct-like necrosis of seromucinous glands. The outlines of the preexistent acini are visible, and there is often rupture of acini with leakage of mucinous material into the surrounding stroma (fig. 15-30). An inflammatory response is invariably present. Over time, the infarcted acini become repopulated with metaplastic squamous epithelial cells. These may show considerable

nuclear variability and mitotic activity, leading to confusion with squamous cell carcinoma (fig. 15-31). The presence of residual mucinous epithelial cells may also mimic mucoepidermoid carcinoma (fig. 15-32). In addition, if there is an overlying mucosal ulcer, its healing may be associated with considerable pseudoepitheliomatous hyperplasia which mingles with the necrotizing sialometaplasia, adding to the diagnostic confusion.

The key to the correct diagnosis of necrotizing sialometaplasia is the recognition, at low-power

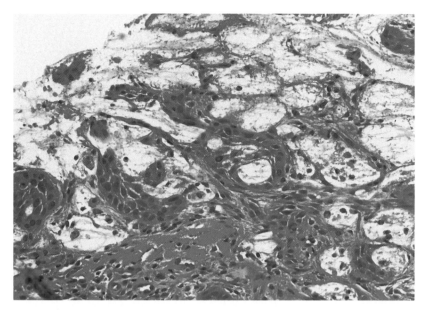

Figure 15-30
NECROTIZING
SIALOMETAPLASIA
The edges of an ulcer due to necrotizing sialometaplasia show infarcted seromucinous glands with rupture and mucin spillage, as well as developing squamous metaplasia.

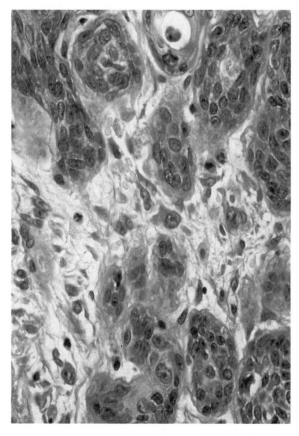

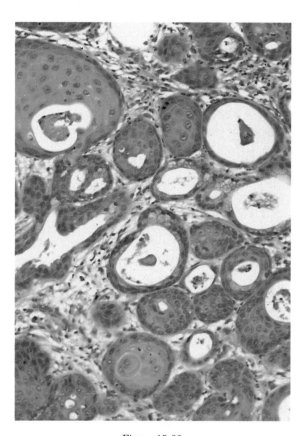

Figure 15-31
NECROTIZING SIALOMETAPLASIA
At higher magnification the proliferating squamous cells in necrotizing sialometaplasia may show considerable nuclear variability, raising the possibility of neoplasia, particularly when encountered in frozen sections.

Figure 15-32
NECROTIZING SIALOMETAPLASIA
Mature squamous cells mixed with residual mucinous cells in necrotizing sialometaplasia may suggest the diagnosis of mucoepidermoid carcinoma. The maintenance of an acinar pattern from the prior seromucinous glands is a helpful diagnostic feature.

magnification, that the lobular architecture of the preexistent acini is preserved. The complex, anastomosing growth pattern typical of squamous cell or mucoepidermoid carcinoma is not present. In addition, residual, obviously necrotic salivary acini may still be present, and the often prominent inflammatory component is also helpful. In our experience, the greatest pitfall occurs at the time of frozen section when the suboptimal tissue preparation and pressure of time add to the diagnostic difficulty. A high index of suspicion regarding the possibility of necrotizing sialometaplasia whenever biopsies are obtained from areas of seromucinous epithelium is of considerable value in avoiding the overdiagnosis of carcinoma.

TEFLON GRANULOMA ("TEFLONOMA")

Since the early 1900s, various foreign substances including paraffin, cartilage, bone paste, tantalum oxide, silicone, and Gelfoam have been injected adjacent to paralyzed vocal cords to improve phonation (118). Currently, a paste of polymerized tetrafluoroethylene or polytef (Teflon) is almost exclusively used for this function (111). Following injection into the thyroarytenoidus muscle, the Teflon produces the desired stiffening of the cord by inducing a localized, fibrotic, foreign body reaction (112,113,118).

Occasionally, the polytef migrates from the vocal cord into the other areas of the larynx, thyroid gland, or neck, and produces a mass lesion which may be subjected to biopsy or fine needle aspiration (fig. 15-33) (109,114,116–118). Polytef is radiolucent in conventional radiographs or computerized tomography (CT) scans (109). Microscopically, polytef consists of shiny, refractile green-yellow particles ranging from 6 to 100 μm and having myriads of shapes (fig. 15-34). The primary bolus becomes surrounded by fibroblasts, and these cells may also penetrate between the particles of polytef. Foreign body giant cells are typically prominent and associated with phagocytosed, irregularly shaped fragments of polytef. Under cross-polarized light, polytef is strongly birefringent. Although not required for routine diagnostic purposes, infrared absorption spectrophotometry clearly documents characteristic carbon to fluorine bonds, and energy dispersive X ray analysis shows a strong peak corresponding to the presence of fluorine (118).

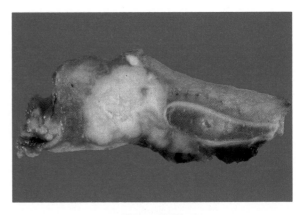

Figure 15-33
TEFLON GRANULOMA
This vertical laryngeal section shows a white nodule of polytef (Teflon) paste in the region of the vocal cords.

Although it may mimic a neoplasm clinically, the distinctive microscopic appearance of a Teflon granuloma allows ready recognition. Polytef injection has also been used as a "tissue stiffener" at other anatomic sites such as the bladder outlet, where it may aid in the control of stress urinary incontinence. Except for granuloma formation, no other adverse reactions have been associated with polytef injection, even though the material may be encountered in small blood vessels and lymphatics (110,115). There is no association with subsequent malignancy. In the larynx, symptomatic "Teflonomas" have been successfully removed by laser ablation (116).

MYOSPHERULOSIS

Petrolatum-based hemostatic packing material is often placed in the paranasal sinuses and nasal cavity following a surgical procedure. Occasionally, this stimulates a fibroinflammatory reaction which may produce a symptomatic mass (123). Microscopically, the mass consists of dense fibrous tissue containing cystic spaces (fig. 15-35); the latter once contained petrolatum extracted during tissue processing. This appearance is thus similar to that of a so-called paraffinoma or sclerosing lipogranuloma. In myospherulosis, however, closer inspection of the cystic spaces demonstrates structures that somewhat mimic yeast forms or algae. There is typically a large "parent body" filled with smaller round spherules said to resemble a "bag of marbles" (fig. 15-36) (121).

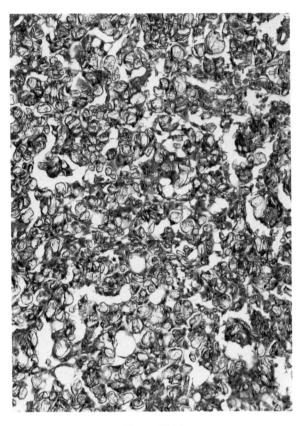

Figure 15-34
TEFLON GRANULOMA
Microscopically, the nodule seen in figure 15-33 consists of highly birefringent, yellow-green fragments of polytef with an associated histiocytic reaction.

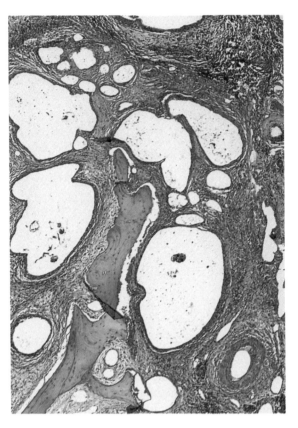

Figure 15-35
MYOSPHERULOSIS
The presence of cystic spaces previously filled with lipid material prior to removal during processing, and surrounded by stromal fibrosis, points to the prior use of oil- or lipid-based packing material. Search of the cystic spaces often demonstrates "myospherules."

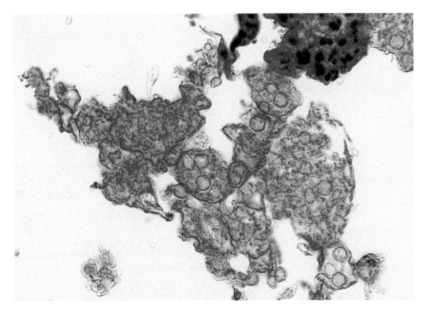

Figure 15-36
MYOSPHERULOSIS
Myospherulosis consists of large, often irregular sac-like structures containing large numbers of smaller myospherules. Both the larger "sacs" and smaller myospherules are now known to represent altered red blood cells.

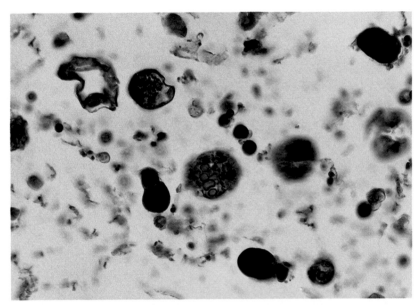

Figure 15-37
MYOSPHERULOSIS
In some instances, the myospherules are densely pigmented, such that their inner structure is more difficult to discern.

The term, myospherule, has been applied to these structures and the overall process has been termed myospherulosis, because identical structures were first described as intramuscular masses under somewhat different clinical conditions (124). Myospherules vary considerably in color, ranging from light pink-red to dark brown (fig. 15-37).

The exact nature of the myospherule was controversial for several years. They were initially suspected to represent a previously undescribed organism (119,120,123). However, recent studies have convincingly documented that myospherules represent altered red blood cells surrounded by fused red blood cell membranes (122,125,128,129). Recognition of the associated sclerosis and consideration of this entity usually allows rapid diagnosis. If fungal or algal forms are suspected, the lack of staining of the myospherule with periodic acid–Schiff or methenamine silver stains aids in their distinction (126). Myospherules are also positive for erythrocyte-related markers such as hemoglobin (127).

REFERENCES

Nasal Polyps

1. Berman JM, Colman BH. Nasal aspects of cystic fibrosis in children. J Laryngol Otol 1977;91:133–9.
2. Chandra RK, Abrol BM. Immunopathology of nasal polypi. J Laryngol Otol 1974;88:1019–24.
3. Drake-Lee AB, Lowe D, Swanston A, Grace A. Clinical profile and recurrence of nasal polyps. J Laryngol Otol 1984;98:783–93.
4. Frazer JP. Allergic rhinitis and nasal polyps. Ear Nose Throat J 1984;63:172–6.
5. Kelly AB. Naso-antral polypus. Lancet 1909;1:89–91.
6. Oppenheimer EH, Rosenstein BJ. Differential pathology of nasal polyps in cystic fibrosis and atopy. Lab Invest 1979;40:445–9.
7. Patriarca G, Nucera E, Di Rienzo V, Schiavino D, Pellegrino S, Fais G. Nasal provocation test with lysine acetylsalicylate in aspirin-sensitive patients. Ann Allergy 1991;67:60–2.
8. Rejowski JE, Caldarelli DD, Campanella RS, Penn RD. Nasal polyps causing bone destruction and blindness. Otolaryngol Head Neck Surg 1982;90:505–6.
9. Settipane GA, Chafee FH. Nasal polyps in asthma and rhinitis. A review of 6,037 patients. J Allergy Clin Immunol 1977;59:17–21.
10. Smith MP. Dysfunction of carbohydrate metabolism as an element in the set of factors resulting in the polysaccharide nose and nasal polypi. Laryngoscope 1971;81:636–44.
11. Wilson JA. Nasal polypi [Editorial]. Clin Otolaryngol 1976;1:4–6.
12. Yazbak PA, Phillips JM, Ball PA, Rhodes CH. Benign nasal polyposis presenting as an intracranial mass: case report. Surg Neurol 1991;36:380–3.

Respiratory Epithelial Adenomatoid and Glandular (Seromucinous) Hamartomas

13. Baillie EE, Batsakis JG. Glandular (seromucinous) hamartoma of the nasopharynx. Oral Surg 1974;38:760–2.
14. Graeme-Cook F, Pilch BZ. Hamartomas of the nose and nasopharynx. Head Neck 1992;14:321–7.
15. Wenig BM, Heffner DK. Respiratory epithelial adenomatoid hamartomas of the sinonasal tract and nasopharynx: a clinicopathologic study of 31 cases. Ann Otol Rhinol Laryngol 1995;104:639–45.
16. Zarbo RJ, McClatchey KD. Nasopharyngeal hamartoma: report of a case and review of the literature. Laryngoscope 1983;93:494–7.

Antrochoanal Polyp

17. Compagno J, Hyams VJ, Lepore ML. Nasal polyposis with stromal atypia. Review and follow-up study of 14 cases. Arch Pathol Lab Med 1976;100:224–6.
18. Hardy G. The choanal polyp. Ann Otol Rhinol Laryngol 1957;66:306–26.
19. Heck WE, Hallberg OE, Williams HL. Antrochoanal polyp. Arch Otolaryngol 1950;52:538–48.
20. Kelly AB. Naso-antral polypus. Lancet 1909;1:89–91.
21. Killian G. The origin of choanal polypi. Lancet 1906;2:81–2.
22. Klenoff BH, Goodman ML. Mesenchymal cell atypicality in inflammatory polyps. J Laryngol 1977;91:751–6.
23. Nakayama M, Wenig BM, Heffner DK. Atypical stromal cells in inflammatory nasal polyps: immunohistochemical and ultrastructural analysis in defining histogenesis. Laryngoscope 1995;105:127–34.
24. Sirola R. Choanal polyps. Acta Otolaryngol 1966;61:42–8.
25. Smith CJ, Echevarria R, McLelland CA. Pseudosarcomatous changes in antrochoanal polyps. Arch Otolaryngol 1974;99:228–30.
26. Wilson JA. Nasal polypi [Editorial]. Clin Otolaryngol 1976;1:4–6.

Vocal Cord Nodule/Polyp

27. Dikkers FG, Nikkels PG. Benign lesions of the vocal folds: histopathology and phonotrauma. Ann Otol Rhinol Laryngol 1995;104:698–703.
28. Gray SD, Hammond E, Hanson DF. Benign pathologic responses of the larynx. Ann Otol Rhinol Laryngol 1995;104:13–8.
29. Kambic V, Radsel A, Zargi M, Acko M. Vocal cord polyps: incidence, histology and pathogenesis. J Laryngol Otol 1981;95:609–18.
30. Strong MS, Vaughan CW. Vocal cord nodules and polyps—the role of surgical treatment. Laryngoscope 1971;81:911–23.

Contact/Intubation Ulcer of the Larynx

31. Donnelly WH. Histopathology of endotracheal intubation. An autopsy study of 99 cases. Arch Pathol 1969;1969:511–20.
32. Fechner RE, Cooper PH, Mills SE. Pyogenic granuloma of the larynx and trachea. A causal and pathologic misnomer for granulation tissue. Arch Otolaryngol 1980;107:30–2.
33. Wenig BM, Heffner DK. Contact ulcers of the larynx. A reacquaintance with the pathology of an often underdiagnosed entity. Arch Pathol Lab Med 1990;114:825–8.

Dermoid Cyst

34. Cauchois R, Testud R, Laccourreye O, Kuffer R, Bremond D, Monteil JP. Nasal dermoid sinus cyst. Ann Otol Rhinol Laryngol 1994;103:615–8.
35. Hacker DC, Freeman JL. Intracranial extension of a nasal dermoid sinus cyst in a 56-year-old man. Head Neck 1994;16:366–71.
36. McAvoy JM, Zuckerbraun L. Dermoid cysts of the head and neck in children. Arch Otolaryngol 1976;102:529–31.
37. McCaffrey TV, McDonald TJ, Gorenstein A. Dermoid cysts of the nose: review of 21 cases. Otolaryngol Head Neck Surg 1979;87:52–9.
38. New GB, Erich JB. Dermoid cysts of the head and neck. Surg Gynecol Obstet 1937;65:48–55.
39. Shafer WG, Hine MK, Levy BM. Development disturbances of oral and paraoral structures. In: A textbook of oral pathology. 4th edition. Philadelphia: WB Saunders, 1983:78–9.
40. Taylor BW, Erich JB. Dermoid cysts of the nose. Mayo Clinic Proc 1967;42:488–94.
41. Taylor SW, Erich JB, Dockerty MB. Dermoids of the head and neck. Minn Med 1966;9:1535–40.

Hairy Polyp

42. Chaudhry AP, Lore JM Jr, Fisher JE, Gambrino AG. So-called hairy polyps or teratoid tumors of the nasopharynx. Arch Otolaryngol 1978;104:517–25.
43. Heffner DK, Schall DG, Thompson LD, Anderson V. Pharyngeal dermoids ("hairy polyps") as accessory auricles. Ann Otol Rhinol Laryngol 1996;105:819–24.

Amyloid Deposition

44. Barnes EL Jr, Zafar T. Laryngeal amyloidosis: clinicopathologic study of seven cases. Ann Otol Rhinol Laryngol 1977;86:3856–63.
45. Bennett JD, Chowdhury CR. Primary amyloidosis of the larynx. J Laryngol Otol 1994;108:339–40.
46. Berg AM, Troxler RF, Grillone G, et al. Localized amyloidosis of the larynx: evidence for light chain composition. Ann Otol Rhinol Laryngol 1993;102:884–9.
47. Chow LT, Chow WH, Shum BS. Fatal massive upper respiratory tract haemorrhage: an unusual complication of localized amyloidosis of the larynx. J Laryngol Otol 1993;107:51–3.
48. Eliachar I, Lichtig C. Local amyloid deposits of the larynx. Electron microscopic studies of three cases. Arch Otolaryngol 1970;92:163–6.
49. Godbersen GS, Leh JF, Hansmann ML, Rudert H, Linke RP. Organ-limited laryngeal amyloid deposits: clinical, morphological, and immunohistochemical results of five cases. Ann Otol Rhinol Laryngol 1992;101:770–5.
50. Lewis JE, Olsen KD, Kurtin PJ, Kyle RA. Laryngeal amyloidosis: a clinicopathologic and immunohistochemical review. Otolaryngol Head Neck Surg 1992;106:372–7.
51. McAlpine JC, Fuller AP. Localized laryngeal amyloidosis: a report of a case with a review of the literature. J Laryngol Otol 1964;78:296–314.
52. Mufarrij AA, Busaba NY, Zaytoun GM, Gallo GR, Feiner HD. Primary localized amyloidosis of the nose and paranasal sinuses. A case report with immunohistochemical observations and a review of the literature. Am J Surg Pathol 1990;14:379–83.
53. Raymond AK, Sneige N, Batsakis JG. Amyloidosis in the upper aerodigestive tracts. Ann Otol Rhinol Laryngol 1992;101:794–6.
54. Ryan RE, Pearson BW, Weiland LH. Laryngeal amyloidosis. Trans Am Acad Ophthalmol Otolaryngol 1977;84:872–7.
55. Schindel J, Ben-Bassat H. Amyloid tumor of the larynx. Case report with electron microscope study. Ann Otol Rhinol Laryngol 1972;81:438–43.

Laryngeal Rheumatoid Arthritis and Nodules

56. Bienenstock H, Lanyi VF. Cricoarytenoid arthritis in a patient with ankylosing spondylitis. Arch Otolaryngol 1977;103:738–9.
57. Bridger MW, Jahn AF, van Nostrand AW. Laryngeal rheumatoid arthritis. Laryngoscope 1980;90:296–303.
58. Dockery KM, Sismanis A, Abedi E. Rheumatoid arthritis of the larynx: the importance of early diagnosis and corticosteroid therapy. South Med J 1991;84:95–6.
59. Friedman BA, Rice DH. Rheumatoid nodules of the larynx. Arch Otolaryngol 1975;101:361–3.
60. Schwartz IS, Grishman E. Rheumatoid nodules of the vocal cords as the initial manifestation of systemic lupus erythematosus. JAMA 1980;244:2751–2.

Rhinoscleroma

61. Andraca R, Edson RS, Kern EB. Rhinoscleroma: a growing concern in the United States? Mayo Clinic experience. Mayo Clin Proc 1993;68:1151–7.
62. Attia OM. Rhinoscleroma and malignancy. Two cases of rhinoscleroma associated with carcinoma. J Laryngol Otol 1958;72:412–5.
63. Barbary A, Fouad H, Fatt-Hi A. Scleroma affecting the middle ear cavity with report of 3 cases. Ann Otol Rhinol Laryngol 1974;83:107–10.
64. Busch RF. Rhinoscleroma occurring with airway obstruction. Otolaryngol Head Neck Surg 1993;109:933–6.
65. Goldberg SN, Canalis RF. Rhinoscleroma as a cause of airway obstruction. Ear Nose Throat J 1980;59:145—9.
66. Gumprecht TF, Nichols PW, Meyer PR. Identification of rhinoscleroma by immunoperoxidase technique. Laryngoscope 1983;93:627–9.
67. Maher AI, El-Kashlan HK, Soliman Y, Galal R. Rhinoscleroma: management by carbon dioxide laser therapy. Laryngoscope 1990;100:783–8.
68. Stiernberg CM, Clark WD. Rhinoscleroma—a diagnostic challenge. Laryngoscope 1983;93:866–70.
69. Trautmann M, Held T, Ruhnke M, Schnoy N. A case of rhinoscleroma cured with ciprofloxacin. Infection 1993;21:403–6.

Rhinosporidiosis

70. Batsakis JG, El-Naggar AK. Rhinoscleroma and rhinosporidiosis. Ann Otol Rhinol Laryngol 1992;101:879–82.
71. Gori S, Scasso A. Cytologic and differential diagnosis of rhinosporidiosis. Acta Cytol 1994;38:361–6.
72. Lasser A, Smith HW. Rhinosporidiosis. Arch Otolaryngol Head Neck Surg 1976;102:308–10.
73. Mears T, Amerasinghe C. Rhinosporidiosis. J Laryngol Otol 1992;106:468.
74. Satyanarayana C. Rhinosporidiosis with a record of 225 cases. Acta Otolaryngol 1960;51:348–56.

Laryngocele/Laryngeal Cyst

75. Benke TT, Zitsch RP III, Nashelsky MB. Bilateral oncocytic cysts of the nasopharynx. Otolaryngol Head Neck Surg 1995;112:321–4.
76. Canalis RF. Observations on the simultaneous occurrence of laryngocele and cancer. J Otolaryngol 1976;5:207–12.

77. Canalis RF, Maxwell DS, Hemenway WC. Laryngocele—an updated review. J Otolaryngol 1977;6:191–9.

78. Celin SE, Johnson J, Curtin H, Barnes L. The association of laryngoceles with squamous cell carcinoma of the larynx. Laryngoscope 1991;101:529–36.

79. Close LG, Merkel M, Burns DK, Deaton CW Jr, Schaefer SD. Asymptomatic laryngocele: incidence and association with laryngeal cancer. Ann Otol Rhinol Laryngol 1987;96:393–9.

80. DeSanto LW. Laryngocele, laryngeal mucocele, large saccules and laryngeal saccular cysts: a developmental spectrum. Laryngoscope 1974;84:1291–6.

81. DeSanto LW, Devine KD, Weiland LH. Cysts of the larynx—classification. Laryngoscope 1970;5:145–76.

82. Holinger LD, Barnes DR, Smid LJ, Holinger PH. Laryngocele and saccular cysts. Ann Otol Rhinol Laryngol 1978;87:675–85.

83. Macfie D. Asymptomatic laryngoceles in wind-instrument bandsmen. Arch Otolaryngol 1966;83:270–5.

84. Micheau C, Luboinski B, Lanchi P, et al. Relationship between laryngoceles and laryngeal carcinomas. Laryngoscope 1978;88:680–8.

85. Morin GV, Shank EC, Burgess LP, Heffner DK. Oncocytic metaplasia of the pharynx. Otolaryngol Head Neck Surg 1991;105:86–91.

86. Murray SP, Burgess LP, Burton DM, Gonzalez C, Wood GS, Zajtchuk JT. Laryngocele associated with squamous carcinoma in a 20-year-old nonsmoker. Ear Nose Throat J 1994;73:258–61.

87. Newman BH, Taxy JB, Laker HI. Laryngeal cysts in adults: a clinicopathologic study of 20 cases. Am J Clin Pathol 1984;81:715–20.

Median Rhomboid Glossitis

88. Burkes EJ, Lewis JR. Carcinoma arising in an area of median rhomboid glossitis. Oral Surg 1976;41:649–52.

89. Crockett DN, O'Grady JF, Reade PC. Candida species and Candida albicans morphotypes in erythematous candidiasis. Oral Surg Oral Med Oral Pathol 1992;73:559–63.

90. Delemarre JF, van der Waal I. Clinical and histopathologic aspects of median rhomboid glossitis. Int J Oral Surg 1973;2:203–8.

91. Gorsky M, Raviv M, Taicher S. Squamous cell carcinoma mimicking median rhomboid glossitis region: report of a case. J Oral Maxillofac Surg 1993;51:798–800.

92. Kolokotronis A, Kioses V, Antoniades D, Mandraveli K, Doutsos I, Papanayotou P. Median rhomboid glossitis. An oral manifestation in patients infected with HIV. Oral Surg Oral Med Oral Pathol 1994;78:36–40.

93. Walsh LJ, Cleveland DB, Cumming CG. Quantitative evaluation of Langerhans cells in median rhomboid glossitis. J Oral Pathol Med 1992;21:28–32.

Juxtaoral Organ of Chievitz

94. Chievitz JH. Beiträge zur Entwicklungsgeschichte der Speicheldrusen. Arch Anat Physiol Abt 1885;9:401–36.

95. Krammer EB, Zenker W. Comments on neuroepithelial structures [Letter]. Am J Clin Pathol 1974;61:571–4.

96. Lutman GB. Epithelial nests in intraoral sensory nerve endings simulating perineural invasion in patients with oral carcinoma. Am J Clin Pathol 1974;61:275–84.

97. Mandl L, Nerlich A, Pankratz H, Hubner G. [The juxta-oral organ (Chievitz organ)—a sensory organ in the bucco-temporal area?]. Pathologe 1993;14:205–9.

98. Ramsay AJ. Persistence of the organ of Chievitz in the human. Anat Record 1935;63:281–93.

99. Tschen JA, Fechner RE. The juxtaoral organ of Chievitz. Am J Surg Pathol 1979;3:147–50.

Necrotizing Sialometaplasia

100. Abrams AM, Melrose R, Howell FV. Necrotizing sialometaplasia. A disease simulating malignancy. Cancer 1973;32:130–5.

101. Brannon RB, Fowler CB, Hartman KS. Necrotizing sialometaplasia. A clinicopathologic study of sixty-nine cases and review of the literature. Oral Surg Oral Med Oral Pathol 1991;72:317–25.

102. Ellis GL, Auclair PL. Tumors of the salivary glands. Atlas of Tumor Pathology, 3rd Series, Fascicle 17. Washington, D.C.: Armed Forces Institute of Pathology, 1995.

103. Fechner RE. Necrotizing sialometaplasia: a source of confusion with carcinoma of the palate. Am J Clin Pathol 1977;67:315–7.

104. Gad A, Willén H, Willén R, Thorstensson S, Ekman L. Necrotizing sialometaplasia of the lip simulating squamous cell carcinoma. Histopathology 1980;4:111–21.

105. Matsumoto T, Kuwabara N, Shiotsu H, Fukuda Y, Yanai A, Ichikawa G. Necrotizing sialometaplasia in the mouth floor secondary to reconstructive surgery for tongue carcinoma. Acta Pathol Jpn 1991;41:689–93.

106. Schroeder WA Jr. Necrotizing sialometaplasia. Otolaryngol Head Neck Surg 1994;111:328–9.

107. Walker GK, Fechner RE, Johns ME, Teja K. Necrotizing sialometaplasia of the larynx secondary to atheromatous embolization. Am J Clin Pathol 1982;77:221–3.

108. Wenig BM. Necrotizing sialometaplasia of the larynx. A report of two cases and a review of the literature. Am J Clin Pathol 1995;103:609–13.

Teflon Granuloma ("Teflonoma")

109. Benjamin B, Robb P, Clifford A, Eckstein R. Giant Teflon granuloma of the larynx. Head Neck 1991;13:453–6.
110. Dedo HH, Carlsöö B. Histologic evaluation of Teflon granulomas of human vocal cords: a light and electron microscopic study. Acta Otolaryngol (Stockh) 1982;93:475–84.
111. Dedo HH, Urrea RD, Lawson L. Intracordal injection of teflon in the treatment of 135 patients with dysphonia. Ann Otol Rhinol Laryngol 1973;82:661–7.
112. Lewy RB. Responses of laryngeal tissue to granular teflon in-situ. Arch Otolaryngol Head Neck Surg 1966;83:355–9.
113. Lewy RB, Millet D. Immediate local tissue reactions to teflon vocal cord implants. Laryngoscope 1978;88:1339–42.
114. Sanfilippo F, Shelburne J, Ingram P. Analysis of a polytef granuloma mimicking a cold thyroid nodule 17 months after laryngeal injection. Ultrastruct Pathol 1980;1:471–5.
115. Schmidt PJ, Wagenfeld D, Bridger MW, et al. Teflon injection of the vocal cord: a clinical and histopathologic study. J Laryngol 1980;9:297–302.
116. Varvares MA, Montgomery WW, Hillman RE. Teflon granuloma of the larynx: etiology, pathophysiology, and mangement. Ann Otol Rhinol Laryngol 1995;104:511–5.
117. Walsh FM, Castelli JB. Polytef granulomas clinically simulating carcinoma of the thyroid. Arch Otolaryngol Head Neck Surg 1975;101:262–3.
118. Wenig BM, Heffner DK, Oertel YC, Johnson FB. Teflonomas of the larynx and neck. Hum Pathol 1990;21:617–23.

Myospherulosis

119. De Schryver-Kecskemeti K, Kyriakos M. The induction of human myospherulosis in experimental animals. Am J Pathol 1977;87:33–46.
120. De Schryver-Kecskemeti K, Kyriakos M. Myospherulosis. An electron-microscopic study of a human case. Am J Clin Pathol 1977;67:555–61.
121. Dunlap CL, Barker BF. Myospherulosis of the jaws. Oral Surg 1980;50:238–43.
122. Kakizaki H, Shimada K. Experimental study of the cause of myospherulosis. Am J Clin Pathol 1993;99:249–56.
123. Kyriakos M. Myospherulosis of the paranasal sinuses, nose and middle ear. A possible iatrogenic disease. Am J Clin Pathol 1977;67:118–30.
124. McClatchie S, Warambo MW, Bremner AD. Myospherulosis. A previously unreported disease. Am J Clin Pathol 1969;51:699–704.
125. Rosai J. The nature of myospherulosis of the upper respiratory tract. Am J Clin Pathol 1978;69:475–81.
126. Shimada K, Kobayashi S, Yamadori I, Ohmori M. Myospherulosis in Japan. A report of two cases and an immunohistochemical investigation. Am J Surg Pathol 1988;12:427–32.
127. Travis WD, Chin-Yang L, Weiland LH. Immunostaining for hemoglobin in two cases of myospherulosis. Arch Pathol Lab Med 1986;110:763–5.
128. Wheeler TM, McGavran MH. Myospherulosis—further observations. Am J Clin Pathol 1980;73:685–6.
129. Wheeler TM, Sessions RB, McGavran MH. Myospherulosis. A preventable iatrogenic nasal and paranasal entity. Arch Otolaryngol 1980;106:272–4.

16

TUMORS OF THE EAR

ANATOMY

The ear is traditionally divided into external, middle, and internal segments (fig. 16-1). The inner ear is not considered here due to the anatomic complexity and infrequency of primary neoplasia in this area.

External Ear

The external ear is composed of the auricle (pinna), the external auditory meatus, and the canal, the medial aspect of which is bounded by the tympanic membrane. The external auditory canal is divided into an outer cartilaginous portion and an inner osseous portion. The outer cartilaginous component is in continuity with the cartilage of the auricle and accounts for one third of the canal whereas the inner osseous portion is bounded medially by the tympanic membrane and comprises the remaining two thirds of the canal length. The cartilaginous portion is not completely encircled by cartilage but is characterized by a defect in the superior and posterior aspect of the canal. The defect is filled with fibrous tissue and imparts a degree of flexibility to the outer portion. In contrast, the inner osseous canal is formed from a continuous bony sleeve that evolves and extends from the tympanic ring during childhood.

Middle Ear

The middle ear (middle ear cleft, tympanic cavity) lies between the tympanic membrane and the internal ear. Contents include the three ossicles (malleus, incus, and stapes), eustacian tube, tympanic cavity proper, epitympanic recess (attic), and the mastoid cavity (fig. 16-1). Within the tympanic cavity, the malleus is attached to the tympanic membrane whereas the stapes is connected by a ligament to the oval opening (fenestra vestibuli); the incus connects the latter two ossicles. The tympanic cavity extends above the level of the drum as the epitympanic recess. Posteriorly, the epitympanic recess is contiguous with the mastoid antrum

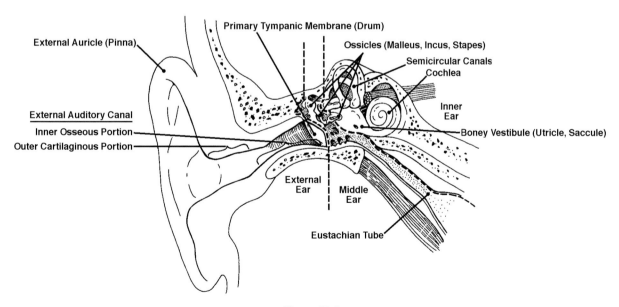

Figure 16-1
ANATOMY

The external (auricle, external auditory canal), middle (eustachian tube, mesotympanum, epitympanum, mastoid), and inner (membranous, osseous labyrinth) ear are the three main divisions separated by the dotted lines in this drawing. (Fig. 271 from Fascicle 25, 2nd Series.)

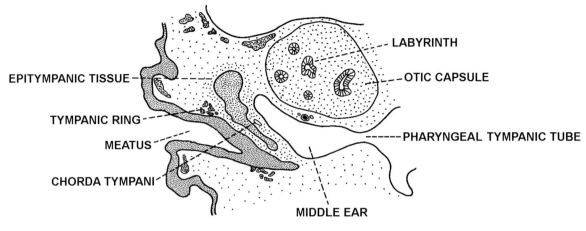

Figure 16-2
EMBRYOLOGY

This drawing elaborates the arrangement of the first external cleft forming the external auditory canal (meatus) and first branchial pouch (pharyngeal tympanic tube) forming the early middle ear space. The relationship of the inner (labyrinth and otic capsule) and the mesenchymal and neuroectodermal structures (ossicle, tympanic ring, chorda tympani) are shown. (Fig. 39 from Davies J. Embryology of the head and neck in relation to the practice of otolaryngology. Washington, D.C.: American Academy of Otolaryngology, 1957.)

and air cells within the petrous portion of the temporal bone. The eustachian tube opens into the anterior wall of the middle ear cleft.

EMBRYOLOGY

Between the fourth and sixth weeks of human embryonic development the paired branchial arches appear as ridges on each side of the future head and neck region (1). The arches have a mesodermal core and are covered externally by ectoderm and internally by endoderm. The arches are separated by ectodermal branchial grooves or clefts. Following the appearance of these grooves, the lateral walls of the endodermal pharynx form a corresponding series of pharyngeal pouches. The endoderm of the pouches contacts the ectoderm of the branchial grooves, forming a double-layered branchial membrane.

External Ear

The external auricle develops from the dorsal aspect of the first branchial groove. The tragus arises from the first branchial arch whereas the remainder of the pinna originates from the mesoderm of the second arch. The dorsal portion of the first branchial groove persists to form the external acoustic meatus. The ventral portion normally disappears, although incomplete obliteration of the ventral groove or persistence of

buried ectodermal cell rests in this area may lead to subsequent developmental abnormalities.

Middle Ear

During the eighth week of development the dorsal portion of the first pouch expands to form the tympanic cavity (middle ear cleft) (fig. 16-2). The mesodermal core of the first branchial arch transforms into a cartilaginous bar (Meckel's cartilage) which extends dorsally into the tympanic cavity to form most of the malleus and incus as well as the tensor tympani muscle. The second branchial arch forms another cartilaginous bar (Reichert's cartilage), which gives rise to the stapes, the remainder of the incus and malleus, the posterior bony canal wall, and the styloid process of the temporal bone. As the tympanic cavity expands, the endodermal epithelium envelopes the ossicles, tendons, and ligaments; thus the latter structures receive a complete epithelial investment (4). The proximal, unexpanded portion of the first pharyngeal pouch elongates to form the eustachian tube. Finally, the tympanic membrane arises from the first branchial membrane between the first branchial and pharyngeal pouches.

Late in fetal development further expansion of the tympanic cavity gives rise to the mastoid antrum and air cells. Mastoid air cells begin to

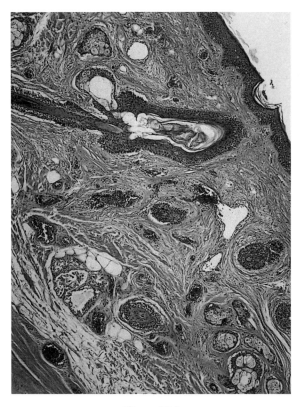

Figure 16-3
EXTERNAL AURICLE
A section of the external auricle emphasizes the adnexa in the dermis and subcutaneous tissue. (Fig. 275 from Fascicle 25, 2nd Series.)

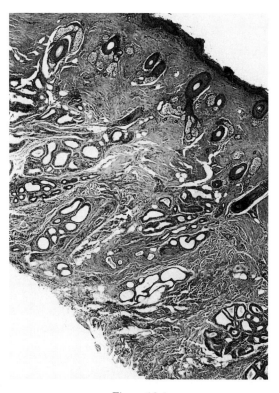

Figure 16-4
EXTERNAL AUDITORY CANAL
The surface of the outer third of the external auditory canal consists of keratinizing squamous cell epidermis. Hair follicles, sebaceous glands, and abundant apocrine ceruminal glands replace the exocrine sweat glands that are present in the subcutaneous tissue of the external auricle. (Fig. 276 from Fascicle 25, 2nd Series.)

develop during fetal life, but most form after birth. The endodermally derived epithelium of the tympanic cavity invades and erodes the surrounding bone and lines the air spaces thus formed ("pneumatization"). The mucous membrane lining the air cells is in continuity with the both the mastoid antrum and tympanic cavity proper.

HISTOLOGY

External Ear

The external ear (pinna) consists of an elastic cartilaginous plate with overlying keratinizing, stratified squamous epithelium. The underlying dermis is essentially identical to that of normal skin and contains hair follicles, sebaceous glands, eccrine (sweat) glands, and a few apocrine glands (fig. 16-3). The fibrofatty subcutaneous tissue layer is virtually absent in the external ear except in the ear lobe, which is little more than a pad of adipose tissue sandwiched between two layers of skin. The cartilage of the pinna, which is continuous with the cartilaginous portion of the external auditory canal, is composed of chondrocytes embedded in a basophilic matrix containing interwoven elastic fibers.

External Auditory Canal. The keratinizing epithelium of the external ear is continuous with the cartilaginous and bony portions of the external ear canal. In the outer, cartilaginous portion the epithelial lining shows prominent rete ridges and adnexal structures (fig. 16-4). In contrast, the epithelium of the inner bony portion is flat, directly adherent to the underlying periosteum, and extends medially to form the outermost layer of the tympanic membrane. Adnexal structures are concentrated in the outer third of the canal, although a few may be found in the superior aspect of the inner canal.

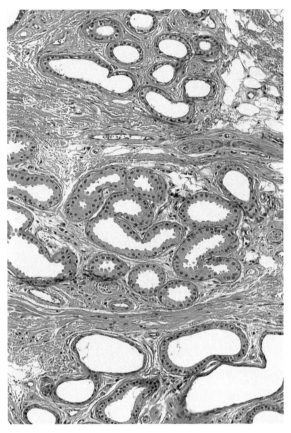

Figure 16-5
CERUMINAL GLANDS
On scanning magnification, normal ceruminal glands
are grouped in well-defined lobules bound by fibrous tissue.

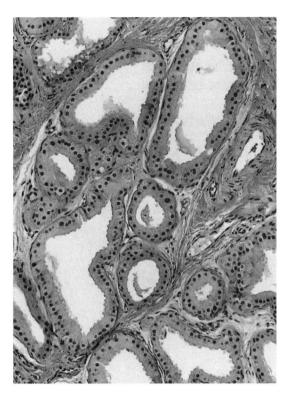

Figure 16-6
CERUMINAL GLANDS
On high magnification, ceruminal glands are composed
of tall "secretory" apocrine-type epithelial cells with secretory droplets on the apical surface. Myoepithelial cells are
occasionally evident at the base of the secretory cell layer.
(Fig. 277 from Fascicle 25, 2nd Series.)

Ceruminal Glands. The ceruminal glands of
the external canal give rise to most of the adenomatous neoplasms of the external ear and thus
merit special attention. The ceruminal glands
closely resemble apocrine glands found elsewhere in the skin and are typically arranged in
lobules and clusters in the deep dermis below the
level of the sebaceous glands (fig. 16-5) (3). The
glands are composed of two cell types, an inner
secretory cell layer and an outer layer of
myoepithelial cells (fig. 16-6). The secretory cells
are cuboidal to low columnar, and contain abundant, brightly eosinophilic cytoplasm with occasional golden pigment granules and distinct
cellular borders (3). Cytoplasmic buds in varying
stages of decapitation (apocrine snouts) are frequently seen on the luminal surface. Nuclei are
usually centrally placed, small, and vesicular.

The outer myoepithelial cells are spindled, with
eosinophilic cytoplasm and elongated nuclei.
The ceruminous glands are connected to the
surface by attenuated ducts lined by a dual layer
of small, darkly staining cuboidal cells which
empty into the luminal portion of a hair follicle.

Tympanic Membrane. The tympanic membrane (pars tensa) is composed of fibrous connective tissue covered externally (external ear canal
side) by a thin layer of keratinizing squamous
epithelium and internally (middle ear side) by a
single layer of low cuboidal cells (figs. 16-7, 16-8).
The external epithelium is continuous with that
lining the inner bony canal, and lacks both rete
pegs and adnexal structures. The epithelial layers cover a central connective tissue zone consisting of two outer (external) layers of radially
arranged collagenous fibers and an inner (internal) layer of circular fibers.

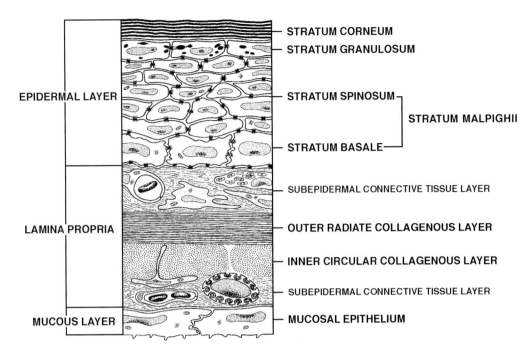

Figure 16-7
PRIMARY TYMPANIC MEMBRANE

A schematic microscopic view of a cross section of the pars tensa of the primary tympanic membrane (ear drum). The epidermal layer faces the external auditory canal. The pars flaccida (Schrapnell's membrane) portion of the drum consists of a similar histological makeup minus the outer and inner collagenous layer. (Fig. 1 from Lim DJ. Tympanic membrane. Electron microscopic observation. Part I. Pars tensa. Part II. Pars flaccida. Acta Otolaryngol 1968;66:181–98, 515–32.)

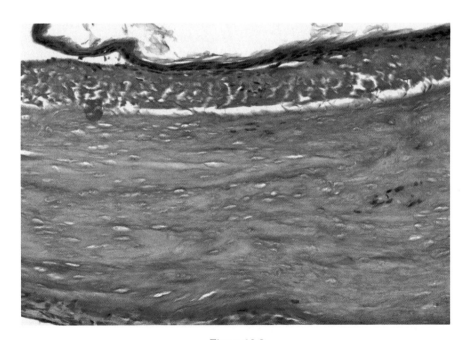

Figure 16-8
TYMPANIC MEMBRANE

The tympanic membrane shown was excised from a 19-year-old male with a history of chronic otitis media. The drum itself is composed of fibrous tissue, which in the specimen shown is markedly thickened and sclerotic. The outer squamous and inner cuboidal covering epithelial layers are evident at the top and bottom of the specimen, respectively.

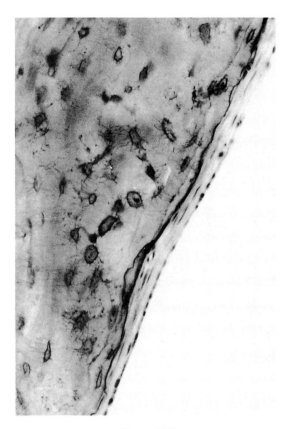

Figure 16-9
MIDDLE EAR

A microscopic view of the normal middle ear mucosa with a flattened, single layered, epithelial mucosal surface and narrow fibrous submucosal layer. (Fig. 280 from Fascicle 25, 2nd Series.)

Middle Ear

The eustachian tube and a variable proportion of the tympanic cavity anterior to the drum are lined by respiratory-type, pseudostratified, ciliated epithelium (2–6). Respiratory-type epithelium may extend along the floor and roof of the middle ear cleft to variably involve the middle ear cleft posterior to the drum as well (2,5). Most of the posterior tympanic cavity, as well as the ossicles, epitympanic recess (attic), and mastoid air cells are lined by a single layer of simple squamous or cuboidal epithelium (fig. 16-9)(4,5). The extent to which the middle ear is lined by respiratory-type or simple cuboidal epithelium, however, is unclear. Sade (2) found that ciliated epithelium involved from one third to two thirds of the middle ear lining. In contrast, Michaels (6) reported that most of the middle ear is predom-

inantly lined by simple cuboidal epithelium, whereas respiratory-type epithelium is only found on portions of the anterior wall and in small patches interspersed among areas of cuboidal epithelium. In all areas the submucosal layer is thin and composed of fibrous tissue containing small vessels and nerves.

Mastoid Air Cells. The mastoid air cells are an interconnecting network of spaces located within the petrous portion of the temporal bone, posterior to the external auditory canal. The air cells are continuous with the middle ear, eustachian tube, and ultimately, the outer air. The air spaces are separated by thin plates of lamellar bone covered by periosteum and an outer layer of simple cuboidal epithelium, similar to that lining the posterior aspect of the middle ear cleft.

TUMORS OF THE EXTERNAL EAR AND AUDITORY CANAL

In the following discussion, only tumors and tumor-like lesions that exclusively occur in, or have a predilection for, the external ear or ear canal are considered (Table 16-1). Other lesions, such as osteomas and seborrheic keratosis, which occur more commonly elsewhere but cause considerable diagnostic confusion when encountered in the external ear, are also discussed. Common, benign cutaneous lesions that may involve the skin surface of the external auricle but are commonly found on other skin surfaces, such as actinic keratosis and keratoacanthoma, are thoroughly detailed elsewhere and are not covered here.

Chondrodermatitis Nodularis Chronica Helicis

Definition. This small, non-neoplastic lesion of the external ear is characterized by a central area of fibrinoid necrosis surrounded by granulation tissue and peripheral epithelial hyperplasia.

General Features. Chondrodermatitis nodularis chronica helicis (CNCH) is a discrete, non-neoplastic, inflammatory lesion of the external ear (7–16). The lesion is currently assumed to result from localized dermal ischemia due to the combined effects of limited blood supply, solar damage, and local trauma. Patients often give a history of sleeping on the affected side, repeatedly compressing the affected area. Thus CNCH

Table 16-1

CLASSIFICATION OF TUMORS AND TUMOR-LIKE LESIONS OF THE EXTERNAL EAR

Tumor-like lesions
Chondrodermatitis nodularis chronica helicis
Keratosis obturans; cholesteatoma; keratin
 granuloma
Angiolymphoid hyperplasia with eosinophilia
Accessory tragus (supernumerary auricle)
Keloid
Osteoma and exostosis

Cystic lesions
Idiopathic cystic chondromalacia (pseudocysts)
First branchial cleft anomalies (congenital cysts)

Benign neoplasms
Ceruminal gland adenoma
Ceruminal gland pleomorphic adenoma
Ceruminal gland syringocystadenoma papilliferum
Seborrheic keratosis
Squamous cell papilloma
Atypical fibroxanthoma

Malignant neoplasms
Ceruminal gland adenocarcinoma
Ceruminal gland adenoid cystic carcinoma
Basal cell carcinoma
Squamous cell carcinoma
Malignant melanoma

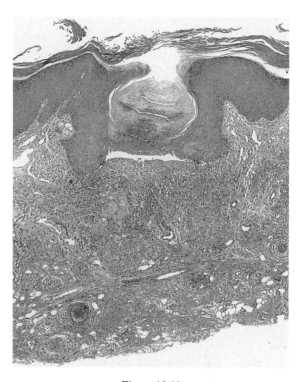

Figure 16-10
CHONDRODERMATITIS
NODULARIS CHRONICA HELICIS
Low magnification examination emphasizes the surface ulceration, centrally located channel, and adjacent pseudoepitheliomatous hyperplasia.

probably represents the transepidermal elimination of underlying degenerated, ischemic tissue (13).

Clinical Features. CNCH usually presents as a tender nodule on the superior helix of the external ear of older individuals. Lesions usually measure less than 1 cm in diameter and frequently show central ulceration. Approximately 70 percent of cases occur in males, and multiple lesions are not uncommon (11). The lesions are painful, particularly on manipulation. Most cases are clinically diagnosed as carcinoma. In one study of 43 cases of CNCH in which a clinical diagnosis was recorded, only 5 were correctly identified; other diagnoses included basal cell carcinoma (25 cases), nonspecified carcinoma (4 cases), squamous cell carcinoma (3 cases), and several miscellaneous benign entities (6 cases) (11).

Pathologic Findings. Lesions are typically small, tan-white, cutaneous nodules measuring less than 1.5 cm in diameter. Central erosion or crusting is often seen. Microscopically, the overlying epidermis shows a central cup-shaped de-

pression or ulceration with marked acanthosis and hyperkeratosis at the margins (fig. 16-10). Lesions are often covered by a hyperkeratotic and parakeratotic crust. The underlying dermal collagen is usually abnormal, and may show edema, homogenization, and fibrinoid necrobiotic necrosis. The necrobiotic collagen is usually surrounded by granulation tissue with acute and chronic inflammation (12,14). The ulcerated center may form a well-defined channel filled with necrotic debris, acute inflammatory cells, and fibrin (fig. 16-11) (8). The channel or the inflammation usually reaches the perichondrium of the underlying auricular cartilage, which may show reactive alterations in the basophilic chondroid matrix, such as hypercellularity, focal disappearance of chondrocytes, fibrosis, or sclerosis (fig. 16-12). Reactive perichondrial cells appear to migrate superficially into the area of dermal necrosis. Degenerative changes in the underlying cartilage, such as focal calcification and ossification, may be seen (7).

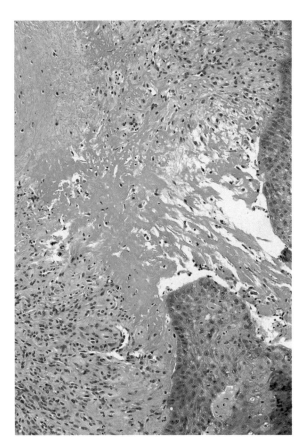

Figure 16-11
CHONDRODERMATITIS
NODULARIS CHRONICA HELICIS
Note the well-defined central channel containing fibrinoid
and necrotic debris and surrounded by granulation tissue.

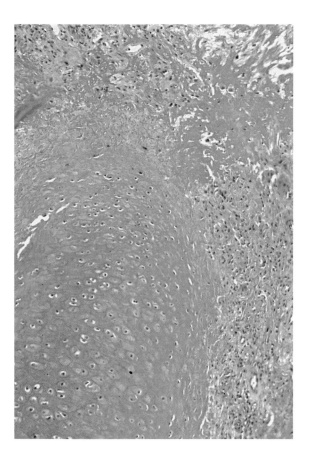

Figure 16-12
CHONDRODERMATITIS
NODULARIS CHRONICA HELICIS
In most lesions the ulcerated channel usually extends to
the underlying cartilage, which in this example shows reactive changes including hypercellularity and pericartilagen-
ous fibrosis.

Differential Diagnosis. Due to the squamous epithelial proliferation and necrobiotic foci
commonly seen in CNCH, the differential diagnosis includes actinic keratosis, squamous cell
carcinoma, and necrobiotic granulomatous lesions such as granuloma annulare. The presence
of a centrally located transepidermal channel in
combination with marginal acanthosis, fibrinoid
dermal necrosis, and transepidermal elimination of necrotic debris, however, is characteristic
and not seen in any of the latter lesions.

Treatment and Prognosis. Simple excision
or curettage of the lesion and the underlying
cartilaginous "bump" is usually curative (9,10).
Most authors advocate an initial intralesional
injection of glucocorticoids, for which a 50 percent curative rate has been reported (11,15).
Recurrent lesions are usually excised.

Keratosis Obturans, Cholesteatoma, and Keratin Granulomas of the External Auditory Canal

Definition. These are benign, non-neoplastic, keratinaceous lesions of the external auditory canal composed of either exfoliated keratin
(keratosis obturans), an enlarging squamous epithelial-lined sac (cholesteatoma), or a foreign
body granulomatous response to the presence of
keratin within the subepithelial tissues (keratin
granuloma) (17–19).

General and Clinical Features. Keratosis
obturans results when exfoliated keratinocytes
from the external canal epithelium are retained
and eventually aggregate to form a solid
keratinaceous plug (19). Continual enlargement

of the lesion may cause mucosal ulceration and canal widening. Bilateral lesions may occur and secondary infection of the plug contents is a frequent complication. Patients are typically young and present with hearing loss and pain (19). Clinically, the lesion appears as a layered plug of white-tan debris within the ear canal. The lesion is thought to result from a deficiency in the normal self-cleaning mechanism of the canal, in which desquamated material is laterally extruded.

Cholesteatomas usually occur in the middle ear (see the middle ear portion of this chapter for a complete discussion of these lesions) but may infrequently originate in the external canal as well. External canal cholesteatomas are unilateral, non-neoplastic lesions composed of an epithelial-lined sac derived from the external canal epidermis. Patients are usually older and present with otorrhea and dull, chronic pain (19).

Keratin implantation granulomas may also develop in the external canal in response to keratinaceous material implanted within the canal mucosa, and are often associated with cholesteatomas (17). It is thought that the keratin gains entrance into the underlying tissue by either unrelenting local pressure exerted by an associated cholesteatoma or following traumatic laceration.

Pathologic Findings. Grossly and histologically, keratosis obturans appears as a solid, concentric mass of desquamated keratinaceous debris arranged in a lamellar, onionskin-like fashion (fig. 16-13). Cholesterol clefts may be present. Secondary bacterial infection with associated acute and chronic inflammation may occur. Large lesions produce ulceration, inflammation, or bony necrosis of the canal wall.

Cholesteatomas are thoroughly covered in the section on middle ear lesions. Briefly, they grossly appear as white, pearly, cystic masses containing creamy or flake-like material. Histologically, the lesions consist of an intact or ruptured thin-walled cyst distended by keratinaceous debris and lined by keratinizing squamous epithelium (18).

Keratin implantation granulomas consist of foreign body type giant cells and associated keratinaceous debris, as well as variable degrees of mixed inflammation with granulation tissue (fig. 16-14). Engulfed keratinaceous fragments are often seen within the giant cell cytoplasm.

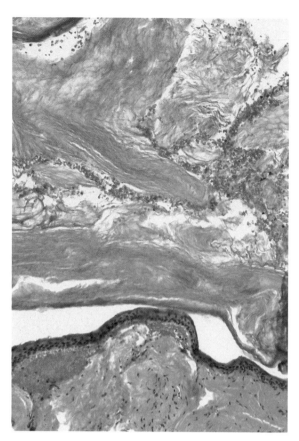

Figure 16-13
KERATOSIS OBTURANS
A rare example of keratosis obturans necessitating surgical excision from the external ear canal. The lesion consists of densely packed orthokeratin arranged in an onion skin, lamellar fashion indicative of successive layers of desquamation. The underlying squamous epithelium of the external ear canal is also present.

Differential Diagnosis. Keratosis obturans, cholesteatomas, and implantation granulomas are often confused with each other clinically. Fortunately, these lesions are easily distinguished histologically, as the keratotic plug of keratosis obturans and the epithelial-lined, keratin-distended sac of cholesteatoma are diagnostic and not seen in other processes. Implantation granulomas may be misinterpreted as inflammatory lesions of infectious etiology if the keratin flakes are rare or overlooked.

Treatment and Prognosis. Keratosis obturans and implantation granulomas are localized, self-limited, inflammatory lesions for which curettage or excision is adequate treatment. Cholesteatomas are benign but may become

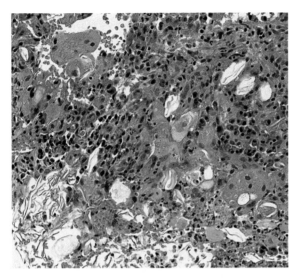

Figure 16-14
KERATIN IMPLANTATION GRANULOMA
A representative lesion excised from the external ear canal showing keratin flakes engulfed by foreign body type giant cells and associated granulation tissue.

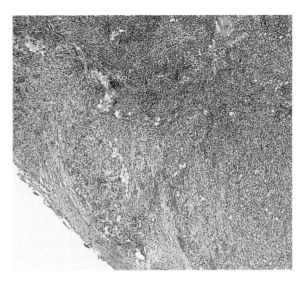

Figure 16-15
ANGIOLYMPHOID HYPERPLASIA
WITH EOSINOPHILIA
On low-power magnification these lesions appear as large, tumor-like masses with an inflammatory and vascular component. Angiolymphoid hyperplasia with eosinophilia is typically confined to the dermis or subcutaneous tissue but ulceration of the overlying epidermis may be seen.

progressively destructive and lead to widespread bony erosion, hearing loss, or abscess formation. Complete surgical excision is advocated, as recurrence frequently follows incomplete removal.

Angiolymphoid Hyperplasia with Eosinophilia

Definition. This is a benign inflammatory vascular proliferation of the external ear composed of small, arborizing vessels lined by plump, epithelioid endothelial cells and an associated chronic inflammatory infiltrate with prominent eosinophils.

General Features. Angiolymphoid hyperplasia with eosinophilia (ALHE), also known as *histiocytoid/epithelioid hemangioma* and *benign angiomatoid nodules* of face and scalp, is a rare, benign, inflammatory vascular lesion occurring in young to middle-aged adults (20–27). Lesions reported as Kimura's disease are widely believed to represent a different clinicopathologic entity (21, 23,27). Angiolymphoid hyperplasia may occur anywhere in the skin, particularly in the scalp and face, with a predilection for the external auricle and auditory canal (24,26). Extrafacial, soft tissue and bony lesions may also occur (25). The precise etiology is unknown, but at least a proportion of lesions are thought to be reactive.

Clinical Features. Tumors usually present as slow-growing, red nodules measuring from a few millimeters to 1 cm in diameter (20,23). Females are affected slightly more often than males. Most patients are young to middle-aged adults, although ALHE may occur at any age. Lesions commonly involve the external ear, external auditory canal, or periauricular tissue; extrafacial tumors are rare. Multiple lesions are common and may coalesce to form subcutaneous plaques measuring up to 10 cm in diameter. Local pruritus is common, and superficial excoriation and bleeding may occur from scratching.

Pathologic Findings. On scanning magnification, ALHE often appears nodular and is usually confined to the dermis or subcutaneous tissue (fig. 16-15). Occasional lesions may appear to arise from vessels, and intravascular forms may occur. Histologically, ALHE is characterized by a proliferation of branching vessels lined by plump, epithelioid endothelial cells and an associated chronic inflammatory infiltrate with eosinophils. The endothelial cells have large vesicular nuclei and abundant, occasionally vacuolated, eosinophilic cytoplasm (fig. 16-16). The epithelioid

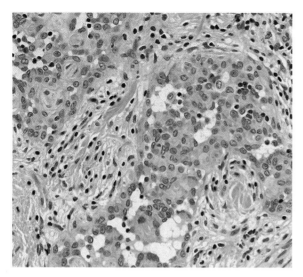

Figure 16-16
ANGIOLYMPHOID HYPERPLASIA
WITH EOSINOPHILIA
Many examples of this entity show the branching vessels lined by plump epithelioid endothelial cells, with little to no accompanying inflammation.

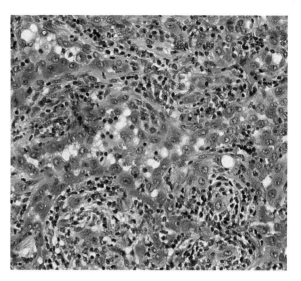

Figure 16-17
ANGIOLYMPHOID HYPERPLASIA
WITH EOSINOPHILIA
Other examples of this lesion may show a prominent chronic inflammatory component complete with scattered eosinophils. (Figures 16-17 and 16-18 are from the same patient.)

cells may show a convex luminal border and project into the vascular lumen in a "tombstone-like" pattern. Mitotic figures are unusual. The chronic inflammatory infiltrate, which may be sparse or dense, consists predominantly of lymphocytes with mast cells, plasma cells, and variable numbers of eosinophils (fig. 16-17). Lymphocytic aggregates may form germinal centers. Most areas contain identifiable vessels, although focally, sheets of plump epithelioid cells with only focal evidence of vascular differentiation may be seen (fig. 16-18). Regional lymph nodes may be enlarged and hyperplastic with an eosinophilic component (27).

Immunohistochemical Findings. As the diagnosis primarily depends on routine histologic examination, few cases of ALHE have been studied immunohistochemically. In those cases, the epithelioid endothelial cells were variably positive for several endothelial markers, including factor VIII–related antigen, CD31, CD34, and *Ulex europeaus* agglutinin (UEA)-I lectin (27).

Differential Diagnosis. ALHE should be distinguished from Kimura's disease, a chronic inflammatory condition that commonly affects Asians but occurs infrequently in Westerners. Clinically, Kimura's disease occurs most often in males, who

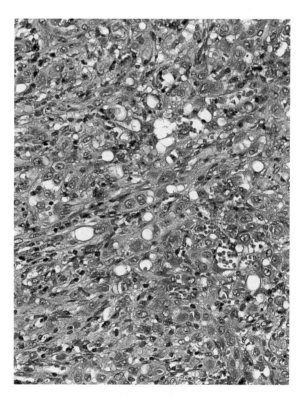

Figure 16-18
ANGIOLYMPHOID HYPERPLASIA
WITH EOSINOPHILIA
Occasional lesions show areas composed of sheets of plump endothelial cells with little to no inflammation.

present with cervical lymphadenopathy with or without associated subcutaneous or soft tissue lesions in the head and neck area. Histologically Kimura's disease is a dermal inflammatory process with markedly dense lymphoid aggregates, germinal center formation, interspersed eosinophils, and thin-walled postcapillary venules. The germinal centers contain spindled, IgE-bearing dendritic reticulum cells, leading to speculation that the disease represents an immunologic reaction to an unidentified stimulus (21,23,27). Both Kimura's disease and ALHE show a marked chronic inflammation with eosinophils. Kimura's disease is distinguished by inconspicuous vessels lined by typical spindled endothelial cells, and not plump, epithelioid cells as in ALHE (21,23,27).

AHLE may be confused with several other entities, including granulation tissue, eosinophilic granuloma, insect bites, malignant lymphoma, and angiosarcoma. The features of a vascular proliferation combined with a dense, polymorphous lymphoid infiltrate and eosinophils excludes most of the latter entities. Occasionally ALHE may show endothelial atypia, but the young age of affected patients, the nodular configuration, lack of interanastomosing vascular channels, presence of eosinophils, and relative absence of mitotic figures and necrosis help to exclude angiosarcoma in virtually all cases.

Treatment and Prognosis. Angiolymphoid hyperplasia is a benign inflammatory lesion without serious sequelae. Local excision is usually curative, although recurrence may develop in a minority of cases.

Accessory Tragus

Definition. This is a benign, pedunculated, preauricular cutaneous lesion characterized by squamous, epithelial-lined fibroconnective tissue with a centrally placed bar of mature hyaline cartilage.

General Features. Accessory tragus, also known as *accessory auricle,* is a congenital anomaly arising from the first branchial cleft, which normally gives rise to the external auditory meatus. Accessory tragus usually presents as an isolated anomaly but may also be associated with cleft lip, cleft palate, and mandibular hypoplasia. Histologically, it often recapitulates the normal anatomy of the external ear.

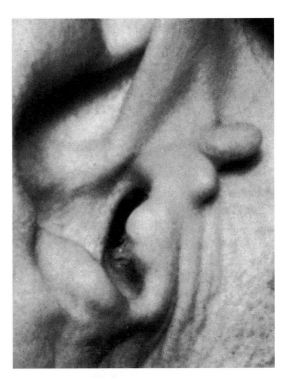

Figure 16-19
ACCESSORY TRAGUS
This 32-year-old woman stated that she had had bilateral nontender growths in the preauricular area ever since she could remember. (Fig. 288 from Fascicle 25, 2nd Series.)

Clinical Features. Accessory tragi are asymptomatic, cutaneous lesions that invariably present at birth (28). The appearance and location is variable, and the lesion may be solitary or multiple, unilateral or bilateral, sessile or pedunculated. Most lesions are located in the preauricular region, slightly above or below the level of the tragus (fig. 16-19).

Pathologic Findings. Accessory tragi typically appear as soft or firm, skin-covered nodules or pedunculated lesions measuring less than 1 cm. Microscopically, the architectural configuration is that of a sessile or pedunculated polyp, with a fibrovascular core covered by stratified squamous epithelium. Most contain a centrally placed lobe or bar of mature hyaline cartilage (fig. 16-20). Adipose tissue, eccrine sweat glands, and pilosebaceous units may be present (28). Lesions without cartilage are often misinterpreted as fibroepithelial papillomas or cutaneous tags.

Treatment and Prognosis. Simple excision is curative.

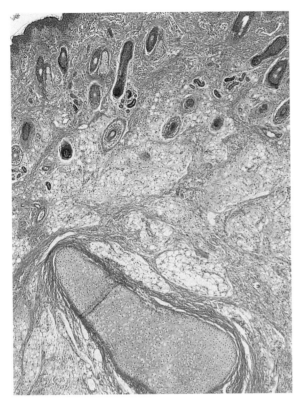

Figure 16-20
ACCESSORY TRAGUS
On histologic section most accessory tragi appear as a polypoid protuberance of mature hyaline cartilage covered by normal-appearing skin, complete with adipose tissue and adnexal structures.

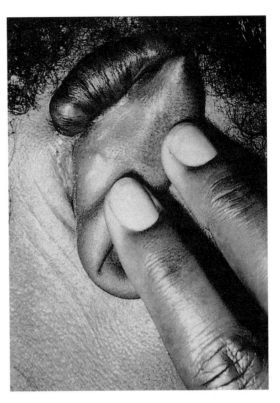

Figure 16-21
KELOID
This 18-year-old black woman had worn glasses for 4 years, and for the past 3 months had noted this slow growing, right-sided, retroauricular tumor. She knew of no specific trauma, except for the irritation of the glasses resting on the ear. (Fig. 285 from Fascicle 25, 2nd Series)

Keloid

Definition. This is a benign, self-limited proliferation of mature collagen, commonly found on the external ear or earlobe, and thought to arise following local trauma.

General and Clinical Features. Keloids are benign, post-traumatic collagenous lesions occurring in predisposed persons, particularly those of the black race (29–31). Lesions classically develop following earlobe piercing for earring insertion.

Keloids may be found on any skin surface, but are predisposed to occur on the external ear, particularly the earlobe (fig. 16-21) (29). Extra-auricular keloids are readily diagnosed as firm, red, raised nodules covered by taut normal skin. Keloids may persist for years, occasionally extending beyond the site of original injury (31).

Pathologic Findings. Lesions are firm, raised nodules covered by normal-appearing skin. Histologically, the dermis and subcutaneous tissue are expanded by thick, hyalinized bundles of collagen admixed with fibroblasts (fig. 16-22). The collagenous bundles are arranged concentrically and focally assume a nodular configuration (fig. 16-23) (30). Adjacent adnexae are atrophic. Depending upon whether the condensation of collagen impinges upon the papillary dermis, the overlying epidermis may appear either flattened or normal.

Differential Diagnosis. By their nodular configuration keloids are distinguished from hypertrophic scar, which may initially appear nodular but mature into lesions with irregular bundles of collagen lying parallel to the skin surface.

Treatment and Prognosis. Surgical excision is the usual treatment but often results in local recurrence. Postoperative low-dose radiation or

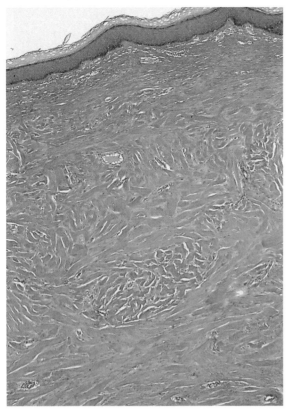

Figure 16-22
KELOID
Keloids typically show an unremarkable or thinned epidermis overlying a marked proliferation of thick, hyalinized bundles of collagen with admixed fibroblasts.

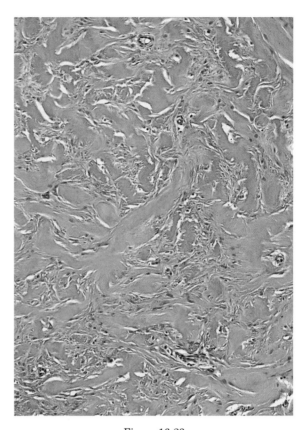

Figure 16-23
KELOID
The proliferating collagenous bundles are hypocellular and often arranged in a poorly defined, concentric, nodular configuration.

glucocorticoid injections have been advocated to prevent recurrence.

Osteoma and Exostosis

Definition. These benign, bony abnormalities of the external ear canal and elsewhere are composed of either a pedunculated (osteoma) or broad-based (exostosis) mass of histologically normal bone.

General Features. Two types of bony deformity within the external ear canal are recognized: osteomas and exostoses (32,33). Osteomas are solitary, localized masses of dense, histologically normal bone attached by a bony pedicle to the tympanosquamous or tympanomastoid suture line (fig. 16-24). These lesions commonly occur in the skull, paranasal sinuses, and facial bones, but may also be found in the external ear canal.

Exostoses are broad-based lesions that are often multiple, bilateral, and symmetric. They typically arise in the external ear canal and probably represent a reactive process (33).

Clinical Features. Osteomas present as pedunculated tumors attached by a bony pedicle to the outer half of the ear canal (33). In one study of 16 osteomas of the external ear, most patients were under 50 years of age (range, 12 to 62 years), with a male to female ratio of 4 to 1 (33). Lesions may obliterate the canal lumen, and symptoms are related to such obstruction.

Exostoses present as broad-based lesions, often located in the medial half of the bony outer ear canal, and often in proximity to the tympanic ring. Most patients are male and under the age of 50 years. In one study intermittent obstruction was the initial symptom in 50 percent of patients (33).

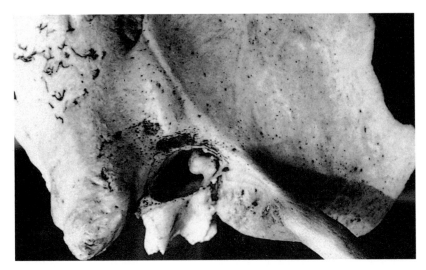

Figure 16-24
OSTEOMA
This temporal bone specimen demonstrates the typical anatomic location of the osteoma at the tympanomastoid suture line. (Fig. 302 from Fascicle 25, 2nd Series.)

Pathologic Findings. Both lesions may appear as small, cigar- to club-shaped masses of compact bone covered by canal mucosa. Histologically, osteomas are composed of interconnecting fascicles of compact, normal-appearing lamellar bone with an inner marrow area filled with fibrovascular connective tissue (fig. 16-25) (32). Lesions occasionally show an outer cortical and an inner cancellous architecture. Rarely, osteomas with a mixture of cortical and medullary bone are encountered. Osteomas are usually covered by periosteum and the normal squamous epithelium of the external canal (fig. 16-26).

Exostoses are composed of parallel layers of dense lamellar bone. In contrast to osteomas, interlamellar spaces are very small or absent (fig. 16-27) (32). Lesions have a heaped up appearance suggestive of a reactive, bony hyperplasia rather than a true neoplasm. Exostoses are covered by periosteum located immediately beneath the squamous lining epithelium of the external canal.

Differential Diagnosis. Clinically, osteomas and exostoses of the external canal may be confused with ossifying fibroma, densely ossified fibrous dysplasia, or osteosarcoma. The presence of concentrically arranged, microscopically normal bone, however, without unusual ("Chinese letter") trabeculae or cytologic atypia excludes the latter possibilities.

Treatment and Prognosis. Surgical excision is recommended for osteomas, whereas extirpation is recommended for exostosis only if the lesion causes symptoms. Local recurrence following excision has not been reported (33).

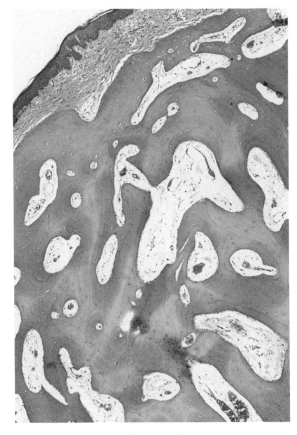

Figure 16-25
OSTEOMA
An osteoma arising from the osseous portion of the external ear canal, projecting into the lumen. The lesion consists of normal-appearing bony cortex and marrow spaces filled with fibrovascular tissue.

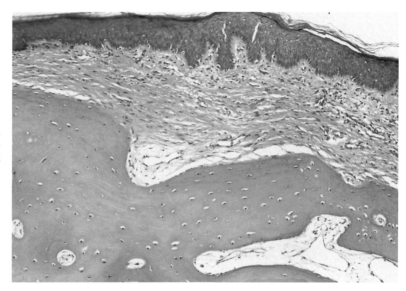

Figure 16-26
OSTEOMA
On high magnification the compact nature of the lamellar bone and the squamous epithelium overlying the external ear canal are better appreciated.

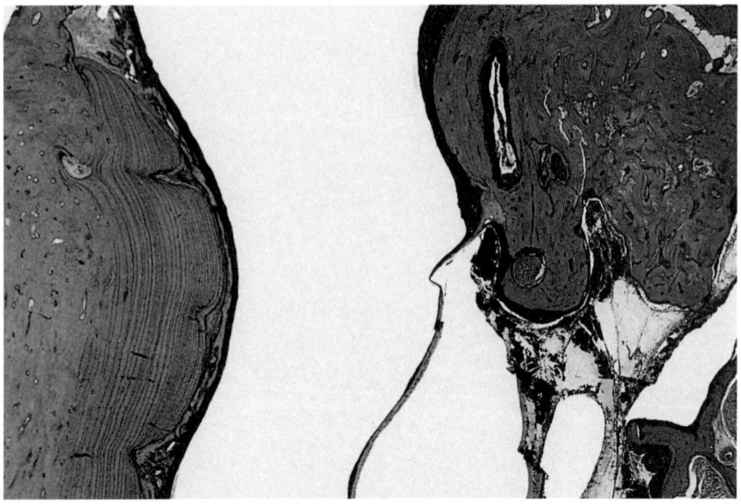

Figure 16-27
EXOSTOSIS
A low-power view of the inner osseous auditory canal shows an exostosis on the left and a smaller one on the right. The suggested "heaped up" bone forming the mass suggests irritation of the periosteal layer of the normal bone. (Fig. 304 from Fascicle 25, 2nd Series.)

Idiopathic Cystic Chondromalacia

Definition. This is a benign, cystic degenerative lesion of cartilage predilected to occur within the auricular cartilage of the outer ear.

General and Clinical Features. Idiopathic cystic chondromalacia (ICC), also known as *pseudocyst of the auricle,* is an unusual, idiopathic lesion characterized by cystic degeneration of the auricular cartilage (34,35). ICC appears clinically as a localized area of swelling (fig. 16-28) (34,35). Lesions typically affect males more often than females (34); young and middle-aged adults are affected most frequently. Lesions may occur along any portion of the auricle, al-though the most common site is immediately adjacent to the helix.

Pathologic Findings. The lesion is typically a well-defined, cystic cavity within the auricular cartilage, filled with clear to yellow fluid. Histologically, ICC appears as simple, unilocular, intracartilagenous cysts without a detectable lining epithelium (fig. 16-29) (34,35). The cysts may be immediately adjacent to, and appear to arise directly from, the auricular cartilage or may be focally surrounded by an intervening layer of fibrovascular granulation tissue (fig. 16-30).

Differential Diagnosis. Distinction from relapsing polychondritis, which may initially present as a localized external ear swelling, is accomplished

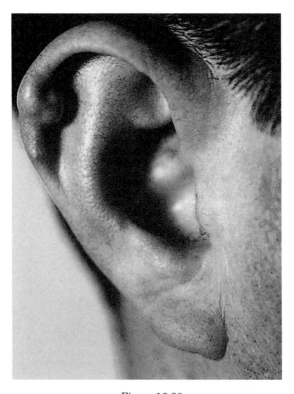

Figure 16-28
IDIOPATHIC CYSTIC CHONDROMALACIA
A 28-year-old man noted a slowly enlarging cyst on the helix of his right ear, which recently had become slightly tender. (Fig. 289 from Fascicle 25, 2nd Series.)

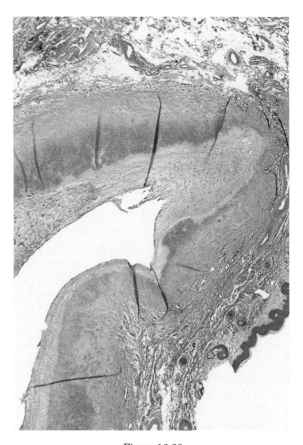

Figure 16-29
IDIOPATHIC CYSTIC CHONDROMALACIA
On low magnification lesions appear as simple, unilocular cysts arising within the auricular cartilage. (Figures 16-29 and 16-30 are from the same patient.)

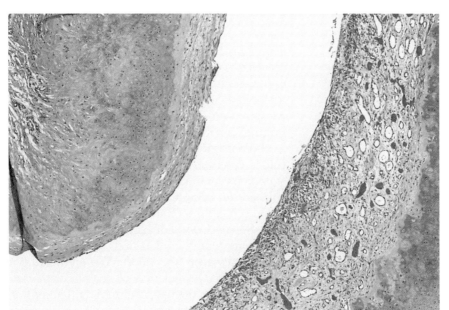

Figure 16-30
IDIOPATHIC CYSTIC
CHONDROMALACIA
The cyst wall is devoid of a lining epithelium and may appear to arise directly from the surrounding cartilage or contain an intervening layer of fibrovascular tissue.

by the multifocal involvement of other body cartilages and systemic symptomatology typical of the latter and not found in ICC.

Treatment and Prognosis. Surgical excision or curettage is usually curative.

Anomalies of the First Branchial Cleft

Definition and General Features. First branchial cleft anomalies are also known as *branchial cleft cysts, congenital cysts, preauricular sinuses,* or *preauricular pits.* Olsen et al. (37) classified first branchial cleft anomalies into three categories: cysts, sinuses, and fistulas. Cystic lesions occur two times more frequently than sinuses and fistulas combined, and are thought to result from either duplication of the first branchial cleft or cystic enlargement of buried cell rests within the ventral portion thereof (fig. 16-31). In contrast, incomplete obliteration of the ventral cleft may result in either sinus anomalies or a fistulous tract opening to the external cutaneous surface or external ear canal (36).

Clinical Features. First branchial cleft cysts appear as solitary cystic lesions, without an associated sinus tract, anterior to the ear. Most cysts arise within or juxtaposed to the parotid gland and are often clinically misdiagnosed as parotid gland tumors. In the study of Olsen et al. (37), cysts arose in three distinct anatomic locations: intraparotid, paraparotid, and infraparotid. The patients ranged in age from 13 to 81 years and females outnumbered males 2 to 1. Symptoms varied from a feeling of fullness to intermittent pain.

Sinus anomalies occur in much younger patients (range, 1 to 13 years) without gender predilection. These anomalies are often associated with cysts and the sinus usually extends from the associated cystic mass to the overlying skin or external canal. Fistulous tracts also may be associated with a cyst. The tract itself often communicates between the cyst (if present) and two external surfaces, usually the overlying skin and the external auditory canal. Fistulas are also almost exclusively encountered in children and are more common on the left than on the right side. The anatomic location of both sinuses and fistulas are highly variable, but both tend to develop along several well-defined tracts (fig. 16-32). Sinuses and fistulous tracts are most

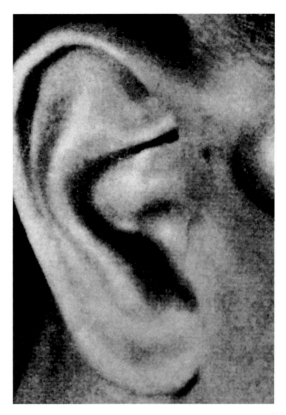

Figure 16-31
CYST OF FIRST BRANCHIAL CLEFT

The anterior auricular cyst represents a branchial cleft cyst, thought to arise from duplication of the first branchial cleft or from cystic expansion of buried cell rests within the ventral portion of the first cleft. (Fig. 19 from Becker W, Buckingham RA, Holinger PH, Korting GW, Lederer FL. Atlas of otorhinolaryngology and broncho-esophagology. Philadelphia: WB Saunders, 1969:6.)

commonly found within or between the following structures: the postauricular region, parotid gland, angle of the jaw, external auditory canal, and middle ear space. They are often infected on presentation and appear as tender, slowly enlarging, erythematous cystic masses.

Pathologic Findings. Cysts, sinuses, or fistulous tracts may be lined by either stratified squamous or ciliated, respiratory-type columnar epithelium. Lymphoid aggregates that form germinal centers are often present within the cystic wall. Subepithelial adnexal structures, including sebaceous glands and islands of cartilage, are occasionally seen (fig. 16-33). The epithelial lining of infected lesions may be necrotic with variable degrees of acute and chronic inflammation and granulation tissue.

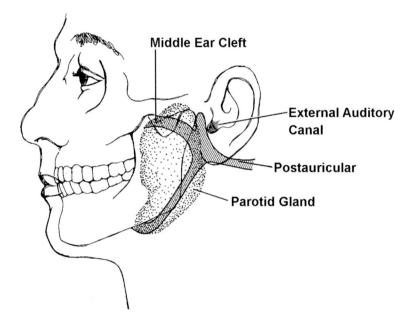

Middle Ear Cleft

External Auditory Canal

Postauricular

Parotid Gland

Figure 16-32
CYST OF FIRST
BRANCHIAL CLEFT
This drawing represents the possible
pathways that the sinuses and fistulas can
follow in relation to the external auricle.
The cutaneous openings can occur anywhere along these tracts. (Adapted from
reference 30.)

Figure 16-33
CYST OF FIRST
BRANCHIAL CLEFT
A sinus draining anterior to the
auricle that duplicates the histology of
the external auditory canal (X25).
(Fig. 294 from Fascicle 25, 2nd Series.)

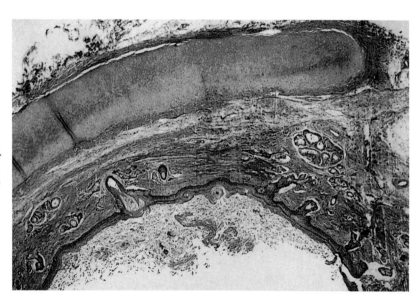

Differential Diagnosis. The anatomic location, epithelial lining, lack of keratinaceous debris,
and occasional presence of adnexal structures
serves to distinguish these lesions from epidermal (retention) cysts, cholesteatoma, idiopathic
cystic chondromalacia, and other cystic lesions.

Treatment and Prognosis. First branchial
cleft anomalies are congenital, benign lesions, although significant enlargement and infection of the
cystic or sinus contents may occur. Complete surgical excision is recommended. During removal of a
cystic lesion, an effort should be made to identify
and remove any associated sinus or fistulous tract.

Ceruminal Adenoma

Definition. This is a benign ceruminal gland
neoplasm characterized by a tubuloglandular
proliferation of apocrine epithelial cells with an
underlying myoepithelial cell layer.

General Features. Ceruminal adenoma, also
known as *ceruminoma,* is a benign tumor arising
from the modified apocrine ceruminal glands of
the external ear. Ceruminal glands are normally
located in the dermis of the cartilaginous portion
of the external auditory canal, thus ceruminal
gland tumors typically arise in this area as well.

401

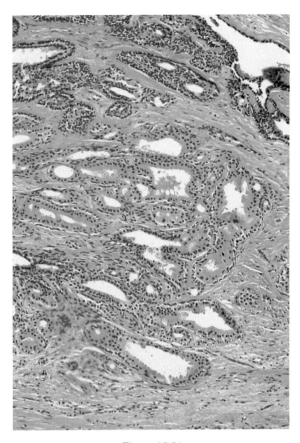

Figure 16-34
CERUMINAL ADENOMA
Adenomas of ceruminal gland derivation typically show a circumscribed proliferation of well-differentiated glands and tubular structures in a variably cellular connective tissue stroma. (Figures 16-34 and 16-35 are from the same patient.)

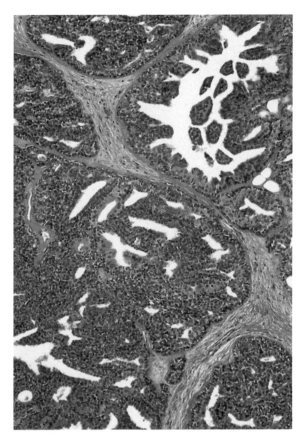

Figure 16-35
CERUMINAL ADENOMA
Occasional adenomas may also show well-defined nests containing "back-to-back" glands and papillations.

Clinical Features. Most ceruminal adenomas present as a painless nodule in the outer half of the external auditory canal. Patients may complain of unilateral hearing loss. There is a male predilection of approximately 2 to 1. Tumors occur over a wide age range but are most common in the fifth and sixth decades.

Gross Findings. Lesions appear as circumscribed, polypoid masses covered by normal skin (38–42). Due to their anatomic location, ceruminal adenomas are usually small, measuring less than 1 cm in diameter, and often appear cystic on cut section (39). Superficial ulceration may be present in a proportion of cases.

Microscopic Findings. Ceruminal adenomas appear as circumscribed but unencapsulated, predominantly glandular proliferations. Most tu-

mors are composed of glands, tubules, and cysts separated by a hyalinized fibrovascular stroma (fig. 16-34) (38,39,42). Back-to-back glandular structures and papillations may also be seen (fig. 16-35). Two distinct cell layers are usually present: an inner, cuboidal, epithelial (apocrine) cell layer and an outer, spindled to cuboidal, myoepithelial layer (fig. 16-36). In occasional tumors a proliferation of myoepithelial cells or an abundant connective tissue stroma may focally obscure or obliterate the two-cell layer architecture (figs. 16-37, 16-38). The inner epithelial cells resemble normal cerumen-secreting, apocrine-type epithelium, with intensely eosinophilic cytoplasm, well-defined cell borders, and luminal secretory droplets ("apocrine snouts") (39). Nuclei are round to oval with finely granular chromatin and occasional nucleoli. The outermost myoepithelial cells are small, attenuated and spindled or cuboidal, with

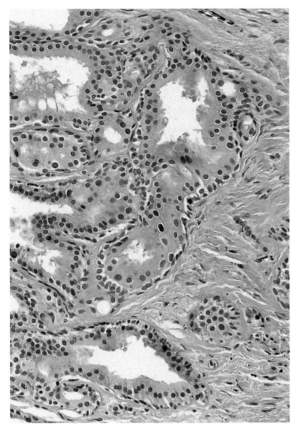

Figure 16-36
CERUMINAL ADENOMA
The glandular structures are lined by an inner layer of eosinophilic, apocrine-like epithelial cells and an outer layer of cuboidal to spindled, clear myoepithelial cells.

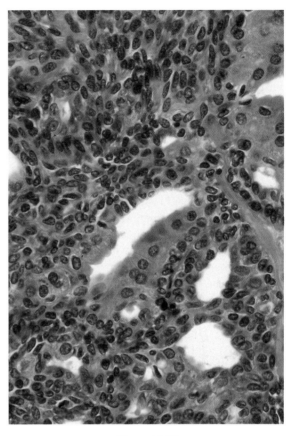

Figure 16-37
CERUMINAL ADENOMA
Occasional tumors may show areas composed of sheets and nests of proliferating myoepithelial cells with a minimal epithelial component.

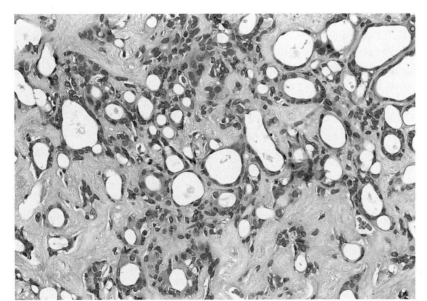

Figure 16-38
CERUMINAL ADENOMA
Rare ceruminal adenomas may contain abundant connective tissue stroma, which may obscure or obliterate the underlying dual epithelial-myoepithelial architecture.

clear cytoplasm and dark-staining nuclei. Nuclear pleomorphism and mitotic activity are typically absent (39,42).

Differential Diagnosis. The primary differential diagnostic consideration is ceruminal adenocarcinoma, which is distinguished from adenoma by the presence of cellular pleomorphism, stromal invasion, and a desmoplastic stromal response. Ceruminal adenomas also show a biphasic epithelial-myoepithelial cellular architecture, whereas carcinomas are composed of a single epithelial cell type. Middle ear adenomas may present in the external canal via a perforated tympanic membrane, but are composed of smaller, low cuboidal cells without apocrine features. Metastatic adenocarcinomas from other sites must be excluded as well.

Treatment and Prognosis. Surgical excision is the modality of choice. Local recurrence may follow incomplete excision, but to our knowledge metastatic dissemination has not been reported (38,42).

Pleomorphic Adenoma of Ceruminal Gland

Definition and General Features. Pleomorphic adenomas (mixed tumors) of ceruminal glands are benign neoplasms composed of both epithelial and mesenchymal elements embedded in a collagenous to myxoid ("chondroid") stroma (43–47). They are common in the major and minor salivary glands and skin (chondroid syringomas), but may occur in the external ear canal as well. Despite earlier proposals that auricular pleomorphic adenomas may arise from the adjacent parotid salivary gland (46) or ectopic salivary gland tissue (44), most investigators believe these lesions arise from the ceruminal glands of the external ear canal. The lesions are rare: in a recent review of the English literature, Dehner et al. (43) found only nine pathologically documented cases arising in the external ear canal.

Clinical Features. Auricular pleomorphic adenoma is a solitary, slow-growing lesion that occurs more frequently in women, aged 27 to 66 years (43,47). The lesion typically presents as a firm, sessile or polypoid mass covered by intact external canal epithelium without ulceration. Symptoms are often related to partial external canal obstruction.

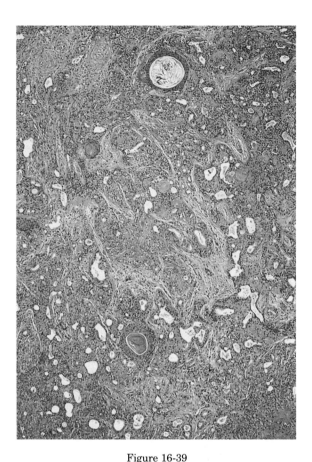

Figure 16-39
PLEOMORPHIC ADENOMA OF CERUMINAL GLAND
Similar to pleomorphic adenomas (mixed tumors) arising elsewhere, those in ceruminal glands are composed of epithelial and myoepithelial cells arranged in tubules, cords, and nests. In the field depicted the stroma is collagenous with only focal myxoid changes. Note the areas of squamous metaplasia.

Pathologic Findings. Reported cases have measured from 1 to 2 cm in greatest diameter (43,45). Similar to pleomorphic adenomas arising in the salivary glands, the auricular variety are microscopically circumscribed but unencapsulated tumors that vary widely in appearance depending upon the amount and type of epithelium and stroma present. The epithelial component consists of a proliferation of both epithelial and myoepithelial cells arranged in tubules, cords, and nests (fig. 16-39). Most of the tubular structures are composed of an inner epithelial and an outer myoepithelial cell layer, but groupings of either cell type alone may be present as well (fig. 16-40). The epithelial cells are oval to polygonal, with centrally placed nuclei and eosinophilic cytoplasm. In tubular areas the inner

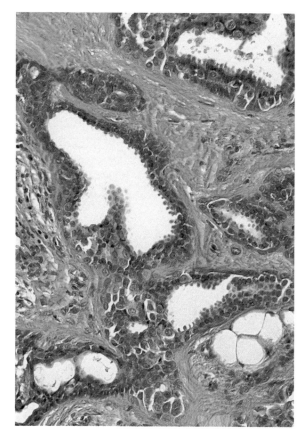

Figure 16-40
PLEOMORPHIC ADENOMA OF CERUMINAL GLAND
On high magnification, the constituent glands are lined by both an outer myoepithelial and an inner epithelial cell layer. The inner epithelial cells show apocrine snouts, reminiscent of normal ceruminal gland epithelium. (Figures 16-40 and 16-41 are from the same patient.)

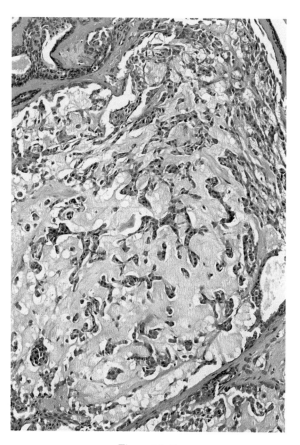

Figure 16-41
PLEOMORPHIC ADENOMA OF CERUMINAL GLAND
In other areas cords of epithelial cells are embedded within a chondromyxoid stroma.

epithelial cells may recapitulate the decapitation secretion pattern characteristic of ceruminous glands. The myoepithelial cells are spindled to cuboidal, with clear to eosinophilic cytoplasm and small, variably hyperchromatic nuclei. The stroma may appear collagenous to myxoid. Dislodged epithelial cells arranged in cords or as single cells may be seen in the myxoid areas, resulting in a "chondromyxoid" appearance (fig. 16-41). Squamous metaplasia may also be seen. Nuclear pleomorphism and mitotic activity are absent.

Differential Diagnosis. Histologically, the admixture of benign epithelial and mesenchymal elements is diagnostic and not recapitulated by other neoplasms. The possibility that an external canal

lesion may originate in the juxtaposed parotid gland, however, should always be considered.

Treatment and Prognosis. Wide local excision is the recommended treatment (45). All lesions reported to date have been benign, although local recurrence may follow incomplete resection.

Syringocystadenoma Papilliferum of Ceruminal Gland

Definition. This benign ceruminal gland neoplasm is characterized by a dermal invagination, into which project fibrovascular papillations lined by apocrine-type glandular epithelium with underlying myoepithelial cells.

General and Clinical Features. Syringocystadenoma papilliferum is a benign cutaneous tumor of apocrine origin most commonly found on the scalp and face (48). Rare examples may

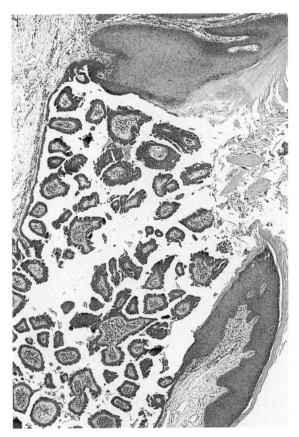

Figure 16-42
SYRINGOCYSTADENOMA PAPILLIFERUM

Similar to lesions arising in the skin, syringocyst-adenoma papilliferum arising in ceruminal glands presents as a cystic invagination from the skin surface lined by papillomatous projections from the cyst wall. (Figures 16-42 and 16-43 are from the same patient.)

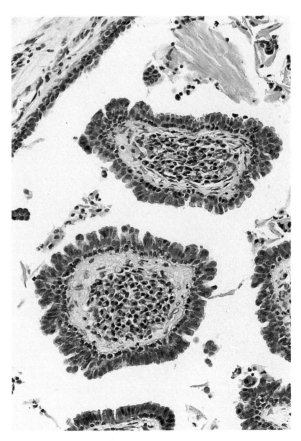

Figure 16-43
SYRINGOCYSTADENOMA PAPILLIFERUM

The papillations and cyst wall are lined by a double cell layer, composed of an inner layer of myoepithelial and outer layer of apocrine-like epithelial cells, complete with secretory snouts. The underlying stroma typically contains a plasma cell-predominant chronic inflammatory infiltrate.

also occur on the external auricle or within the ear canal; the latter are of probable ceruminous gland origin. Clinically, syringocystadenoma papilliferum appears as a nodule or plaque, with or without an overlying crust. Scalp lesions are frequently associated with a nevus sebaceous, an association that has not been documented in the ear. Of six patients with auricular syringocystadenoma papilliferum, there were two men and four women, ranging in age from 22 to 75 years (49).

Pathologic Findings. Lesions are characterized by a cystic dermal invagination, the lower aspect of which gives rise to numerous papillations that project into the cystic lumen (fig. 16-42) (48,49). Tubular lumina may be seen within the papillations or the underlying dermis. The upper aspect of the invagination is usually lined by ke-

ratinizing squamous epithelium contiguous with the overlying skin. The lower aspect of the cyst and the papillations are lined by glandular epithelium of two cell layers, similar to that seen in the normal apocrine gland (fig. 16-43). The inner (secretory) layer is composed of columnar cells with abundant eosinophilic cytoplasm, apical snouts, and bland, oval nuclei. The outer (myoepithelial) layer consists of smaller, cuboidal cells with round nuclei and scant cytoplasm. A characteristic, variably dense, plasma cell infiltrate is usually present within the papillations and, less commonly, the surrounding tumoral stroma. Rarely, the papillations give rise to variably sized epithelial "tufts" without a fibrovascular core (fig. 16-44).

Treatment and Prognosis. Surgical excision is curative.

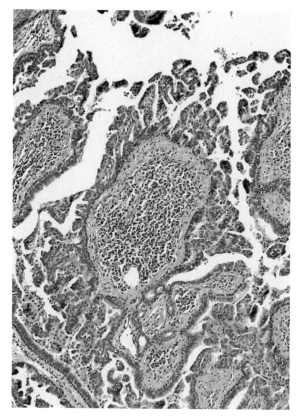

Figure 16-44
SYRINGOCYSTADENOMA PAPILLIFERUM

Rare lesions, such as the tumor depicted, may be architecturally complex, and show variably sized papillations that give rise to epithelial cell "tufts" without a fibrovascular core.

Seborrheic Keratosis

Definition. This is a benign squamous proliferation composed of normal-appearing squamous epithelial cells and smaller basaloid cells, with accompanying hyperkeratosis, acanthosis, and papillomatosis.

General and Clinical Features. Also known as *basal cell papilloma,* seborrheic keratosis is a common, benign, pigmented cutaneous neoplasm (50–54). Seborrheic keratoses are very common cutaneous lesions that may also, albeit rarely, occur in the external auditory canal. To our knowledge only two cases have been reported in this location (51,52), although we have occasionally encountered additional examples.

Tumors characteristically appear as sharply demarcated, verrucous plaques that appear to be stuck onto normal skin. Patients are usually middle-aged or elderly, and there is no sex predilection. On cutaneous surfaces the lesions may be single, but are often multiple. Both reported cases involving the external ear presented as large, exophytic masses that filled the ear canal (51,52).

Pathologic Findings. Lesions are light yellow to dark brown, elevated plaques with a verrucous surface and a soft, greasy consistency. Occasional lesions may appear smooth or pedunculated. Most measure from a few millimeters to 1 cm, although tumors measuring up to several centimeters have been described. Seborrheic keratoses show a variety of histologic appearances, and six histologic subtypes are recognized: acanthotic, hyperkeratotic, reticulated, clonal, irritated, and melanoacanthoma variants. The two reported external ear canal cases were both acanthotic lesions, composed of thick, interanastomosing cords of basaloid cells with interspersed horn cysts. All types show hyperkeratosis, acanthosis, and papillomatosis (fig. 16-45) (54). The lesions project upwards such that the entire proliferation rests above the plane of the surrounding skin. Two types of cells are usually present: normal-appearing squamous cells and smaller, uniform basaloid cells, with relatively large nuclei and darkly staining cytoplasm (fig. 16-46). Both true horn cysts (orthokeratotic foci within the tumor) and pseudo-horn cysts (surface invaginations of keratinaceous debris that appear cystic on cross section) may be seen.

Differential Diagnosis. Seborrheic keratosis may be clinically and histologically mistaken for basal cell and squamous cell carcinomas. It is distinguished from the latter neoplasms by the lack stromal invasion and a lower tumor border that remains on an even plane with the surrounding normal epidermis. Unfortunately, the latter features may not be evident on limited biopsy specimens. Accordingly, a definitive diagnosis of seborrheic keratosis should probably be reserved for excisional specimens. Irritated variants may show a downward proliferation of atypical squamoid cells and thus simulate a squamous cell carcinoma, but to date, irritated variants have not been described in the external canal.

Treatment and Prognosis. All types of seborrheic keratosis are benign lesions and surgical excision is curative. Formation of an in situ carcinoma (bowenoid transformation) may

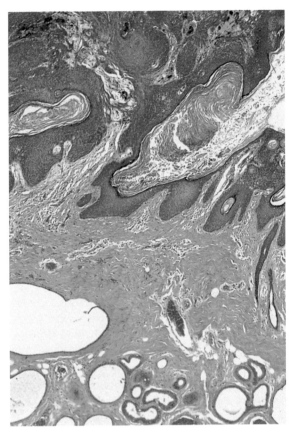

Figure 16-45
SEBORRHEIC KERATOSIS

This lesion within the external ear canal is histologically identical to seborrheic keratoses found elsewhere on the skin, showing hyperkeratosis, acanthosis, and papillomatosis. An apocrine-type ceruminous gland is seen underlying the proliferation, which rests above the plane of the adjacent epidermis. (Figures 16-45 and 16-46 are from the same patient.)

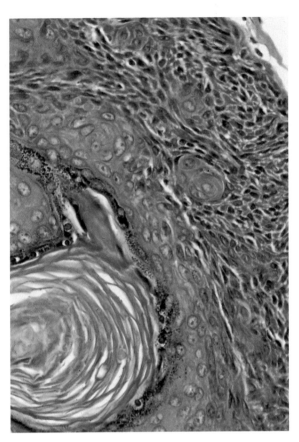

Figure 16-46
SEBORRHEIC KERATOSIS

Histologically, all variants of seborrheic keratosis are composed of small, uniform basaloid cells and normal-appearing squamous cells. Interspersed horn cysts may occasionally be seen.

rarely be seen, particularly in lesions arising in sun-exposed areas (50,53).

Squamous Cell Papilloma

Definition and General Features. Squamous cell papilloma is a benign, exophytic proliferation which may occur on the external auricle or external ear canal.

Clinical Features. Squamous cell papillomas appear as thin, polypoid lesions attached to the underlying skin surface by a narrow stalk. Symptoms are usually minimal or absent. All ages may be affected; there is no sex predilection (55).

Pathologic Findings. Squamous cell papillomas grossly appear as exophytic, tan-white lesions

with a cauliflower-like appearance. Histologically, they are composed of typically narrow, branching, fibrovascular fronds covered by one to several layers of mature, benign-appearing squamous epithelium (fig. 16-47). A variable degree of parakeratosis or orthokeratosis is often seen. Mitotic activity and nuclear pleomorphism are absent.

Treatment and Prognosis. Surgical excision is curative, and is the treatment modality of choice.

Atypical Fibroxanthoma

Definition. Atypical fibroxanthoma is a cutaneous lesion of low-grade malignancy which histologically resembles malignant fibrous histiocytoma.

General Features. Atypical fibroxanthoma was first described by Helwig in 1963 (57) and was

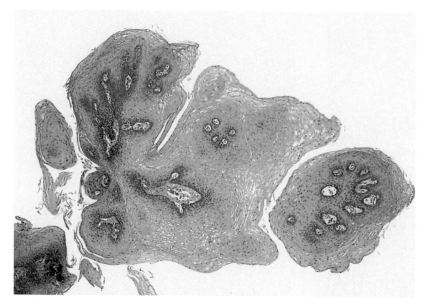

Figure 16-47
SQUAMOUS CELL PAPILLOMA
A typical squamous papilloma of
the external auricle is composed of
thin, uniform fibrovascular papillations covered by multiple layers of benign squamous epithelium.

initially considered to represent a benign, probably reactive lesion. Subsequent reports of metastases to regional lymph nodes and elsewhere,
however, indicated that this is a tumor of low-
grade malignancy (56,58). The tumor may represent the cutaneous equivalent of malignant
fibrous histiocytoma, which it resembles histologically (56).

Clinical Features. Atypical fibroxanthoma
commonly presents as a raised, nodular lesion
on sun-exposed areas of skin, including the external auricle, in elderly individuals (56–59).
Lesions are typically small, often less than 2 cm.
Most are covered by normal skin, whereas a
minority may appear ulcerated and clinically
simulate a carcinoma.

Pathologic Findings. Histologically, atypical fibroxanthoma is a cellular dermal infiltrate
that typically extends to the overlying epidermis
and subcutaneous fat (fig. 16-48) (59). The infiltrate is composed of an admixture of different
cells, predominated by oval to spindled cells with
hyperchromatic or vesicular, pleomorphic nuclei
and lightly eosinophilic, tapered cytoplasm. The
spindled cells may be arranged in small bundles
or haphazardly. Epithelioid, histiocyte-like cells
with abundant, foamy cytoplasm and large, multinucleated giant cells containing multiple pleomorphic nuclei are often present (fig. 16-49). The
degree of giant cell and foamy cell change is
variable; these cell types may predominate in

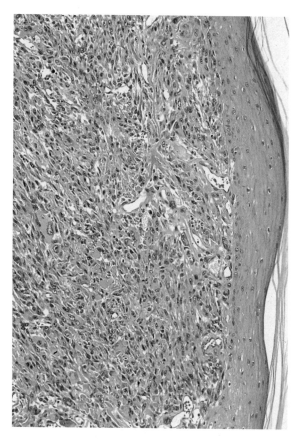

Figure 16-48
ATYPICAL FIBROXANTHOMA
The lesion appears as a hypercellular dermal infiltrate
which extends to the overlying epidermis and into the underlying subcutaneous fat.

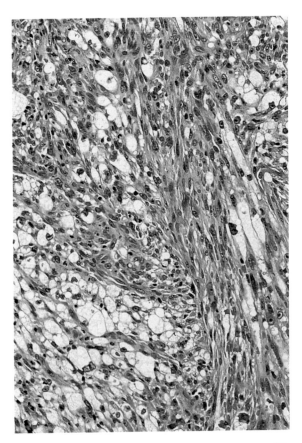 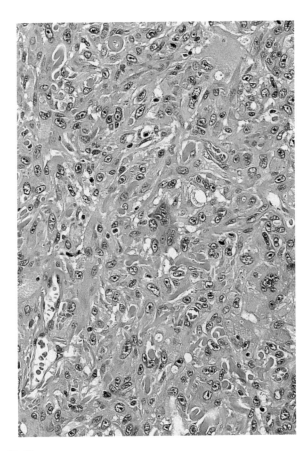

Figure 16-49
ATYPICAL FIBROXANTHOMA

Left: Most tumors are composed of oval to spindled cells with eosinophilic cytoplasm and hyperchromatic, pleomorphic nuclei. Larger epithelioid cells with abundant, foamy cytoplasm are often present as well.

Right: Other lesions may be entirely composed of oval to spindled cells, with only negligible foamy cell change. Multinucleated giant cells (center) are pathognomonic of this lesion.

some lesions but be difficult to find or absent in others. Multiple mitoses are usually present, some of which may be atypical. On immunohistochemical examination the neoplastic cells are strongly positive for vimentin and variably positive for muscle-specific actin (60). Reactivity for alpha-1-antitrypsin and alpha-1-antichymotrypsin may also be seen. Staining for cytokeratin, S-100 protein, and HMB-45 is uniformly negative, although most cases contain non-neoplastic S-100–positive dendritic cells within the lesion or overlying epidermis (60).

Differential Diagnosis. Atypical fibroxanthomas must be differentiated from spindle cell variants of squamous cell carcinoma and malignant melanoma. Most cases of the former are distinguished by the presence of multinucleated

giant cells. Lesions without giant cells may require immunohistochemical examination. On immunostaining the distinction is not difficult, as the neoplastic cells of atypical fibroxanthomas are positive for vimentin and occasionally muscle-specific actin but not keratin, S-100 protein, or HMB-45 (60). In contrast, squamous carcinomas usually stain at least focally for cytokeratin, and melanomas invariably react for S-100 protein and HMB-45. In addition, muscle-specific actin is typically not positive in either of the latter lesions.

Treatment and Prognosis. Most atypical fibroxanthomas are cured by local excision. Rare cases of regional lymph node and pulmonary metastases, however, have been reported (60). To date there are no clinical or histologic predictors of aggressive biologic behavior (56–60).

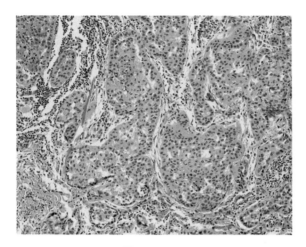

Figure 16-50
CERUMINAL ADENOCARCINOMA
A low-power view of a low-grade ceruminal adenocarcinoma. Note the glandular configuration and focal presence
of a desmoplastic and lymphocytic stromal response. (Figures 16-50 and 16-51 are from the same patient.)

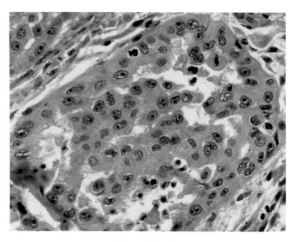

Figure 16-51
CERUMINAL ADENOCARCINOMA
A high-power view of the lesion depicted in figure 16-50.
The tumor cells are polygonal, with eosinophilic cytoplasm
and oval, vesicular nuclei with occasionally prominent nucleoli. Moderate nuclear pleomorphism and occasional mitotic
figures are present. The tumor is composed of a single cell
type; the biphasic epithelial-myoepithelial cell population
typical of ceruminal adenoma is absent.

Ceruminal Adenocarcinoma

Definition, General and Clinical Features.
Ceruminal adenocarcinoma is a malignant glandular neoplasm composed of apocrine-type epithelial cells and originating in the apocrine
ceruminal glands of the external ear canal. The
age range of affected patients is wide (26 to 71
years), although most patients are in their fifth
or sixth decades of life (61–64). There is no apparent predilection for either sex. Clinically,
most patients present with pain, discharge,
hearing loss, or a sensation of blockage in the
external auditory canal (62,64). A mass lesion is
usually present within the external canal or
periauricular soft tissues with associated erosion or ulceration. Ceruminous adenocarcinomas are locally aggressive lesions. In many cases
the tumor extends into the middle ear, petrous
and temporal bones, and results in extensive
bony destruction (64).

Pathologic Findings. Tumor localized to the
external canal is a firm, solid nodular mass with
superficial ulceration. Locally invasive tumors
are firm and white-tan, with a homogeneous,
infiltrative cut surface.

Dehner and Chen (61) separated ceruminal
adenocarcinomas into low-grade and high-grade
types based on microscopic findings. Histologically, low-grade tumors often recapitulate the
histology of the normal ceruminal gland, with
glandular, tubular, or cribriform structures lined
by one to multiple layers of epithelial cells (61).
Low-grade tumors may appear cytologically similar to benign adenomas but are distinguished
from the latter by the presence of stromal invasion and a desmoplastic stromal response (fig.
16-50)(64). The neoplastic cells are low columnar
to cuboidal with variable amounts of eosinophilic
or clear cytoplasm and oval, hyperchromatic to
vesicular nuclei with occasional nucleoli. Apical
cytoplasmic snouts may be seen. Mild to moderate nuclear pleomorphism and scattered mitotic
figures are usually present.

High-grade lesions are composed of smaller,
ovoid to polygonal neoplastic cells arranged in
irregular glands, cords, and sheets, which extensively infiltrate the surrounding, often desmoplastic stroma (fig. 16-51). Notably, high-grade
tumors may show minimal or no evidence of apocrine derivation and must be distinguished from
metastatic adenocarcinomas originating from
other sites. The neoplastic cells are recognizably
epithelial but poorly differentiated, with moderate
to scant amounts of cytoplasm and enlarged,
hyperchromatic nuclei with prominent nucleoli
(fig. 16-52). Marked nuclear pleomorphism and
abundant mitotic figures are commonly seen.

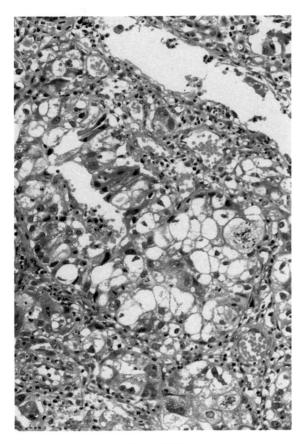

Figure 16-52
CERUMINAL ADENOCARCINOMA

A high-grade, anaplastic ceruminal adenocarcinoma is composed of both eosinophilic and clear cells arranged in cords and sheets. Marked nuclear pleomorphism and abnormal mitotic figures are readily evident.

Differential Diagnosis. Ceruminal adenocarcinomas, particularly low-grade lesions, should be carefully distinguished from ceruminal adenomas by noting the absence of a biphasic epithelial-myoepithelial cellular population and the presence of unequivocal stromal invasion. A metastasis from an adenocarcinoma arising in a distant primary site must also be considered.

Treatment and Prognosis. Due to the aggressive nature of these tumors, an initial en bloc surgical resection is recommended. For tumors that extend into the middle ear or temporal bone, resection of the temporal bone and contiguous structures is advised (62). Routine postoperative radiation has been advocated (62,63). Despite these and other measures, however, local recurrence develops in up to 50 percent of cases (64). Death from uncontrolled local disease occurs in

a small proportion of patients. Regional lymph node and pulmonary metastases have been reported but are extremely rare (63).

Adenoid Cystic Carcinoma of Ceruminal Gland

Definition. This is a malignant ceruminal gland neoplasm composed of small, basaloid-type cells arranged in either a cribriform, tubular-trabecular, or solid configuration.

General Features. Adenoid cystic carcinoma is a malignant epithelial tumor that usually occurs within the major or minor salivary glands but may also arise from the ceruminous glands of the external auditory canal (65–74). In one series of 37 external auditory canal glandular tumors, adenoid cystic carcinoma was the most common neoplasm, comprising 65 percent of cases (70). Interestingly, despite the proposed origin from the ceruminal gland, morphologically comparable tumors hardly ever arise from apocrine glands elsewhere in the skin. Direct extension from a primary parotid gland tumor should be excluded in all cases.

Clinical Features. Localized ear pain, often for several years' duration, is the most common presenting complaint, and may be related to the propensity of these tumors for perineural invasion. The age range of affected patients is wide, but most patients are in the sixth decade of life (69, 70). Physical examination commonly reveals a localized mass or nodule within the external canal.

Pathologic Findings. Similar to their salivary gland counterparts, external ear canal adenoid cystic carcinomas are architecturally variable lesions which may be divided into three histologic subtypes: cribriform, tubular-trabecular, and solid. To our knowledge, a relationship between histologic type and prognosis has not been established for adenoid cystic carcinoma arising from ceruminal glands.

Histologically, cribriform variant tumors contain cellular nests or sheets with numerous cribriform, cylindric ("pseudo-luminal") spaces occupied by either a periodic acid–Schiff (PAS)-positive, mucopolysaccharide secretion or hyalinized collagenous cylinders (figs. 16-53, 16-54). Trabecular-tubular type tumors are composed of elongated epithelial strands, some of which contain duct-like or tubular lumina, surrounded by hyalinized connective tissue (fig. 16-55). Solid

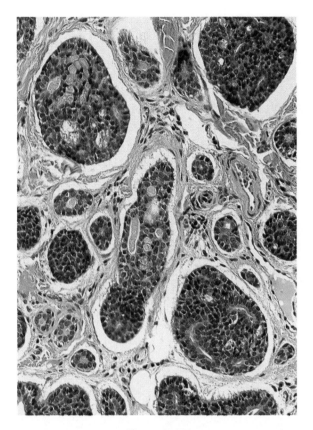

Figure 16-53
ADENOID CYSTIC CARCINOMA
A cribriform or "classic" variant of adenoid cystic carcinoma is composed of tumor cell nests surrounding cylindrical to ovoid spaces. The punched-out spaces contain either a basophilic mucopolysaccharide substance or a hyalinized, collagenous plug.

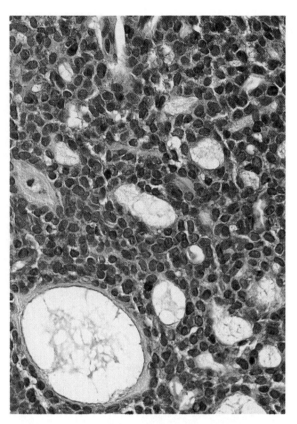

Figure 16-54
ADENOID CYSTIC CARCINOMA
Other cribriform variants may be composed of tumor cell sheets containing cylindrical, pseudoluminal spaces.

variants are characterized by solid epithelial islands or sheets devoid of cribriform or cylindric spaces (fig. 16-56). In all three variants, the nests, sheets, and trabeculae are composed of a single cell type: a small, cuboidal, basaloid cell with scant amounts of basophilic cytoplasm and dark-staining nuclei with a granular chromatin pattern (65,66,68–70,72–74). Nuclear pleomorphism is rarely present. Mitotic activity varies considerably; most tumors show few mitotic figures. Perineural invasion by tumor cells is a frequently noted hallmark of this neoplasm (fig. 16-57).

Differential Diagnosis. Adenoid cystic carcinomas, particularly solid variants, may be misinterpreted as cutaneous basal cell carcinomas on biopsy specimens. In contrast to basal cell carcinomas, however, adenoid cystic tumors typically show cribriform foci and perineural invasion and lack both peripheral pallisading and

continuity with the overlying epidermis. The possibility of a primary origin in the parotid gland must also be considered.

Treatment and Prognosis. Wide radical surgical excision is the treatment of choice. The value of adjuvant radiation is unknown (66,68). Despite the treatment modality, however, patients typically experience a protracted but relentless clinical course, marked by local recurrence and distant metastases, usually to the lungs (65). In the salivary gland, perineural invasion, bone involvement, a solid histologic pattern, and local recurrence have been associated with a worse prognosis (66–72). In one study of 21 patients with adenoid cystic carcinoma of the external canal, who had surgical resection, 10 were dead of disease 6 to 29 years after diagnosis, 4 were alive with locally recurrent disease and pulmonary metastases, and 7 were alive without disease 1 to 12 years after treatment (71).

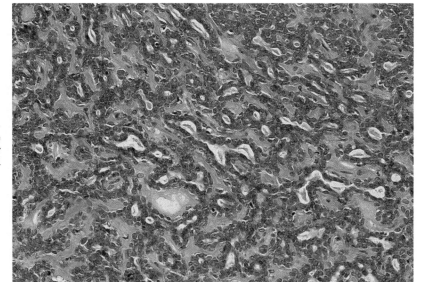

Figure 16-55
ADENOID CYSTIC CARCINOMA
A trabecular-tubular variant of adenoid cystic carcinoma, in which the neoplastic cells form duct-like, tubular structures surrounded by a hyalinized collagenous stroma.

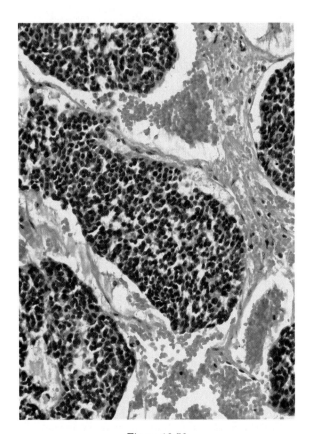

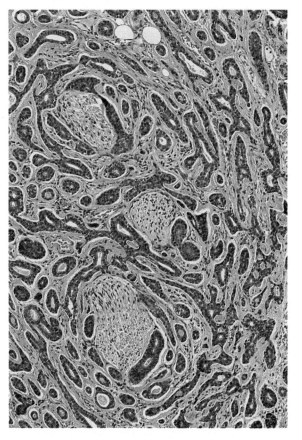

Figure 16-56
ADENOID CYSTIC CARCINOMA
A solid adenoid cystic carcinoma showing nests of neoplastic cells without collagenous cylinder or tubular lumina formation.

Figure 16-57
ADENOID CYSTIC CARCINOMA
Perineural invasion is a hallmark of this lesion.

Basal Cell Carcinoma of the External Ear

Definition and General Features. Basal cell carcinomas (BCCs) are low-grade malignant epithelial tumors that arise from the basal cells of normal epidermis, almost exclusively on hair-bearing skin. The neoplastic cells strongly resemble the basal cells of the normal epidermis. Sun exposure is considered to be the major predisposing factor to tumor development, hence the head and neck, including the external ear, is frequently involved (75–81). In one series of 122 cutaneous tumors of the external ear, 90 percent were BCCs and 10 percent were squamous cell carcinomas (68). Overall, BCCs account for 21 percent of all neoplasms of the ear and temporal bone.

Clinical Features. Patients of all ages are affected but most are in the sixth decade of life or older. Most are Caucasian, with a 2 to 1 male predominance. Most external ear BCCs arise on sun-exposed areas, but tumors occur behind the auricle as well. BCCs often have a pearly white, translucent, telangiectatic border; large lesions usually show central ulceration with crusting (fig. 16-58). In the series of 71 BCCs of the external ear, 29 were on the posterior surface, 22 on the helix and antihelix, 10 on the concha, and 10 on the anterior pinna and lobule (80). Large lesions often appear ulcerated and may extend to the underlying mastoid, temporal bone, or cranial cavity.

Gross Findings. In general, five types of BCC are recognized: 1) nodulo-ulcerative or solid (the most common); 2) morphea-like or fibrosing; 3) adenoid; 4) superficial; and 5) fibroepithelioma types. Adenoid variants are classified either alone or with nodulo-ulcerative lesions. Nodulo-ulcerative lesions begin as small, pearly nodules which may show central ulceration with progressive growth. Morphea-like tumors are commonly poorly defined, flat, indurated plaques which infrequently if ever ulcerate.

Microscopic Findings. Although all histologic variants of BCC may occur in the external ear, the nodulo-ulcerative and morphea-like variants are the most common. Of the 496 external ear BCCs reported by Bailin et al. (75), 53 percent were nodulo-ulcerative and 27 percent were morphea-like. Nodulo-ulcerative variants typically appear as variably sized, smoothly contoured nests of neoplastic cells within the dermis, focally attached to the overlying epidermis (fig. 16-59). Peripheral

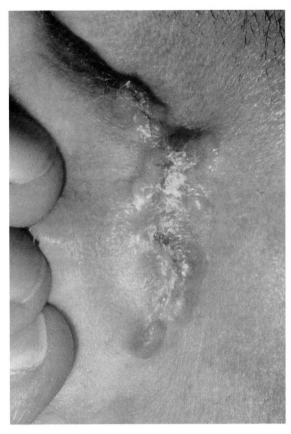

Figure 16-58
BASAL CELL CARCINOMA
A patient presenting with a large basal cell carcinoma behind the auricle. Note the central ulceration and the pearly, translucent border typical of these lesions.

palisading of tumor cells is frequently seen. Areas of stromal retraction are often present around tumoral islands on both fixed and frozen sections (fig. 16-60). Intracellular melanin deposition ("pigmented BCC") or horn cysts ("keratotic basal cell carcinoma") may be present. Morphea-like lesions consist of rows and narrow strands of neoplastic cells surrounded by a dense, desmoplastic stroma. Only a single layer or "indian file" of neoplastic cells may be present and largely obscured by the fibrotic stroma (fig. 16-61). Peripheral pallisading is usually not seen. In general, tumors tend to hug the epidermis and spread laterally along the cutaneous surface.

Irrespective of the architectural type, the neoplastic cells are invariably small and monotonous, with ovoid dark nuclei and scant cytoplasm. Nuclei may be vesicular but nuclear pleomorphism and

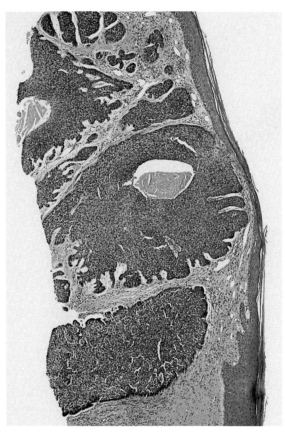

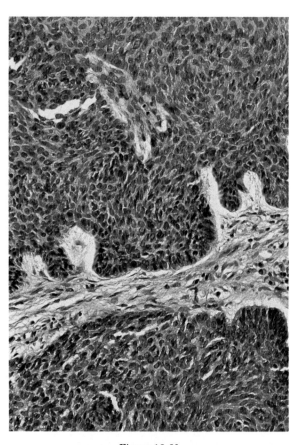

Figure 16-59
BASAL CELL CARCINOMA
Shave biopsy of a nodulo-ulcerative variant showing smoothly contoured nests of small, basaloid cells extending into the underlying dermis.

Figure 16-60
BASAL CELL CARCINOMA
The tumor nests are composed of small, monotonous cells with dark nuclei and scant basophilic cytoplasm. Peripheral pallisading of tumor cells and foci of stromal retraction, two hallmark findings of these lesions, are present.

Figure 16-61
BASAL CELL CARCINOMA
Morphea-like variants appear as rows and strands of neoplastic cells surrounded, and compressed by, a dense desmoplastic stroma.

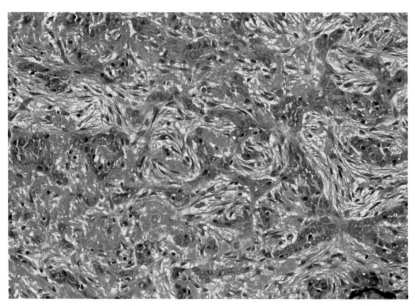

mitotic figures are rarely observed. The surrounding stroma may appear either desmoplastic or, less commonly, mucinous.

Differential Diagnosis. BCCs must be distinguished from seborrheic keratoses, which may also show a proliferation of small, basaloid cells extending into the dermis. In seborrheic keratoses, however, the entire lesion generally lies on a plane above that of the surrounding epidermis. Peripheral pallisading and stromal retraction are usually absent. Solid BCCs may be confused with adenoid cystic carcinoma, although the latter lesion is not connected with the overlying epidermis and often shows cribriform areas and perineural invasion.

Treatment and Prognosis. Most BCCs are indolent neoplasms that are largely cured by complete surgical excision, which is the modality of choice. The most common reason for treatment failure is incomplete resection, thus surgical margin assessment is mandatory (78). Morphealike variants tend toward insidious subcutaneous infiltration not appreciated on clinical or gross examination. Metastases are exceedingly rare but may spread by either hematogenous or lymphatic routes (76,81).

Squamous Cell Carcinoma of the External and Middle Ear

Definition and General Features. Squamous cell carcinoma is a malignant epithelial neoplasm composed of squamous cells and originating from the lining epithelium of the auricle, auditory canal, middle ear, or mastoid. It accounts for approximately 10 to 15 percent of all primary cutaneous carcinomas of the external ear, whereas basal cell carcinoma comprises virtually all of the remaining 85 percent (82–84,86,90,92,94–96). Squamous cell carcinomas are much more common on the external auricle or external canal than in the middle ear or mastoid. Primary middle ear lesions are unusual and may be difficult to distinguish from tumors of the external canal involving the middle ear by direct extension, thus these lesions are considered together (84). In one study of 136 patients with malignant neoplasms of the external ear and temporal bone, 85 were squamous cell carcinomas (86). Of these, 46 tumors (54 percent) arose on the external auricle or cartilaginous ear canal, 12 (14 percent) arose in the osseous portion of the external canal

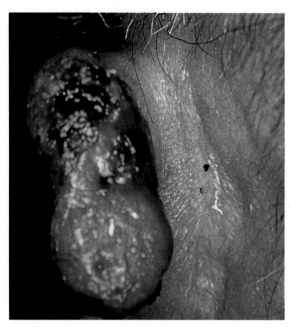

Figure 16-62
SQUAMOUS CELL CARCINOMA
A squamous cell carcinoma presenting as a nodular, ulcerated, hemorrhagic mass on the external auricle of an elderly white male.

or mastoid cortex, and 27 (32 percent) were found in the middle ear, facial canal, or mastoid air cells. Of 116 cases of primary squamous cell carcinoma of the ear, reported by Lewis (92), 18 (15 percent) arose in the middle ear cleft.

Clinical Features. Squamous cell carcinoma of the external ear and auditory canal is a disease of elderly white males, who usually complain of a mass with pain and otorrhea (fig. 16-62) (82,86, 95). Tumors appear as an elevated plaque, an ulcer, or a friable, granular mass. Similar to basal cell carcinoma, sun exposure is the major risk factor for disease development and more than 95 percent of reported patients are white (83,92). Of tumors arising on the external ear, the helix is the most common anatomic site (53 percent of patients), followed by the antihelix and triangular fossa (19 percent), the posterior pinna (14 percent), the lobule or concha (5 percent each), and the tragus (4 percent) (83). The age range is wide although most patients are in the sixth to seventh decade of life (82,84,89). For external ear tumors, males usually predominate: one study reported a male to female ratio of nearly 50 to 1 (94). In contrast, auditory canal tumors

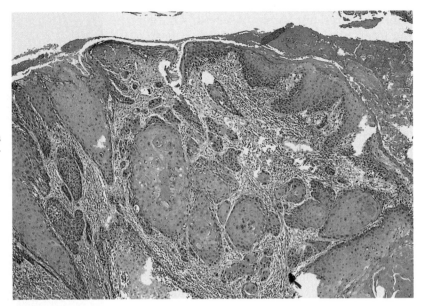

Figure 16-63
SQUAMOUS CELL CARCINOMA
A well-differentiated tumor extends tongues of keratinizing squamous epithelium into the underlying stroma.

show a mild to moderate female predominance (89,90,92). For auditory canal tumors, complete canal occlusion is commonly seen (89). Tumors arising in the cartilaginous portion of the external canal spread easily, as the cartilaginous walls offer little resistance. Lesions of the inner, osseous canal, which is surrounded by an effective barrier of dense bone, often spread laterally into the outer canal or middle ear (96).

Squamous carcinoma of the middle ear is similarly a disease of adults in the sixth decade of life or older, most of whom have a history of chronic otitis media (90,96). In contrast to external ear lesions, squamous cell cancer of the middle ear appears to have an almost even sex distribution (90,92). Patients often present with hearing loss or discharge (90,92,96). Tumors may present as deceptively bland polypoid or "granulation tissue-like" lesions in the middle ear or external canal (90,92,96). Due to the often simultaneous presence of chronic otitis media and the nonspecific symptoms, patients may be treated empirically and remain undiagnosed for months or even years after initial presentation (90,92). Middle ear tumors may cause widespread bony destruction, with frequent penetration into the mastoid or through the middle ear roof into the middle cranial fossa (90,96). Invasion into the eustachian tube or inferiorly into the skull base or soft tissues of the neck is common. Middle cranial

fossa involvement or extension into the skull base may result in functional palsies and spread along the seventh and eighth or ninth through twelfth cranial nerves, respectively (90,96).

Pathologic Findings. Squamous cell carcinomas may are well, moderately, or poorly differentiated (84). Well-differentiated tumors cytologically resemble the stratified squamous epithelium from which these lesions theoretically arise (fig. 16-63). The neoplastic cells are arranged in sheets and nests, which (at least focally) appear to arise from the overlying epidermis. Intercellular bridge formation, keratinization, and horn cyst formation may be seen. Moderately differentiated tumors usually infiltrate in nests, cords, or as single cells, with little to no evidence of keratinization. Poorly differentiated lesions often show diffuse, single cell stromal invasion and may be difficult to recognize as squamous in nature. Most studies of external and middle ear squamous cell carcinomas report an even distribution of well-, moderately, and poorly differentiated variants (82–84,86,89,90,92, 94–96); spindle cell variants may be seen as well. The exact incidence of spindled variants is unclear, as most are admixed under the category of poorly differentiated tumors (84). One study of 486 patients with squamous carcinoma of the external ear reported that 2 percent of the lesions were spindle cell variants (83).

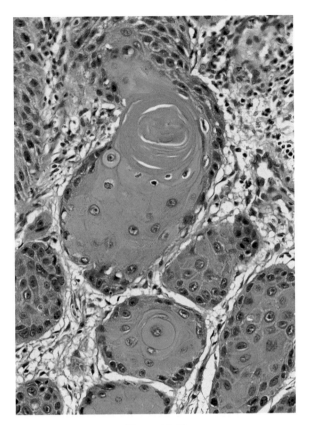

Figure 16-64
SQUAMOUS CELL CARCINOMA
On high magnification, well-differentiated tumors show tongues and well-defined nests of large, polygonal squamous cells with fibrillary, eosinophilic cytoplasm and well-defined cell borders. Keratinization is often present. The nuclei are vesicular, centrally located, and minimally pleomorphic.

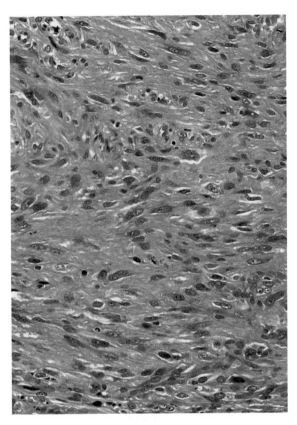

Figure 16-65
SQUAMOUS CELL CARCINOMA
Poorly differentiated tumors are often not recognizable as squamous in nature, and may be composed of polygonal, round, or, as in the case shown, spindled cells with nuclear pleomorphism.

The neoplastic cells in well-differentiated tumors are polygonal, with moderate to abundant eosinophilic cytoplasm and well-defined cell borders. Nuclei are commonly vesicular, with variably prominent nucleoli but minimal pleomorphism (fig. 16-64). Moderately to poorly differentiated tumor cells are smaller and have a high nuclear to cytoplasmic ratio, nuclear pleomorphism, and mitotic activity. Moderately differentiated tumor cells often retain an epithelioid shape, eosinophilic fibrillar cytoplasm, and well-defined cell borders, and thus are still recognizably squamous in nature. In poorly differentiated lesions, however, the neoplastic cells may appear small, large, bizarre or multinucleated (fig. 16-65). Tumors composed predominantly or solely of spindled cells occur.

Differential Diagnosis. Squamous cell carcinoma of the external ear may be clinically confused with "malignant" external otitis, chronic otitis externa, cholesteatoma, actinic keratosis, and basal cell carcinoma. Irritated seborrheic keratoses and inflammatory lesions with pseudoepitheliomatous hyperplasia may also simulate squamous cell cancer. The latter entities, however, are noninvasive, inflammatory or reactive lesions. Accordingly, the presence of a cytologically atypical or frankly malignant squamous epithelial proliferation with unequivocal stromal invasion is specific for carcinoma and excludes the latter lesions. Predominantly or exclusively spindle cell variants may be mistaken for malignant melanoma or atypical fibroxanthoma. Unlike squamous cell carcinomas, atypical fibroxanthomas are characterized by an admixture of cell types, including foamy cells and bizarre multinucleated giant cells immunohistochemically positive for vimentin but not cytokeratin (85,87,88,91,93). Malignant melanoma is often distinguished by the presence of melanin and the presence of a junctional component. The neoplastic cells are immunoreactive for vimentin, S-100 protein, and with HMB-45. They are negative for cytokeratin.

Treatment and Prognosis. In early studies, most squamous cell carcinomas of the external ear were advanced at presentation (79,81). Extensive local invasion was commonly seen although metastases to regional lymph nodes or distant sites were rare. In a series of 486 patients with squamous cell carcinoma of the external ear, 6 percent presented with suspected nodal metastases, whereas another 6 percent developed nodal dissemination in the subsequent 24 months; distant metastases developed in only 1 percent (83). Middle ear and mastoid squamous cell carcinomas have a somewhat worse prognosis since tumors are advanced at presentation; regional lymph node metastases develop in approximately 15 percent of patients, but distant metastases are rare (90,92, 96). Mortality usually results from complications of local disease rather than distant spread. In one study, after 5 years of follow-up death from tumor occurred in only 1 of 17 patients with auricular tumors in contrast to 11 of 21 (52 percent) patients with auditory canal neoplasms (84). In other studies of auditory canal and middle ear squamous cell carcinomas considered together, the 5-year survival rate is under 30 percent (86,90).

Complete surgical excision with radiation therapy is the modality of choice. Locally advanced disease may require resection of the pinna, parotid gland, temporomandibular joint, mandible, or en bloc resection of the temporal bone. The histologic findings (i.e., level of differentiation), size, and anatomic site of the tumor does not closely correlate with the development of metastases (83).

Malignant Melanoma of the External Ear

Definition and General Features. Malignant melanoma is a highly aggressive tumor arising from intraepidermal melanocytes or their antecedents, on or near a cutaneous surface. Malignant melanoma of the external ear accounts for 7 to 14 percent of all head and neck melanomas (97–106). In one review, melanoma of the external ear

comprised 6.7 percent of 2,824 melanomas diagnosed from all anatomic sites over a 35-year period (105). Thus the incidence of melanoma on the external ear appears to be proportional to the anatomic area involved.

Clinical Features. The patient age range varies from 7 to 83 years, with an average of 50 to 56 years (99,105). In most series, males predominate: Pack et al (105) reported a male to female ratio of 3 to 1. The auricle is involved in most cases; lesions arising in the external canal or middle ear are exceedingly rare. In one series, tumors arose on the helix in 43 percent of patients, the antihelix in 24 percent, the lobe and tragus in 7 percent, and the posterior helix, posterior ear, and preauricular region in 5 percent each (105). Most patients present with a pigmented, asymptomatic mass of the auricle.

Four major types of malignant melanoma have been described: 1) superficial spreading melanoma; 2) nodular melanoma; 3) acral lentiginous melanoma; and 4) lentigo maligna melanoma. In one series of 75 patients with malignant melanoma of the external ear in whom the histologic subtype was known, 44 lesions (59 percent) were superficial spreading and 31 (41 percent) were nodular (99). Other series confirm that, similar to malignant melanoma in other sites, the superficial spreading type is by far the most common variant arising on the external ear (106).

Gross Findings. Nodular melanoma is characterized by vertical growth and clinically appears as an elevated, deeply pigmented nodule that may show central ulceration. Superficial spreading tumors appear as variably elevated, plaque-like or scaly lesions that appear pink, tan-brown, or black (fig. 16-66).

Microscopic Findings. The microscopic features of malignant melanoma are described in detail elsewhere. Briefly, all major types originate from the dermal-epidermal junction and irregularly spread laterally and/or downward into the underlying dermis; upward extension into the epidermis may also be seen. Tumors invariably show irregular junctional activity and infiltrate the underlying dermis in nests, cords, alveolar formations, or individual cells (fig. 16-67). The tumor cells vary in both size and shape but two major types are generally recognized: an epithelioid and a spindled cell type. In nodular and superficial spreading variants the neoplastic

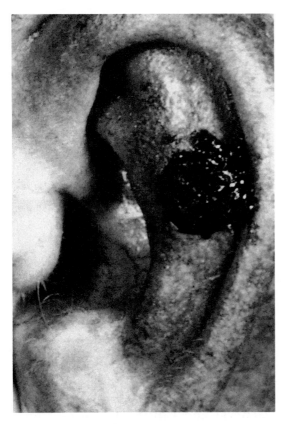

Figure 16-66
MALIGNANT MELANOMA

This external auricle melanoma is of the superficial spreading type with early satellitosis. (Fig. 321 from Fascicle 25, 2nd Series.)

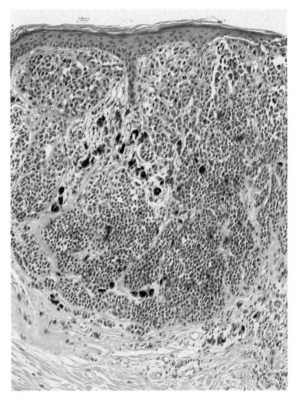

Figure 16-67
MALIGNANT MELANOMA

A typical nodular malignant melanoma of the external auricle invading the underlying reticular dermis. (Figures 16-67 and 16-68 are from the same patient.)

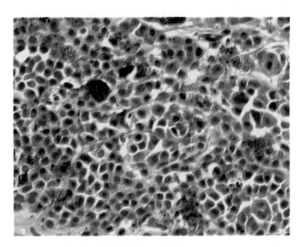

Figure 16-68
MALIGNANT MELANOMA

Both superficial spreading and nodular melanomas, the most common types found on the external ear, are composed largely of epithelioid cells. The nodular melanoma shown is composed entirely of epithelioid cells lying in nests and loose alveolar formations. Melanin production is readily evident within the neoplastic cells.

cells are predominantly epithelioid, although spindled foci may be seen (fig. 16-68). The tumor cells may be large or small, with variable amounts of basophilic, eosinophilic, or amphophilic cytoplasm. Nuclei may appear small and darkly stained, medium sized with clumped chromatin, or large and vesicular with prominent nucleoli. Mitotic activity is variable. The amount of melanin varies: epithelioid lesions may show extensive melanin production, whereas melanin is scant to absent in most spindled variants. Pigment may be identified in dermal histiocytes ("melanophages") as well.

Immunohistochemical Findings. Malignant melanomas of the ear and other sites are usually immunohistochemically positive for vimentin, S-100 protein, and, in most cases, with HMB-45 (102,104). Rare melanomas negative for S-100 protein have been described (97).

Treatment and Prognosis. As with melanomas arising in other sites, the features best related to tumor behavior are the stage of disease and the depth of invasion (98,100,101,106). Tumor thickness is the most important prognostic factor in stage 1 tumors, determined either by the Clark level or absolute thickness as proposed by Breslow et al. (98,100,103). These systems are described in detail elsewhere. Nevertheless, one study described patients with external ear melanomas as having an unusually poor prognosis not readily explained by the classic risk factors (106). In one study, 10-year survival rates for patients with tumors less than 1 mm, 1 to 3 mm, and greater than 3 mm thick were 65, 55, and 25 percent, respectively (99). Metastases, when they occur, are usually to regional lymph nodes; hematogenous dissemination is rare. Recommended treatment varies from wedge excision to partial or full amputation of the ear for stage 1 lesions. Elective parotidectomy and regional lymph node dissection are usually performed in patients with known nodal metastases (99,105).

TUMOR-LIKE LESIONS AND NEOPLASMS OF THE MIDDLE EAR

The following section covers those tumors and tumor-like lesions that preferentially involve the middle ear (Table 16-2). Selected lesions that usually occur elsewhere but may also arise in the middle ear or temporal bone and cause diagnostic confusion, such as inverted papilloma, meningioma, and rhabdomyosarcoma, are also mentioned. This section also includes aggressive papillary tumors of the temporal bone and endolymphatic sac, which primarily arise in the endolymphatic sac area of the inner ear but often present as middle ear or mastoid lesions. Acoustic neurilemomas are covered in chapter 7 and are not reiterated here. Squamous cell carcinoma of the middle ear is covered in conjunction with that of the external ear and auditory canal in the previous section. Other lesions that may rarely involve the middle ear by direct extension, such as parotid gland or nasopharyngeal tumors, are not considered. Primary osteogenic and cartilaginous lesions that may affect the temporal bone are covered in the Third Series Fascicle, Tumors of Bones and Joints (107).

Table 16-2

CLASSIFICATION OF MIDDLE EAR AND MASTOID TUMORS

Tumor-like lesions
 Inflammatory polyps
 Cholesteatoma
 Choristoma

Neoplasms
 Paraganglioma
 Middle ear adenoma
 Inverted papilloma of middle ear and mastoid
 Aggressive papillary tumor of temporal bone
  and endolymphatic sac
 Meningioma of temporal bone
 Metastatic carcinoma to the middle ear/
  temporal bone
 Rhabdomyosarcoma of middle ear

Inflammatory (Aural) Polyp

Definition. Inflammatory polyp is a non-neoplastic, polypoid proliferation of granulation tissue and inflammatory cells arising in the setting of longstanding local inflammation.

General and Clinical Features. Chronic middle ear inflammation (otitis media) can stimulate a proliferation of fibrous granulation tissue that can result in the formation of a polypoid tissue mass. These lesions, termed inflammatory polyps, may perforate the tympanic membrane and present in the external canal (108). Partial or total destruction of the ossicles may occur in longstanding cases (108). Inflammatory polyps usually arise in a background of chronic otitis media, thus an infectious etiology should always be sought with proper culturing techniques and histologic stains.

Pathologic Findings. Inflammatory polyps of the middle ear are essentially polypoid accumulations of granulation tissue, and thus do not represent true polyps. Similar to granulation tissue in other body sites, recently developed lesions appear as hypercellular proliferations of arborizing capillaries and fibroblasts with admixed acute and chronic inflammatory cells. Older lesions may be hypocellular and fibrous with few vessels and inflammatory cells. Cholesterol clefts or granulomata with a foreign body type giant cell reaction may be seen.

Inflammatory polyps are frequently covered by a single layer of cuboidal to columnar, often

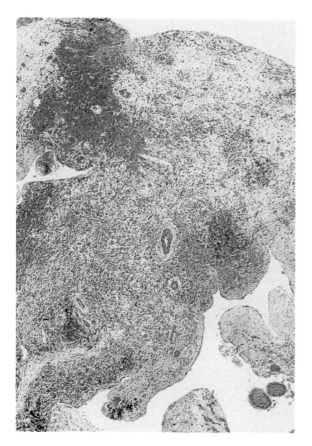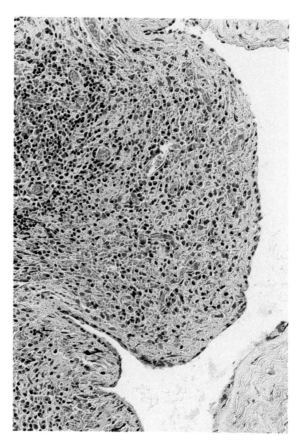

Figure 16-69
INFLAMMATORY POLYP OF THE MIDDLE EAR
Left: Inflammatory polyps consist of a polypoid proliferation of granulation tissue with admixed chronic inflammatory cells.
Right: Granulation tissue polyps are often lined by an attenuated layer of squamous metaplastic or cuboidal middle ear epithelium.

ciliated epithelium, similar to that present in the surrounding middle ear mucosa (fig. 16-69). In chronic cases the polypoid protrusions may be covered by squamous metaplastic epithelium. Cystic, gland-like epithelial inclusions may be present in the underlying stroma (fig. 16-70). These glandular inclusions, which presumably result from either tangential sectioning or invagination of an irregular lining membrane or stromal overgrowth with epithelial entrapment, should not be mistaken for adenomatous neoplasia.

Differential Diagnosis. The gland-like inclusions characteristic of inflammatory polyps may be confused with an adenoma or carcinoma. Instead of the abundant "back-to-back" arrangement typical of adenomatous neoplasms, however, glandular inclusions in inflammatory polyps are randomly distributed and widely separated by granulation tissue stroma.

Treatment and Prognosis. Effective treatment requires identification of the (usually infectious) etiologic agent. Complications of inflammatory polyps are extremely rare and include connective tissue obliteration of the attic or middle ear cleft, tympanic membrane scarring, ossicle damage or destruction, obliteration of the oval and round windows, and mastoiditis (108).

Cholesteatoma

Definition. Cholesteatoma is a non-neoplastic but potentially aggressive lesion characterized by the presence of keratin-producing squamous epithelium in the middle ear space or mastoid.

General Features. Cholesteatomas, also known as *epidermal cysts* and *keratomas,* may be viewed as epidermal inclusion cysts involving the middle ear or mastoid bone (109–113). They

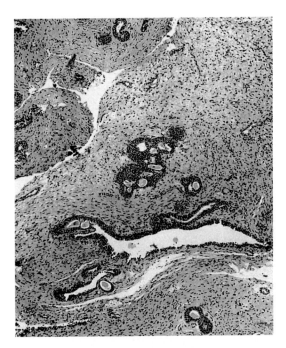 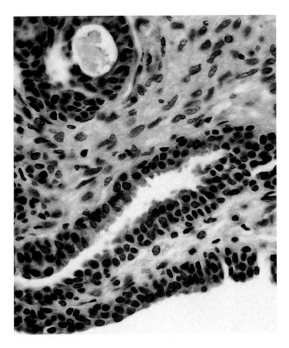

Figure 16-70
INFLAMMATORY POLYP OF THE MIDDLE EAR

Left: Inflammatory polyps may rarely contain variable numbers of simple gland-like inclusions. The inclusions, which may result either from tangential sectioning or invagination of an irregular lining epithelium or mucosal entrapment by stromal overgrowth, should not be confused with adenomatous neoplasia. (Fig. 322 from Fascicle 25, 2nd Series; both figures are from the same patient.)

Right: The gland-like inclusions are composed of cuboidal to low columnar, often ciliated epithelium similar to that present in the surrounding middle ear mucosa. (Fig. 323 from Fascicle 25, 2nd Series.)

may be congenital or acquired and have been classified as either "closed," in which a cystic mass is present, or open, in which aberrant stratified squamous lining epithelium sheds keratinaceous debris directly into the middle ear cavity.

Congenital cholesteatomas are usually found in children with no history of ear disease, behind an intact tympanic membrane in the upper anterior aspect of the middle ear cleft (113). Most congenital lesions have been attributed to the proliferation of aberrant epithelial remnants (110,112,113). In partial support of this theory is the finding of epithelial cell rests in the epithelium of the fetal middle ear at its junction with the eustachian tube (110). The clinical behavior of congenital cholesteatomas is identical to that of acquired lesions.

In contrast to congenital lesions, most acquired cholesteatomas are associated with a perforated eardrum and a history of either chronic otitis media, trauma, or surgical manipulation. Acquired lesions may result from several mechanisms: 1) the proliferation of the basal cell layer of the external canal epithelium under the subtympanic membrane fibrous tissue into the middle ear cleft; 2) the localized retraction of the superior, pars flaccida portion of the eardrum into the middle ear cleft; 3) the aberrant lateral migration of stratified squamous epithelium from the external ear canal or external surface of the drum into the middle ear via a tympanic membrane perforation; or 4) implantation or entrapment of stratified squamous epithelium within the middle ear cleft following eardrum trauma or a surgical procedure. Probably any one of these proposed mechanisms may contribute to cholesteatoma formation in a given patient.

Clinical Features. Age at diagnosis can range from birth to over 80 years, but adults in the third and fourth decades of life are most commonly affected. There is no apparent predilection for either sex and the left and right ears are equally affected. Cholesteatomas often remain localized to the middle ear but may extend into the mastoid air cells, epitympanic space, or petrous portion of the temporal bone. In longstanding cases, the continuing accumulation of keratinaceous debris often causes a slowly progressive erosion of the ossicles and surrounding bone (109).

Congenital lesions are usually discovered in children with no history of ear disease as pearly gray, cystic lesions located behind an intact eardrum (113). Acquired lesions have been described clinically as pearly gray to yellow, irregular structures, usually seen in conjunction with chronic otitis media or tympanic membrane perforation (109). Definitive diagnosis is usually made during clinical examination.

Pathologic Findings. Grossly, most cholesteatomas appear as variably sized, soft, spherical lesions with a white, pearly sheen (110,111). Congenital lesions are histologically identical to acquired ones, with the exception that acquired lesions are usually more often of the "open" variety. On cut section, most cholesteatomas are "closed" cystic lesions containing waxy, white or creamy, granular material and surrounded by a thin capsule. Histologically, closed cholesteatomas usually appear as simple cysts distended with keratinaceous debris and lined by keratinizing, stratified squamous epithelium containing all the layers of normal epidermis (fig. 16-71) (110,112). Open cholesteatomas often appear as rare foci of keratinizing squamous epithelium lining the middle ear. The membrane may be thin and only several cell layers thick, or may show an organized, rete peg type architecture. The epithelial lining sheds layers of keratin in a concentric, radial fashion, which accumulate in an onion skin-like fashion and can be seen grossly. In curettage specimens, cholesteatomas may appear as rare free-floating fragments of keratinizing squamous epithelium or keratinaceous material alone (fig. 16-72). Areas of chronic inflammation, fibrosis, and dystrophic calcification may be present in the surrounding tissue.

Treatment and Prognosis. Complete surgical excision is the recommended treatment, since incompletely or partially removed lesions often recur. Untreated lesions may erode surrounding bone and extend into adjacent structures.

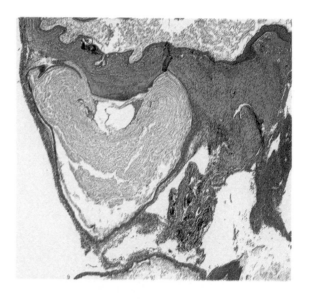

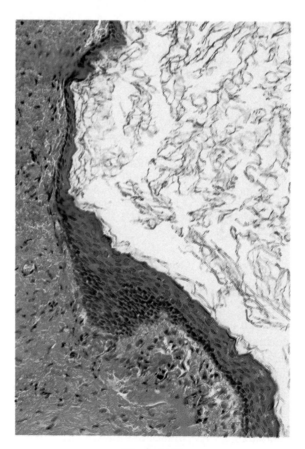

Figure 16-71
MIDDLE EAR CHOLESTEATOMA

Top: A representative closed cholesteatoma is lined by stratified squamous epithelium which sheds keratinaceous debris in a radial, concentric fashion.

Bottom: The lining epithelium contains all the layers of normal squamous epithelium.

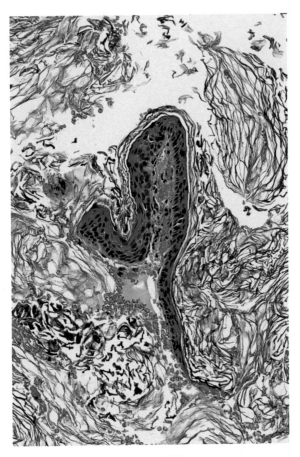

Figure 16-72
MIDDLE EAR CHOLESTEATOMA
Curettage specimens may consist of rare, detached ("free-floating") fragments of keratinizing squamous epithelium and associated keratinaceous debris.

Choristoma

Definition and General Features. Choristomas, or the presence of histologically normal tissue in a body site where such tissues are not normally found, are generally considered to represent developmental defects. Virtually all middle ear choristomas reported to date have been composed of either salivary gland or glial tissue (114,116,117,119,120–126,128).

Many lesions cited in the literature as glial choristomas were, in fact, associated with a defect in the adjacent temporal bone and thus represent encephaloceles rather than true choristomas (115, 118,127). Other glial choristomas were associated with local destruction of bone by a cholesteatoma, chronic otitis media, meningitis, or previous surgery, and may have been connected to the cranial vault (119). True glial choristomas without an associated bony defect or connection to the central nervous system are rare (117,120,125).

Clinical Features. Reported patients with middle ear choristomas tend to be either children or young adults who present with unilateral hearing loss or discharge (122,124). Either ear may be involved but there is a marked left ear preponderance (114,122,124). Clinically, choristomas often appear as lobulated, nonpulsatile tissue masses behind an intact eardrum. They may be positioned anywhere in the middle ear cleft but are commonly found in the posterior-superior region, and range from only millimeters in size to lesions that completely fill the tympanic cavity (122, 124). A single salivary gland choristoma that extended from the middle ear into the mastoid air cells has been described (128). Most salivary gland choristomas have been intimately associated with the seventh cranial nerve (116,121,124,126). Absence of the oval window and developmental abnormalities of the ossicles, external ear, or face may also be present (122,124).

Pathologic Findings. Salivary gland choristomas are composed of well formed, serous and mucinous glands, usually complete with ducts and fibroadipose tissue (121,122,124,128). The glands may be arranged in a haphazard or lobular fashion similar to that seen in the normal submandibular gland (fig. 16-73) (121,122,124,128). Glial choristomas are composed predominantly of astrocytes with an abundant fibrillary background (fig. 16-74).

Treatment and Prognosis. Choristomas are benign, nonprogressive lesions adequately treated by local excision. Only a single case of a salivary gland-type tumor (presumably) arising from a middle ear choristoma has been reported (122). A proportion of salivary gland choristomas have been associated with the facial nerve, thus biopsy without surgical resection has been advocated (121).

Jugulotympanic Paraganglioma

Definition. This is a benign neoplasm arising from branchiomeric paraganglia and composed of histologically bland epithelioid chief cells surrounded by smaller, spindled, often inapparent "sustentacular" cells.

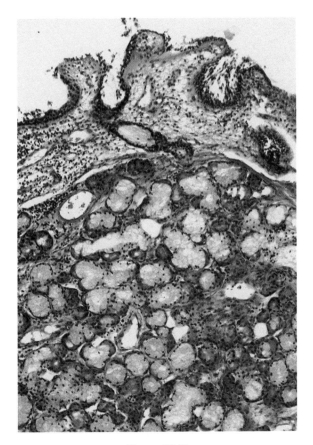

Figure 16-73
SALIVARY GLAND-TYPE CHORISTOMA
An isolated, subepithelial focus of seromucinous salivary gland-type tissue found in the middle ear of a middle-aged female who presented with a feeling of fullness in the affected ear. The finding of normal-appearing salivary gland tissue in an abnormal location qualifies as a choristoma.

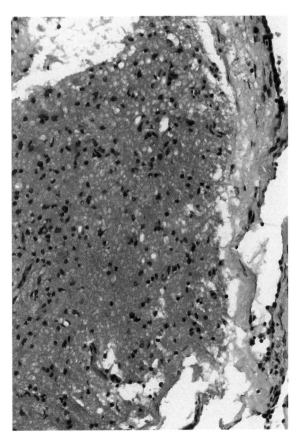

Figure 16-74
GLIAL-TYPE CHORISTOMA
The lesion depicted was found behind an intact tympanic membrane in the middle ear cleft of a middle-aged male with a prolonged history of unilateral hearing loss. The mass consists of a proliferation of astrocytes in a fibrillary background. Simple gland-like epithelial inclusions are also present, probably due to tangential sectioning of the irregular, overlying epithelium. Clinical studies failed to demonstrate associated bony defects or a connection with the central nervous system, thus the lesion was considered to represent a glial choristoma.

General Features. Jugulotympanic paragangliomas, also referred to as *glomus jugulare* and *glomus tympanicum,* are true neoplasms of varying aggressiveness that arise from the branchiomeric group of paraganglia (129–138). The branchiomeric group, so named because of their intimate relationship to the branchial arches, includes the jugulotympanic, intercarotid, subclavian, laryngeal, coronary, aorticopulmonary, and pulmonary paraganglia. Virtually all paragangliomas in the middle ear or temporal bone are of jugulotympanic derivation. An average of two or three jugulotympanic paraganglia may normally be found in the middle ear and temporal bone; anatomic sites include the jugular bulb, within the middle ear cavity over the cochlear promontory, and along the course of Jacobsen's (tympanic branch of the ninth) or Arnold's (auricular branch of the tenth) nerves. One survey found that approximately 85 percent of jugulotympanic paragangliomas arose in the jugular bulb area, followed by the middle ear cleft (12 percent), and the external ear canal (3 percent); the latter are derived from those paraganglia associated with Arnold's nerve (fig. 16-75) (132).

Clinical Features. Jugulotympanic paraganglia are the most common neoplasms of the middle ear and temporal bone. Most patients are adults between the ages of 30 and 65, with an average age of 50 years. Approximately three

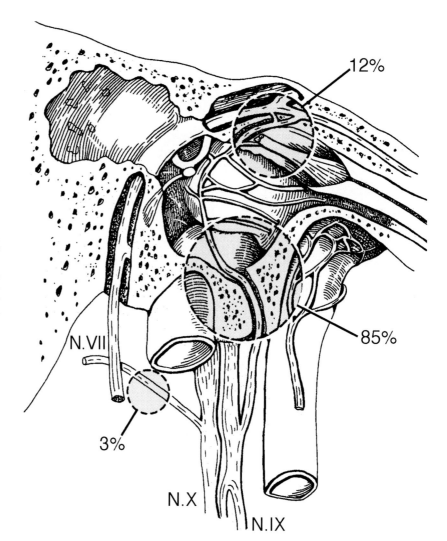

Figure 16-75
JUGULOTYMPANIC
PARAGANGLIOMA

The schematic depicts the anatomic location of 90 jugulotympanic paragangliomas in the AFIP files from 1940 through 1975. Note that the great majority of tumors (about 85 percent) arise in association with the wall of the jugular bulb. (Fig. 327 from Fascicle 25, 2nd Series.)

fourths of affected patients are female (129,130, 138). Most patients present with hearing loss, although otic discharge, pain, or tinnitus may also be present. Symptom duration may range from weeks to years (130,138). Occasional paragangliomas are functional, with signs or symptoms of excess catecholamine secretion (131). Otologic examination usually reveals a red-brown, polypoid mass presenting either behind a bulging eardrum or protruding into the external canal. Extensive hemorrhage on manipulation is often noted. Radiologic studies reveal a soft tissue middle ear mass with variable degrees of bony erosion. Angiographically, paragangliomas are invariably hypervascular.

The clinical behavior is typically that of slow but progressive growth with eventual infiltra-

tion of adjacent bone. An approximately 2 percent rate of metastasis has been reported for jugulotympanic paragangliomas (129). There are no clinical or histologic features that consistently correlate with aggressive clinical behavior.

Pathologic Findings. Jugulotympanic paraganglioma specimens are soft, homogeneous tissue fragments measuring up to 1 cm in aggregate dimension. Histologically, they are composed of uniform, epithelioid chief cells often arranged in distinct cell nests (zellballen), cords, and trabeculae, separated by indistinct sustentacular cells and a prominent capillary network (fig. 16-76) (134). The cells are arranged haphazardly within the cellular nests, with no evidence of polarization or lumen formation. Stromal fibrosis and hemorrhage are often present and may be extensive.

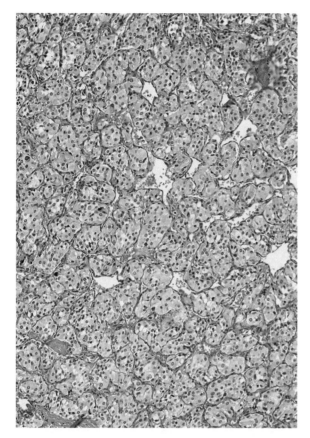

Figure 16-76
JUGULOTYMPANIC PARAGANGLIOMA
On low magnification paragangliomas are predominantly composed of well-defined nests of neoplastic cells (zellballen) with a prominent intervening capillary and venous network.

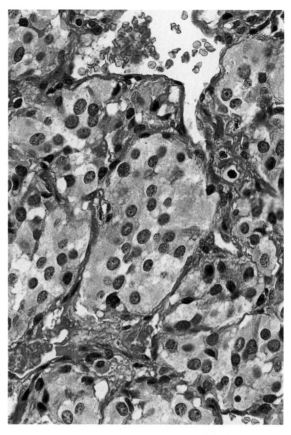

Figure 16-77
JUGULOTYMPANIC PARAGANGLIOMA
The neoplastic chief cells are uniform and oval to polygonal, with moderate amounts of eosinophilic cytoplasm and inapparent cell borders. The nuclei are evenly contoured and contain finely granular chromatin. The sustentacular cells surrounding the cell nests are inapparent and rarely appreciated on routine stains.

The nesting pattern may be indistinct in sclerotic tumors but is easily highlighted by reticulin staining. The chief cells are oval to polygonal, with moderate amounts of eosinophilic cytoplasm and indistinct cellular borders (fig. 16-77). In occasional tumors the chief cells may contain abundant, deeply eosinophilic (oncocytic) cytoplasm. Nuclei are uniform and centrally placed, with finely granular chromatin and inconspicuous nucleoli. Cells with large, bizarre, or pleomorphic nuclei may be seen but are not indicative of increased biologic aggressiveness (fig. 16-78). Mitotic figures and tumor necrosis are rare. The supportive sustentacular cells, which show spindled to stellate nuclei and elongated indistinct cytoplasmic processes, are usually difficult to discern on hematoxylin and eosin stains.

Immunohistochemical Findings. The neoplastic cells of jugulotympanic paragangliomas, similar to paragangliomas elsewhere, are immunohistochemically positive for vimentin, neuron-specific enolase, synaptophysin, and chromogranin (fig. 16-79) (133,135). Most tumors are positive for serotonin as well (133). The presence of vimentin- and S-100 protein-positive encircling sustentacular cells is a hallmark of paragangliomas in general (fig. 16-80). Cytokeratin positivity in jugulotympanic paragangliomas is rare but has been reported (133).

Electron Microscopic Findings. Ultrastructurally, a mixture of "light" and "dark" neoplastic cells is often seen. Both types of cells show extended, intertwining cytoplasmic processes

429

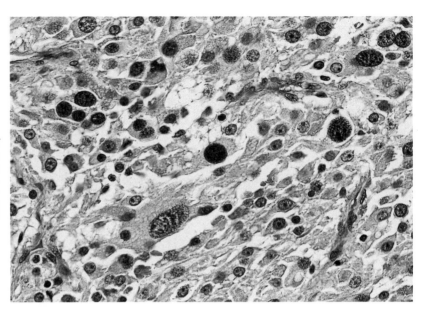

Figure 16-78
JUGULOTYMPANIC
PARAGANGLIOMA

Occasional tumors show foci of marked nuclear pleomorphism, with nuclear enlargement, chromatin clumping, and prominent nucleoli. Despite their striking appearance, tumors with these nuclear changes do not have an increased risk of local recurrence or distant metastasis.

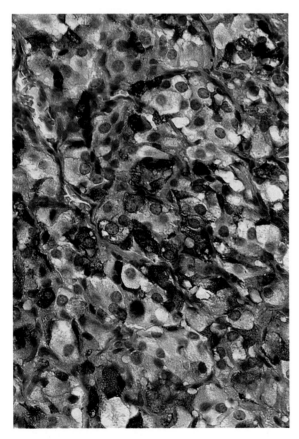

Figure 16-79
JUGULOTYMPANIC PARAGANGLIOMA

A representative jugulotympanic paraganglioma showing diffuse intracytoplasmic positivity for chromogranin in the neoplastic chief cells. (Figures 16-79 and 16-80 are from the same patient.)

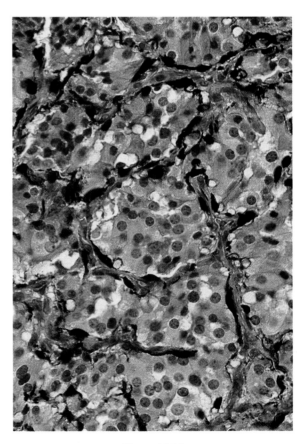

Figure 16-80
JUGULOTYMPANIC PARAGANGLIOMA

The supportive sustentacular cells are strongly immunoreactive for S-100 protein.

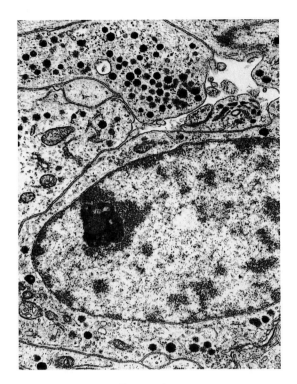

Figure 16-81
JUGULOTYMPANIC PARAGANGLIOMA
The most characteristic ultrastructural feature of jugulotympanic paraganglioma is the presence of intracytoplasmic, electron-dense neurosecretory-type granules measuring from 120 to 200 nm in diameter. (Fig. 330 from Fascicle 25, 2nd Series.)

joined by rudimentary cellular attachments. The most characteristic ultrastructural finding is the presence of numerous membrane-bound, electron-dense, neurosecretory type granules, which are largely uniform and range in diameter from 120 to 200 nm (fig. 16-81) (134). Sustentacular cells are difficult to identify ultrastructurally and are not seen in most preparations.

Differential Diagnosis. Paragangliomas may be clinically confused with other polypoid mass lesions arising in the middle ear such as cholesteatoma, middle ear adenoma, and aggressive papillary tumors, the last of which may also appear hypervascular on angiography. Histologically, however, the epithelioid cells and nesting pattern of paragangliomas distinguish these lesions from keratotic cholesteatomas, glandular adenomas, or papillary neoplasms. Middle ear lesions that may histologically simulate paraganglioma include metastatic renal cell carcinoma, metastatic follicular thyroid carcinoma, meningothelial

meningioma, and granular cell tumor, all of which are extremely rare in the middle ear or temporal bone. In addition, the latter tumors lack neuroendocrine features, whereas paragangliomas are immunohistochemically positive for neuron-specific enolase, chromogranin, and synaptophysin. The presence of an S-100 protein-positive sustentacular cell population is also highly characteristic, given the appropriate clinical and cytologic features.

Treatment and Prognosis. Complete surgical resection is the treatment of choice (138). Localized middle ear tumors are often amenable to local excision alone, whereas radical mastoidectomy may be required for locally invasive or jugular bulb lesions (136). Local recurrence rates of up to 50 percent have been reported following attempted surgical resection (134,137). About 15 percent of patients die, usually from either tumoral extension into the cranial vault or metastases to regional lymph nodes, lungs, liver, and bone (134,137).

Middle Ear Adenoma

Definition. This is a benign, nonaggressive, exclusively glandular neoplasm arising from the flattened to cuboidal epithelial cells lining the middle ear.

General Features. Primary (nonsalivary) neoplasms arising from the lining epithelium of the middle ear or mastoid are rare. The pertinent literature is difficult to assess as middle ear adenomas have been variably (and erroneously) labeled as ceruminous adenomas (144), adenocarcinomas (145,151,153,154), and carcinoid tumors (148), as well as other terms. A proportion of these reports fail to exclude metastases or middle ear extension from an adjacent site; others show little to no pathologic documentation, further adding to the confusion. Designations utilizing the term ceruminous or ceruminoma are particularly erroneous, since ceruminous glands are found only in the lateral two thirds of the external auditory canal, and ectopic ceruminal glands have not been identified in the middle ear. The earlier practice of labeling all glandular middle ear tumors as adenocarcinoma is also unfortunate, as virtually all middle ear adenomas are nonaggressive, nonmetastasizing lesions.

Middle ear adenomas may show variable degrees of neuroendocrine differentiation, leading several investigators to report otherwise typical examples of middle ear adenoma as carcinoid tumors. Manni et al. (148) reviewed 17 published cases of middle ear "carcinoid" tumors, some of which showed trabecular growth patterns, the presence of neurosecretory-like granules on electron microscopy, or immunohistochemical positivity for cytokeratin, neuron-specific enolase, chromogranin, and various polypeptide hormones. Neuroendocrine cells do not normally exist in the middle ear mucosa; thus the emergence of such tumors probably results from the neuroendocrine differentiation of a pluripotential stem cell. As typical middle ear adenomas may show trabecular growth and the presence of rare neurosecretory-type granules on electron microscopy, we are of the opinion that middle ear adenomas and carcinoids represent variants of a single entity showing varying degrees of neuroendocrine differentiation. Importantly, distinguishing middle ear carcinoids from middle ear adenomas, based on the relative degree of neuroendocrine differentiation, is of no biologic significance, as both tumor "types" are resectable, nonrecurrent, nonaggressive neoplasms. As such, we agree with El-Naggar et al. (143) that distinguishing middle ear carcinoids from adenomas is of little clinical utility and, as far as the current authors are concerned, not recommended.

It is important, however, to distinguish middle ear adenomas from aggressive papillary tumors which may rarely arise in the middle ear but more commonly develop in the endolymphatic sac or temporal bone and involve the middle ear by local extension (vide infra).

Clinical Features. Affected patients are usually adults with a mean age of 39 years (150). Patients commonly present with unilateral conductive hearing loss or tinnitus (147,150,156). Sex distribution and laterality are approximately equal (147,150). On radiologic examination, virtually all middle ear adenomas present as soft tissue density lesions confined to the middle ear, without evidence of bony erosion or destruction (142,150). Most cases are diagnosed preoperatively as either paraganglioma (66 percent) or cholesteatoma (16 percent) (147,150). The correct diagnosis is rarely, if ever, made prior to histologic examination.

Intraoperatively, the tumor is well defined, encapsulated, tan-gray to yellow, and lobulated; most observers note the absence of prominent

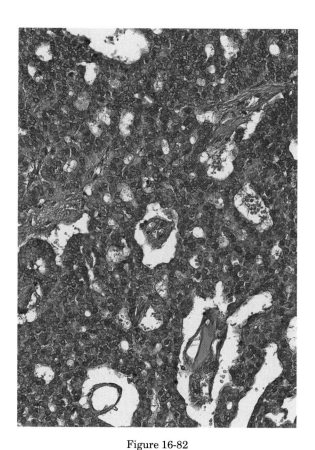

Figure 16-82
MIDDLE EAR ADENOMA
A typical middle ear adenoma showing back-to-back glandular structures formed by small, uniform, cuboidal cells.

vascularity. The ossicles are often encased by tumor although involvement of the mastoid antrum, attic, hypotympanum, and eustachian tube orifice is rare (150,152). Ossicle erosion and microscopic involvement of the facial nerve have been encountered, but bony invasion or extension beyond the middle ear cavity is typically absent (140,150,152).

Pathologic Findings. Middle ear adenomas are often removed piecemeal and received as multiple fragments of light tan, soft tissue measuring less than 1 cm in aggregate dimension. Histologically, they are typically composed of cytologically bland, cuboidal to columnar epithelial cells arranged in glands, sheets, cords, and nests (140,142, 150,156). Most tumors are predominantly glandular, although cellular cords and trabeculae may be seen (fig. 16-82). The glands are usually lined by a single cell layer, without evidence of underlying myoepithelial cells, and may contain an

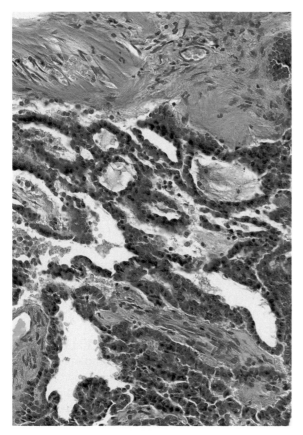

Figure 16-83
MIDDLE EAR ADENOMA
Occasional middle ear adenomas show glandular structures and cellular cords separated by varying amounts of fibrotic stroma. (Figures 16-83 and 16-84 are from the same patient.)

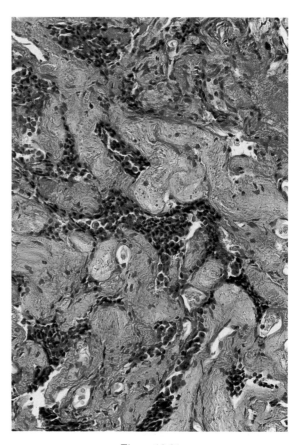

Figure 16-84
MIDDLE EAR ADENOMA
Rare middle ear adenomas show a marked desmoplastic response with trabeculae of neoplastic cells and little to no glandular formation.

eosinophilic, PAS-positive secretion. The intervening collagenous stroma is variable in amount but typically paucicellular (fig. 16-83). Rare tumors may show large areas of hypocellular collagen alternating with compressed trabeculae of neoplastic cells; gland formation in these lesions may be focal or absent (fig. 16-84). Tumors may also show evidence of recent and remote hemorrhage, with cholesterol clefts, foreign body giant cells, and foamy or hemosiderin-laden macrophages.

Cytologically, the neoplastic cells strongly resemble the normal epithelium of the middle ear. The cells are cuboidal, polygonal to ovoid, and contain centrally placed nuclei, eosinophilic, finely granular cytoplasm, and indistinct cell borders (142,147,150). The nuclei are round, uniform, and often hyperchromatic without detectable nucleoli. Cases predominantly composed of

"plasmacytoid" tumor cells with eccentric nuclei containing finely granular chromatin may also be seen (151). Mild nuclear pleomorphism may be present but mitotic figures are rare to absent.

To our knowledge, all pathologically documented cases of middle ear adenoma have lacked clinical, gross, or microscopic evidence of overt bony invasion. Adenomas may erode the ossicles or, in about one fourth of cases, penetrate the tympanic membrane (150).

Immunohistochemical Findings. Few middle ear adenomas have been studied immunohistochemically. Those tumors examined have been consistently immunoreactive for keratin, epithelial membrane antigen, and vimentin; neuron-specific enolase, S-100 protein, chromogranin, and synaptophysin may also be positive (149,151,156).

Electron Microscopic Findings. Ultrastructurally, the tumors are composed of cuboidal tumor cells with prominent apical microvilli. The cells often show a basal lamina and are joined by tight junctions and desmosomes (140, 147,149,152). Nuclei are oval with clumped chromatin and variably prominent nucleoli. An unusual characteristic, possibly unique to this neoplasm, is that two distinct types of secretory granules may be present: apically oriented mucous granules and basally located, electron-dense neurosecretory-type granules (149,152, 156). Typically cells contain one or the other granule type, but not both.

Differential Diagnosis. Middle ear adenomas must be distinguished from paraganglioma, ceruminous tumors from the outer ear canal, aggressive papillary tumors of the temporal bone and endolymphatic sac, and metastatic neoplasms. Paragangliomas contain a highly vascular stroma and a cellular nesting (zellballen) pattern, features not present in middle ear adenomas. Furthermore, the glandular architecture and keratin positivity characteristic of middle ear adenomas are absent in paragangliomas. Ceruminal gland adenomas and adenocarcinomas of the outer ear canal may occasionally involve the middle ear by direct extension and, similar to middle ear adenomas, are glandular tumors composed of brightly eosinophilic cells (139). However, the glands in ceruminal gland adenomas are composed of two cell layers, with an inner secretory and outer myoepithelial cell layer. Ceruminal gland adenocarcinomas are typically pleomorphic tumors that usually show evidence of bony invasion and involve the external canal.

Perhaps the most important distinction is to separate middle ear adenomas from the aggressive papillary tumors of the temporal bone and endolymphatic sac, as the latter lesions have a marked tendency to invade bone and extend intracranially. As the neoplastic cells in the two lesions may appear morphologically similar, the distinction is usually made by the presence or absence of papillations, which are at least focally present in aggressive papillary tumors but absent in middle ear adenomas. We are aware of only a single reported case of a papillary middle ear tumor arising in a patient without evidence of bony destruction (141); the tumor recurred locally, however, and extended follow-up was not provided. Otherwise, virtually all other reported papillary middle ear tumors are aggressive, locally destructive lesions, the majority of which probably arise in the endolymphatic sac and involve the middle ear secondarily.

Metastases to the temporal bone that may cause potential confusion with middle ear adenoma are rare (139,146,155). Metastatic carcinomas to the middle ear are usually (but not invariably) histologically pleomorphic and show evidence of necrosis, neither of which are present in middle ear adenoma. Metastatic renal cell carcinoma, particularly granular cell variants, may initially appear similar to middle ear adenomas but lack glandular elements (146,155). Furthermore, these and other metastatic lesions are rarely confined to the middle ear cavity, and often involve other portions of the temporal bone with evidence of bone destruction.

Treatment and Prognosis. Middle ear adenomas are usually treated by complete local excision with tympanoplasty, mastoidectomy, or both (142,147,150,156). Surgical excision is curative in most patients although local recurrence has been reported (142,147).

Schneiderian-Type (Inverted) Papilloma of Middle Ear and Mastoid

Definition. This is a benign papillary epithelial neoplasm arising from the lining epithelium of the middle ear and mastoid. These lesions are histologically identical to the schneiderian-type inverted papillomas arising from the sinonasal tract (157).

General and Clinical Features. Schneiderian-type papillomas of the middle ear and mastoid are rare; to the best of our knowledge only seven cases have been reported in the English literature (158–161). Similar to their sinonasal counterparts, middle ear and mastoid inverted papillomas are nonmetastasizing lesions that often recur following excision (160,161). Due to differences in terminology and variable pathologic documentation, it is difficult to subcategorize those cases reported thus far as either inverted, fungiform (exophytic), or oncocytic (cylindrical cell). There is a single report of a middle ear inverted papilloma with an associated squamous cell carcinoma, but the pathologic documentation of the latter case is equivocal (160).

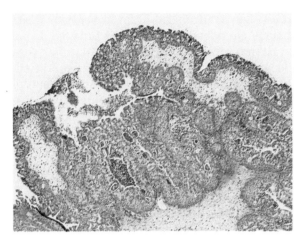

Figure 16-85
INVERTED SCHNEIDERIAN PAPILLOMA
OF THE MIDDLE EAR

A rare example of a primary middle ear inverted schneiderian papilloma removed from a 19-year-old woman who presented with a 1-year history of progressive unilateral hearing loss and otalgia. (Courtesy of Dr. J.L. Ward, Columbia, SC and Dr. E.L. Barnes, Pittsburgh PA.)

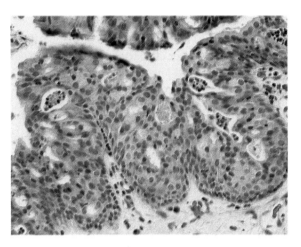

Figure 16-86
INVERTED SCHNEIDERIAN PAPILLOMA
OF THE MIDDLE EAR

On high-power microscopy the lesion is composed of multiple layers of uniform epithelial cells with scattered mucocytes and intraepithelial microcysts containing mixed inflammatory cells. (Courtesy of Dr. J.L. Ward, Columbia, SC and Dr. E.L. Barnes, Pittsburgh, PA.)

Six of the seven reported patients were women ranging in age from 19 to 77 years (mean, 42 years). Presenting complaints included otalgia, unilateral hearing loss, and discharge. The left ear was involved in five cases, the right ear in two cases. In four cases the lesion was discovered as a polypoid mass protruding through a perforated tympanic membrane; one of these also showed tumoral invasion and destruction of the adjacent mastoid, temporal bone, and inner ear (158–161). The remaining cases were confined to the middle ear (161). Two patients had a previous history of a sinonasal schneiderian papilloma excised 1.5 and 9 years earlier (158,160). While the middle ear papilloma in these cases occurred on the same side and was the same histologic type as the earlier sinonasal lesions, the two sites were not anatomically contiguous. In addition, there was no evidence of sinonasal or nasopharyngeal papillomas in either patient when the middle ear lesions were discovered. Thus the relationship (if any) between the middle ear and schneiderian tumors is unclear (158,160).

Pathologic Findings. Intraoperatively and grossly the tumors are described as multilobulated, grape-like, or polypoid masses within and often filling the middle ear cleft. Most middle ear schneiderian-type papillomas are predomi-

nantly exophytic but focally contain inverted (endophytic) regions as well (fig. 16-85). Histologically, most lesions appear as papillary neoplasms composed of arborizing papillary fronds with a fibrovascular core lined by multiple layers of uniform, cytologically bland, squamous, transitional, or ciliated columnar cells (fig. 16-86) (158–161). Intercellular bridges may be identified but keratinization is absent (161). Papillomas may be composed of a single cell type or, more commonly, an admixture of cell types. Mitoses are present but usually limited to the basal layers. Similar to their schneiderian counterparts, most tumors have acute and chronic inflammatory cells, scattered mucocytes with abundant basophilic cytoplasm, and intraepithelial microcysts containing mucous or inflammatory cells scattered throughout the epithelium (161).

Differential Diagnosis. Schneiderian papillomas may be confused with middle ear adenomas, which occasionally have a predominant sheet-like growth pattern. Middle ear adenomas, however, show at least focal evidence of glandular formation and lack the fibrovascular papillations, interspersed inflammatory cells, mucocytes, and intraepithelial microcysts typical of schneiderian-type papillomas. Aggressive papillary tumors of the temporal bone and endolymphatic sac may initially simulate a schneiderian papilloma, but the former tumors are composed of papillations lined by a single layer of epithelial cells and almost invariably show evidence of bony destruction. A well-differentiated squamous cell or basal cell carcinoma extending from the external ear canal must also be excluded.

Treatment and Prognosis. The preferred treatment is complete surgical excision, usually by tympanomastoidectomy. Limited efforts at conservative excision usually result in tumor recurrence. In one study, four of five patients had from one to seven episodes of local tumor recurrence over a period of 15 years (161). Despite multiple recurrences, however, at last follow-up all five patients were alive without evidence of disease at 6 to 144 months (median, 84 months) after diagnosis.

Aggressive Papillary Tumor of Temporal Bone and Endolymphatic Sac (Low-Grade Adenocarcinoma of Endolymphatic Sac Origin)

Definition. This is a nonmetastasizing but locally aggressive, destructive papillary epithelial proliferation arising in the endolymphatic sac or elsewhere in the temporal bone.

General Features. The origin and precise nature of aggressive papillary tumors of the temporal bone and endolymphatic sac are vigorously contested issues (162–180). Most lesions have been found in the region of the endolymphatic sac, an epithelial lined, terminal saccular enlargement of the vestibular aqueduct that lies between the inner and outer layers of the dura on the posterior surface of the petrous portion of the temporal bone (162,168,170,171,174,176,177,179,180). Rare papillary tumors, however, have been described arising from the area of the jugular bulb (176), middle ear, and mastoid (166,169,178) without radiologic evidence of endolymphatic sac involvement. Further complicating the issue, most reported lesions are advanced tumors involving the middle ear, mastoid, petrous portion of the temporal bone, and posterior cranial fossa, thus obscuring the site of origin (162). The debate over the cell and site of origin is beyond the scope of this Fascicle. Nonetheless, pathologists and clinicians alike should recognize that papillary tumors arising in the endolymphatic sac or elsewhere in the temporal bone are almost always aggressive lesions that

must be distinguished from biologically inert middle ear adenomas and other tumors.

Standardization of nomenclature has also been problematic. The inherent vagaries of scientific reporting and the debate over the site of origin has resulted in these tumors being variably labeled as *aggressive papillary middle ear tumors, low-grade adenocarcinomas of endolymphatic sac origin, endolymphatic sac tumors, papillary endolymphatic sac tumors, aggressive papillary tumor of temporal bone,* and *papillary adenomas,* among others (162,164,165,168–171, 173,174,176,177,179,180). To emphasize the aggressive but nonmetastasizing clinical behavior of these tumors, papillary architecture, and potential sites of origin elsewhere in the temporal bone, we favor the term "aggressive papillary tumor of temporal bone and endolymphatic sac" for these lesions, but fully recognize acceptable alternative designations, such as papillary neoplasm (or adenocarcinoma) of endolymphatic sac.

Clinical Features. Aggressive papillary tumors of temporal bone and endolymphatic sac affect a wide age range, with a median of 42 years (165,168,174). Sex distribution is equal, and a similar number of tumors have occurred on the right and left side. Bilateral tumors are extremely rare but may occur (164,175,179). Virtually all patients are symptomatic and commonly present with unilateral hearing loss and vertigo. At the time of presentation, most patients have a blue or red discolored mass behind an intact tympanic membrane, and some have perforated eardrums (165). All papillary neoplasms show some degree of local invasion with bony destruction, but distant metastases have not been reported to date.

Radiologically, papillary tumors present as soft tissue (osteolytic) masses with destruction of the posterior aspect of the petrous bone, middle ear cleft, and mastoid air cells. Most smaller lesions are located around the posterior aspect of the petrous portion of the temporal bone, near the expected location of the endolymphatic sac (174). Advanced tumors may extend posteriorly into the cranial fossa, anteriorly into the cavernous sinus, or inferiorly to involve the skull base in the vicinity of the jugular foramen (fig. 16-87) (174). Bilateral lesions are strongly associated with von Hippel-Lindau disease (164,171,179). The statistical association is sufficiently strong that a diagnosis of a papillary tumor of the temporal bone or

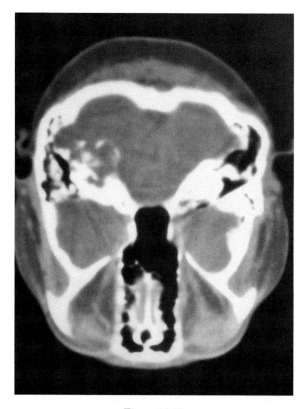

Figure 16-87
AGGRESSIVE PAPILLARY TUMOR OF
MIDDLE EAR/TEMPORAL BONE

Computerized tomographic scan of an aggressive papillary tumor arising in the left petrous bone and extending into the posterior cranial fossa.

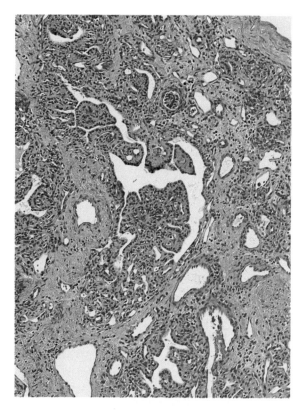

Figure 16-88
AGGRESSIVE PAPILLARY TUMOR
OF MIDDLE EAR/TEMPORAL BONE

Most aggressive papillary tumors are composed of small, blunt, fibrotic papillations of variable width surrounded by a desmoplastic stromal response.

endolymphatic sac, particularly for bilateral lesions, should stimulate an investigation for the other manifestations of von Hippel-Lindau disease (164).

Pathologic Findings. Papillary tumor specimens are usually fragments of red-brown gritty tissue measuring 2 cm or less. Histologically, tumors are predominantly papillary and composed of variably sized fibrovascular septa lined by a single layer of cuboidal to low columnar cells (165,169). The extent of papillary change is variable: some tumors are composed of tall, thin, well-formed papillations with a minimal fibrotic response, whereas others show smaller, variably fibrotic papillations admixed with an accompanying desmoplastic response (figs. 16-88, 16-89). Cellular cords and trabeculae may also be seen. The neoplastic cells contain moderate amounts of clear, vacuolated, or eosinophilic cytoplasm

with discernable cell borders. The nuclei are oval, mildly irregular, and centrally placed, with coarsely granular chromatin and small, inconspicuous nucleoli (fig. 16-90). Marked nuclear pleomorphism and mitotic figures are not seen. A hypocellular desmoplastic stromal response with hemorrhage and cholesterol clefts is often present, with extensive infiltration of adjacent fibrous tissue and bone. Rare tumors may show acinar structures or microcysts containing an eosinophilic, strongly PAS-positive proteinaceous material resembling colloid; such lesions may simulate a metastatic papillary carcinoma of the thyroid (166,168).

Immunohistochemical Findings. Almost all cases reported have been immunoreactive for cytokeratin, epithelial membrane antigen, and vimentin (165,168,170). Variable positivity for neuron-specific enolase, Leu-7, glial fibrillary

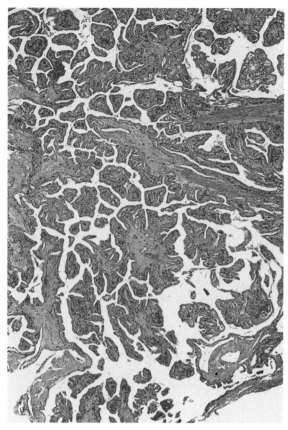

Figure 16-89
AGGRESSIVE PAPILLARY TUMOR
OF MIDDLE EAR/TEMPORAL BONE

Rarely, aggressive papillary tumors show an exuberant proliferation of tall, thin, epithelial-lined fibrovascular septa with little to no desmoplastic response.

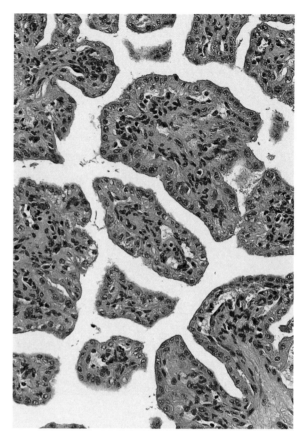

Figure 16-90
AGGRESSIVE PAPILLARY TUMOR OF
MIDDLE EAR/TEMPORAL BONE

On high magnification the papillations are lined by a single layer of eosinophilic, cuboidal epithelial cells with minimal nuclear pleomorphism.

acidic protein, and S-100 protein has also been reported. Staining for lysozyme, actin, synaptophysin, chromogranin, desmin, and thyroglobulin is usually negative.

Electron Microscopic Findings. On electron microscopic examination, papillary tumors show a single layer of epithelial cells with short, interdigitating cytoplasmic processes joined by desmosomes (165,168). The apical cytoplasm often displays microvilli, whereas the basal portion is lined by a basal lamina. The tumor cells contain moderate amounts of intercytoplasmic organelles and rare, electron-dense, neurosecretory-type granules measuring 200 to 350 μm.

Differential Diagnosis. Aggressive papillary tumors of temporal bone and endolymphatic sac must be distinguished from their less aggressive middle ear adenoma counterparts. On biopsy

material, both are composed of histologically bland, cuboidal epithelial cells with a desmoplastic stromal response. Papillary tumors, however, are predominantly papillary lesions often composed of clear cells, whereas middle ear adenomas are glandular-trabecular (nonpapillary) neoplasms composed of epithelial cells with eosinophilic cytoplasm. Clinically, papillary tumors are usually widely destructive lesions centered around the endolymphatic sac, whereas middle ear adenomas are typically confined to the middle ear.

Another differential diagnostic consideration is metastatic papillary carcinoma of the thyroid, as rare papillary tumors may contain glandular or cystic areas with a PAS-positive, proteinaceous substance resembling colloid. The nuclei in papillary tumors of the temporal bone and endolymphatic sac usually lack the nuclear grooves, stratification, and overlapping typical of papillary thyroid carcinoma. Immunohistochemical staining for thyroglobulin, which is invariably present in papillary thyroid lesions but absent in primary temporal bone and endolymphatic sac tumors, may be used in problematic cases.

The literature also contains reports of papillary epithelial tumors involving the cerebellopontine angle and temporal bone, some of which were described as choroid plexus papillomas (163), whereas others were designated papillary endolymphatic sac neoplasms with cerebellopontine angle extension (173). Distinguishing these lesions is problematic, as there is a marked morphologic similarity between the lining cells of the endolymphatic sac and the choroid plexus (163,172,173). Megerian (172) reported that transthyretin expression could be used to distinguish choroid plexus papillomas, which are transthyretin positive, from papillary tumors of the temporal bone and endolymphatic sac, which are transthyretin negative.

Treatment and Prognosis. The only known effective treatment for papillary tumors of the temporal bone and endolymphatic sac is complete surgical resection. Adjunct radiation or chemotherapy is of no known benefit. In patients in whom total surgical resection is possible the prognosis is good. In the study of Heffner (168), of 12 patients who underwent total tumor resection as initial therapy, 11 were free of disease from 2 to 12 years later. In contrast, of 7 patients who received incomplete resection, 6 had local recurrence an average of 6 years after resection and 2 died of tumor.

Meningioma of Temporal Bone

Definition. This is a benign but occasionally locally invasive proliferation of arachnoid cells, originating from the meninges covering the central nervous system.

General Features. Extracranial meningiomas are rare but have been reported in numerous sites, including the head and neck (181–194). Head and neck extracranial meningiomas, similar to their intracranial counterparts, are also thought to arise from arachnoid cells. Ectopic arachnoidal villi may be found in several areas throughout the temporal bone, including: the internal auditory meatus, the jugular foramen, the geniculate ganglion region, and the sulcus of the

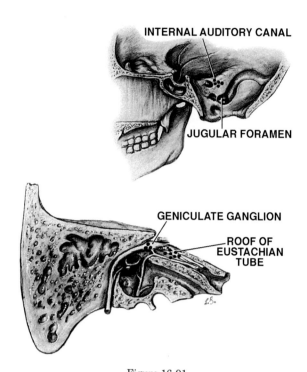

Figure 16-91
MENINGIOMA OF MIDDLE EAR/TEMPORAL BONE

The schematic indicates the most common sites of extracranial meningiomas involving the temporal bone. (Fig. 54 from Nager GT. Meningiomas involving the temporal bone. Springfield, IL: Charles C. Thomas, 1964:159.)

greater and lesser superficial petrosal nerves in the roof of the eustachian tube (fig. 16-91) (187,189). Thus meningiomas may either arise from the posterior or middle cranial fossa and involve the middle ear by direct extension or arise primarily within the temporal bone. Most reported cases of temporal bone meningioma have an intracranial component; primary tumors without a detectable intracranial component are rare (183,192). In a 1982 review, Salama and Stafford (192) found 18 primary temporal bone middle ear meningiomas in the English and French literature.

Clinical Features. The few primary temporal bone meningiomas reported to date show clinical features similar to their intracranial counterparts, with a patient age range of 17 to 68 years and a marked female predominance (192). Patients present with hearing loss, headaches, vertigo, or otorrhea (183,184,187,192). Clinical examination often reveals a soft tissue mass filling the middle ear or the external ear canal.

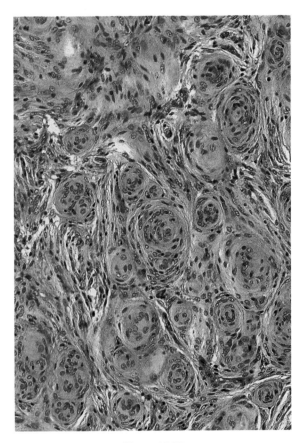

Figure 16-92

MENINGIOMA OF MIDDLE EAR/TEMPORAL BONE

A meningothelial ("syncytial") meningioma resected from the temporal bone of a 51-year-old male. An intracranial component was not present. The tumor is composed of nests and whorls of uniform, oval tumor cells with eosinophilic cytoplasm and inapparent cell borders.

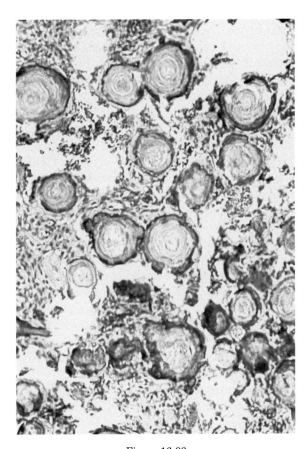

Figure 16-93

MENINGIOMA OF MIDDLE EAR/TEMPORAL BONE

A psammomatous meningioma removed from the middle ear of a 42-year-old female. Psammomatous variants are characterized by syncytial whorls of neoplastic cells interspersed with numerous concentrically laminated calcifications known as psammoma bodies.

Pathologic Findings. Gross pathologic descriptions of temporal meningiomas are rare; the few tumors described were received as multiple fragments of granular or gritty tan-brown tissue (187,189,192). Meningiomas have traditionally been divided into several morphologic subtypes: meningotheliomatous, fibroblastic, transitional, psammomatous, angiomatous, papillary, secretory, and anaplastic variants. Temporal bone/middle ear meningiomas may assume any of the latter forms, although the meningothelial type appears to be the most common, followed by the transitional and psammomatous variants (181,183,186, 188,189). Meningothelial tumors, also known as *syncytial variants,* are composed of uniform, oval to focally spindled tumor cells arranged in nests, whorls, and lobules encompassed by thin fibrovascular septa (fig. 16-92). The tumor cells have moderate amounts of eosinophilic cytoplasm with poorly defined cell borders, imparting a syncytial appearance to the lesion. Nuclei are round and centrally placed, with finely granular, pale chromatin and inconspicuous nucleoli. Intranuclear cytoplasmic invaginations are frequently present. Nuclear pleomorphism is rare and mitotic figures are uncommon. Transitional variants are characterized by concentric whorls of elongated to spindled tumor cells with ill-defined eosinophilic cytoplasm and bland nuclei. The central aspect of the cellular whorls often contains a capillary blood vessel. Lesions in which the whorls are largely replaced by concentric laminae of calcium salts or psammoma bodies are referred to as *psammomatous variants* (fig. 16-93).

Immunohistochemical Findings. To our knowledge none of the temporal bone meningiomas reported to date has been studied immunohistochemically. Meningiomas in general, however, are invariably immunoreactive for vimentin and epithelial membrane antigen (182, 190,193,194). A minority of tumors may also stain for cytokeratin and S-100 protein.

Electron Microscopic Findings. Ultrastructurally, meningiomas are characterized by ovoid to spindled cells with long, interdigitating cytoplasmic processes connected by desmosomes (191). Prominent, occasionally whorled bundles of intracytoplasmic intermediate filaments may be seen, with moderate numbers of mitochondria, golgi apparatti, and endoplasmic reticulum.

Differential Diagnosis. Meningothelial meningiomas may superficially resemble paragangliomas, as both may present as variably sized lobules of epithelioid cells surrounded by a delicate fibrovascular stroma. Paragangliomas, however, lack cellular whorls, contain a second, sustentacular cell population and, in contradistinction to meningiomas, stain for neuroendocrine markers but not epithelial membrane antigen. Predominantly spindled transitional meningiomas may also be confused with schwannoma. Meningiomas, however, lack the pointed, wavy nuclei, alternating hypocellular and hypercellular areas, and nuclear pallisading typical of schwannomas.

Treatment and Prognosis. The treatment for extracranial meningioma is surgical excision. Radiation and chemotherapy are ineffective, perhaps due to the slow growth characteristic of these lesions (184). The prognosis is good to excellent following complete resection (184,187, 188,192). Patients with extensive or intracranial disease, however, have a guarded outlook. Surgical resection in such cases is seldom complete, and tumors often occur.

Metastatic Neoplasms to the Middle Ear

Metastases to the temporal bone are rare. The literature contains sporatic reports of metastatic neoplasms to the middle ear or temporal bone, primarily in the form of case reports. To our knowledge, the only significant series of temporal bone metastases are those of Adams, Belal, Hill, Jahn, Maddox, and Schuknecht et al. (195–200). Unfortunately, pathologic documentation

in these reports is scant at best. The most comprehensive report was published in 1976 by Hill and Kohut (197) who found 102 previously reported cases of metastatic carcinoma involving the temporal bone. Metastatic tumors involving the temporal bone most commonly arose from, in descending order of frequency, the breast (18 percent), lung (12 percent), kidney (10 percent), stomach (8 percent), and larynx (5 percent). Not surprisingly, the most common metastatic tumors to the temporal bone, i.e., carcinomas of the breast, lung, and kidney, all have a known predilection for metastasizing to bone. Metastatic melanoma frequently involved the temporal bone as well (6 percent of cases). The temporal bone area most involved was the petrous portion or the osseous labyrinth of the inner ear; the middle ear was involved in only a minority of cases (195,196).

Most patients with temporal bone metastases had a known primary tumor at the time of presentation (197,198,200). In some patients, however, the temporal bone metastasis was the initial presentation of an unknown primary malignancy (199). Patient age and gender distribution are characteristic of the underlying tumor and are thus nonspecific. Presenting symptomatology is also variable. In most cases recognition of the lesion as a metastasis was unknown prior to resection.

Rhabdomyosarcoma of the Middle Ear

Definition. Rhabdomyosarcoma is a malignant neoplasm showing histologic, immunohistochemical, and ultrastructural evidence of skeletal muscle differentiation.

General Features. Rhabdomyosarcomas are highly malignant neoplasms that constitute the most frequent sarcoma arising in the head and neck area in children (201,203,205,206,209,210). Of 558 rhabdomyosarcomas evaluated at the Armed Forces Institute of Pathology (AFIP), 44 percent arose in the head and neck, with 3 percent originating in the ear or mastoid bone (203). A recent literature review of 777 head and neck rhabdomyosarcomas reported that 14 percent of tumors arose from the middle ear or mastoid (201).

Rhabdomyosarcomas vary in histologic appearance depending on the growth pattern and degree of cellular differentiation (201,203,205,206,209). Most tumors can be classified as either embryonal

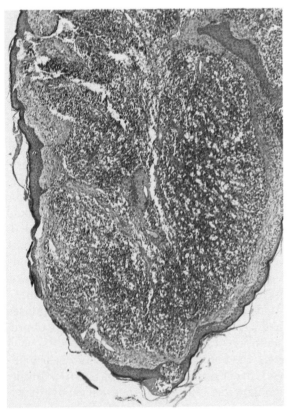

Figure 16-94
RHABDOMYOSARCOMA OF THE MIDDLE EAR
An embryonal rhabdomyosarcoma discovered in the middle ear of a 2-year-old boy. The lesion is covered with metaplastic squamous epithelium and was clinically diagnosed as an aural polyp. (Courtesy of Dr. J.L. Ward, Columbia, SC and Dr. E.L. Barnes, Pittsburgh, PA.) (Figures 16-94 through 16-96 are from the same patient.)

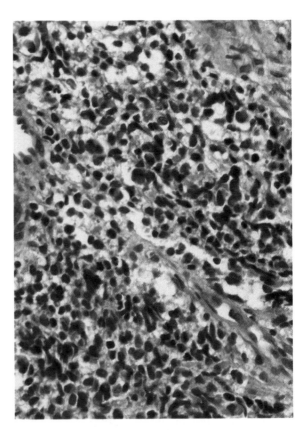

Figure 16-95
RHABDOMYOSARCOMA OF THE MIDDLE EAR
The tumor is composed of closely packed tumor cells embedded in a variably myxoid stroma.

(including spindle cell tumors), botryoid, alveolar, or pleomorphic; patients with spindle cell and botryoid tumors have the best prognosis (204). Undifferentiated variants may also occur. Diagnosis may be difficult due to extensive overlapping between groups.

Clinical Features. Rhabdomyosarcoma of the ear almost exclusively occurs in children under 12 years of age (mean, 4.4 years); both sexes are equally affected (205). Tumors usually arise in the middle ear or mastoid, but are typically advanced at presentation, thus obscuring the precise site of origin. Patients present with hearing loss, pain, and hemorrhagic discharge from the affected ear. Tumors usually present as a polypoid, friable mass in the external ear canal. Metastases to the lungs, bones, or regional lymph nodes are present in 20

to 35 percent of patients at presentation, and up to two thirds of patients show signs of meningeal involvement (205,209,210). Tumor extension inferiorly into the soft tissues of the neck, laterally into the petrous temporal bone and posterior cranial fossa, and medially into the nasopharyngeal region is often seen (205).

Pathologic Findings. Almost all rhabdomyosarcomas of the ear are of the embryonal or botryoid type (201,203,205,206,209,210). Embryonal variants are usually either polypoid or widely infiltrative tumor masses ranging in size from 1 to 6 cm (median, 1.3 cm) (fig. 16-94) (205,209). Botryoid variants often appear polypoid and gelatinous. Histologically, embryonal rhabdomyosarcomas show areas of varying cellularity, with regions of closely packed tumor cells alternating with areas in which the tumor cells are separated by a myxoid or edematous stroma (fig. 16-95) (206). Tumors consist of a variable admixture of undifferentiated

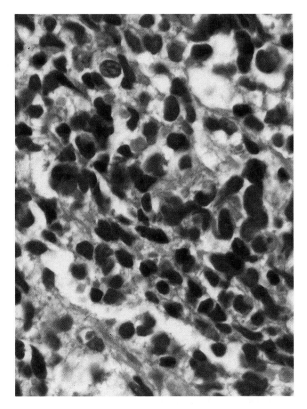

Figure 16-96
RHABDOMYOSARCOMA OF THE MIDDLE EAR
The tumor is predominantly composed of small undifferentiated cells and rare, larger differentiated cells (rhabdomyoblasts) with eosinophilic cytoplasm.

and differentiated cells (rhabdomyoblasts). Undifferentiated tumor cells appear small, round or spindled, with inapparent or small amounts of cytoplasm and dense hyperchromatic nuclei containing one or two small nucleoli. Mitoses are usually abundant. Differentiated cells are typically large and round, with eosinophilic cytoplasm and centrally placed, dense nuclei (fig. 16-96). The cytoplasm may appear granular and contain perinuclear arrays of deeply eosinophilic fibrillary material. Definitive cross-striations are seen in about 50 percent of cases (206). Classic strap-, tadpole-, and racquet-shaped rhabdomyoblasts are uncommon and usually seen in embryonal variants with a predominant spindle cell component (206). The proportion of undifferentiated and rhabdomyoblast-like cells varies from tumor to tumor and in different areas of the same tumor, but most lesions show a predominance of undifferentiated cells. Tumors largely composed of differentiated cells are rare but may occur, particularly after polychemotherapy (207).

Immunohistochemical Findings. Rhabdomyosarcomas are immunohistochemically positive for vimentin, desmin, muscle-specific actin, myoglobin, and myosin (201,203). The degree and extent of staining for muscle-related markers is proportional to the degree of differentiation, with primitive tumors showing only focal reactivity, whereas staining is prominent in tumors with recognizable rhabdomyoblasts. A proportion of rhabdomyosarcomas may express other muscle-related markers such as fetal heavy chain skeletal myosin and myoD1, but the specificity of these markers has yet to be demonstrated (202,204).

Ultrastructural Findings, Special Techniques, and Differential Diagnosis. These features are adequately covered in the rhabdomyosarcoma section in chapter 12 and are not reiterated here.

Treatment and Prognosis. As with rhabdomyosarcomas arising in other sites, current treatment is multimodal, usually with chemotherapy (typically vincristine, dactinyomycin, and cyclophosphamide or adriamycin) followed by surgical resection, with or without radiation (209). Prognosis is variably affected by histologic type, anatomic site of origin, and clinical stage (203,205,206). Treatment is initiated only after definitive pathologic diagnosis (usually by biopsy) and a careful assessment of clinical stage via both radiologic and clinical techniques. For parameningeal tumors, including rhabdomyosarcomas of the middle ear and mastoid, the presence or absence of meningeal involvement is an important consideration (210). Parameningeal rhabdomyosarcomas with meningeal involvement are usually treated with extensive radiation and intrathecal chemotherapy, followed by surgery (206). Following multidisciplinary treatment, the Intergroup Rhabdomyosarcoma Study I reported that 9 of 19 patients (47 percent) with middle ear or mastoid tumors were alive without disease from 2.2 to 6.5 years after diagnosis (209). The Intergroup Rhabdomyosarcoma Study II reported that patients with cranial parameningeal rhabdomyosarcomas, including those with ear tumors, had an overall 5-year survival rate of approximately 70 percent (206). Clinical outcome is primarily dependent upon the presence or absence of meningeal involvement.

REFERENCES

Anatomy, Embryology, Histology

1. Dayal VS, Farkashidy J, Kokshanian A. Embryology of the ear. Can J Otolaryngol 1973;2:136–42.
2. Friedmann I, Arnold W. Gross anatomy, development, histology of the ear and ossicles. In: Pathology of the ear. Edinburgh: Churchill Livingstone, 1993:3–19.
3. Michaels L. The ear. In: SS Sternberg, ed. Histology for pathologists. New York: Raven Press, 1992:925–50.
4. Michaels L. The normal ear. In: Ear, nose, and throat histopathology. London: Springer Verlag, 1987:3–24.
5. Sade J. Middle ear mucosa. Arch Otolaryngol 1966;84:137–43.
6. Wetli CV, Pardo V, Millard M, Gerston K. Tumors of ceruminous glands. Cancer 1972;29:1169–78.

Chondrodermatitis Nodularis Chronica Helicis

7. Garcia E, Silva L, Martins O, Da Silva Picoto A. Bone formation in chondrodermatitis nodularis helicis. J Dermatol Surg Oncol 1980;6:582–5.
8. Goette DK. Chondrodermatitis nodularis chronica helicis: a perforating necrobiotic granuloma. J Am Acad Dermatol 1980;2:148–54.
9. Haber H. Chondrodermatitis nodularis chronica helicis. Hautarzt 1960;11:122–7.
10. Kromann N, Hoyer H, Reymann F. Chondrodermatitis nodularis chronica helicis treated with curettage and electrocauterization. Acta Derm Venereol (Stockholm) 1983;63:85–7.
11. Metzger SA, Goodman ML. Chondrodermatitis helicis. A clinical re-evaluation and pathological review. Laryngoscope 1976;86:1402–12.
12. Newcomer VD, Steffen CG, Sternberg TH, et al. Chondrodermatitis nodularis chronica helicis. Arch Dermatol 1953;68:241–55.
13. Santa Cruz DJ. Chondrodermatitis nodularis helicis: a transepidermal perforating disorder. J Cutan Pathol 1980;7:70–6.
14. Shuman R, Helwig EB. Chondrodermatitis nodularis chronica helicis. Am J Clin Pathol 1954;24:126–44.
15. Wade TR. Chondrodermatitis nodularis helicus. Cutis 1979;24:406–8.
16. Winkler M. Knotchenformige Erkrankung am Helix (Chondermatitis Nodularis Chronica Helicis). Arch Dermatol Syph 1915;12:278–85.

Keratosis Obturans, Cholesteatoma, and Keratin Granulomas

17. Hawke M, Jahn AF. Keratin implantation granuloma in external ear canal. Arch Otolarygol Head Neck Surg 1974;100:317–8.
18. Michaels L. Pathology of cholesteatomas: a review. JR Soc Med 1979;72:366–9.
19. Piepergerdes MC, Kramer BM, Behnke EE. Keratosis obturans and external auditory canal cholesteatoma. Laryngoscope 1980;90:383–91.

Angiolymphoid Hyperplasia with Eosinophilia

20. Barnes L, Koss W, Nieland D. Angiolymphoid hyperplasia with eosinophilia: a disease that may be confused with malignancy. Head Neck Surg 1980;2:425–34.
21. Googe PB, Harris NL, Mihm MC Jr. Kimura s disease and angiolymphoid hyperplasia with eosinophilia: two distinct histopathologic entities. J Cutan Pathol 1987;14:263–71.
22. Grimwood R, Swinehart SM, Aeling JL. Angiolymphoid hyperplasia with eosinophilia. Arch Dermatol 1979;115:205–7.
23. Kuo TT, Shih LY, Chan HL. Kimura's disease: involvement of regional lymph nodes and distinction from angiolymphoid hyperplasia with eosinophilia. Am J Surg Pathol 1988;12:843–54.
24. Olsen TG, Helwig EB. Angiolymphoid hyperplasia with eosinophilia. A clinicopathologic study of 116 patients. J Am Acad Dermatol 1985;12:781–96.
25. Rosai J, Gold J, Landy R. The histiocytoid hemangioma. A unifying concept embracing several previously described entities of skin, soft tissues, large vessels, bone, and heart. Hum Pathol 1979;10:707–30.
26. Thompson JW, Colman M, Williamson C, Ward PH. Angiolymphoid hyperplasia with eosinophilia of the external ear canal. Arch Otolaryngol 1981;107:316–9.
27. Urabe A, Tsuneyoshi M, Enjoji M. Epitheloid hemangioma versus Kimura's disease: a comparative clinicopathologic study. Am J Surg Pathol 1987;11:758–66.

Accessory Tragus

28. Brownstein MH, Wanger NH, Helwig EB. Accessory tragi. Arch Dermatol 1971;104:625–31.

Keloid

29. Cheng LH. Keloid of the ear lobe. Laryngoscope 1972;82:673–81.
30. Mancini RE, Quaife JV. Histogenesis of experimentally produced keloids. J Invest Dermatol 1962;38:143–81.
31. Murray JC, Pollack SV, Pinnel SR. Keloids: a review. J Am Acad Dermatol 1981;4:461–70.

Osteoma and Exostosis

32. Graham MD. Osteomas and exostosis of the external auditory canal. A clinical, histopathological, and scanning electron microscopic study. Ann Otol Rhinol Laryngol 1979;88:566–72.

33. Sheehy JL. Diffuse exostoses and osteomata of the external auditory canal: a report of 100 operations. Otolarygol Head Neck Surg 1982;90:337–42.

Idiopathic Cystic Chondromalacia

34. Hansen JE. Pseudocysts of the auricle in Caucasians. Arch Otolaryngol Head Neck Surg 1967;85:13–4.

35. Heffner DK, Hyams VJ. Cystic chondromalacia (endochondral pseudocyst) of the auricle. Arch Pathol Lab Med 1986;110:740–3.

Branchial Cleft Anomalies

36. Brownstein MH, Wanger NH, Helwig EB. Accessory tragi. Arch Dermatol 1971;104:625–31.

37. Olsen KD, Maragos NE, Weiland LH. First branchial cleft anomalies. Laryngoscope 1980;90:423–36.

Ceruminal Gland Adenoma

38. Batsakis JG, Hardy GC, Hishiyama RH. Ceruminous gland tumors. Arch Otolaryngol 1967;86:66–9.

39. Dehner LP, Chen KT. Primary tumors of the external and middle ear: benign and malignant glandular neoplasms. Arch Otolaryngol Head Neck Surg 1980;106:13–9.

40. Habib MA. Ceruminoma in association with other sweat gland tumors. J Laryngol Otol 1981;95:415–20.

41. Hicks GW. Tumors arising from glandular structures of the external auditory canal. Laryngoscope 1983;93:326–40.

42. Hyams VJ, Michaels L. Benign adenomatous neoplasms (adenoma) of the middle ear. Clin Otolaryngol 1976;1:17–26.

Ceruminal Gland Pleomorphic Adenoma

43. Dehner LP, Chen KT. Primary tumors of the external and middle ear. Benign and malignant glandular neoplasms. Arch Otolarygol 1980;106:13–9.

44. Goldenberg RA, Block BL. Pleomorphic adenoma manifesting as an aural polyp. Arch Otolaryngol 1980;106:440–1.

45. Hicks GW. Tumors arising from the glandular structures of the external auditory canal. Laryngoscope 1983;93:326–40.

46. Pulec JL. Glandular tumors of the external auditory canal. Laryngoscope 1977;10:1601–12.

47. Weitl CV, Pardo V, Millard M, Gerston K. Tumors of ceruminous glands. Cancer 1972;29:1169–78.

Ceruminal Gland Syringocystadenoma Papilliferum

48. Lever WF, Schaumburg-Lever G. Tumors of the epidermal appendages. In: Histopathology of the skin, 7th ed. Philadelphia: JB Lippincott, 1990:578–650.

49. Nager GT. Neoplasms and other lesions of the external ear. In: Pathology of the ear and temporal bone. Baltimore: Williams & Wilkins, 1993:387–412.

Seborrheic Keratosis

50. Baer RL, Garcia RL, Partsalidou V, Ackerman AB. Papillated squamous cell carcinoma in situ arising in a seborrheic keratosis. J Am Dermatol 1981;5:561–5.

51. Deutsch HJ. Tumors of the ear canal. Seborrheic keratosis. Arch Otolaryngol 1970;91:80–1.

52. Lambert PR, Fechner RE, Hatcher CP. Seborrheic keratosis of the ear canal. Otolaryngol Head Neck Surg 1987;96:198–201.

53. Rahbari H. Bowenoid transformation of seborrheic verrucae (keratoses). Br J Dermatol 1979;101:459–73.

54. Sanderson KV. The structure of seborrheic keratoses. Brit J Dermatol 1968;80:588–93.

Squamous Cell Papilloma

55. Nager GT. Neoplasms and other lesions of the external ear. In: Pathology of the ear and temporal bone. Baltimore: Williams & Wilkins, 1993:387–412.

Atypical Fibroxanthoma

56. Enzinger FM. Atypical fibroxanthoma and malignant fibrous histiocytoma. Am J Dermatopathol 1979;1:185.

57. Helwig EB. Atypical fibroxanthoma. Tex State Med J 1963;59:664–7.

58. Helwig EB, May D. Atypical fibroxanthoma of the skin with metastases. Cancer 1986;57:368–76.

59. Kroe DJ, Pitcock JA. Atypical fibroxanthoma of the skin. Report of ten cases. Am J Clin Pathol 1969;51:487–92.

60. Ma CK, Zarbo RJ, Gown AM. Immunohistochemical characterization of atypical fibroxanthoma and dermatofibrosarcoma protruberans. Am J Clin Pathol 1992;97:478–83.

Ceruminal Gland Adenocarcinoma

61. Dehner LP, Chen KT. Primary tumors of the external and middle ear. Benign and malignant glandular neoplasms. Arch Otolaryngol 1980;106:13–9.
62. Hicks GW. Tumors arising from the glandular structures of the external auditory canal. Laryngoscope 1983;93:326–40.
63. Pulec JL. Glandular tumors of the external auditory canal. Laryngoscope 1977;87:1601–12.
64. Wetli CV, Pardo V, Millard M, Gerston K. Tumors of ceruminous glands. Cancer 1972;29:1169–78.

Ceruminal Gland Adenoid Cystic Carcinoma

65. Dehner LP, Chen KT. Primary tumors of the external and middle ear. Benign and malignant glandular neoplasms. Arch Otolaryngol 1980;106:13–9.
66. Eby LS, Johnson DS, Baker HW. Adenoid cystic carcinoma of the head and neck. Cancer 1972;29:1160–8.
67. Hicks GW. Tumors arising from the glandular structures of the external auditory canal. Laryngoscope 1983;93:326–40.
68. Matsuba HM, Simpson JR, Mauney M, et al. Adenoid cystic salivary gland carcinoma: a clinicopathologic correlation. Head Neck Surg 1986;8:200–4.
69. Perzin KH, Gullane P, Conley J. Adenoid cystic carcinoma involving the external auditory canal. A clinicopathologic study of 16 cases. Cancer 1982;50:2873–83.
70. Pulec JL. Glandular tumors of the external auditory canal. Laryngoscope 1977;87:1601–12.
71. Pulec JL, Parkhill EM, Devine KD. Adenoid cystic carcinoma (cylindroma) of the external auditory canal. Trans Am Acad Opthalmol Otolaryngol 1963;67:673–94.
72. Santucci M, Bondi R. New prognostic criterion in adenoid cystic carcinoma of salivary gland origin. Am J Clin Pathol 1989;91:132–6.
73. Spiro RH. Salivary neoplasms: overview of a 35 year experience with 2,807 patients. Head Neck Surg 1986;8:177–84.
74. Spiro RH, Huvos AG, Strong EW. Adenoid cystic carcinoma of salivary gland origin: a clinicopathologic study of 242 cases. Am J Surg 1974;128:512–20.

Basal Cell Carcinoma

75. Bailin PH, Levine HL, Wood BG, Tucker HM. Cutaneous carcinoma of the auricular and periauricular region. Arch Otolaryngol Head Neck Surg 1980;106:692–6.
76. Conley J, Sachs NE, Romo T, Labay G. Metastatic basal cell carcinoma of the head and neck. Otolaryngol Head Neck Surg 1985;93:78–85.
77. Gellin GA, Kopf AW, Garfinkel L. Basal cell epithelioma. Arch Dermatol 1965;91:38–45.
78. Goodwin WJ, Jesse RH. Malignant neoplasms of the external auditory canal and temporal bone. Arch Otolaryngol 1980;106:675–9.
79. Levine HL, Bailin PL. Basal cell carcinoma of the head and neck: identification of the high risk patient. Laryngoscope 1980;50:955–61.
80. Metcalf PB Jr. Carcinoma of the pinna. N Engl J Med 1954;251:91–5.
81. von Domarus H, Stevens PJ. Metastatic basal cell carcinoma. Report of five cases and review of 170 cases in the literature. J Am Acad Dermatol 1984;10:1043–60.

Squamous Cell Carcinoma

82. Bailin PL, Levine HL, Wood BG, Tucker HM. Cutaneous carcinoma of the auricular and periauricular region. Arch Otolaryngol 1980;106:692–6.
83. Byers R, Kesler K, Redmon B, Medina J, Schwarz B. Squamous carcinoma of the external ear. Am J Surg 1983;146:447–50.
84. Chen KT, Dehner LP. Primary tumors of the external and middle ear. I. Introduction and clinicopathologic study of squamous cell carcinoma. Arch Otolaryngol 1978;104:247–52.
85. Enzinger FM. Atypical fibroxanthoma and malignant fibrous histiocytoma. Am J Dermatopathol 1979;1:185.
86. Goodwin WJ, Jesse RH. Malignant neoplasms of the external auditory canal and temporal bone. Arch Otolaryngol 1980;106:675–9.
87. Helwig EB. Atypical fibroxanthoma. Tex State Med J 1963;59:664–7.
88. Helwig EB, May D. Atypical fibroxanthoma of the skin with metastases. Cancer 1986;57:368–76.
89. Johns ME, Headington JT. Squamous cell carcinoma of the external auditory canal. Arch Otolaryngol 1974;100:45–9.
90. Kenyon GS, Marks PV, Scholtz CL, Dhillon R. Squamous cell carcinoma of the middle ear. A 25-year retrospective study. Ann Otol Rhinol Laryngol 1985;94:273–7.
91. Kroe DJ, Pitcock JA. Atypical fibroxanthoma of the skin. Report of ten cases. Am J Clin Pathol 1969;51:487–92.
92. Lewis JS. Squamous cell carcinoma of the ear. Arch Otolaryngol 1973;97:41–2.
93. Ma CK, Zarbo RJ, Gown AM. Immunohistochemical characterization of atypical fibroxanthoma and dermatofibrosarcoma protuberans. Am J Clin Pathol 1992;97:478–83.
94. Metcalf PB Jr. Carcinoma of the pinna. N Engl J Med 1954;251:91–5.
95. Shiffman NJ. Squamous cell carcinomas of the skin of the pinna. Can J Surg 1975;18:279–83.
96. Stell PM. Carcinoma of the external auditory meatus and middle ear. Clin Otolaryngol 1984;9:281–99.

Malignant Melanoma

97. Argenyi ZB, Cain C, Bromley C, Nguyen AV, Abraham AA, Kerschmann R, LeBoit PE. S-100 protein negative malignant melanoma: fact or fiction? Am J Dermatopathol 1994;16:233–40.

98. Breslow A. Tumor thickness, level of invasion and node dissection in stage I cutaneous melanoma. Ann Surg 1975;182:572–5.

99. Byers RM, Smith JL, Russell N, Rosenberg V. Malignant melanoma of the external ear. Review of 102 cases. Am J Surg 1980;140:518–21.

100. Clark WH, From K, Bernadino EA, Mihm MC. The histogenesis and biologic behavior of primary human malignant melanomas of the skin. Cancer Res 1969;29:705–27.

101. Donnellan MJ, Seemayer T, Huvos AG, Mike V, Strong EW. Clinicopathologic study of cutaneous melanoma of the head and neck. Am J Surg 1972;124:450–5.

102. Gown AM, Vogel AM, Hoak D, Gough F, McNutt MA. Monoclonal antibodies specific for melanocytic tumors distinguish subpopulations of melanocytes. Am J Pathol 1986;123:195–203.

103. Hansen MG, McCarten AB. Tumor thickness and lymphocytic infiltration in malignant melanoma of the head and neck. Am J Surg 1974;128:557–61.

104. Ordónez NG, Xialong JI, Hickey RC. Comparison of HMB-45 monoclonal antibody and S-100 protein in the immunohistochemical diagnosis of melanoma. Am J Clin Pathol 1988;90:385–90.

105. Pack GT, Conley J, Oropeza R. Melanoma of the external ear. Arch Otolaryngol 1970;92:106–13.

106. Wanebo HJ, Cooper PH, Young DV, Harpole DH, Kaiser DL. Prognostic factors in head and neck melanoma: effect of lesion location. Cancer 1988;62:831–7.

Inflammatory Polyps

107. Fechner RE, Mills SE. Tumors of the bones and joints. Atlas of Tumor Pathology, 3rd Series, Fascicle 8. Washington, D.C.: Armed Forces Institute of Pathology, 1992.

108. Nager GT. Acute and chronic otitis media (tympanomastoiditis) and their regional and endocranial complications. In: Pathology of the ear and temporal bone. Baltimore: Williams & Wilkins, 1993:220–97.

Cholesteatoma

109. Kreutzer EW, DeBlanc GB. Extra-aural spread of acquired cholesteatoma. Arch Otolaryngol 1982;108:320–3.

110. Michaels L. An epidermoid formation in the developing middle ear: possible source of cholesteatoma. J Otolaryngol 1986;15:169–74.

111. Michaels L. Pathology of cholesteatoma: a review. J R Soc Med 1979;72:366–9.

112. Nager GT. Epidermoids involving the temporal bone: clinical, radiological, and pathological aspects. Laryngoscope 1975;85(Suppl):1–22.

113. Peron DL, Schuknecht HF. Congenital cholesteatoma with other abnormalities. Arch Otolaryngol 1975;101:498–505.

Middle Ear Choristomas

114. Batsakis JG. Adenomatous tumors of the middle ear. Ann Otol Rhinol Laryngol 1989;98:749–52.

115. Gavilan J, Trujillo M, Gavilan C. Spontaneous encephalocele of the middle ear. Arch Otolaryngol 1984;110:206–7.

116. Hociota D, Ataman T. A case of salivary gland choristoma of the middle ear. J Laryngol Otol 1975;89:1065–8.

117. Klein MV, Schwaighofer BW, Sobel DF, Fantozzi RD, Hesselink JR. Heterotopic brain in the middle ear: CT findings. J Comput Assist Tomogr 1989;13:1058–60.

118. Levy RA, Platt N, Aftalion B. Encephalocele of the middle ear. Laryngoscope 1971;81:126–30.

119. McGregor DH, Cherian R, Kepes JJ, Kepes M. Heterotopic brain tissue of middle ear associated with cholesteatoma. Am J Med Sci 1994;308:180–3.

120. Michaels L. Neoplasms and similar lesions of the middle ear. In: Ear, nose, and throat histopathology. Berlin: Springer-Verlag, 1987:67–76.

121. Mischke RE, Brackmann DE, Gruskin P. Salivary gland choristoma of the middle ear. Arch Otolaryngol 1977;103:432–4.

122. Moore PJ, Benjamin BN, Kan AE. Salivary gland choristoma of the middle ear. In J Pediatr Otorhinolaryngol 1984;8:91–5.

123. Quaranta A, Mininni F, Resta L. Salivary gland choristoma of the middle ear. J Laryngol Otol 1981;95:953–6.

124. Saeger KL, Gruskin P, Carberry JN. Salivary gland choristoma of the middle ear. Arch Pathol Lab Med 1982;106:39–40.

125. Slater DN, Timperley WR, Smith CM. Heterotopic middle ear gliomatosis [Letter]. Histopathology 1988;12:230–1.

126. Steffen PM, House WF. Salivary gland choristoma of the middle ear. Arch Otolaryngol 1962;76:64–75.

127. Williams DC. Encephalocele of the middle ear. J Laryngol Otol 1986;100:471–3.

128. Wine CJ, Metcalf JE. Salivary gland choristoma of the middle ear and mastoid. Arch Otolaryngol 1977;103:435–6.

Jugulotympanic Paraganglioma

129. Alford BR, Guilford FR. A comprehensive study of tumors of the glomus jugulare. Laryngoscope 1962;72:765–87.

130. Chen KT, Dehner LP. Primary tumors of the external and middle ear. II. A clinicopathologic study of 14 paragangliomas and three meningiomas. Arch Otolaryngol 1978;104:253–9.

131. Farrior JB Jr, Hyams VJ, Benke RH, Farrior JB. Carcinoid apudoma arising in a glomus jugulare tumor: review of endocrine activity in glomus jugulare tumors. Laryngoscope 1980;90:110–9.

132. Hyams VJ, Batsakis JG, Michaels L. Tumors of the upper respiratory tract and ear. Atlas of Tumor Pathology, 2nd series, Fascicle 25, Washington, D.C.: Armed Forces Institute of Pathology, 1988:306.

133. Johnson TL, Zarbo RJ, Lloyd RV, Crissman JD. Paragangliomas of the head and neck: immunohistochemical neuroendocrine and intermediate filament typing. Mod Pathol 1988;1:216–23.

134. Lack EE, Cubilla AL, Woodruff JM. Paragangliomas of the head and neck region. A pathologic study of tumors from 71 patients. Hum Pathol 1979;10:191–218.

135. Linnoila RI, Keiser HR, Steinberg SM, Lack EE. Histopathology of benign versus malignant sympathoadrenal paragangliomas: clinicopathologic study of 120 cases including unusual histologic features. Hum Pathol 1990;21:1168–80.

136. McCabe BF, Fletcher M. Selection of therapy for glomus jugulare tumors. Arch Otolaryngol 1969;89:182–5.

137. Rossenwasser H. Long-term results of therapy of glomus jugulare tumors. Arch Otolaryngol 1973;97:49–54.

138. Spector GJ, Ciralsky RH, Ogura JH. Glomus tumors in the head and neck: III. Analysis of clinical manifestations. Ann Otol Rhinol Laryngol 1975;84:73–9.

Middle Ear Adenoma

139. Adams GL, Paparella MM, El Fiky FM. Primary and metastatic tumors of the temporal bone. Laryngoscope 1971;81:1273–85.

140. Bailey QR, Weiner JM. Middle ear adenoma: a case report with ultrastructural findings. J Laryngol Otol 1986;100:467–70.

141. Batsakis JG. Pathology consultation: adenomatous tumors of the middle ear. Ann Otol Rhinol Laryngol 1989;98:749–52.

142. Benecke JE, Noel FL, Carberry JN, House JW, Patterson M. Adenomatous tumors of the middle ear and mastoid. Am J Otol 1990;11:20–6.

143. El-Naggar AK, Pflatz M, Ordonez NG, Batsakis JG. Tumors of the middle ear and endolymphatic sac. Path Ann 194;29(Pt 2):199–231.

144. Gillanders DA, Worth AJ, Honore LH. Ceruminous adenoma of the middle ear. Can J Otolaryngol 1974;3:194–201.

145. Harrison K, Cronin J, Greenwood N. Ceruminous adenocarcinoma arising in the middle ear. J Laryngol Otol 1974;88:363–8.

146. Hill BA, Kohut RI. Metastatic adenocarcinoma of the temporal bone. Arch Otolaryngol 1976;102:568–71.

147. Hyams VJ, Michaels L. Benign adenomatous neoplasm (adenoma) of the middle ear. Clin Otolaryngol 1976;1:17–26.

148. Manni JJ, Faverly DR, Van Haelst UJ. Primary carcinoid tumors of the middle ear. Report of four cases and a review of the literature. Arch Otolaryngol Head Neck Surg 1992;118:1341–7.

149. McNutt MA, Bolen JW. Adenomatous tumor of the middle ear. A cytologically uniform neoplasm displaying a variety of architectural patterns. An ultrastructural and immunocytochemical study. Am J Clin Pathol 1985;84:541–7.

150. Mills SE, Fechner RE. Middle ear adenoma. Am J Surg Pathol 1984;8:677–85.

151. Ribe A, Fernandez PL, Ostertarg H, et al. Middle-ear adenoma (MEA): a report of two cases, one with predominant plasmacytoid features. Histopathology 1997;30:359–64.

152. Riches WG, Johnston WH. Primary adenomatous neoplasms of the middle ear. Light and electron microscopic features of a group distinct from the ceruminomas. Am J Clin Pathol 1982;77:153–61.

153. Siedentop KH, Jeantet C. Primary adenocarcinoma of the middle ear. Report of three cases. Ann Otol Rhinol Laryngol 1961;70:719–33.

154. Stone H, Lipa M, Bell R. Primary adenocarcinoma of the middle ear. Arch Otolaryngol 1975;101:702–5.

155. Taxy JB. Renal adenocarcinoma presenting as a solitary metastasis: contribution of electron microscopy to diagnosis. Cancer 1981;48:2056–62.

156. Wassef M, Kanavaros P, Polivka M, et al. Middle ear adenoma: a tumor displaying mucinous and neuroendocrine differentiation. Am J Surg Pathol 1989;13:838–47.

Schneiderian Papilloma of Middle Ear and Mastoid

157. Hyams VJ. Papillomas of the nasal cavity and paranasal sinuses. A clinicopathologic study of 315 cases. Ann Otol Rhinol Laryngol 1971;80:192–206.

158. Kaddour HS, Woodhead CJ. Transitional papilloma of the middle ear. J Laryngol Otol 1992;106:628–9.

159. Roberts WH, Dinges DL, Hanly MG. Inverted papilloma of the middle ear. Ann Otol Rhinol Laryngol 1993;102:890–2.

160. Stone DM, Berktold RE, Ranganathan C, Wiet RJ. Inverted papilloma of the middle ear and mastoid. Otolaryngol Head Neck Surg 1987;97:416–8.

161. Wenig BM. Schneiderian-type mucosal papillomas of the middle ear and mastoid. Ann Otol Rhinol Laryngol 1996;105:226–33.

Aggressive Papillary Tumor Of Temporal Bone and Endolymphatic sac

162. Batsakis JG, El-Naggar AK. Papillary neoplasms (Heffner's tumors) of the endolymphatic sac. Ann Otol Rhinol Laryngol 1993;102:648–51.

163. Blamires TL, Friedmann I, Moffat DA. Von Hippel-Lindau disease associated with an invasive choroid plexus tumor presenting as a middle ear mass. J Laryngol Otol 1992;106:429–35.

164. Gaffey MJ, Mills SE, Boyd JC. Aggressive papillary tumor of middle ear/temporal bone and adnexal papillary cystadenoma. Manifestations of von Hippel-Lindau disease. Am J Surg Pathol 1994;18:1254–60.

165. Gaffey MJ, Mills SE, Fechner RE, Intemann SR, Wick MR. Aggressive papillary middle-ear tumor: a clinicopathologic entity distinct from middle ear adenoma. Am J Surg Pathol 1988;12:790–7.

166. Goebel JA, Smith PG, Kemink JL, Graham MD. Primary adenocarcinoma of the temporal bone mimicking paragangliomas: radiographic and clinical recognition. Otolaryngol Head Neck Surg 1987;96:231–8.

167. Hassard AD, Boudreau SF, Cron CC. Adenoma of the endolymphatic sac. J Otolaryngol 1984;13:213–6.

168. Heffner DK. Low-grade adenocarcinoma of probable endolymphatic sac origin. A clinicopathologic study of 20 cases. Cancer 1989;64:2292–302.

169. Lavoie M, Morency RM. Low-grade papillary adenomatous tumors of the temporal bone: report of two cases and review of the literature. Mod Pathol 1995;8:603–8.

170. Levin RJ, Feghali JG, Morganstern N, Llena J, Bradley MK. Aggressive papillary tumors of the temporal bone: an immunohistochemical analysis in tissue culture. Laryngoscope 1996;106:144–7.

171. Megerian CA, McKenna MJ, Nuss RC, et al. Endolymphatic sac tumors: Histopathologic confirmation, clinical characterization, and implication in von Hippel-Lindau disease. Laryngoscope 1995;105:801–8.

172. Megerian CA, Pilch BZ, Bhan AK. McKenna MJ. Differential expression of transthyretin in papillary tumors of the endolymphatic sac and choroid plexus. Laryngoscope 1997;107:216–21.

173. Meyer JR, Gebarski SS, Blaivas M. Cerebellopontine angle invasive papillary cystadenoma of endolymphatic sac origin with temporal bone involvement. AJNR Am J Neuroradiol 1993;14:1319–23.

174. Mukherji SK, Albernaz V, Castillo M, et al. Papillary endolymphatic sac tumors: CT, MR, and angiographic findings in 20 cases. Radiology (in press).

175. Poe DS, Tarlov EC, Thomas CB, Kveton JF. Aggressive papillary tumors of temporal bone. Otolaryngol Head Neck Surg 1993;108:80–6.

176. Pollak A, Bohmer A, Spycher M, Fisch U. Are papillary adenomas endolymphatic sac tumors? Ann Otol Rhinol Laryngol 1995;104:613–9.

177. Shambaugh GE, Clemis JD, Arenberg IK. Endolymphatic duct and sac in Meniere's disease. Arch Otolaryngol 1969;89:816–25.

178. Stone HE, Lipa M, Bell RD. Primary adenocarcinoma of the middle ear. Arch Otolaryngol 1975;101:702–5.

179. Thomas CB, Kveton JF, Poe DS, Zamani AA, Tarlov EC. Aggressive papillary tumor of temporal bone in von Hippel-Lindau disease. Surg Pathol 1993;5:63–71.

180. Watzke D, Bast TH. The development and structure of the otic (endolymphatic) sac. Anat Rec 1950;106:361–79.

Meningioma of Middle Ear and Temporal Bone

181. Alguacil-Garcia A, Pettigrew NM, Sima AA. Secretory meningioma: a distinct subtype of meningioma. Am J Surg Pathol 1986;10:102–11.

182. Artlich A, Schmidt D. Immunohistochemical profile of meningiomas and their histological subtypes. Hum Pathol 1990;21:843–9.

183. Chen KT, Dehner LP. Primary tumors of the external and middle ear. II. A clinicopathologic study of 14 paragangliomas and three meningiomas. Arch Otolaryngol 1978;104:253–9.

184. Granich MS, Pilch BZ, Goodman ML. Meningiomas presenting in the paranasal sinuses and temporal bone. Head Neck Surg 1983;5:319–28.

185. Maniglia AJ. Intra and extracranial meningiomas involving the temporal bone. Laryngoscope 1978;88(Suppl 12):1–58.

186. Michaels L. Neoplasms and similar lesions of the middle ear. In: Ear, nose and throat histopathology. London: Springer-Verlag, 1987:67–76.

187. Nager GT. Meningiomas. In: Pathology of the ear and temporal bone. Baltimore: Williams & Wilkins, 1993:620–70.

188. Nager GT. Meningiomas involving the temporal bone, clinical and pathological aspects. Springfield: Charles C. Thomas, 1964:62–76.

189. Nager GT, Heroy J, Hoeplinger M. Meningiomas invading the temporal bone with extension to the neck. Am J Otolaryngol 1983;4:297–324.

190. Radley MG, Di Sant Agnese PA, Eskin TA, Wilbur DC. Epithelial differentiation in meningiomas. An immunohistochemical, histochemical, and ultrastructural study—with review of the literature. Am J Clin Pathol 1989;92:266–72.

191. Rubenstein LJ. Tumors of the central nervous system. Atlas of Tumor Pathology, 2nd series, Fascicle 6. Washington, D.C.: Armed Forces Institute of Pathology, 1972:169.

192. Salama N, Stafford N. Meningiomas presenting in the middle ear. Laryngoscope 1982;92:92–7.

193. Schnitt SJ, Vogel H. Meningiomas. Diagnostic value of immunoperoxidase staining for epithelial membrane antigen. Am J Surg Pathol 1986;10:640–9.

194. Theaker JM, Gatter KC, Esiri MM, Fleming KA. Epithelial membrane antigen and cytokeratin expression by meningiomas: an immunohistochemical study. J Clin Pathol 1986;39:435–9.

Metastatic Neoplasms to the Middle Ear

195. Adams GL, Paparella MM, El Fiky FM. Primary and metastatic tumors of the temporal bone. Laryngoscope 1971;81:1273–85.

196. Belal A. Metastatic tumors of the temporal bone. A histopathologic report. J Laryngol Otol 1985;99:839–46.

197. Hill BA, Kohut RI. Metastatic adenocarcinomas of the temporal bone. Arch Otolaryngol 1976;102:568–71.

198. Jahn AF, Farkashidy J, Berman JM. Metastatic tumors in the temporal bone: a pathophysiologic study. J Otolaryngol 1979;8:85–95.

199. Maddox HE. Metastatic tumors of the temporal bone. Ann Otol Rhinol Laryngol 1967;76:149–65.

200. Schuknecht HF, Allam AF, Murakami Y. Pathology of secondary malignant tumors of the temporal bone. Ann Otol Rhinol Laryngol 1968;77:5–22.

Rhabdomyosarcoma of Middle Ear and Temporal Bone

201. Barnes L. Tumors and tumor-like lesions of the soft tissues. In: Barnes L, ed. Surgical pathology of the head and neck. New York: Marcel Dekker, 1985:725–880.

202. Dias P, Parham DM, Shapiro DN, Webber BL, Houghton PJ. Myogenic regulatory protein (MyoD1) expression in childhood solid tumors: diagnostic utility in rhabdomyosarcoma. Am J Pathol 1990;137:1283–91.

203. Enzinger FM, Weiss SW. Rhabdomyosarcoma. In: Soft tissue tumors. 3rd ed. St. Louis: Mosby, 1995:539–77.

204. Eusebi V, Rilke F, Ceccarelli C, Fedeli F, Schiaffino S, Bussolati G. Fetal heavy chain skeletal myosin. An oncofetal antigen expressed by rhabdomyosarcoma. Am J Surg Pathol 1986;10:680–6.

205. Jaffe RB, Fox JE, Batsakis JG. Rhabdomyosarcoma of the middle ear and mastoid. Cancer 1971;27:29–37.

206. Maurer HM, Gehan EA, Beltangady M, et al. The Intergroup Rhabdomyosarcoma Study-II. Cancer 1993;71:1904–22.

207. Molenaar WM, Oosterhuis JW, Kamps WA. Cytologic differentiation in childhood rhabdomyosarcomas following polychemotherapy. Hum Pathol 1984;15:973–9.

208. Newton WA Jr, Gehan EA Webber BL, et al. Classification of rhabdomyosarcomas and related sarcomas. Pathologic aspects and proposal for a new classification—an Intergroup Rhabdomyosarcoma Study. Cancer 1995;76:1073–85.

209. Raney RB, Lawrence W, Maurer HM, et al. Rhabdomyosarcoma of the ear in childhood. A report from the Intergroup Rhabdomyosarcoma Study. Cancer 1983;51:2356–61.

210. Tefft M, Fernandez C, Donaldson M, Newton W, Moon TE. Incidence of meningeal involvement by rhabdomyosarcoma of the head and neck in children: a report of the Intergroup Rhabdomyosarcoma Study (IRS). Cancer 1978;42:253–8.

Index*

Upper Aerodigestive Tract

*Numbers in boldface indicate table and figure pages.

The Ear